The
ROY
ADAPTATION
MODEL

second edition

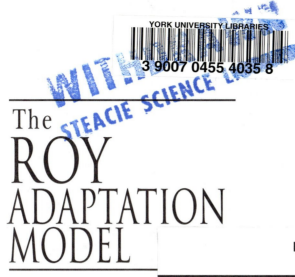

The
ROY ADAPTATION MODEL

second edition

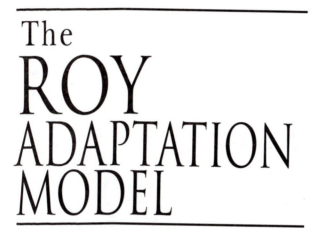

Sister Callista Roy, PhD, RN, FAAN
Professor and Nurse Theorist
School of Nursing
Boston College
Chestnut Hill, Massachusetts

Heather A. Andrews, PhD, RN
Principal Partner
Quality Leadership Associates
Sherwood Park, Alberta, Canada

APPLETON & LANGE
Stamford, Connecticut

Notice: The authors and the publisher of this volume have taken care to make certain that the doses of drugs and schedules of treatment are correct and compatible with the standards generally accepted at the time of publication. Nevertheless, as new information becomes available, changes in treatment and in the use of drugs become necessary. The reader is advised to carefully consult the instruction and information material included in the package insert of each drug or therapeutic agent before administration. This advice is especially important when using, administering, or recommending new or infrequently used drugs. The authors and the publisher disclaim all responsibility for any liability, loss, injury, or damage incurred as a consequence, directly or indirectly, of the use and application of any of the contents of this volume.

Copyright © 1999 by Appleton & Lange
A Simon & Schuster Company
© 1991 by Appleton & Lange
© 1986 by Appleton-Century-Crofts
© 1984 by Prentice Hall
© 1976 by Prentice Hall

All rights reserved. This book, or any parts thereof, may not be used or reproduced in any manner without written permission. For information, address Appleton & Lange, Four Stamford Plaza, PO Box 120041, Stamford, Connecticut 06912-0041.

www.appletonlange.com

99 00 01 02 03 / 10 9 8 7 6 5 4 3 2 1

Prentice Hall International (UK) Limited, *London*
Prentice Hall of Australia Pty. Limited, *Sydney*
Prentice Hall Canada, Inc., *Toronto*
Prentice Hall Hispanoamericana, S.A., *Mexico*
Prentice Hall of India Private Limited, *New Delhi*
Prentice Hall of Japan, Inc., *Tokyo*
Simon & Schuster Asia Pte. Ltd., *Singapore*
Editora Prentice Hall do Brasil Ltda., *Rio de Janeiro*
Prentice Hall, *Upper Saddle River, New Jersey*

Library of Congress Cataloging-in-Publication Data
Roy, Callista.
    The Roy adaptation model / Callista Roy, Heather A.
Andrews.
        p.   cm.
    Rev. ed. of: The Roy adaptation model / [edited by]
Callista Roy, Heather A. Andrews. c1991.
    Includes bibliographical references and index.
    ISBN 0-8385-8248-6 (pbk.)
    1. Roy adaptation model.   2. Nursing—Psychological
aspects.   3. Nurse and patient.   I. Andrews, Heather
A.   II. Title.
    [DNLM: 1. Nursing Process.   2. Adaptation,
Psychological.   3. Models, Nursing.   WY 100R888r
1999]
RT84.5.R66   1999
610.73'01'9—dc21
DNLM/DLC
for Library of Congress   98-33477
                                        CIP

ISBN 0-8385-8248-6

90000

9 780838 582480

Acquisitions Editor: David P. Carroll
Production Editor: Karen Davis
Designer: Mary Skudlarek

PRINTED IN THE UNITED STATES OF AMERICA

Dedicated to the loving memory of Mrs. Pirth Irene Roy, LVN
Wife, mother, nurse, and extraordinary woman of deep faith, hope, and love.

CONTENTS

CONTRIBUTORS

Kathleen Connerley, MS, RN
Assistant Administrator of Patient Care Services
St. Joseph Regional Medical Center
Lewiston, Idaho

Susanna Ristau, RN
Program Director
Patient Care Services
St. Joseph Regional Medical Center
Lewiston, Idaho

Coralee Lindberg, RN, BSN
Director Medical/Surgical Departments
St. Joseph Regional Medical Center
Lewiston, Idaho

Mary McFarland, PhD, RN
Dean and Professor of Professional Studies
Gonzaga University
Spokane, Washington

PREFACE

The Roy Adaptation Model is an introduction to the Roy Adaptation Model for nursing education and clinical nursing practice based on the model developed by Sister Callista Roy. The purpose of this second edition of the definitive text is to provide an update that (1) maintains the essential concepts of the model while reflecting new developments and enhanced integration of the model elements; (2) focuses on contemporary issues of health care delivery with social and cultural sensitivity; (3) provides for clarity of basic content, while at the same time expanding the theoretical basis for the adaptive modes; and (4) incorporates applications to both individuals and groups.

Many textbooks have continued to discuss nursing models as significant for professional nursing practice, particularly in guiding the nursing process. Some texts assess the philosophical, theoretical, and conceptual bases for the views of particular nurse theorists. There are additional textbooks that review the work of nurse theorists and provide analysis and critique or application to practice, education, research, or administration. No other text on a nursing model has the vantage point of unifying and presenting model-based knowledge that derives from 30 years of conceptual development and implementation in practice, education, and research.

The model was implemented as the basis of the nursing curriculum at Mount St. Mary's College in Los Angeles in March 1970. The program became the laboratory for the development of the model, with faculty and graduates working with Dr. Roy to develop and publish the elements of the model. Today the faculty and campus at Mount St. Mary's College provide the flagship implementation of the model in nursing education that is recognized throughout the world. In addition, faculty continue to be friends and colleagues who have provided significant input for this revision.

This book builds on the first edition and on four previous books on the Roy Adaptation Model authored by Roy, with contributions by colleagues at Mount St. Mary's. A significant development for the Roy model publications was Roy's collaboration with Dr. Heather Andrews in 1986 and 1991. Dr. Andrews brought a wealth of knowledge and experience as an educator using the Roy Adaptation Model and also the perspective of a nursing administrator in complex health care systems in Canada.

The essentials of the model are used to organize this second edition, and much of the basic content from the first edition has been included. However, there are significant changes in both content and organization. Each chapter on the adaptive modes has been reorganized to include three levels of adaptive processes—integrated life processes, compensatory processes, and compromised processes. Content is provided for assessment of the processes, using relevant behaviors and stimuli that lead to making nursing judgments about adaptation levels. Information from the first edition that illustrates these levels has been retained with updated references, and new content has been added to complete each chapter. Theoretical content has been expanded to include the adaptive processes of groups as well as individuals. Presentation of nursing care planning provides case applications related to both. The process of nursing diagnosis has been simplified and tables are included that relate Roy's typology of positive indicators of adaptation and adaptation problems to the work of the North American Nursing Diagnosis Association. Key definitions, figures, and tables have been retained and new ones have been added as they relate to the expanded content.

A particular feature of this edition is the introduction of Roy's definition of adaptation for the 21st century. Relevant scientific and philosophical assumptions are discussed as they derive from a synthesis of Roy's earlier work with her thinking about cosmic knowledge in the new millennium. The aim is to update content, but also to look to the future of nursing knowledge development based on the model.

The text is now divided into three parts. Part I serves as a three-chapter introduction. The first chapter reintroduces and updates earlier works related to the development of nursing and nursing models. Chapters 2 and 3 present the major concepts of the model and their application to the nursing process.

Part II deals with all four adaptive modes, now defined as physiologic–physical, self-concept–group identity, role function, and interdependence, to encompass the group perspective. Chapter 4 introduces the modes and offers application to the group physical system. As in previous editions, one chapter is dedicated to each of the components of the physiologic mode for the individual. For each of the remaining three modes, content has been incorporated into one comprehensive chapter. The content and organization of each of these chapters build a strong theoretical knowledge base for assessment on the two levels described by Dr. Roy. Then individual and group situations are used to illustrate nursing diagnosis, goal setting, intervention, and evaluation.

In Part III, Chapter 17 describes a recent implementation project of the Roy Model at St. Joseph's Regional Medical Center in Lewiston, Idaho. This project was of particular interest to Dr. Roy because leaders of the project were former master's students she taught at the University of Portland. Further, the medical center is one of the institutions operated by the Sisters of St. Joseph of Carondelet of which she has been a member for more than 40 years. On two occasions Dr. Roy has practiced nursing at St. Joseph's, first on the medical–surgical units, and then as acting director of nursing.

Finally, Chapter 18 is a significant addition to the literature on applications of the model in nursing research. In addition to updated content on Roy's research, it provides a summary of a major project designed to analyze, critique, and synthesize the first 25 years of research based on the Roy Adaptation Model. The project was planned, conducted, and published by the Boston-based Adaptation Research in Nursing Society, a group of seven dedicated colleagues who worked with Dr. Roy on the four-year project.

This text is intended primarily for use in agencies and educational institutions that are using the Roy Adaptation Model as the basis for nursing practice and education. It provides essential content for entry-level nursing students, new nursing service personnel, and faculty. Master's level students will find the clarity of presentation and the updated content an efficient method to become acquainted with the essentials and recent developments of the model as a basis for further analysis and application of the model concepts. Doctoral students and other nurse scholars can find within the elements of the model the basis for significant research questions and for adding to basic and clinical knowledge development. In addition, the text serves as an illustration of major strategies for knowledge development in nursing. Derivations of new applications to all nursing specialties, including independent practice, are implied from the essentials described here and from the references cited.

This text provides a clear articulation of the essence of nursing to the profession, to other health care disciplines, and to the public. Every effort has been made to focus on the essential nature of nursing, its unique perspective, role, and the implications of what that role means as the systems of health care are shifting. This clarity about nursing can help to facilitate the transitions to effective systems that meet the needs of individuals and societal groups of the 21st century.

The authors are indebted to those who have assisted with the development of this text. We appreciate greatly those who have contributed to and offered stimulation to the development of the model through the years, especially, as noted earlier and in the special acknowledgments, our colleagues at Mount St. Mary's College. Nurses in practice, students at all levels, and audiences throughout the world have provided insightful observations and questions that are a great source of stimulation in this ongoing work.

We acknowledge particularly Janice Tracey, the editorial and staff assistant to Dr. Roy, who is funded by a grant from the Sisters of St. Joseph of Carondelet. Janice's eye for English composition and diligence in handling many details made it possible to complete this second edition during a heavy school year. She contributed greatly to the quality of the work. Both of us have a long list of those who have contributed in some way to us personally and to our work. To each we are grateful.

We appreciate the staff at Appleton & Lange, particularly David Carroll, editor, and Karen Davis, production editor, who were patient with our efforts to complete this major revision, after an earlier work plan had to be suspended unexpectedly in 1995. Sister Callista Roy is grateful to colleagues at Boston College, her religious community, her friends and family, and especially her dear mother, who supported and prayed for her through a second craniotomy, this time for a ninth cranial nerve swannoma. We believe that the delay itself contributed to the content and quality of this work. It is with great joy that we offer the fruits of these 30 years to our publics.

Sister Callista Roy
Heather A. Andrews

ACKNOWLEDGMENTS

We would like to acknowledge in a special way the authors of previous versions of this text (1976, 1984, and 1991) who contributed to the development of many of the basic concepts of the Roy Adaptation Model and provided the basis for the flagship implementation of the model in nursing education at Mount St. Mary's College, Los Angeles, California, which is recognized around the world today.

- Faculty from Mount St. Mary's College, Los Angeles, California:

  Sue Ann Brown
  Marjorie Buck
  Zona Chalifoux
  Joan Seo Cho
  Edda Coughran
  Marjorie Clowry Dobratz
  Marie Driever
  Sheila Driscoll
  Jeannine R. Dunn
  Janet Dunning
  Edythe Ellison
  Barbara Gruendemann
  Joan Hansen
  C. Margaret Henderson
  Mary Hicks
  Mary Howard
  Karen Jensen

  Sonja Liggett
  Sister Theresa Marie McIntier
  Nancy Malaznik
  Kathleen Anschutz Nuwayhid
  Nancy Zewen Perley
  Brooke Randell
  Marsha Milton Roberson
  Marsha Keiko Sato
  Ann Macaluso Schofield
  Jane Servonsky
  Mary Sloper
  Nancy Taylor
  Mary Poush Tedrow
  Catherine Rivera Thompson
  Sharon Vairo
  Joyce Van Landingham

- Graduates of Mount St. Mary's College:

  Lorraine Ann Marshall
  Cecilia Martinez
  Sally Valentine

- Colleagues of Sister Callista Roy:

  Joanne Gray
  Donna Romyn

I PART

INTRODUCTION TO THE ROY ADAPTATION MODEL

The Roy Adaptation Model is currently one of the most highly developed and widely used conceptual descriptions of nursing. Formal development of the model began in the late 1960s and, since that time, nurses in the United States and around the world have helped Roy to clarify, refine, and extend the basic concepts to the stage of development presented in this text. The major concepts associated with nursing models—recipient of care, the environment, health, the goal of nursing, and nursing activities—are introduced in this section and discussed in further detail throughout the text.

Part I of this text provides the foundation for more detailed exploration of the Roy Adaptation Model. In Chapter 1, the reader is introduced to the profession of nursing and the associated knowledge base, including the manner in which nursing models fit into the picture. Chapter 2 focuses specifically on the Roy Adaptation Model and describes it according to the major concepts associated with nursing models in general. Chapter 3 provides the reader with an overview of the nursing process according to the model. This introductory section leads to Part II, where the specific components of the Roy Adaptation Model are addressed individually.

1

DEVELOPMENT OF NURSING MODELS

Nursing is a profession that meets health care needs in society. All professions have two characteristics. First, professions are developed to contribute to the good of society. Second, professions use specialized knowledge to meet specific social needs. Health and well-being are major needs for individuals, families, nations, and the world as a whole. This chapter focuses on the specific nature of nursing as a knowledge-based health care profession. The kind of knowledge that serves as the foundation for the nursing profession is identified. Conceptual models for nursing practice are a particular approach to developing nursing knowledge and several nursing models are described and illustrated. This chapter provides background for further study of the Roy Adaptation Model.

► OBJECTIVES

After studying this chapter, the reader will be able to do the following:

1. Identify two characteristics of professions.

2. Name three common concerns of nursing as a profession.

3. Identify the domain of the nursing profession.

4. Name three major concepts that constitute the focus of nursing.

5. List three approaches to knowledge development for the science of nursing.

6. Identify the essential elements of a conceptual model for nursing.

7. Associate specified elements of a conceptual model with the model's author.

► KEY CONCEPTS DEFINED

Conceptual model for nursing: A set of concepts or images that identify and relate the essential elements of nursing, such as recipient of care, environment, health, goal of nursing, nursing activities.

Domain: The area of social concern that represents the focus of responsibility for a profession.

Environment: In the domain of nursing, all that influences people and their health including physical surroundings, other people, and the earth and its life-giving, but limited, resources.

Health: In general, the person's total well-being and human integrity.

Holistic: The philosophic assumption pertaining to the unified expression of physical, thinking, and feeling processes in human behavioral patterns.

Model: A description or analogy used to help visualize something that cannot be observed directly.

Nursing: A health care profession that focuses on human life processes and patterns, and emphasizes promotion of health for individuals, families, groups, and society as a whole.

Philosophic assumptions: The values and beliefs that are the foundation of nursing knowledge and practice.

Profession: A scholarly discipline that uses its specialized knowledge for a social good.

► NATURE OF NURSING

Nursing is a *profession* that uses specialized knowledge to contribute to the needs of society for health and well-being. All professions develop to meet particular needs in society. Law professionals aim to maintain justice and civil order. Clergy are expected to meet spiritual needs and to interpret religious doctrine and practice. Among the needs of society, health and well-being are basic. Without health and well-being, the person cannot live a satisfying and productive life. Human potential may be limited by lack of health and inadequate fulfillment of health care needs. When people in a society are not using their full human capabilities, the society itself is threatened.

Several professions have developed to contribute to health and well-being. Medicine emerged to heal illness and injury. Pharmacy developed to prepare and dispense medicinal preparations. What is the particular need for which nursing is accountable? Throughout history, there have been persons, both men and women, who tended to the sick, injured, and children. This was particularly the case in times of war and other threats such as plague or famine. Modern nursing looks to the efforts of Florence Nightingale during the Crimean War and after, in Britain, for the inspiration and general principles to identify nursing's place in society.

Characteristics of Modern Nursing

Florence Nightingale was committed to accomplishing good for those who suffered. She came from the privileged class in Victorian England. However, she was touched by the needs she saw around her, particularly of poor children who were ill. Nightingale was determined to do more than live a life of security and comfort, supported by her family, as women of her class did in the 19th century. When her country went to war in Eastern Europe, she organized women to go with her to provide nursing care to injured and ill soldiers. Other courageous people have similarly provided nursing care in difficult situations. In civil wars in both the United States and France, women, particularly those who were in religious groups, went to the battlefields to provide care and comfort. However, in addition to her extensive health care work, Nightingale also left a legacy of writings about the nature of nursing and of her actions to improve health in her society.

In her influential writings, Nightingale emphasized that nursing was more than administering medications and applying poultices. Rather, nursing aims to promote health by the proper use of the environment to aid the natural reparative processes. The essentials of nursing, according to Nightingale, include fresh air, light, warmth, cleanliness, quiet, and the proper selection and administration of diet. She strongly advocated that mothers, teachers, and nurses be educated in the laws of life, that is, understanding what makes for "healthy existences" (Nightingale, 1859, p. 7). Nightingale declared that nursing was a significant way to improve the health of the British nation. In the schools of nursing that she established, nurses were educated to understand health and how to use the environment, both to promote health and to provide energy for the person's natural healing processes. The Nightingale approach to nursing education came to North America in the founding of three schools in 1873, Bellevue Training School in New York City, the Connecticut Training School in New Haven, and Boston Training School (Donahue, 1996).

Writings of nurses in the last two decades of the 20th century expanded richly on the characteristics of nursing that Nightingale articulated. The understanding of nursing at the turn of the 21st century is challenged by the health care demands of recent decades. In an era of massive use of technology in health care, authors emphasize that nursing is characterized by much more than procedures and medical assistant functions. Allan and Hall (1988) noted that the medical model has not worked very well as a clinical framework because it ignores environment, holism, and process. Nursing today has a strong focus on each of these, and on health rather than disease. This is noted in the nursing models used as illustrations in this chapter and in the discussion of health as a major concept of the Roy Adaptation Model presented in Chapter 2.

Newman (1994) and Pender (1996) are two contemporary writers in nursing who explore ways of looking at health as the pattern of one's life. Today nurses have increasing knowledge about how physical and social environments affect the person and health. Nurses study major developments in biobehavioral sciences using knowledge about biologic life systems, from cell physiology to ecosystem science. They learn about human behavior from disciplines such as cultural anthropology, sociology, and psychology. In addition, many nurse-scientists are contributing to a broad understanding of the interactions of people with the environment and of the effect of these interactions on the health of individuals, social groups, and the earth itself. Rogers (1980 and 1990a) explored this theme in her view of unitary human beings and their integral and mutual interaction with environmental fields. For this significant nurse-leader of the 20th century, the human field and the environmental field are coextensive with the universe. Leininger (1991), a nurse-anthropologist, examined environment from the perspective of cultural care.

The theme of an active role for nurses in changing standards of health care is reflected by nursing organizations and by individual nurse authors. Aiken (1992) noted that nurses in the United States during the 1980s gained a foothold in national, state, and local public policy arenas and entered the 1990s ever more optimistic about public policy as a vehicle to advance nursing's professional agenda and to improve health care. In the early 1990s, the National League for Nursing (NLN) and the American Nurses Association (ANA) presented a nursing-sponsored national health plan. Features of the plan included provision of access to needed services; an emphasis on the economic advantages of direct reimbursement for nursing, both outpatient and inpatient; and the specific designation of nurses as providers for certain services (Maraldo & Fagin, 1992). Nurses in all levels of professional organizations continue to work to affect the political process to reform health care.

The American Academy of Nursing was founded in 1973 (McCarthy, 1985) to provide the nursing profession with visionary leadership, facilitate the contributions of nursing leaders, advance scientific knowledge, and influence the development of effective health care policies and practice. In its first decade, the Academy issued four major policy statements covering topics such as long-term care and nurses in primary care. More recently, it has issued position papers related to health policy concerning AIDS and care of the elderly. Scientific sessions of the Academy in the late 1990s have focused on enabling Academy Fellows and other nurse-leaders to contribute to policy documents related to the health care of global citizens and to identify the role of informatics as the infrastructure for health and for quality.

Lynaugh (1992) assessed nursing's history in relation to society and noted that today the profession is more pragmatic and confrontational, and less deferential and altruistic, than it used to be. In this sense, it is more integrated and less isolated from the larger society. Kerr (1996) cited the example of nursing's influence during the drafting of legislation leading to the 1984 Canada Health Act. Through persistent and intense lobbying by the Canadian Nurses Association, the legislation ultimately "ended practices of extra billing [by physicians] and user fees and with the introduction of a statement that provided federal funding for services provided by 'health practitioners'" (Kerr 1996, p. 223). This was a first step toward better utilization of health care professionals and more cost-effective health care. In the United States, nurses have been leaders in the privately funded national program All Kids Count Childhood Immunization Initiative. The purpose of the program is to establish immunization monitoring and follow-up systems. When combined with other local, state, and federal immunization efforts, this system will help increase immunization rates among preschool children and reduce rates of illness, disability, and death from vaccine-preventable diseases. The initiative takes a simple idea and deals with the complexities of the intersecting public- and private-sector responsibilities for child health care. It has played a role in setting national policy for the development of immunization registry and follow-up systems (Isaacs & Knickman, 1997).

Two characteristics of nursing that have received much attention in recent literature are the focus on caring and clinical reasoning. Nightingale (1859) alluded to these characteristics in her persuasive discussion about the importance of observation. She noted that the nurse "must be a sound, and close, and quick observer; and she must be a woman of delicate and decent feeling" (Nightingale, 1859, p. 71). It is current nurse-authors, however, who have thoroughly explored the concept of caring as central to the nature of nursing (Leininger, 1991; Morse, Solberg, Neader, Bottorff, & Johnson, 1990; Watson, 1985). Similarly, authors such as Gordon, Murphy, Candee, and Hiltunen (1994) have derived a model of nursing clinical judgment. They distinguish three types of clinical reasoning: diagnostic, ethical, and therapeutic.

Thus, the characteristics of modern nursing can be summarized based on the rich heritage of nursing and on the scholarly work and clinical practice of contemporary nurses. Nursing is a health care profession that focuses on the life patterns of persons. The emphasis is on health and how mutual interactions of the person and environment promote health. As a profession, nursing has a commitment to promote health and full life-potential for individuals, families, groups, and society as a whole. Caring is a key aspect of the nursing commitment, and clinical reasoning skills are foremost in the practice of professional nursing. This contemporary view of nursing was reflected in an influential article by Donaldson and Crowley (1978) two decades ago. These authors identified the commonalities of nursing as the following.

1. Concern with principles and laws that govern life processes, well-being, and optimum functioning of human beings, sick or well.
2. Concern with the pattern of human behavior in interaction with the environment in critical life situations.
3. Concern with the processes by which positive changes in health status are effected.

Nature of Knowledge

As a health care profession, nursing uses specialized knowledge. Specialized knowledge has both substance (What is it about?) and method (How is it developed?). Nursing's social commitment is to contribute to health by focusing on life processes of persons in their environments. This goal directs the development of specialized nursing knowledge.

Knowledge for professional practice depends on the profession's area of responsibility in society. An area of responsibility is referred to as the *domain* of the profession. The domain (area of social concern) of nursing is contributing to health by focusing on life processes of people in their environments. In outlining knowledge needed in the domain of nursing, it has been useful to focus on understanding three major concepts: persons (or recipients of nursing care), environment, and health.

The person is the main focus of nursing. Nurses are involved in the health of persons as individuals and in groups such as families and the communities that form society. Knowledge includes values and beliefs as well as scientific facts and principles. The values and beliefs of nursing are referred to as *philosophic assumptions*. Major philosophic assumptions about the person include:

1. The individual person is of value, and therefore worthy of respect and care.
2. Individual persons are responsible for making decisions that influence their lives.
3. Persons are holistic, that is, their physical, thinking, and feeling processes function together in a unified expression of human behavioral patterns.
4. People function interdependently with other persons in environments of the earth to create societies.

To understand the person, the nurse begins with a strong commitment to values about the person. These beliefs are not enough, however. The nurse will also have knowledge about the science of *holistic* persons. This knowledge will be biobehavioral and will include the understanding of the person as a living system made up of cells and physiologic body systems. Nursing knowledge of persons will also focus on how people behave holistically to influence their health. As is noted later in this chapter, nursing conceptual models further enhance the understanding and knowledge about persons within the domain of nursing.

Since nursing's concern is with persons in interaction with the environment, the second area of content of nursing knowledge relates to environment. *Environment* in the domain of nursing has been described as all that influences people and their health. In particular, environment refers to the person's physical surroundings, warm or cold, comfortable or plain, and the people in one's life, whether they are supportive or indifferent. In addition, a contemporary view of environment includes the earth and its resources that are both life-giving and limited.

As Nightingale noted in her foundational tenets of modern nursing, it is important for the nurse to know the laws of health or what makes for "healthy existence." In general, the concept of *health* refers to the person's total well-being. The laws of health that are part of nursing knowledge refer to the regular patterns noted in people and their environments, which result in the person's maintaining wholeness and integrity. The integrity of the person is defined by what nurses believe about people, that is, that they are valued; are in charge of their lives; have consistency of thinking, feeling, and being; and are in harmony with their world and others in it. Knowledge for nursing, then, includes understanding health.

The content of nursing knowledge focuses on persons and how they interact with their environments to enhance well-being and human integrity, whether sick or well. For example, nurses are concerned with how the developmentally challenged child can reach the highest level of functioning, and how the dying cancer patient can maintain the right to make decisions as long as possible. Nursing knowledge also looks at patterns of human behavior within particular environments, and at various critical periods of life. In each lifetime, there are times that are more significant for the person because of expected gradual changes, such as adolescence, or because of more abrupt or unexpected changes, such as sudden injury or illness. Nurses deal with developing families when a baby is born. They observe how family members prepare themselves and their home when a loved one is returning to them after suffering a disabling illness, such as a stroke.

Finally, nursing knowledge deals with ways in which people can bring about positive changes in their interactions with the environment to promote health. Beyond simply learning about how certain factors threaten a person's health (cigarette smoking, for example), nursing knowledge is more concerned with all aspects of the process of promoting health. In the example of cigarette smoking, nursing knowledge broadens to the understanding of individual processes of habit formation and alteration of underlying needs, attitudes, and learning. In addition, nursing knowledge considers social processes such as regional economic pressures and marketing strategies of involved industries and the opposition of public policy and government regulation.

Knowledge Development in Nursing

As noted at the beginning of the chapter, a profession is a scholarly discipline that uses its knowledge for a social good. Knowledge in nursing involves philosophic assumptions and scientific principles related to persons, environment, and health. Philosophic assumptions and scientific principles are developed by a community of scholars who also practice nursing. Florence Nightingale initially developed the discipline of nursing by writing down her convictions and observations in caring for soldiers affected by war and the environment of war. The person as the primary focus of nursing knowledge has been discussed in detail by Rogers (1990a) and Roy (1996). It is the consensus of nurses, reflected in their writings, that has led to the commonly held values and beliefs about persons. The science of nursing is also developed by the community of scholars and practitioners of nursing. The development of scientific principles, however, also involves a scientific approach and evidence beyond common consensus.

The purpose of science is to observe, classify, and investigate relationships that lead to understanding and provide the ability to deal with natural phenomena. Phenomena are the objects of study in the domain. Basically, a scientific approach observes and classifies phenomena, or objects, according to a particular viewpoint. The relationships between the phenomena, or the parts of any one object, are then identified and the general theories or principles of their interaction are stated and tested. Thus, in biology, living organisms, from the smallest ones, such as invisible viruses, to the complex human being, are arranged in a hierarchy according to their various characteristics. As biologists studied living beings, they identified patterns of the activities of various species, for example, ingestion and reproduction. In this way, general theories or statements of relationships that are believed to hold true under given conditions are established. Thus, the field of biology proposes certain principles about the replication and duplication of genetic material in all living beings.

In the development of scientific knowledge for nursing, nurses observe and classify the processes of the person interacting with the environment to promote health. The relationships between the concepts and the processes are identified and the general theories of their interactions and how nurses can affect them are stated and tested. Nurses believe that their growing knowledge about people's holistic processes for promoting their own well-being can have a significant influence on levels of health status.

The methods that nurses use for developing knowledge of the science of nursing include three approaches: nursing conceptual model development, theory construction, and research to test and develop new theories. In this text, discussion focuses on the first level, and specifically, the Roy Adaptation Model. Each conceptual model for nursing provides a particular focus for the study of life processes as they are viewed in the domain of nursing.

▶ NURSING MODELS

A *model* is defined most simply as a description or analogy used to help visualize something that cannot be observed directly. When scientists work with problems of travel in space, they use models of the galaxies and models of spacecraft. The pieces of the models represent the features of the actual galaxies and spacecraft that are involved. However, these representations are in an abstract form. They can be built with styrofoam and glue to some miniature scale of what they stand for, or they can be further abstracted to mathematical formulas and appear as dots and lines in motion on a computer screen or words in sentences that denote concepts and their relationships.

The scientific body of knowledge associated with the domain of nursing supports the provision of a professional service to society, namely, contributing to health by focusing on life processes of persons in their environments. Just as any model is made up of the essential parts of what it represents, so a nursing model is made up of essential parts, or elements, of the domain of nursing. We define a *conceptual model for nursing* as a set of concepts or images that identify and relate the essential elements of nursing. The essential elements of a model for nursing practice, or concepts to be included, are as follows.

1. A description of the person or groups receiving nursing care.
2. A specified meaning for environment.
3. A definition of health.
4. A statement of the broad goal of nursing.
5. A delineation of approaches to reach the goal of nursing.

A model describes each of these concepts and shows in a general way how the concepts are related to one another. From the time of Florence Nightingale (1820–1910) to the present, the writings of nurses can be analyzed to show various ways of addressing the major domain concepts of nursing. Some authors identify as many as 25 different nursing models in the United States alone (Marriner-Tomey, 1994). Models have been developed in other countries as well (Pearson & Vaughan, 1986). However, for illustration, seven selected models are described in this chapter. This discussion can prepare the reader to pursue the expanding literature in the field. A brief description of the selected authors' views of person, environment, health, and nursing goals and approaches are summarized in Table 1–1 and discussed in the following section.

Selected Examples

Hildegard Peplau

Hildegard Peplau had a significant influence on model development in nursing. With a background in psychiatric nursing, Peplau presented the elements of her model in a 1952 book, *Interpersonal Relations in Nursing*. Peplau's work had an impact, not only on the teaching of psychiatric nursing, but also on the shift in models of nursing from a major focus on the needs of the person to a focus that included the nurse–patient relationship. Peplau remains influential in defining nursing and served on the task force of the Congress for Nursing Practice of the American Nurses Association, which issued a landmark policy statement on the nature and scope of nursing practice (American Nurses Association 1982).

Peplau focused attention on the person receiving nursing care as a *developing personality*. Careful observations and thoughtful insights from clinical work provided the basis for the concepts of this nursing model. In addition, a study of the work of psychoanalytic theorist Harry Stack Sullivan (1953) provided some of the background for understanding the person, and for describing the dynamic interaction that occurs during development in early infancy

TABLE 1–1   **EXAMPLES OF NURSING MODELS**

Person	Environment	Health	Nursing Goal and Approaches
Peplau A developing being pursuing satisfaction and interpersonal security and contact.	Cultural and social context.	A word symbol that implies the forward movement of the personality and other ongoing human processes in the direction of constructive, productive, personal and community living.	Development of personality and other human processes through significant, therapeutic interpersonal relationships, with four phases.
Johnson A behavioral system composed of seven subsystems: affiliative, dependency, ingestive, eliminative, sexual, aggressive, and achievement.	Objects, events, situations, and forces that provide the system's functional requirements of protection, nurturance, and stimulation.	Behavioral system balance and stability that show efficient and effective behavioral functioning.	To restore, maintain, or attain behavioral system balance and dynamic stability at the highest possible level for the individual through assessing behavioral instability and plans to stimulate, protect, defend, inhibit, or facilitate behavior.
Orem An individual with universal, developmental, and health-deviation types of self-care requisites who may vary in power to engage in self-care.	Physical, chemical, biologic, and social conditions relevant to self-care requisites and basic conditioning factors.	A state of the person characterized by soundness or wholeness of developed human structures and of bodily and mental functioning that requires continuous self-care of therapeutic quality.	To help people meet their own and dependent others' self-care demands by helping the patient accomplish therapeutic self-care and move toward independent self-care as well as become competent in providing and managing care requisites.
Rogers A unitary, pandimensional, negentrophic energy field identified by pattern, organization, and manifestation of characteristics and behaviors that are specific to the whole, which cannot be predicted from knowledge of the parts.	An irreducible pandimensional energy field identified by pattern and organization and integral with the human field.	A rhythmic pattern of energy exchange which is mutually enhancing and expresses full life-potential.	To strengthen the integrity of the human–environment energy field by directing and redirecting patterning, primarily by noninvasive modalities.

TABLE 1-1   EXAMPLES OF NURSING MODELS (CONT.)

Person	Environment	Health	Nursing Goal and Approaches
Roy			
An adaptive system with cognator and regulator subsystems acting to maintain adaptation in the four adaptive modes: physiologic–physical, self-concept–group identity, role function, and interdependence.	All conditions, circumstances, and influences surrounding and affecting the development and behavior of persons and groups, with particular consideration of mutuality of person and earth resources.	A state and a process of being and becoming integrated and whole that reflects person and environment mutuality.	To promote adaptation for individuals and groups in the four adaptive modes, thus contributing to health, quality of life, and dying with dignity by assessing behavior and factors that influence adaptive abilities and by intervening to expand those abilities and to enhance environmental interactions.
Newman			
Pattern of consciousness that is expanding and moving through varying degrees of organization and disorganization as one unitary process.	Implicate order, or unseen multidimensional pattern, as ground or basis for all things and the explicate order, or tangibles, that periodically arise as temporary manifestations of the total pattern.	Expanding consciousness, pattern of the whole, encompassing disease and nondisease, regarded as the explication of the underlying pattern of the person and environment.	Pattern identification and expanding consciousness through personal transformations and forming shared consciousness.
Leininger			
Individual in a given cultural context that has learned, shared, and transmitted values, beliefs, norms, and lifeways that guide individual thinking, decisions, and actions in patterned ways.	The context of the totality of an event, situation, or particular experience that give meaning to human expressions, interpretations, and social interactions in particular physical, ecological, sociopolitical, and cultural settings.	A state of well-being that is culturally defined, valued, and practiced, and which reflects the ability of individuals, or groups, to perform their daily role activities in culturally expressed, beneficial and patterned lifeways.	To focus on human care phenomena and activities in order to assist, support, facilitate, or enable individuals and groups to maintain, or regain, their well-being by using cultural care preservation and maintenance, accommodation and negotiation, and repatterning or restructuring.

and childhood. The individual pursues satisfaction of physiologic demands, interpersonal security, and interpersonal contact. In this process, tensions of need, anxiety, and loneliness are created. The energy of these tensions, according to Peplau, can be transformed in positive directions.

Peplau does not define or describe the concept of environment. However, her writing reflects the general notion of environment as including *the cultural and social context*. Particularly, it is the cultural forces, together with the infant's biological constitution, that determine personality.

For Peplau, health is a word symbol that implies *forward movement of personality and other ongoing human processes in the direction of creative, productive, personal and community living.* Her writing emphasizes personality development and nursing as an approach to people rather than describing health or environment in detail.

Given Peplau's view of the person, the specific goal of nursing can be stated most simply as: *to foster forward movement of the personality and other ongoing human processes in the direction of creative, constructive, and productive personal and community living.* Peplau noted that nurses facilitate natural ongoing tendencies in human organisms. The nurse is an educating instrument and a maturing force, aiming at forward movement. Peplau's greatest contribution to the development of nursing science was the delineation of the interpersonal process as the approach used in nursing. The nurse improves the person's social context by therapeutic interaction with the person. Peplau described this process as a series of phases involving different roles for the nurse and the person.

The orientation phase involves learning the nature of the person's difficulty and the extent of the need for help. The identification phase is the time period in which the person is responding to the nurse and feeling a sense of belonging and identification. The exploitation phase occurs when the person identifies with the nurse and proceeds to make full use of the services offered, including the nurse's interpersonal skills. The resolution phase generally concludes the process as old ties and dependencies are relinquished and the person prepares to resume independence. Peplau's emphasis is that the phases, and roles of nurse and patient within the phases, are fluid in nature and tend to flow together or move backward or forward as the person moves forward or regresses. During the fluctuating phases, the nurse can fulfill a variety of roles, including teacher, resource person, counselor, and surrogate. Within the nursing approach of the interpersonal relationship, Peplau emphasized the specific skills of observing, communicating, and recording.

Dorothy Johnson

Toward the end of the 1950s, Dorothy E. Johnson began to write about the nature of a science of nursing and to emphasize the need to clarify the goal of nursing and the scientific knowledge involved (Johnson, 1959). Johnson's writing reflects premises about nursing as a direct service provided to individuals or groups under the stress of illness. By the 1960s, the Johnson nursing model became the basis of the undergraduate nursing curriculum at the University of California at Los Angeles, and in the 1970s, she developed the first graduate course focused on models of nursing. Johnson's teaching, related writing, speaking, sharing of unpublished materials, and consultation with schools of nursing did much to establish the rapid growth of nursing models for education and practice in the decades of the 1960s and 1970s.

Through these decades, Johnson developed and taught a comprehensive view of the person as the recipient of nursing care. This was later published, together with the other elements of the Johnson Behavioral System

Model, in 1980. According to Johnson (1980), the person is *a behavioral system that has a tendency to achieve and maintain stability in patterns of functioning.* Like Nightingale, Johnson observed that similar patterns occur in both health and illness. Johnson postulates that the whole behavioral system of a person is composed of seven subsystems: affiliative, dependency, ingestive, eliminative, sexual, aggressive, and achievement. The goals of the behavioral systems are the survival, reproduction, and growth of the human organism. To maintain the stability of the system, and thus to meet its goal, each subsystem must receive adequate input to meet functional requirements or sustenance imperatives. Johnson defined these inputs as protection, nurturance, and stimulation. Problems arise for the person when there are disturbances in the structure or function of the subsystems, or because the level of behavioral functioning is less than optimal.

Johnson frequently mentioned environment, but did not directly define the term. However, from her writing, one can infer that environment referred to *the objects, events, situations, and forces that provide the system's functional requirements of protection, nurturance, and stimulation.*

Similarly, health is often referred to in Johnson's writing, but not defined. Johnson's concept of health can be inferred from her discussions of the person and of nursing's goal. For Johnson, health can be represented as *behavioral system balance and stability that shows efficient and effective behavioral functioning.*

According to the Johnson Behavioral System Model, the goal of nursing is *to restore, maintain, or attain the person's behavioral stability.* Nursing aims to establish regularities in behavior so that each subsystem can fulfill its goal. Behavioral stability exists when a minimum expenditure of energy is required, continued biologic and social survival is ensured, and some degree of personal satisfaction is accrued. Behavioral stability might be observed either as physiologic changes or as behavioral changes such as the lessening of disorder, purposelessness, or unpredictability.

Johnson defined nursing approaches in terms of the stages of the nursing process: assessment, diagnosis, intervention, and evaluation. The nurse assesses the stability of the behavioral subsystems and diagnoses the dynamics of any instability noted. For intervention, according to this model, the nurse can do any of the following: protect, restrict, defend, inhibit, or facilitate. Johnson described the nurse as an external regulatory force acting to preserve the organization and integration of the person's behavior. The outcome of nursing intervention is evaluated according to the goal of behavioral stability.

Dorothea Orem

Also in the late 1950s, Dorothea Orem was developing another major model of nursing. Orem's initial formulations of a self-care framework stemmed from nursing practice experience and the need to describe the subject matter of nursing. The immediate impetus was the development of a curriculum guideline for practical nurses that Orem undertook as a consultant at the

U.S. Department of Health, Education, and Welfare (Orem, 1959). Later, Orem worked with several work groups of nurse-scholars to further describe the basic concepts of this nursing model. The major text on the self-care framework, *Nursing: Concepts of Practice,* was published in 1971 and has been updated in 1980, 1985, 1991, and 1995. Orem made significant contributions to nursing knowledge by identifying a unique domain and the boundaries of nursing as a science and an art. Orem's model is used extensively in nursing education, practice, and research. A self-care institute has been established in the United States. An International Orem Society for Nursing Science and Scholarship was founded in 1991.

Orem refers to the person as *a self-care agency.* Self-care agency is the power of the person to engage in self-care. This power is a complex, acquired ability to meet one's continuing requirements for care. It regulates life processes; maintains or promotes integrity of human structure, functioning, and human development; and promotes well-being. Self-care requisites, or requirements, include the following.

1. Universal requisites. Those that apply for all persons during all stages of the life cycle and are associated with life processes and the integrity of human structure and functioning.
2. Developmental requisites. Those that are associated with human development processes and with conditions and events occurring during various stages of the life cycle.
3. Health-deviation requisites. Those that are associated with disease, injury, disfigurement, disability, and with medical care measures used for diagnosis and treatment.

The definition of environment used in Orem's conceptual model is the *physical, chemical, biologic, and social conditions relevant to self-care requisites and basic conditioning factors.* Orem's definition of health stems from her concept of person. In this framework, health refers to *the state of the person characterized by soundness or wholeness of developed human structures and of bodily and mental functioning.* Health requires self-care of therapeutic quality.

A major concept of the Orem model is the theory of the nursing system. This theory provides a specific goal and approach for nursing. The goal of nursing is *to help people meet their own and dependent others' self-care demands.* Orem describes three types of nursing approaches. Each approach is made up of a continuing series of actions produced as ways of helping to meet the person's therapeutic self-care demands or to regulate their self-care agency. The particular approach used depends on the person's self-care agency, that is, the ability to meet self-care demands. The wholly compensatory nursing system is used when the person is unable to engage in self-care activities that require ambulation and movement. The partly compensatory system exists when both nurse and patient perform care measures or other actions involving manipulative tasks or ambulation. The third type of nursing approach is the supportive-educative system, which is used when the patient is able to perform, or can and should learn to perform, required measures of externally or internally oriented therapeutic self-care but cannot do so without assistance. The eventual outcome of patient care, based on the Orem model, is that the person is independent and able to manage universal, developmental, and therapeutic self-care requisites.

Martha Rogers

Martha Rogers was involved in the scholarly discussions focused on the need to clarify the nature of nursing that were common in the late 1950s and early 1960s. In her book *Educational Revolution in Nursing,* Rogers (1961) presented the goal of nursing as the movement of the person toward maximum health. In 1970, she described evolving views on the nature of nursing in a book entitled *An Introduction to the Theoretical Basis of Nursing.* Later, Rogers (1980) presented the basics of nursing as the science of unitary human beings. In the last decades of her life, she expanded on earlier themes in both writing (Rogers, 1990a,1992) and speaking (Rogers, 1987, 1990b) and left the legacy of a solid conceptual system and a vision of nursing for the future.

The major contribution of Rogers' work was a revolutionary concept of the human person. Given today's assumption of the holism of the person, it is not easy to recognize the extent of the shift in thinking that Rogers called for in describing the person as *a unitary, four-dimensional, negentropic energy field.* According to Rogers, nursing is the only learned profession that truly deals with a unitary view of the total person, since other sciences study various parts of the person or an addition of parts. She recognized that, for nurses who have been taught other basic sciences, it is difficult to think in terms of unitary patterns rather than parts of the person. However, Rogers energetically insisted on the unitary view of the person and of identifying concepts of holism that were not truly reflecting unitary patterns. Within Rogers' conceptual scheme, there are descriptions of the characteristics of the unitary, four-dimensional person. The human energy field evolves rhythmically along life's nonlinear, spiraling axis. This image led to representing Rogers' conceptual system by the popular child's coiled toy known as "Slinky."

Rogers was specific in the discussion of environment since this is a major concept in her theoretical formulations. Just as the person is unitary, Rogers viewed environment as *irreducible and as a pandimensional energy field.* This field is also identified by pattern and organization, and most particularly is integral with the human field. Rogers' emphasis on the lack of boundaries between the person and environment was a turning point in conceptual thinking in nursing (Newman, 1994). For Rogers, the person–environment field is coextensive with the universe.

Rogers described health as *an expression of the life process.* Rogers maintained that there are no absolute norms for health and that manifestations of human and environmental field patterns deemed to have high value are labeled "wellness" by society, and those deemed to have low value are labeled "illness." However, in the glossary of terms that Rogers frequently used in public presentations of her work, she did not have a specific definition of health. When Rogers was a member of the Nurse Theorist Group of the National Conference on Nursing Diagnosis that met in the late 1970s and early 1980s, the group submitted the following definition of health that is reflective of Rogers' science of unitary human beings. Health is *a rhythmic pattern of energy exchange which is mutually enhancing and expresses full life potential* (Kim & Moritz, 1982, p. 246). It is important to note that Rogers' concept of unitary human–environmental fields calls for replacing the dichotomy between health and disease with a new synthesis. This idea was later expanded by another theorist, Margaret Newman (1994).

The goal of nursing, according to Rogers, is to promote health, or more specifically, to strengthen the integral human–environment energy field. She noted that the human–environment energy fields have diverse manifestations. Nursing approaches begin with pattern manifestation appraisal (Barrett, 1988), that is, the nurse becomes aware of relevant pattern information through sensations, thoughts, feelings, awareness, imagination, memory, introspective insights, intuitive apprehensions, and recurring themes and issues (Crowling, 1990). In later discussions, Rogers noted that this science requires new interventions and that many of these new approaches are noninvasive. Examples of such noninvasive nursing approaches include therapeutic touch, imagery, meditation, relaxation, unconditional love, attitudes of hope and humor, and the use of sound, color, and motion (Rogers, Doyle, Racolin, & Walsh, 1990). The Society of Rogerian Scholars was founded in 1986 to foster the development of the science of unitary human beings.

Sister Callista Roy

Sister Callista Roy began her work on a nursing model while she was a graduate student studying with Dorothy E. Johnson from 1963 to 1966. The first published work on the model was an article in 1970 (Roy, 1970). The same year, the model was implemented as the basis of the baccalaureate curriculum at Mount St. Mary's College in Los Angeles. The major concepts of the model will be discussed in greater detail in the remaining chapters. For the purpose of this chapter, the basic elements are summarized so that they can be seen in perspective with other major nursing models selected as illustrations.

Roy describes the person as *an adaptive system*. As with any type of system, the person has internal processes that act to maintain the integrity of the person. These processes have been broadly categorized as a regulator subsystem and a cognator subsystem. The regulator involves physiologic processes such as chemical, neurologic, and endocrine responses that allow the body to cope with the changing environment. For example, when a person perceives a sudden threat, such as an oncoming car approaching just after stepping off the curb, a rush of energy is available from an increase of adrenal hormones.

The cognator subsystem involves the cognitive and emotional processes of interacting with the environment. In the example of the person who runs from an oncoming car, the cognator acts to process the emotion of fear. The perceptions of the situation are also processed and the person can come to some new decision about where and how to cross the street safely. Both cognator and regulator activity are manifested in four particular ways in each person: in behaviors indicating physiologic–physical function, self-concept–group identity, role function, and interdependence. These four ways of categorizing the effects of cognator and regulator activity are called adaptive modes. Adaptive modes and coping processes for groups of persons are also described by the Roy model.

The Roy model uses a definition of environment as *all the conditions, circumstances, and influences surrounding and affecting the development and behavior of persons and groups.* From the perspective of the person's place in the evolving universe, environment is a biophysical community of beings with complex patterns of interaction, feedback, growth, and decline, constituting periodic and long-term rhythms. Person and environment interactions are input for the person as an adaptive system. This input involves both internal and external factors. Roy used the work of Helson (1964), a physiologic psychologist, to categorize these factors as focal, contextual, and residual stimuli. A specific consideration as a stimulus is adaptation level, which has an internal effect on coping behaviors.

Roy's concept of health is related to the concept of adaptation. Persons are viewed as adaptive systems that interact with the environment and grow and develop. Health is the reflection of person and environment interactions that are adaptive. Adaptive responses promote integrity. According to this model, health is defined as *a process and a state of being, and becoming whole and integrated in a way that reflects person and environment mutuality.*

Roy's view of the goal of nursing was the first major concept of her nursing model to be described. Roy began this work by attempting to identify the unique function of nursing in promoting health. Since a number of health care workers have the goal of promoting health, it seemed important for nursing to identify a unique goal. As a staff nurse in pediatric settings, Roy noted the great resiliency of children in responding to major physiologic and psychological changes. Yet nursing intervention was needed to support and promote this positive coping. It seemed then that the concept of adaptation, or positive coping, might be used to describe the goal or function of nursing. From this initial notion, Roy developed a description of the goal of nursing as: *the promotion of adaptation for individuals and groups in each of the four adaptive modes, thus contributing to health, quality of life, and dying with dignity.*

Nursing approaches, according to the Roy Adaptation Model, involve assessment of behavior and the factors affecting adaptation, and intervention to promote adaptive abilities and enhance environment interactions. Roy's view of adaptation, together with the other major concepts of the model, will be described in greater detail in Chapter 2.

Margaret Newman

Margaret Newman noted that her view of health as expanding consciousness is grounded in personal experience, but was stimulated by Rogers' insistence on the unitary nature of a human being in interaction with the environment (Newman, 1994). Newman first presented these concepts of nursing at a nursing theory conference in New York in 1978. Newman's clinical research, doctoral teaching, and collaboration in practice have been integral to the developing ideas explored in major publications in the 1980s and 1990s.

Since the concept of health is the major focus of Newman's theoretical work, the definitions of person, environment, and the goal and approaches of nursing have been extrapolated from her discussions of health. The person is viewed as *a pattern of consciousness.* Consciousness is defined as the information of the system that provides the capacity to interact with the environment. Newman (1994) noted that in the human system, the capacity for information processing includes not only thinking and feeling, but also all the information embedded in the nervous system, endocrine system, immune system, and genetic code. The human pattern is expanding and life is evolving in the direction of higher levels of consciousness. At the same time, there are complementary forces of order and disorder that maintain a fluctuating field. These fluctuations are what make possible the periodic transformations that shift the person into a higher order of functioning. Organization and disorganization are one unitary process.

Newman cites Bohm's (1980) analogies of the implicate and explicate order as useful in understanding the theory underlying expanding consciousness. Given the meaning of these terms, it seems that they can represent the meaning of environment in this conceptualization of the domain of nursing. The implicate order is described as the multidimensional pattern that is the ground or basis for all things. The explicate order, on the other hand, is the tangibles that periodically arise as temporary manifestations of the total pattern present in the implicate order. Environment is the *patterned basis of all being.* As in Rogers' work, it is not possible to separate the person from environment since the person's pattern is also rooted in the implicate order. Newman (1994) assumed that consciousness is coextensive in the universe and is the essence of all matter.

Newman defined health as *expanding consciousness.* The theorist emphasized seeing health as the pattern of the whole. By whole, she is referring to the pattern of interaction of an individual with the environment. Newman noted that disease is not a separate entity that invades the body, but rather is a manifestation of the evolving pattern of person–environment interaction. From this perspective, health is the pattern of the whole person–environment and encompasses disease and nondisease. Disease is a manifestation of the underlying pattern and, in fact, is one way to envision a general pattern of energy flow of the person. People also are not separate with separate diseases, but are open energy systems constantly interacting and evolving with others. Health includes the greater whole of the person–environment pattern interacting with the family and the community.

Newman questioned the assumption that interventions are aimed at producing a particular result. To intervene with a particular solution in mind assumes that the nurse knows what form the pattern of expanding consciousness will take. Specific goal setting and approaches are not the issue. Rather, Newman (1994) directed the professional "to enter into *partnership* with the client, often at a time of chaos, with the mutual goal of participating in an authentic relationship, trusting that in the process of its unfolding, both will emerge at a higher level of consciousness" (p. 97). The time or event of disorganization represents an opportunity for pattern recognition, that is, the turning point in the evolution of consciousness. People have the capacity for understanding that which enables them to gain insight into their patterns. Insights lead to evolving consciousness with an accompanying gain in freedom of action. Nurses are reflective of their own patterns and go through personal transformations that make it possible to be partners with others in this process.

Madeleine Leininger

Madeleine Leininger is a nurse-anthropologist who places human care at the center of the discipline and profession of nursing. In the mid-1950s, while working in child psychiatric nursing, Leininger observed concerns about cultural factors with which both the staff and contemporary psychodynamic theories were not prepared to deal. Leininger discussed these concerns with Margaret Mead and pursued them in intensive doctoral studies and field research in cultural and social anthropology. During the 1950s and 1960s, Leininger wrote of the common areas of knowledge in nursing and anthropology. From her insights and scholarly pursuits, she developed the field of transcultural nursing, with a national society established in 1974 and the first textbook published in 1978. Leininger has been a leader in graduate education and in developing research methods and resources in many academic institutions in the United States.

Leininger published these ideas as a formal nursing theory in journal articles in 1985 and 1988. In the opening of her 1991 text, *Culture Care Diversity and Universality: A Theory of Nursing,* Leininger provided quotations from writing and public addresses from 1950 to 1991 to demonstrate that during these four decades, she had challenged nurses worldwide to reflect on care as the essence and central focus of nursing. There are other nurse-theorists who focus on care as the central concept of nursing, notably Benner and Wrubel (1989) and Watson (1985). However, given the primacy in time and depth of development of Leininger's work, there is reason to select her theory as an illustration.

The person, for Leininger, is *the individual in a given cultural context that has learned, shared, and transmitted values, beliefs, norms, and lifeways that guide individual thinking, decisions, and actions in patterned ways.* The lifeways patterns by which individuals and groups assist, support, facilitate, or enable another individuals or group to maintain their well-being and health, to improve their human condition and lifeway, or to deal with illness, handicaps, or death, are called cultural care. Human care is a universal phenomenon; caring acts and processes are necessary for human birth, development, growth, survival, and peaceful death. Cultural care involves both diversity and universality. Diversity is the variability and differences in meanings, patterns, values, lifeways, or symbols of care within and among social groups. Universality is the common, similar, or dominant uniform care lifeways or symbols that are manifest among many cultures.

In Leininger's cultural care theory of nursing, environment is *the context of the totality of an event, situation, or particular experiences that give meaning to human expressions, interpretations, and social interactions in particular physical, ecological, sociopolitical, and cultural settings.* Leininger uses a sunrise model to help visualize different dimensions of the theory. In the top half of the rising sun, cultural and social structural dimensions are portrayed. These include technological, religious and philosophic, kinship and social, political and legal, economic, and educational factors, with cultural values and lifeways in the center.

The related definition of health used by Leininger (1991) is as follows: Health refers to *a state of well being that is culturally defined, valued, and practiced, and which reflects the ability of individuals, or groups, to perform their daily role activities in culturally expressed, beneficial and patterned lifeways* (p. 48). Both generic, folk or lay care systems and professional care systems are used to improve health conditions or to deal with handicap and death situations.

The goal of nursing, according to Leininger, is *to focus on human care phenomena and activities in order to assist, support, facilitate, or enable individuals or groups to maintain or regain their well-being or health in culturally meaningful and beneficial ways, or to help people face handicaps or death.* Three approaches are used by nurses using this model to serve people: cultural care preservation and maintenance, cultural care accommodation and negotiation, and cultural care repatterning or restructuring. Nursing care decisions and actions are based on both generic care knowledge learned from the cultural group and professional knowledge obtained from research. Using the cultural care diversity and the universality theory of nursing, according to the elements of the sunrise model, the nurse keeps in mind the total gestalt of diverse influences to describe and explain care, with health and well-being as outcomes.

► SUMMARY

Nursing is a health care profession that focuses on human life patterns and emphasizes promotion of health for individuals, families, groups, and society as a whole. Nursing knowledge is based on a strong commitment to values about the person and strives to understand how people interact with the environment and behave holistically to influence their health. Nurse-authors since the time of Florence Nightingale have been developing concepts and knowledge related to the domain of nursing, that is, person, environment, health, and the goals and approaches of nursing.

This chapter included illustrations of nursing models reflected in the writings of Peplau, Johnson, Orem, Rogers, Roy, Newman, and Leininger. Nursing conceptual models one way of developing nursing knowledge. This knowledge is then tested in research, taught in nursing education, and used to guide nursing practice. The remainder of this text will focus on the Roy Adaptation Model of nursing and on knowledge based on the model and its use in practice.

► EXERCISES FOR APPLICATION

1. What does the concept "health" mean to you personally? Write down phrases that capture your understanding of and beliefs about health and then compare your definition to that provided by one of the theorists discussed in this chapter.

2. Prepare a table comparing the domains of practice of four health care professions with which you are familiar. Are there any overlapping areas of responsibility or duplication of roles?

3. This chapter described "the person," or the recipient of nursing care, from the perspectives of seven nurse-theorists. Choose the one viewpoint that appears to be the furthest from your perception of "the person." What aspect(s) of the theorist's description do not align with your beliefs?

► ASSESSMENT OF UNDERSTANDING

Questions

1. What are the two characteristics of professions?
   (a) _____
   (b) _____

2. From the following statements, select the three that represent the common concerns of nursing as a profession.
   (a) the principles and laws that govern life processes, well-being, and optimum functioning of human beings.
   (b) the healing of illness and injury at all stages of development in human beings.
   (c) the pattern of human behavior in interaction with the environment in critical life situations.
   (d) the processes by which positive changes in health status are effected.
   (e) the physiologic problems that are evidenced in situations of ill health or disease.

3. Which one of the following statements best describes the nursing profession's area of responsibility in society?
   (a) care of persons experiencing illness.
   (b) life processes of persons in their environments.
   (c) psychosocial health of individuals and families.
   (d) health promotion and disease prevention.

4. Name the three major concepts that constitute nursing's focus.
   (a) _____
   (b) _____
   (c) _____

5. List three approaches to knowledge development for nursing science.
   (a) _____
   (b) _____
   (c) _____

6. Which of the following are the five essential elements of a conceptual model for nursing?
   (a) health
   (b) pathophysiology
   (c) environment
   (d) nursing approaches
   (e) nursing's goals
   (f) health promotion
   (g) person

7. Associate the specified element of a nursing model with the name of the nurse-author who developed it.

Element	Author
_____ (a) persons as unitary human beings	1. Newman
_____ (b) health as adaptation	2. Johnson
_____ (c) nursing process with identification phase	3. Rogers
_____ (d) self-care requisites	4. Leininger
_____ (e) behavioral system	5. Orem
_____ (f) health as expanding consciousness	6. Roy
_____ (g) nursing as cultural care	7. Peplau

Feedback

1. (a) developed to contribute to the good of society.
   (b) use specialized knowledge to meet specific social needs.

2. a, c, d

3. b

4. (a) persons
   (b) environment
   (c) health

5. (a) nursing model development
   (b) theory construction
   (c) research to develop and test theories

6. a, c, d, e, g

7. (a) 3, (b) 6, (c) 7, (d) 5, (e) 2, (f) 1, (g) 4

▶ **REFERENCES**

Aiken, L. (1992). Charting nursing's future. In Aiken, L., & Fagin, C. (Eds.), *Charting nursing's future: Agenda for the 1990s* (pp. 3–12). Philadelphia: Lippincott.

Allan, J., & Hall, B. (1988). Challenging the focus on technology: A critique of the medical model in a changing health care system. *Advances in Nursing Science, 10(3),* 22–34.

American Nurses Association. (1982). *Nursing: A social policy statement.* Kansas City, MO: American Nurses Association.

Barrett, E. A. (1988). Using Rogers' science of unitary human beings in nursing practice. *Nursing Science Quarterly, 1,* 50–51.

Benner, P., & Wrubel, J. (1989). *The primacy of caring: Stress and coping in health and illness.* Menlo Park, CA: Addison-Wesley.

Bohm, D. (1980). *Wholeness and the implicate order.* London: Routledge & Kegan Paul.

Crowling, W. R., III. (1990). A template for unitary pattern-based nursing practice. In Barrett, E. A. (Ed.), *Visions of Rogers' science-based nursing* (pp. 45–65). New York: National League for Nursing.

Donahue, M. P. (1996). *Nursing, the finest art: An illustrated history* (2nd ed.). St. Louis: Mosby.

Donaldson, S. K., & Crowley, D. (1978). The discipline of nursing. *Nursing Outlook, 26,* 113–120.

Gordon, M., Murphy, C., Candee, D., & Hiltunen, E. (1994). Clinical judgement: An integrated model. *Advances in Nursing Science, 16(4),* 55–70.

Helson, H. (1964). *Adaptation level theory.* New York: Harper & Row.

Issacs, S. L., & Knickman, J. R. (Eds.). (1997). *To improve health and health care 1997: The Robert Wood Johnson Foundation anthology.* San Francisco: Jossey-Bass.

Johnson, D. E. (1959). A philosophy of nursing. *Nursing Outlook, 7,* 198–200.

Johnson, D. E. (1980). The behavioral system model for nursing. In Riehl, J., & Roy, C. (Eds.), *Conceptual models for nursing practice* (2nd ed., pp. 207–216). New York: Appleton-Century-Crofts.

Kerr, J. R. (1996). The organization and financing of health care: Issues for nursing. In Kerr, J.R., & MacPhail, J. (Eds.), *Canadian nursing: Issues and perspectives* (pp. 216–227). St. Louis: Mosby.

Kim, M., & Moritz, D. (1982). *Classification of nursing diagnosis: Proceedings of the third and fourth national conferences.* New York: McGraw-Hill.

Leininger, M. (1978). *Transcultural nursing: Concepts, theory, and practices.* New York: Wiley.

Leininger, M. (1985). Transcultural care diversity and universality: A theory of nursing. *Nursing and Health Care, 6,* 209–212.

Leininger, M. (1988). Leininger's theory of nursing: Cultural care diversity and universality. *Nursing Science Quarterly, 1(4),* 152–160.

Leininger, M. (1991). *Culture, care, diversity and universality: A theory of nursing.* New York: National League for Nursing.

Lynaugh, J. (1992). Nursing's history: Looking backward and seeing forward. In Aiken, L., & Fagin, C. (Eds.), *Charting nursing's future: Agenda for the 1990s* (pp. 435–447). Philadelphia: Lippincott.

Maraldo, P., & Fagin, C. (1992). The nurses' national health plan. In Aiken, L., & Fagin, C. (Eds.), *Charting nursing's future: Agenda for the 1990s* (pp. 504–515). Philadelphia: Lippincott.

Marriner-Tomey, A. (1994). *Nursing theorists and their work* (3rd ed.). St. Louis: Mosby.

McCarthy, R. (1985). *History of the American Academy of Nursing.* Kansas City, MO: The American Nurses Association.

Morse, J., Solberg, S., Neander, W., Bottorff, J., & Johnson, J. (1990). Concepts of caring and caring as a concept. *Advances in Nursing Science, 13(1),* 1–14.

Newman, M. (1994). *Health as expanding consciousness* (2nd ed.). New York: National League for Nursing.

Nightingale, F. (1859). *Notes on nursing: What it is and what it is not* (facsimile edition). Philadelphia: Lippincott.

Orem, D. E. (1959). *Guides for developing curricula for the education of practical nurses.* Washington, DC, U.S. Dept of Health, Education and Welfare, Office of Education, U.S. Govt. Printing Office.

Orem, D. E. (1971). *Nursing: Concepts of practice.* New York: McGraw-Hill.

Orem, D. E. (1980). *Nursing: Concepts of practice* (2nd ed.). New York: McGraw-Hill.

Orem, D. E. (1985). *Nursing: Concepts of practice* (3rd ed.). New York: McGraw-Hill.

Orem, D. E. (1991). *Nursing: Concepts of practice* (4th ed.). St. Louis: Mosby Yearbook.

Orem, D. E. (1995). *Nursing: Concepts of practice* (5th ed.). St. Louis: Mosby Yearbook.

Pearson, A., & Vaughan, B. (1986). Common characteristics of nursing models: The patient or client. *Nursing Models for Practice, 3,* 26–39.

Pender, N. (1996). *Health promotion in nursing practice* (3rd ed.). Stamford, CT: Appleton & Lange.

Peplau, H. (1952). *Interpersonal relations in nursing.* New York: Putnam.

Rogers, M. (1961). *Educational revolution in nursing.* New York: Macmillan.

Rogers, M. (1970). *An introduction to the theoretical basis of nursing.* Philadelphia: Davis.

Rogers, M. (1980). Nursing: A science of unitary man. In Riehl, J., & Roy, C. (Eds.), *Conceptual models for nursing practice* (pp. 329–337). New York: Appleton-Century-Crofts.

Rogers, M. (1987). Rogers' Framework. Paper presented at Nurse Theorist conference, Pittsburgh.

Rogers, M. (1990a). Nursing: Science of unitary, irreducible, human beings: Update 1990. In Barrett, E. A. (Ed.), *Visions of Rogers' science-based nursing* (pp. 105–113). New York: National League for Nursing.

Rogers, M. (1990b). Space-age paradigm for new frontiers in nursing. In Parker, M. E. (Ed.), *Nursing theories in practice* (pp. 105–113). New York: National League for Nursing.

Rogers, M. (1992). Nursing science and the space age. *Nursing Science Quarterly, 5,* 27–34.

Rogers, M., Doyle, M., Racolin, A., & Walsh, P. (1990). A conversation with Martha Rogers on nursing in space. In Barrett, E. A. (Ed.), *Visions of Rogers' science-based nursing* (pp. 375–386). New York: National League for Nursing.

Roy, C. (1970). Adaptation: A conceptual framework for nursing. *Nursing Outlook, 18,* 42–45.

Roy, C. (1997). Knowledge as universal cosmic imperative. *Proceedings of nursing knowledge impact conference 1996* (pp. 95–118). Chestnut Hill, MA: Boston College Press.

Sullivan, H. (1953). *The independent theory of psychiatry.* New York: Norton.

Watson, J. (1985). *Nursing: Human science and human care: A theory of nursing.* Norwalk, CT: Appleton-Century-Crofts.

2

ESSENTIALS OF THE ROY
ADAPTATION MODEL

The first formal description of the Roy Adaptation Model was made by Sister Callista Roy while a graduate student at the School of Nursing of the University of California at Los Angeles. The roots of the model lie in Roy's personal and professional background. Roy is committed to philosophic assumptions characterized by the general principles of humanism, and by veritivity and cosmic unity, two terms given special meaning by Roy. The scientific foundation for the model was based on assumptions from systems theory and adaptation-level theory. More recently, a redefinition of adaptation for the future has been used to extend the scientific assumptions.

Under the mentorship of Dorothy E. Johnson, Roy became convinced of the importance of defining nursing. She was also influenced by studies in the liberal arts and the natural and social sciences. Clinical practice in pediatric nursing provided experience with the resilience of the human body and spirit. Roy began to seek ways to express these beliefs about nursing and to explore them further in her studies. The first publication on the Roy Adaptation Model appeared in 1970 (Roy, 1970). At that time, Roy was on the faculty of the baccalaureate nursing program of a small liberal arts college. There, she had the opportunity to lead the implementation of this model of nursing as the basis of the nursing curriculum. During the next decade, more than 1,500 faculty and students at Mount St. Mary's College helped to clarify, refine, and develop the basic concepts of the Roy Adaptation Model for nursing. In the 1980s, Roy was influenced by postdoctoral work in neuroscience nursing. During the 1990s, as faculty member and nurse-theorist at Boston College, Roy focused on contemporary movements in nursing knowledge and the continued integration of spirituality with an understanding of nursing's role in promoting adaptation.

This chapter provides an overview of the major concepts of the Roy Adaptation Model of nursing and the associated philosophic and scientific assumptions as they have developed over time.

► OBJECTIVES

After studying this chapter, the reader will be able to do the following:

1. Identify the initial scientific and philosophic assumptions underlying the Roy Adaptation Model and describe directions for the future.

2. Identify the key terms in Roy's description of humans as adaptive systems.

3. State the difference between adaptive and ineffective responses.

4. Differentiate the three classes of stimuli.

5. Define adaptation level and identify three levels described by the Roy Adaptation Model.

6. In a situation involving an individual, identify specific behaviors as indicative of cognator or regulator activity.

7. In a group situation, label identified behaviors as indicative of stabilizer or innovator activity.

8. Define health in terms of the Roy Adaptation Model.

9. Describe the goal of nursing in terms of the Roy Adaptation Model.

► KEY CONCEPTS DEFINED

Adaptation: The process and outcome whereby thinking and feeling persons, as individuals or in groups, use conscious awareness and choice to create human and environmental integration.

Adaptation level: Adaptation level represents the condition of the life processes described on three levels as integrated, compensatory, and compromised.

Adaptive responses: Responses that promote integrity in terms of the goals of human systems.

Behavior: Internal or external actions and reactions under specified circumstances.

Cognator subsystem: For individuals, a major coping process involving four cognitive-emotive channels: perceptual and information processing, learning, judgment, and emotion.

Compensatory process: Adaptation level at which the cognator and regulator have been activated by a challenge to the integrated life processes.

Compromised process: Adaptation level resulting from inadequate integrated and compensatory life processes; an adaptation problem.

Contextual stimuli: All other stimuli present in the situation that contribute to the effect of the focal stimulus.

Coping processes: Innate or acquired ways of responding to the changing environment.

Cosmic unity: A broad term that refers to scientific and philosophic assumptions based on redefining adaptation for the 21st century, which stresses the principle that persons and the earth have common patterns and integral relationships.

Environment: All conditions, circumstances, and influences that surround and affect the development and behavior of humans as adaptive systems, with particular consideration of person and earth resources.

Focal stimulus: The internal or external stimulus most immediately confronting the human system.

Goal of nursing: Promotion of adaptation in each of the four modes.

Health: A state and process of being and becoming integrated and whole.

Humanism: The broad movement in philosophy and psychology that recognizes the person and subjective dimensions of the human experience as central to knowing and valuing (Roy, 1988).

Human adaptive system: As an adaptive system, the human system is described as a whole with parts that function as a unity for some purpose. Human systems include people as individuals or in groups including families, organizations, communities, and society as a whole.

Ineffective responses: Responses that do not contribute to integrity in terms of the goals of the human system.

Innovator subsystem: Pertaining to humans in a group, the internal subsystem that involves structures and processes for change and growth.

Integrated life process: Adaptation level at which the structures and functions of a life process are working as a whole to meet human needs.

Regulator subsystem: For individuals, a major coping process involving the neural, chemical, and endocrine systems.

Residual stimulus: An environmental factor within or without the human system with effects in the current situation that are unclear.

Stabilizer subsystem: For groups, the subsystem associated with system maintenance and involving established structures, values, and daily activities whereby participants accomplish the purpose of the social system.

Stimulus: That which provokes a response, or more generally, the point of interaction of the human system and environment.

System: A set of parts connected to function as a whole for some purpose and that does so by virtue of the interdependence of its parts.

Veritivity: A principle of human nature that affirms a common purposefulness of human existence (Roy, 1988).

► OVERVIEW OF THE ROY ADAPTATION MODEL

Nursing models, as conceptual descriptions of nursing, are based on both philosophic assumptions and scientific principles. Knowledge development for any field reflects and moves forward the philosophic and scientific thinking of the day. So, too, do nurse-theorists identify the beliefs, values, and knowledge on which they base their work. For the Roy Adaptation Model, the concept of adaptation rests on scientific and philosophic assumptions as these have developed over time.

The scientific assumptions initially reflected the von Bertalanffy (1968) general systems theory and Helson's (1964) adaptation-level theory and later included the unity and meaningfulness of the created universe. The philosophic assumptions on which the model is based were originally identified as associated with humanism and veritivity. The further development of the philosophic assumptions focuses on people's mutuality with others, the world, and a god-figure. The manner in which the major concepts of the model have been developed and expanded evidences the pervasive influence of the theorist's scientific and philosophic background. Within the context of the initial scientific and philosophic perspectives, specific assumptions underlying the development of the Roy Adaptation Model can be identified. These assumptions are illustrated in Table 2–1.

In anticipation of nursing in the 21st century, and following work done to mark the quarter-century anniversary of the initial publication of the model, Roy (1997a) provided a redefinition of adaptation and a restatement of the assumptions that are the foundation of the model. Foundational to the Roy Adaptation Model is the goal of enhancing life processes through adaptation. Roy (1997a) defined *adaptation* as the process and outcome whereby

TABLE 2–1 ASSUMPTIONS UNDERLYING THE ROY ADAPTATION MODEL

Scientific

Systems Theory	Adaptation-level Theory
Holism	Behavior as adaptive
Interdependence	Adaptation as a function of stimuli and adaptation level
Control processes	Individual, dynamic adaptation levels
Information feedback	Positive and active processes of responding
Complexity of living systems	

Philosophic

Humanism	Veritivity
Creativity	Purposefulness of human existence
Purposefulness	Unity of purpose
Holism	Activity, creativity
Interpersonal process	Value and meaning of life

thinking and feeling persons, as individuals or in groups, use conscious awareness and choice to create human and environmental integration.

Scientific Assumptions

The scientific assumptions on which the model is based include systems theory and adaptation-level theory. As the concepts associated with the model have evolved, so too has the understanding of the scientific assumptions upon which the model is based.

The contribution of systems theory to the scientific foundation of the Roy Model is evident in the description of humans as adaptive systems. Roy views *human adaptive systems* as functioning with interdependent parts acting in unity for some purpose. Control mechanisms are central to the functioning of human systems. The systems theory concepts related to inputs (stimuli) and outputs (behaviors) also contribute important concepts to the model. Living systems, however, are regarded as nonlinear, multifaceted, and complex phenomena. The process is never viewed as a single stimulus initiating a given response. Rather living systems, particularly human adaptive systems, involve complex processes of interaction.

Adaptation-level theory (Helson, 1964) forms the parent theory for the origin of the Roy adaptation concept and the description of humans as adaptive systems having the capacity to adapt and to create changes in the environment. The ability to respond positively to these changes is a function of the human system's *adaptation level,* a changing point influenced by the demands of the situation and the internal resources. These include capabilities, hopes, dreams, aspirations, motivations, and all that makes humans constantly move toward mastery (Roy, 1990). Three levels of adaptation described in this book are integrated, compensatory, and compromised.

Roy's early description of the inner dynamics of adaptation called the regulator and cognator control subsystems have, over time, enhanced the understanding of central adaptive processes and adaptation levels. This concept has been expanded to encompass humans in groups with the introduction of stabilizer and innovator control processes (Roy & Anway, 1989).

Philosophic Assumptions

Roy (1988) identified eight specific assumptions associated with the two philosophic principles of humanism and veritivity. *Humanism* is defined as the broad movement in philosophy and psychology that recognizes the person and subjective dimensions of human experiences as central to knowing and valuing. It serves as the basis for the following four specific assumptions. In humanism, it is believed that humans, as individuals and in groups, share in creative power; behave purposefully, not in a sequence of cause and effect; possess intrinsic holism; and strive to maintain integrity and to realize the need for relationships.

Veritivity, a term coined by Roy (1988), pertains to the principle of human nature that affirms a common purposefulness of human existence. In veritivity, it is believed that people in society are viewed in the context of the purposefulness of human existence, unity of purpose of humankind, activity and creativity for the common good, and value and meaning of life. Further articulation of the philosophic assumptions underlying the Roy Adaptation Model can be found in Roy (1988) and Roy (1997a, b).

Developing Model Concepts for the Next Century

In addressing the challenge to redefine adaptation for the future, Roy (1997a) combined expanded notions of systems theory and adaptation theory into the one set of scientific assumptions illustrated in Table 2–2. The ideas and language of systems theory is compatible with futurists' views of the universe as progressing in structure, organization, and complexity. Rather than a system acting to maintain itself, the emphasis shifts to the purposefulness of human existence in a universe that is creative. Roy further emphasizes that science does not negate a creator or the meaningfulness of human existence, and that repeatedly in Eastern and Western cultures, human beings maintain a belief in a god-figure. Further understanding of these ideas can be gained from careful reading of Roy's work (Roy, 1997a, b).

In an expansion of the model's philosophic assumptions, Roy (1997a) drew upon the richness of diverse cultures to represent a philosophic theory of reality that is the foundation of the basic concepts of the model (see Table 2–2). This philosophic stance states that "nursing sees persons as co-extensive with their physical and social environments. Nurse scholars take a value-based stance. Rooted in beliefs and hopes about the human person, they fashion a discipline that participates in the well-being of persons" (Roy, 1997a, p. 42). A broad term that Roy uses to refer to scientific and philosophic assumptions based on redefining adaptation for the 21st century is *cosmic unity,* which stresses the principle that person and the earth have common patterns and integral relationships.

TABLE 2–2 **VISION BASIC TO CONCEPTS FOR THE 21ST CENTURY**

Scientific Assumptions

Systems of matter and energy progress to higher levels of complex self-organization.

Consciousness and meaning are constitutive of person and environment integration.

Awareness of self and environment is rooted in thinking and feeling.

Humans by their decisions are accountable for the integration of creative processes.

Thinking and feeling mediate human action.

System relationships include acceptance, protection, and fostering of interdependence.

Persons and the earth have common patterns and integral relationships.

Persons and environment transformations are created in human consciousness.

Integration of human and environment meanings results in adaptation.

Philosophic Assumptions

Persons have mutual relationships with the world and God.

Human meaning is rooted in an omega point convergence of the universe.

God is intimately revealed in the diversity of creation and is the common destiny of creation.

Persons use human creative abilities of awareness, enlightenment, and faith.

Persons are accountable for the processes of deriving, sustaining, and transforming the universe.

Roy (1997a) further drew upon three major characteristics of creation spirituality (Swimme & Berry, 1992) in refining the philosophic assumptions of the Roy Adaptation Model.

1. A focus on awareness and the notion of eliminating false consciousness.
2. Enlightenment to reach self-control, balance, and quietude.
3. The reclamation of earthly creation as the core of faith.

These underlying assumptions and visions for the future have constituted the basis for and are evident in the specific description of the following major concepts of the Roy Adaptation Model—humans as adaptive systems as both individuals and groups, the environment, health, and the goal of nursing.

▶ HUMANS AS ADAPTIVE SYSTEMS

From the perspective of the discipline of nursing, humans are the focus of nursing activities. The view of humans as adaptive systems provides a paradigm for the manner in which nurses relate to and interact with individuals; their families; and the groups, organizations, communities, and societies of which they are a part.

Roy describes humans in terms of holistic adaptive systems (Roy 1984). The term *holistic* stems from the philosophic assumptions underlying the model and pertains to the idea that human systems function as wholes in one unified expression of meaningful human behavior. They are, then, more than the sum of their parts. Persons represent unity in diversity. Similarly, there is diversity among persons and their earth, yet all are united in a common destiny. The term *adaptive* is an integral concept in the scientific assumptions underlying the model. Human systems have thinking and feeling capacities, rooted in consciousness and meaning, by which they adjust effectively to changes in the environment and, in turn, affect the environment. Persons and the earth have common patterns and mutuality of relations and meaning.

To begin an understanding of humans as adaptive systems, it is important to grasp the meaning of the term system. Broadly defined, a *system* is a set of parts connected to function as a whole for some purpose and it does so by virtue of the interdependence of its parts. In addition to having wholeness and related parts, systems can be viewed as experiencing inputs, outputs, and control and feedback processes. This dynamic and multifaceted interaction is simplified for illustrative purposes in Figure 2–1.

Roy has applied this general systems theory in the description of humans as adaptive systems. As illustrated in Figure 2–2, input for humans has been termed stimulus. A *stimulus* has been defined as that which provokes a response. It is the point of interaction of the human system and environment. Stimuli can come externally from the environment (external stimuli) or may originate in the internal environment (internal stimuli). Certain stimuli pool to make up a specific internal input, the adaptation level.

Adaptation level represents the condition of the life processes. Three levels are described: integrated, compensatory, and compromised life processes. Adaptation level affects the human system's ability to respond positively in a situation. The human's behavior (output) is a function of the input stimuli

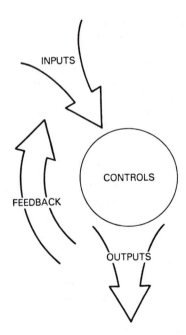

FIGURE 2–1. Diagrammatic representation of a simple system.

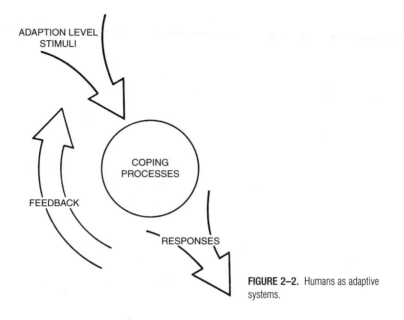

FIGURE 2–2. Humans as adaptive systems.

and the individual or group adaptation level. This changing level is significant as humans and environment are constantly in the process of change. An integrated life process may change to a compensatory process which evokes attempts to reestablish adaptation. If the compensatory processes are not adequate, compromised processes result.

In this model, the major processes for coping are termed the regulator and the cognator subsystems as they apply to individuals, and the stabilizer and innovator subsystems as applied to groups. The cognator–regulator and stabilizer–innovator act to maintain integrated life processes for the person or group. The life processes—integrated, compensated, or compromised— are manifested in behavior. Over time, the behavior of the basic life processes can reoccur in patterns that can be recognized as indicative of a given individual or group.

Behavior as the output of human systems takes the form of adaptive responses and ineffective responses. These responses act as feedback or further input to the system, allowing people to decide whether to increase or decrease efforts to cope with the stimuli. As will be evident, when humans as adaptive systems are explored further, all of the various aspects of human systems are interrelated and anything happening in one aspect will have an effect on the others. Similarly, viewing adaptive systems from different perspectives will allow emphasis on different aspects of the person or group. The image of the kaleidoscope is used to understand how elements change places and reflect different patterns with each turn of the instrument. Another image that provides a similar insight is that of the changing patterns of a computer-generated laser light show. Images are larger or smaller, stand up straight or turn in circles, while colors are changing and lights appear in different places and perspectives. The person is always a unified whole; however, at any given time, one perspective or another may be more apparent to the viewer.

It has been noted that human systems are affected by and, in turn, affect the world around and within. In the broadest sense, this world is called the environment (external and internal). According to the Roy Adaptation Model, the environment is more specifically classified as stimuli: focal, contextual, and residual. At any point in time, adaptation level is a significant internal stimulus. For purposes of developing knowledge to understand adaptive persons and groups, adaptation levels are described as integrated, compensatory, or compromised. The varying adaptation levels significantly affect the ability to cope with the changing environment. Based on the environment and the current adaptation level, humans make a response. Responses are observed as behavior and can be adaptive or ineffective.

The nurse soon learns that persons never act in isolation, but are influenced by the environment and, in turn, affect the environment. Environment is both physical and social. Understanding this ongoing interaction of people with their world and with others in it is important to nursing practice.

Stimuli

The Roy Adaptation Model describes three classes of stimuli that form the environment (Roy 1984b). The names of these stimuli and their original descriptions are based on the work of a physiologic psychologist, Harry Helson (1964). The use of these categories by thousands of nurses has clarified their meaning within the nursing framework.

The *focal stimulus* is the internal or external stimulus most immediately in the awareness of the human system; the object or event most present in consciousness. For example, a person may turn around quickly when a loud noise comes from behind or be annoyed by an internal buzzing sound. The person focuses on the stimulus and spends energy dealing with it. In this example of internal or external noise, the person tries to find its source to decide how to handle it. For a family, a violent act against a member can be an event that commands the attention of the others and elicits energy and action to deal with it. The 1995 bombing of a federal building in Oklahoma City became a focal stimulus for that community as people from throughout the United States were strongly aware of these events and banded together to assist those victimized by the event.

With the environment constantly changing, many stimuli never become focal; that is, they never command the attention of the human system. We generally are not conscious of the weather unless it is particularly pleasant, unpleasant, or changing. Similarly, positive or negative changes in the environment can become focal, and the human system encounters them and is required to make a response.

As the nurse using the Roy Adaptation Model views the patient, many stimuli that may be focal will be noted. For the surgical patient, pain may be a focal stimulus, the one on which the patient focuses attention and energy.

For the pediatric patient, being away from home may be the focal change. When the nurse is working in the home with an elderly patient who is recovering from a stroke, it may be apparent that the person focuses conscious awareness mainly on the fear of another stroke.

Similarly, in a community setting, a polluted water supply may not command the attention of members of the community until several people become severely ill as a result of consuming contaminating substances in the water. An outbreak of malaria becomes a focal stimulus for the entire community.

Contextual stimuli are all other stimuli present in the situation that contribute to the effect of the focal stimulus. That is, contextual stimuli are all the environmental factors that present to the human system from within or without but which are not the center of attention or energy. These factors will influence how the human system can deal with the focal stimulus.

In our common experience with the weather, it is not the temperature alone that makes us react to the heat or cold. When high humidity is added to high temperatures, the heat is less tolerable, and when a wind chill is added to cold temperature, one is more affected by the cold. While more attention is devoted to the focal stimulus, the contextual stimuli are those that also can be identified as affecting the situation.

Just as a patient may have many environmental changes that can be focal, so each of those situations can have many contextual stimuli. The person in pain may be more distressed by pain when the cause of it is unknown. Similarly, pain may be better tolerated when the person knows that it is expected and that it is temporary. A little girl may handle being away from her family more easily when she can have her own toys with her and expects her parents to return. The man who fears another stroke may find that this fear is intensified by memories of his own stroke and of the death of a brother from a stroke. A community with significant economic resources may find it easier to deal with a disastrous situation than a community with few economic advantages. In these examples, it can be seen that the contextual stimuli are also within or outside human systems and that they can be positive or negative factors.

Residual stimuli are environmental factors within or without human systems, the effects of which are unclear in the current situation. There may not be an awareness of the influence of these factors, or it may not be clear to the observer that they are having an effect. For example, a person who is frightened in a storm may have forgotten being lost once in a storm as a child. A friend who observes that the person is very frightened may have a hunch that there has been a bad experience in the past. However, in describing what is causing the fright, the observer can only consider this as a possibility since the person has never mentioned such an experience.

Recent understanding of communities and their development such as that described by Kretzmann and McKnight (1993) suggest that the manner in which society approaches assistance to disadvantaged groups may be one factor (stimulus) that actually exacerbates the problems of the community. The traditional "needs based approach" may be a residual stimulus that ignores capabilities and strengths within the community, thus actually contributing to failure of programs intended to help. This possibility constitutes a residual stimulus with an effect on the community that is yet to be understood.

In looking at what is affecting human systems in a given nursing situation, it is useful for the nurse to consider possible influencing stimuli and, in this way, further describe the situation. For example, a nurse may observe the child's reaction to being away from home and consider that this might be the child's first separation from her family. The nurse frequently uses the category of residual stimuli to place general knowledge about what influences the type of behavior observed. The nurse then gets to know the situation and those involved well enough to decide whether that stimulus is focal, contextual, or perhaps not applicable to the patient. By using the category of residual stimuli, one has a place to include even uncertain influencing stimuli and the nurse's intuitive impressions.

The nurse recognizes that focal, contextual, and residual stimuli change rapidly. The person and environment interaction is constantly changing and the significance of any one stimulus is changing. What is focal at one time soon becomes contextual and what is contextual may slip far enough into the background to become residual, that is, just a possible influence. For example, a person watching a national weather report may be vaguely aware of the weather patterns in another part of the country. However, if that person will be traveling to that area soon, attention is focused on what is said about that location. The relevance of the stimulus draws the person's attention to it. Again, the image of the changing patterns of a kaleidoscope or laser light show is brought to mind in recognizing changing stimuli affecting human experiences.

Just as the adaptation model emphasizes the person's coping abilities as an important stimulus, further exploration of the concept of "capacity focused development" as opposed to focusing on "needs, deficits, and problems" as it relates to community adaptation may prove to be an important contextual or focal stimulus in assisting communities in their responses to the factors affecting them. Throughout this text, there are examples of the three types of stimuli and their importance in providing nursing care according to the Roy Adaptation Model.

Adaptation Level

Among the focal, contextual, and residual stimuli is a significant internal input, the adaptation level. *Adaptation level* is the name given to three possible conditions of the life processes of the human adaptive system: integrated, compensatory, and compromised. The Roy Adaptation Model has always identified adaptation level as a stimulus. However, until now, the concept was defined and described only briefly. In developing knowledge related to basic life processes of each component of the adaptive modes (demonstrated in the chapters in Part II), the model now indicates that these processes will vary at three levels: integrated, compensatory, and compromised. The first adaptation level is termed integrated. The term *integrated* describes the structures and functions of the life process working as a whole to meet human needs.

For example, intact skin acts as a nonspecific defense to protect against infection. Integrated adaptation level thus constitutes a stimulus for the person.

The second adaptation level is the *compensatory* level at which the cognator and regulator have been activated by a challenge to the integrated processes. An example of a compensatory adaptation level is fever, which inhibits the multiplication of bacteria and increases metabolic rate to enhance repair.

The third adaptation level is the *compromised* level. When both integrated and compensatory processes are inadequate, an adaptation problem can result. Such problems become part of the nurse's consideration of the person as having a compromised adaptation level. Disrupted skin integrity and infection are two examples of compromised processes of the basic life process of protection.

Life processes will be discussed further in relation to each adaptive mode. Adaptation level is described by identifying whether the life process is integrated, compensatory, or compromised. As a stimulus, the changing condition of adaptation level affects the human system's ability to respond positively in a situation. Assessment of adaptation level is part of the assessment of stimuli. However, when the nursing process is described in Chapter 3, it will be noted that what is a compromised process affecting the person as a whole may also be the outcome of the assessment and described as a given nursing diagnosis. This shows the characteristic of the model that requires a nurse to look at a human experience from different perspectives, similar to changing patterns of the kaleidoscope or laser lights.

Helson (1964) first used the term adaptation level in a technical sense. The human system's ability to deal with a situation comes from two aspects, the demands of the situation and the current internal conditions. An example from Helson's work pertains to a person lifting a series of varying lead weights and judging their heaviness. The person's response to each weight is influenced by the actual weight of the object and other factors in the situation, physical fitness relative to weight lifting, for example. Thus, ability to respond positively depends on all three types of stimuli and the current condition of relevant life processes of the person. The focal stimulus is judged to have the greatest effect because it will determine which life processes are relevant in describing the current adaptation level. There may also be many related contextual stimuli and any number of residual stimuli that can be considered. The condition of the internal capabilities, described by adaptation level, will be a key factor in the given environment.

Beyond the description given by Helson, the concept of adaptation level has been developed further to identify knowledge for nursing. The notion of adaptation level conveys that the human system is not passive in relation to the environment. The human system and the environment are in constant interaction with each other. A given person, on most days, maintains integrated life processes. According to the Roy Adaptation Model, the regulator and cognator of the individual (innovator and stabilizer for the group) are the internal subsystems for changing adaptation levels from one condition to another. If the ability to deal with a new experience is limited, information and learning about the new situation may be actively sought. For example, in setting up a new household, a young person may choose to take a short course on finances. In this way, individuals change their own adaptation level. Learning creates a compensatory process to reach a new adaptation level. Without such learning, the person's adaptation level could have been compromised, resulting in debt and eventual bankruptcy.

Similarly, persons also change the external environment. For example, if a group of employees finds that a focal concern for them is the unrealistic demands of their employer, they may take positive action together to change the employer's expectations. In this way, the persons are active participants in the dynamic process of interacting purposefully with the environment and adjusting adaptation level.

When thinking of adaptation level in clinical terms, it is important to note that nurses meet people who have varying levels of ability to cope with changing circumstances. Some life processes are integrated, others may be at a compensatory level, and others may be compromised. These varying levels reflect both the challenges and strengths of the internal and external environment. At any given time, people will respond on the basis of the combined effect of the internal and external environment. Adaptation level identifies a key factor of the internal environment. As has been noted, the current internal state includes the effects of the human system's past experiences, even those of which one has little or no awareness. The nurse is impressed often by the extent to which people can cope with potentially overwhelming situations. Many parents and families of children with birth defects respond with love, concern, and appropriate planning. This response is related to the pooled effect of all that these people bring to this demanding situation and to the new levels of adaptation they attain.

Adaptation level, then, describes the condition of the life processes as a significant focal, contextual, or residual stimulus in a situation. The adaptation level and all other stimuli present determine a range of coping for the human system. Many positive life experiences provide a broad range of abilities to deal with life's changes. A changing situation can limit that range. For example, a single parent may have worked very hard to maintain a family and home with a broad range of coping that is an example to friends and colleagues. However, recognizing that he or she is the sole support and parent of that family, the parent may find it unusually difficult to handle an illness that requires even a short hospitalization. Nurses can play an important role in supporting life processes and helping people to use cognator and regulator processes, or stabilizer and innovator processes, to develop integrated and compensatory adaptation levels.

Nurses are aware of both the strengths and limitations of the people with whom they deal, whether they are individual patients, families, groups, communities, or co-workers. Nurses also recognize minor fluctuations in their own changing adaptation levels in situations of fatigue and anxiety. Furthermore, they know that, at times, working with cases of high demand, they must call on all their resources, and sometimes those outside, to deal with the physical and emotional demands of the situation. Nurses do not avoid these experiences, but can see them as new opportunities for growth, further extension of inner resources, and the raising of adaptation levels.

Behavior

As has just been described, stimuli and adaptation level serve as input to human adaptive systems. Simply speaking, processing of this input through control processes results in behavioral responses. Those familiar with the American Nurses Association (ANA, 1995) discussion of the definition of nursing are aware of the emphasis placed on attention to the full range of human experiences and responses to health and illness without restriction to a problem-focused orientation. The Roy Adaptation Model suggests a particular way of viewing human experiences and responses. Within the model, responses are not limited to problems, needs, and deficiencies. Rather, the model reflects all responses of the human adaptive system including capacities, assets, knowledge, skills, abilities, and commitments. These responses are called behavior.

Behavior is defined in the broadest sense as internal or external actions and reactions under specified circumstances. A person who responds to a loud noise by walking toward the noise is making an external response. At the same time, the person's increased heart rate is an internal response.

Human systems such as organizations also demonstrate behavior. In response to fiscal constraints and other environmental factors such as too many hospital beds for the population base, many hospitals are in positions that require responses such as downsizing and mergers with other organizations. In terms of such change, anxiety, conflict, and confusion tend to be behaviors that permeate the organization.

Behaviors, whether individual or collective, can be observed, sometimes measured, or subjectively reported. The ANA's *Social Policy Statement* (1995) notes that nurses integrate objective data with knowledge gained from an understanding of the patient or group's subjective experience. For example, one can see the person walk across the room, a monitor can measure heart rate, or the person can share feelings of being frightened. The "mood" of the organization can be observed in interaction with employees, measured through employee satisfaction surveys, or is evident in the quality of services provided.

As the nurse views a human adaptive system, the output behavior shows how well the system is adapting in interaction with the environment. This observation is key to nursing assessment and intervention. The nurse's assessment of behaviors is discussed in detail in Chapter 3. The reader is also referred to the *Nursing Manual: Assessment Tool According to the Roy Adaptation Model* (Cho, 1998).

An important concern is whether the behavior is adaptive or ineffective. In general, understanding the effectiveness of behaviors can take place only in collaboration with those involved, the individual or those in a group or collective. The understanding is specific to that human system and the inherent conditions and circumstances. However, the Roy Adaptation Model provides broad guidelines for nursing judgments about adaptive behaviors.

Adaptive responses are those that promote the integrity of the human system in terms of the goals of adaptation: survival, growth, reproduction, mastery, and person and environment transformations. To drink water when one's body fluids are depleted is an adaptive response contributing directly to survival. Similarly, to seek out new educational experiences contributes to growth, mastery, and higher levels of adaptation. Reproduction includes the continuation of the human species by having children, but it also involves the many ways that people extend themselves in time and space by creative works and moral presence.

From a societal perspective, the Native American grandfather lives on in the life of his grandchild by instilling the values of the tribe in the child. One's personal contributions are propagated both through individuals and to the whole society. The cultural heritage left by poets and artists can be viewed as their own adaptive responses related to reproduction.

Human systems, as individuals, families, groups, organizations, or communities, must sense changes in the environment and make adaptations in the way they function to accommodate new environmental requirements. In some situations and at some developmental stages, the appropriate response may be discontinuation of the system, or death, as it relates to the individual.

Adaptive responses, then, promote the goals of adaptation and promote the integrity of the human system. In turn, the human system's adaptation has an effect on the broader society. Based on Roy's definition of adaptation for the 21st century (Roy, 1997a), new knowledge can be developed related to higher levels of complex self-organization; consciousness and meaning; integration of creative processes; common person and earth patterns; diversity and destiny; convergence and transformation of the universe; and human creative abilities of awareness, enlightenment, and faith.

Ineffective responses, on the other hand, are those that neither promote integrity nor contribute to the goals of adaptation and the integration of persons with the earth. That is, they can, in the immediate situation or if continued over a long time, threaten the human system's survival, growth, reproduction, mastery, or person and environment transformations. To refuse to eat for one day may not be a serious threat to survival, but to continue such a fast over many weeks may be a serious threat and is ineffective for survival. Inability of an organization such as a hospital to respond to environmental changes may result in its closure or reconstitution into a different entity.

In judging effectiveness, then, one looks at the effect of the behavior on the general goals of adaptation and a broad understanding of the term as it pertains to human systems. At the same time, the system's individual goals are a major consideration. On the personal level, for example, there has been much discussion of the right to die. In certain stages of illness, sheer survival may not be the person's highest goal. Rather, the person may choose to be free from medical intervention to enter the final developmental stage of life, that is, preparation for death. One author (Dobratz, 1984) has described this developmental stage according to the Roy model as life closure. Goals of reproduction, in the sense of legacy of self, and mastery are more prominent at this time. The total integrity of the person may be at its highest point as all of the experiences of life are brought together in this closure. Using the words of the philosophic assumptions for the 21st century, the person strives for an omega point and God as the common destiny of creation. Ineffective responses in this situation would be those that do not contribute to the person's own adaptive goals.

Another example is a family situation. At a certain stage in the life of a dysfunctional family, it may be appropriate for the members to consider pursuing different directions, particularly if that response promotes adaptation for other family members. Such may be the case in the situation of an abusive parent who is threatening the integrity of the children.

In addition to these broad guidelines for determining adaptive and ineffective responses, the nurse's understanding of the coping processes (regulator and cognator subsystems for the individual, stabilizer and innovator subsystems for the group) can offer further guidelines. In general, indications of adaptive difficulty for an individual can be observed in pronounced regulator activity and cognator ineffectiveness. For example, a person can have a rapid pulse and tense muscles, but deny any concern. The nurse recognizes that the body is automatically responding to some threat, but the person is not effectively using cognitive and emotional processes to deal with the situation. The response that there is no concern is ineffective in handling the threat.

Indication of adaptive difficulty in groups can be observed in situations of pronounced stabilizer activity with innovator ineffectiveness. Malphurs (1993) described this phenomenon in declining churches. He suggests that many churches become stagnant because their members are intent on preserving the status quo and refuse to respond to environmental factors that necessitate adaptation and change. Attempts at revitalization are strongly resisted. The group is exhibiting pronounced stabilizer activity with innovator ineffectiveness.

Chapter 3 includes further discussion of the nurse's assessment of adaptive and ineffective behavior and how the basic concepts of the Roy Adaptation Model are used in conjunction with established norms.

▶ COPING PROCESSES

In applying the notion of a simplified system's control processes to human adaptive systems, the Roy model conceptualizes the complex dynamics within the person as the coping processes. Broadly categorized, these processes are the regulator subsystem and the cognator subsystem as the concept pertains to individuals, and the stabilizer and innovator subsystems when referring to groups.

Coping processes are defined as innate or acquired ways of interacting with (responding to and influencing) the changing environment. Innate coping processes are genetically determined or common to the species and are generally viewed as automatic processes; humans do not have to think about them. An example of an innate coping process is the ability to concentrate hemoglobin. When a person moves to a high altitude where the oxygen saturation of the air is less, hemoglobin concentration in the blood gradually increases. This automatically permits sufficient oxygen to be carried to the organs of the body. This response is automatic, unconscious, and innate.

Acquired coping processes are developed through strategies such as learning. The experiences encountered throughout life contribute to customary responses to particular stimuli. A child soon learns an appropriate response to a ringing telephone; the ringing (stimulus) activates acquired coping processes that result in a series of actions to answer the phone (response). This response is deliberate, conscious, and acquired.

Cognator and Regulator Coping Subsystems

In consideration of the individual as a human adaptive system, the Roy model further categorizes these innate and acquired coping processes into two major subsystems, the regulator and the cognator. A basic type of adaptive process, termed the *regulator subsystem,* responds automatically through neural, chemical, and endocrine coping channels. Stimuli from the internal and external environment (through the senses) act as inputs to the nervous system and affect the fluid, electrolyte, and acid–base balance, and the endocrine system. The information is channeled automatically in the appropriate manner and an automatic, unconscious response is produced. At the same time, inputs to the regulator subsystem have a role in forming perceptions.

A mother in labor provides an example of regulator subsystem activity. During the birth process, internal stimuli, both chemical and neural, initiate endocrine and central nervous system activity to produce physiologic responses of labor such as uterine contractions and the opening of the cervix to permit birth of the baby. External stimuli, such as medications administered during labor (for example, a drug with an action that intensifies uterine contractions), also affect regulator subsystem activity and, subsequently, body response.

All aspects of the regulator subsystem are so interrelated that one cannot isolate any one system as being the only active system in a particular process. As in the labor example, both chemical and neural processes are involved. These complex interrelationships are further evidence of the holistic and integrated nature of the person.

The second major coping process pertaining to the individual is termed the *cognator subsystem.* This subsystem responds through four cognitive-emotive channels: perceptual and information processing, learning, judgment, and emotion. Perceptual and information processing includes the activities of selective attention, coding, and memory. This component of the cognator is discussed further in Chapter 12. Learning involves imitation, reinforcement, and insight whereas the judgment process encompasses such activities as problem solving and decision making. Through the person's emotions, defenses are used to seek relief from anxiety and to make affective appraisal and attachments.

An example that illustrates all four cognitive-emotive channels is that of a person driving a car. Learning (imitation, reinforcement, and insight) is involved in mastering the skills needed to operate the vehicle. When gear shifting is required, insight as to the position and function of the various gear ratios and correct positioning of the gearshift are essential. The "rules of the road" and their application are handled by perceptual and information processing, and the judgment process is continuously active, although at some times it may be more effective than at others. Even the emotions are called into action, especially when another driver has suddenly cut into the line of traffic.

As with the regulator subsystem, internal and external stimuli including psychological, social, physical, and physiologic factors act as inputs to the cognator subsystem. This information is processed through the four channels mentioned previously and responses are produced.

Thinking again of the driver, the traffic light ahead has just turned yellow. The driver is already 10 minutes late for an appointment (external and internal stimuli). Through the judgment process, the driver decides to go through the yellow light instead of stopping. The response would probably be to step a little harder on the accelerator.

Stabilizer and Innovator Control Processes

Just as control processes are central to the functioning of individuals, so control processes are inherent in the functioning of human social systems. With respect to groups, Roy (Roy & Anway, 1989) categorizes the control mechanisms as the stabilizer and the innovator subsystems to coincide with the regulator and cognator subsystems associated with the individual.

Groups, in this perspective, have two overriding goals, one related to stability, the other to change. Thus, the term stabilizer is used to refer to the structures and processes aimed at system maintenance. Just as the adaptive individual has neural-chemical-endocrine activities and engages in processes that act to maintain homeostasis, equilibrium, and growth potential, so the group, as an adaptive system, has strategies and engages in processes that act to stabilize. The *stabilizer subsystem* involves the established structures, values, and daily activities whereby participants accomplish the primary purpose of the group and contribute to common purposes of society. For example, within a family unit, specified members fulfill wage earning activities; others may be primarily responsible for nurturance and education of children. The family members possess values that influence the way in which they respond to their environment and fulfill their daily responsibilities to each other and society. The same can be said for other social clusters such as community groups, organizations, and society as a whole.

The second control process described by Roy relative to humans in groups is the *innovator subsystem.* This subsystem involves the structures and processes for change and growth in human social systems. Just as the cognator for the person involves cognitive and emotional channels for responding to a changing environment, the aggregate has parallel information and human processes for innovation and change. The innovator dynamism involves cognitive and emotional strategies for change to higher levels of potential. Both established long-term and short-term strategies are included. For example, in organizations, strategic planning activities, "think tanks," team-building sessions, and social functions constitute innovator strategies. When the innovator subsystem of a group is intact and operating well, new goals emerge and new growth and mastery are achieved, as well as person and environment transformation.

These examples have been simplified for the purposes of illustration. Roy and Roberts (1981) have described possible ways to conceptualize the interrelationships of the regulator and cognator subsystems. The complex relationships within and between the two dimensions of the individual system and a group system further illustrate the holistic nature of humans as adaptive systems.

▶ THE ADAPTIVE MODES

Although it has been possible to identify specific processes inherent in the regulator–cognator and stabilizer–innovator subsystems, it is not possible to observe directly the functioning of these systems. Only the responses that are created can be observed. The behaviors that result from the control processes can be observed in four categories or adaptive modes for individuals developed by Roy to serve as a framework for assessment (Roy, 1984). These four modes, initially developed for human systems as individuals, have been expanded to encompass groups. These are now termed the physiologic–physical, self-concept–group identity, role function, and interdependence modes. It is through these four major categories that responses to and interaction with the environment are carried out and adaptation can be observed. The four adaptive modes are discussed in greater detail in the chapters of Part II; however, a definition of each is provided here.

The category of behavior pertaining to physical aspects of human systems is termed the *physiologic–physical mode* for individuals and groups. The physiologic part of the mode in the Roy Adaptation Model is associated with the way humans as individuals interact as physical beings with the environment. Behavior in this mode is the manifestation of the physiologic activities of all the cells, tissues, organs, and systems comprising the human body. For the individual, the physiologic mode has nine components. There are five basic needs: oxygenation, nutrition, elimination, activity and rest, and protection. In addition, four complex processes are involved in physiologic adaptation. These are the senses; fluid, electrolyte, and acid–base balance; neurologic function; and endocrine function. The underlying need for the physiologic mode is physiologic integrity. For humans in groups it is more appropriate to use the term *physical* in referring to the first adaptive mode. At the group level, this mode pertains to the manner in which the collective human adaptive system manifests adaptation relative to basic operating resources, that is, participants, physical facilities, and fiscal resources. The basic need associated with the physical mode for the group is resource adequacy, or wholeness achieved by adapting to change in physical resource needs.

Some fluctuations in the quality and strength of any one or more physiologic or physical factors over time are expected; however, prolonged ineffectiveness or compromised state of functioning could have dramatic and negative consequences for the person or group as a whole. For example, if a community continues to permit pollution of its rivers from industries in its environment, the physical health of the community members will be affected. The individual may not show the effects of pollutants immediately, but gradually will show vague symptoms, then a more defined pattern of illness.

The category of behavior pertaining to the personal aspects of human systems is termed the self-concept–group identity mode. The basic need underlying the self-concept mode for the individual has been identified as psychic and spiritual integrity, the need to know who one is so that one can be or exist with a sense of unity. Self-concept is defined as the composite of beliefs and feelings that a person holds about him- or herself at a given time. Formed from internal perceptions and perceptions of others, self-concept directs one's behavior. Components of the self-concept mode are the physical self, including body sensation and body image; and the personal self, comprised of self-consistency, self-ideal, and moral-ethical-spiritual self.

Group identity is the relevant term to use for the second mode related to groups. Identity integrity is the need underlying this group adaptive mode. The mode is comprised of interpersonal relationships, group self-image, social milieu, and culture.

Nurses in a unit can have self-concepts whereby they see themselves as physically capable of the work involved. In addition, they feel comfortable meeting their own expectations of being a caring professional. In a social system, such as a nursing care unit, an associated culture can be described. There is a social environment experienced by the nurses, administrators, and other staff that is reflected by those who are part of the nursing care group. As such, the self-concept–group identity mode can reflect adaptive or ineffective behaviors associated with an individual nurse or the nursing care unit as an adaptive system.

The category of behavior pertaining to roles in human systems is termed the role function mode for both the individual and the group. From the perspective of the individual, the role function mode focuses on the roles that the individual occupies in society. A role, as the functioning unit of society, is defined as a set of expectations about how a person occupying one position behaves toward a person occupying another position. The basic need underlying the role function mode has been identified as social integrity, the need to know who one is in relation to others so that one can act.

Roles within a group are the vehicle through which the goals of the social system are actually accomplished. They are the action components associated with group infrastructure. Roles are designed to contribute to the accomplishment of the group's mission, or the tasks or functions associated with the group. The role mode includes the functions of administrators and staff, the management of information, and systems for decision making and maintaining order. The basic need associated with the group role function mode is termed role clarity, the need to understand and commit to fulfill expected tasks, so that the group can achieve common goals.

The category of behavior pertaining to interdependent relationships of individuals and groups is termed the interdependence mode. The interdependence mode is the final adaptive mode Roy describes. For the individual, the mode focuses on interactions related to the giving and receiving of love, respect, and value. The basic need of this mode is termed relational integrity, the feeling of security in nurturing relationships. For groups, the interdependence mode pertains to the social context in which the group operates. This involves both private and public contacts both within the group and with those outside the group.

Two specific relationships are the focus within the interdependence mode for the individual: significant others, persons who are the most important to the individual, and support systems, others contributing to meeting interdependence needs. For the group, the components include context, infrastructure, and resources.

Individual and group behavior is viewed in relation to the four adaptive modes. The modes provide a particular form or manifestation of cognator–regulator and stabilizer–innovator activity within human adaptive systems. In the chapters that follow, the adaptive modes are described separately, in-

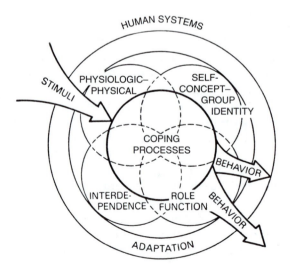

FIGURE 2–3. Diagrammatic representation of human adaptive systems.

cluding their theoretical basis and guidelines for assessment and the other steps of the nursing processes. However, as has been noted several times, the nurse is aware that the person or group is to be viewed as a whole and cannot be separated into parts. The four modes are depicted as four overlapping circles in Figure 2–3. At the center of the figure is a circle representing the coping processes. An illustration of the interrelationship of the modes is noted by the intersection of the physiologic–physical mode in the diagram by each of the other three modes. Behavior in the physiologic–physical mode can have an effect on or act as a stimulus for one or all of the other modes. In addition, a given stimulus can affect more than one mode, or a particular behavior can be indicative of adaptation in more than one mode. Such complex relationships among modes further demonstrate the holistic nature of humans as adaptive systems.

► ENVIRONMENT

Environment is the second major concept of a nursing model and it is understood as the world within and around humans as adaptive systems. According to the Roy Adaptation Model, human systems interact with the changing environment and make adaptive responses. For human beings, life is never the same. It is constantly changing and presenting new challenges. The human system has the ability to make new responses to these changing conditions. As the environment changes, humans have the continued opportunity to grow, develop, and transform the meaning of life for everyone. One example of a positive response to changing circumstances is the patient who reorders life's priorities after suffering a near-fatal heart attack. Altering a style of living can provide a more satisfying life for the person and the family. For example, the person may make a decision to spend more time with a spouse and children and less time at work.

Another example illustrates the group perspective. In response to an increasing incidence of HIV infection and AIDS in native Canadians, the Atlantic First Nations AIDS Task Force has undertaken a program to teach native people about HIV and AIDS and the effect it could have on their communities and their people as a whole. Native communities across Canada are involved in the effort. This constitutes a creative response of a human adaptive system (a societal group) to changing circumstances in the environment.

In describing the environment, Roy has drawn upon the work of Helson (1964). This physiologic psychologist describes adaptation as a function of the degree of change taking place and the human system's adaptation level. The three types of stimuli described previously pool to make up the adaptation level. Adaptation level has been described previously as part of the internal environment of integrated, compensatory, or compromised life processes. Stimuli immediately confronting the human system are termed focal stimuli. All other stimuli present that can be identified as influencing the situation are called contextual stimuli. The residual stimuli are those that may influence the adaptation level, but whose effect has not been confirmed.

Thus, *environment* includes all conditions, circumstances, and influences that surround and affect the development and behavior of humans as adaptive systems, with particular consideration of person and earth resources. Another definition compatible with broad notions of person and environment interactions from the perspective of an evolving universe is the description of the environment as a biophysical community of beings with complex patterns of interaction, feedback, growth, and decline, constituting periodic and long-term rhythms (Swimme & Berry, 1992).

► HEALTH

As an understanding of health has been sought over the past decades by both professionals and the public, the complexity of the concept has become increasingly apparent. No consistent view of health exists in the literature and only recently has published research dealing with perceptions of health been available. It is generally agreed that an understanding of the complex nature of health continues to evolve.

Traditionally, health was viewed as a concept anchoring one end of a health–illness continuum. This view of health is now seen as simplistic and unrealistic since it does not accommodate the coexistence of wellness and illness and excludes individuals with chronic disabilities or terminal illness who, in spite of their condition, are dealing effectively with life's challenges.

Health, defined as the absence of disease, is a Western biomedical perspective with a biologic focus. Thus, the diagnosis and treatment of disease have become widely synonymous with health care. This perspective, however, excludes consideration of cultural, social, and psychological constructs of health as perceived by individuals and their families and friends. It does not emphasize health promotion as an important approach to improving health or the use of complementary therapies as effective health treatments.

Some views of health have come to be accepted by both the lay public and health care professionals. One of the more common perspectives on health is that published by the World Health Organization (United Nations, 1968) and reaffirmed in the 1986 Ottawa Charter. Health is "a state of complete physical, mental and social well-being and not merely the absence of disease or infirmity" (World Health Organization et al., 1986). Fitzgerald (1994, p. 197) expressed concern about the widespread acceptance of this definition by stating, "We now act as if we really believe that disease, aging, and death are unnatural acts and all things are remediable. All we have to do, we think, is know enough (or spend enough), and disease and death can be prevented or fixed." Fitzgerald endorsed the notion of health as presented by Illich (1994). Illich maintained that health is not freedom from the inevitability of death, disease, unhappiness, and stress, but the ability to cope with them in a competent way.

Health is defined by Pender (1987, p. 27) as "the actualization of inherent and acquired human potential through goal-directed behavior, competent self-care, and satisfying relationships with others while adjustments are made as needed to maintain structural integrity and harmony with the environment." The American Nurses Association notes in *Nursing's Social Policy Statement* (1995) that health and illness are human experiences, but that the presence of illness does not preclude health nor does optimal health preclude illness.

Many authors have emphasized the contextual nature of health. For example, Watson (1985) viewed health as an individually defined phenomenon. McCormack and Gooding (1993) illustrated the essence of health as described by homeless persons while Sorrell and Smith (1993, p. 336) portrayed the Navajo view of health as "a holistic state, where harmony and balance between individual's physical, social, and spiritual state and the physical, social, and spiritual environment are achieved." Fryback (1993) provided a perspective on health in terms of terminal and chronic disease. Each of these presentations emphasizes the importance of contextual factors when defining health.

The United States Public Health Service presented national health goals for the year 2000. Three broad goals for the health of all Americans were presented as the major health challenges and opportunities for health gains in the decade of the 1990s. These include increasing the span of healthy life, reducing health disparities among Americans, and achieving access to preventive services. In the mid-1990s, data were reviewed to evaluate these goals. Burrell, Gerlach, and Pless (1997) report that related to health promotion priorities, good progress has been made in reducing adult use of tobacco products and in alcohol-related automobile deaths. Gains have been less apparent in exercising regularly, eating less fatty diets, and decreasing stress-related problems. The proportion of the population that is overweight has increased. Health protection data show that the number of motor vehicle deaths has declined, work-related deaths have declined, and there has been a decline in outbreaks of illness caused by *Salmonella*. The improvements in preventive service priorities are noted by significant progress in reducing cholesterol levels, controlling hypertension, and increasing the use of cancer screening services. The problems for all three priorities remain for the most vulnerable populations, that is, those who lack health insurance and do not have the financial resources to pay for health care and preventive services.

An understanding of the description of health as presented in the Roy Adaptation Model is contingent on an understanding of the concepts of the human adaptive system and the environment as presented earlier in this chapter. This understanding of health is also deeply rooted in the scientific and philosophic assumptions that are the foundation of the model. It is recognized that, with further consideration of the model from the theoretical perspective and its increasing use in practice, the clarity with which this concept can be described will be enhanced.

Earlier in the chapter, human beings were described as adaptive systems constantly growing and developing within changing environments. Health for human adaptive systems can be described as a reflection of this interaction or adaptation.

In earlier discussion, adaptation was viewed as a positive response of human systems that promotes survival, growth, reproduction, mastery, and person and environment transformations. Adaptive responses were said to promote integrity or wholeness relative to these goals, with the use of integrity to mean soundness or an unimpaired condition leading to wholeness. Health is viewed in light of human goals and the purposefulness of human existence. The fulfillment of this purpose in life is reflected in becoming integrated and whole. Thus, in the Roy Adaptation Model, *health* is defined as a state and a process of being and becoming an integrated and whole human being. Lack of integration represents lack of health (Roy 1984).

Consider the following two situations. In the first case, a 29-year-old woman, as a result of an accident, is quadriplegic. Although confined to a wheelchair and assisted by mechanical devices, she has developed a fruitful and meaningful life as a wife, author, and painter. Her perspective on life is an encouragement to all those with whom she comes in contact.

In the second case, a 20-year-old male college student is becoming increasingly dependent on drugs to see him through his academic year. Where initially he was using them during stressful periods of examination, now he is finding that he cannot function on a day-to-day basis without their assistance. His grades are falling and he is considering withdrawing from school.

In considering health as a reflection of adaptation with a goal of becoming integrated and whole, it is the first situation that exemplifies health. The woman is demonstrating the integration indicative of successful adaptation while the young man is responding ineffectively to his changing environment. The need for intervention is apparent.

▶ GOAL OF NURSING

Generally speaking, nursing's goal is to contribute to the overall goal of health care, that is, to promote the health of individuals and society. According to the American Nurses Association (1995, p. 3), "People seek services of nurses to obtain information and treatment in matters of health and illness. They use nursing care to resolve problems or manage health-promoting behaviors. Nurses help people identify both short- and long-term goals and act as advocates for people dealing with barriers encountered in obtaining health care."

The ANA (1995) specified that the aim of nursing actions is "to assist patients, families, and communities to improve, correct or adjust to physical, emotional, psychosocial, spiritual, cultural, and environmental conditions for which they seek help." To be meaningful within the context of a nursing model, the goal of nursing must be described in terms of the related concepts of the model.

The discipline of nursing focuses on human and environment interactions that promote maximum human development and well-being. As discussed in depth in Chapter 3, nursing activities in terms of the Roy Adaptation Model involve assessment of behavior and the stimuli that influence adaptation. Nursing judgments are based on this assessment and interventions are planned to manage these stimuli. The goal of nursing is to promote adaptation.

Consider the situation of a first-time mother hospitalized for the birth of her child. Following the birth, nursing care for the mother would be directed toward helping her adapt to her new role. In addition to physiologic concerns such as nutrition, elimination, and protection from infection, goals would relate to the mother's ability to care for the child, the support systems that she may have in place when help is required, and the integrity of her self-concept throughout the adjustment period. In this case, the goal of nursing care is to assist the new mother in all aspects of adaptation. The nurse will identify the mother's adaptation level and coping abilities, identify difficulties, and intervene where necessary to promote the mother's adaptation. In this manner, the integrity of the newborn child is maintained as well.

In nursing situations involving advanced practice, nurses are involved in providing care to people in groups, whether they be families, organizations, communities, or society as a whole. Again, nursing activities involve the assessment of group behaviors and the stimuli that influence adaptation of the group. Nursing judgments are based on this assessment and interventions are planned to manage these stimuli. Again, the goal of nursing is to promote adaptation.

Another example of this goal is a nurse who is involved as an occupational health nurse for employees in a hospital. When the incidence of needle-stick injuries is observed to be increasing, that nurse will work with employees to determine what factors appear to be influencing this trend. The interventions in this instance are focused on addressing the matters that are contributing to the problem.

Thus, Roy defines the *goal of nursing* as the promotion of adaptation in each for the four modes, thereby contributing to health, quality of life, or dying with dignity. It must be recognized that complete physical, mental, and social well-being, the common understanding of optimal health, is not possible for every human system. It is the nurse's role to promote adaptation in situations of health and illness and to enhance the interaction of human systems with the environment, thereby promoting health. In keeping with the assumptions of the model developed for the 21st century, nurses aim to enhance system relationships through acceptance, protection, and fostering of interdependence and to promote personal and environmental transformations.

▶ SUMMARY

In summary, the Roy Adaptation Model defines humans, both individually and in groups, as human adaptive systems, with coping processes acting to maintain adaptation with respect to four adaptive modes. The concept of humans as adaptive systems was depicted in Figure 2–3. Stimuli from the internal and external environment activate the coping processes—the regulator and cognator subsystems of individuals, and the stabilizer and innovator subsystems of groups—which in turn produce behavioral responses relative to the physiologic–physical, self-concept–group identity, role function, and interdependence modes for individuals and groups. These responses can be either adaptive, and thus promote the integrity or wholeness of the human system (as depicted by the arrow remaining within the adaptation circle), or ineffective, and not contributing to the goals of the human system (as shown by arrows extending beyond the adaptation circle). Although, for descriptive purposes, it has been necessary to present each aspect of the human adaptive system as a separate entity, the model is based on the belief that human systems function in a holistic manner with each aspect related to and affected by the others.

Health, according to Roy Adaptation Model, is a state and a process of being and becoming integrated and whole. It is a reflection of adaptation, that is, the interaction of the human adaptive system and the environment. Nurses act to promote this adaptation. The goal of nursing is stated as the promotion of adaptation in each of the four modes. In promoting adaptation, the nurse contributes to the health of the human adaptive system, the quality of life, and dying with dignity.

The scientific and philosophic assumptions that form the basis for these ideas are systems theory, adaptation-level theory, humanism, veritivity, and cosmic unity. As the major concepts of the model are explored in more depth, the influence of these foundational assumptions will become increasingly evident.

► EXERCISES FOR APPLICATION

1. Imagine yourself in rush-hour traffic approaching an intersection at which the light for your direction of traffic has just turned to yellow. Suggest focal, contextual, and residual stimuli that might have an effect on your judgment as to what action to take.

2. From your personal experience of writing an important examination, suggest focal, contextual, and residual stimuli that serve (a) to broaden your adaptation level or range of coping abilities, and (b) to limit that range.

3. In considering your own behavioral responses during the last minute, suggest two responses that can be (a) observed, (b) measured, and (c) subjectively reported.

4. Suggest two behavioral responses that would be considered adaptive in promoting your mastery of the content presented in this chapter and two that would be considered ineffective. An example of an adaptive response would be "underlining important concepts"; an ineffective response would be "daydreaming."

5. Jot down phrases that are descriptive of your personal perception of health. Compare them to the definition of health identified in the Roy Adaptation Model.

6. Identify several examples of nursing situations in which health care is provided for groups. An example would be an occupational health nurse in an industrial situation.

▶ ASSESSMENT OF UNDERSTANDING

Questions

1. Associate the specific assumptions in Column A with the appropriate major scientific and philosophic perspectives in Column B (note all that apply).

Column A	**Column B**
_____(a) human systems possess intrinsic holism	1. systems theory
	2. adaptation-level theory
_____(b) control processes are central to human functioning	3. humanism
	4. veritivity
_____(c) human systems behave purposefully	5. cosmic unity
_____(d) there is unity of purpose of humankind	
_____(e) environmental changes can be focal, contextual, or residual	
_____(f) persons and the earth have common patterns and integral relationships	

2. Fill in the missing words.
In human systems, inputs have been termed _____ and _____ _____. The controls, or _____ _____, are central to function and their activity is manifest by _____, which act as feedback and further input to the system.

3. Label each of the following descriptions according to whether it indicates an adaptive (A) or ineffective (I) response.
(a) _____ disrupts integrity
(b) _____ does not contribute to survival, growth, reproduction, mastery, or transformations
(c) _____ promotes integrity
(d) _____ contributes to the goals of the human system

4. *Situation:* A four-year-old child is having a plaster cast changed. He has been wearing casts on his left ankle since he was 6 months old to correct a

congenital problem. The second the plaster saw comes into view, he begins to scream, calling for his mother. On previous occasions, the staff doing the procedure have had to restrain him and proceed as quickly as possible with their task.

Label the following stimuli as focal (F), contextual (C), or residual (R).

(a) _____ past experience with cast removal
(b) _____ the sight of the plaster saw
(c) _____ previous cut due to saw blade

5. Which of the following statements apply to *adaptation level?*
   (a) It represents the condition of the life processes.
   (b) It is a person's state of health.
   (c) It affects human system's ability to respond positively.
   (d) It can be described as integrated, compensated, or compromised.

6. Classify the underlined behaviors in the following situation as being indicative of regulator or cognator activity.

   As a young woman was <u>driving calmly down the street</u>, smelling fresh spring air, a small child suddenly ran out in front of her car. She <u>slammed on the brakes</u> and <u>swerved to the left</u> to avoid hitting him. As the child ran off, oblivious to the near accident, she was left in silence with fierce <u>pounding of her heart</u> in her chest and her <u>body shaking</u> with fright.

7. Classify the underlined behaviors in the following group situation as indicative of stabilizer or innovator activity.

   The staff of the Pregnancy Crisis Center has recently had a <u>change in leadership</u> and, in an effort to <u>develop new direction</u> for the agency, is <u>holding a day-long retreat</u> for all staff. Karen, a long-time employee, has been appointed to arrive early to save seats at a table so that <u>"the gang" can sit together.</u> She and her friends are <u>critical of the decision to devote an entire day to planning activities.</u> The Center has been <u>working well in the same fashion for years.</u> "This business of <u>strategic planning</u> is a waste of time."

8. Insert the appropriate words in the following description of health according to the Roy Adaptation Model.

   Health is a _____ and a _____ of being and becoming _____ and _____.

9. Which of the following statements pertain to the goal of nursing as described in the Roy Adaptation Model?
   (a) to achieve the health of individuals and groups in society
   (b) to enhance the interaction of human systems and the environment
   (c) to promote adaptation
   (d) to promote complete physical, mental, and social well-being for every person

Feedback

1. (a) 1 and 3
   (b) 1
   (c) 3 and 4
   (d) 4
   (e) 2
   (f) 5

2. stimuli, adaptation level, coping processes, responses or behaviors

3. (a) I
   (b) I
   (c) A
   (d) A

4. (a) C
   (b) F
   (c) R

5. a, c, d

6. Behaviors indicative of regulator activities: pounding of her heart, body shaking. Behaviors indicative of cognator activity: driving calmly down the street, slammed on the brakes, swerved to the left.

7. Behaviors indicative of stabilizer activity: "the gang" can sit together, critical of the decision to devote an entire day to planning activities, working well in the same fashion for years. Behaviors indicative of innovator activity: change in leadership, develop new direction, holding a day-long retreat, strategic planning.

8. state, process, integrated, whole

9. b, c

► REFERENCES

American Nurses Association. (1995). *Nursing's social policy statement.* Kansas City, MO: American Nurses Association.

Burrell, L. O., Gerlach, M. J. M., & Pless, B. S. (1997). *Adult nursing: Acute and community care* (2nd ed.). Stamford, CT: Appleton & Lange.

Cho, J. (1998). *Nursing manual: Assessment tool according to the Roy Adaptation Model.* Glendale, CA: Polaris Publishing.

Dobratz, M. C. (1984). Life closure. In Roy, Sr. C. (Ed.), *Introduction to nursing: An adaptation model* (2nd ed., pp. 497–518). Englewood Cliffs, NJ: Prentice Hall.

Fitzgerald, F. T. (1994). The tyranny of health. *New England Journal of Medicine, 331,* 196–198.

Fryback, P. B. (1993). Health for people with a terminal diagnosis. *Nursing Science Quarterly, 6(3),* 147–159.

Helson, H. (1964). *Adaptation level theory.* New York: Harper & Row.

Illich, I. (1974). Medical nemesis. *Lancet, 1*(7863), 918–921.

Kretzmann, J. P., & McKnight, J. L. (1993). *Building communities from the inside out.* Evanston, IL: Center for Urban Affairs and Policy Research, Northwestern University.

Malphurs, A. (1993). *Pouring new wine into old wineskins: How to change a church without destroying it.* Grand Rapids, MI: Baker Books.

McCormack, D., & Gooding, B. A. (1993). Homeless persons communicate their meaning of health. *Canadian Journal of Nursing Research, 25,* 33–50.

Pender, N. (1987). *Health promotion in nursing practice* (2nd ed.). Norwalk, CT: Appleton & Lange.

Roy, Sr. C. (1970). Adaptation: A conceptual framework for nursing. *Nursing Outlook, 18,* 42–45.

Roy, Sr. C. (1984). *Introduction to nursing: An adaptation model* (2nd ed.). Englewood Cliffs, NJ: Prentice Hall.

Roy, Sr. C. (1988). An explication of the philosophical assumptions of the Roy Adaptation Model. *Nursing Science Quarterly, 1(1),* 26–34.

Roy, Sr. C. (1990). Theorist's response to "Strengthening the Roy Adaptation Model through conceptual clarification." *Nursing Science Quarterly, 3(2),* 64–66.

Roy, Sr. C. (1997a). Future of the Roy model: Challenge to redefine adaptation. *Nursing Science Quarterly, 10(1),* 42–48.

Roy, Sr. C. (1997b). Knowledge as universal cosmic imperative. *Proceedings of nursing knowledge impact conference 1996* (pp. 95–118). Chestnut Hill, MA: Boston College Press.

Roy, Sr. C., & Anway, J. (1989). Roy's Adaptation Model: Theories and propositions for administration. In Henry, B., Arndt, C., DeVincenti, M., & Marriner-Tomey, A. (Eds.), *Dimensions and issues of nursing administration.* St. Louis: Mosby.

Roy, Sr. C., & Roberts, S. (1981). *Theory construction in nursing: An adaptation model.* Englewood Cliffs, NJ: Prentice Hall.

Sorrell, M. S., & Smith, B. A. (1993). Navajo beliefs: Implications for health professionals. *Journal of Health Education, 24(6),* 336–338.

Swimme, B., & Berry, T. (1992). *The universe story.* San Francisco: Harper.

United Nations (1968). *Everyman's United Nations* (8th ed., p. 509). New York: UN Office of Public Information (UN publication E.67.I.2).

von Bertalanffy, L. (1968). *General systems theory.* New York: Braziller.

Watson, J. (1985). *The philosophy and science of caring.* Boulder: Colorado Associated University Press.

World Health Organization, Health and Welfare Canada, Canadian Public Health Association. (1986). *Ottawa charter for health promotion.* Ottawa, Canada: WHO, HWC, CPHA.

► **ADDITIONAL REFERENCES**

Roy, Sr. C. (1983). Roy Adaptation Model and application to the expectant family and the family in primary care. In Clements, J., & Roberts, F. (Eds.), *Family health: A theoretical approach to nursing care* (pp. 255–278, 298–303, 375–378). New York: Wiley.

Roy, Sr. C. (1984). The Roy Adaptation Model in nursing: Applications in community health nursing. Paper presented at the eighth annual Community Nursing Conference, Chapel Hill, NC.

Roy, Sr. C., & Corliss, C. (1993). The Roy Adaptation Model: Theoretical update and knowledge for practice. In Parker, M. (Ed.), *Patterns of nursing theories in practice* (pp. 215–229). New York: National League for Nursing.

3

THE NURSING PROCESS ACCORDING TO THE ROY ADAPTATION MODEL

The goal of nursing is to contribute to the overall aim of health care, that is, to promote the health of individuals and society. To accomplish this goal, nurses involve the full and active participation of the patient (American Nurses Association [ANA], 1995) and collaborate with other health care professionals to develop a composite plan of health care. Each health care discipline has its own area of independent practice but also functions in overlapping and interdependent areas. In a rapidly changing health care system, nurses recognize that "nursing's scope of practice has a flexible boundary that is responsive to the changing needs of society and the expanding knowledge base of its theoretical and scientific domains" (ANA, 1995, p. 12). It is the domain of nursing and the nursing process related to nursing's social concern that distinguishes it from other health-related disciplines.

Current discussions of the definition of nursing are based on an earlier statement that referred to nursing as "the diagnosis and treatment of human responses to health and illness" (quoted in ANA, 1995, p. 6). Another feature noticed in current definitions is that emphasis is placed on the full range of human experiences and responses to health and illness without restriction to a problem-focused orientation (ANA, 1995). The Roy Adaptation Model suggests a particular way of viewing human experiences and responses. Within the model, responses are not limited to problems, needs, and deficiencies. Rather, the model reflects all responses of the human adaptive system including capacities, assets, knowledge, skills, abilities, and commitments. These responses are called behavior.

The recipients of nursing care are human beings as individuals and as collectives such as families, groups, organizations, communities, and society as a whole. Nursing practice is conducted through the vehicle of the *nursing process,* a problem-solving approach for gathering data, identifying capacities and needs, establishing goals, selecting and implementing approaches for nursing care, and evaluating the outcomes of care provided.

Each theoretical perspective of nursing presents the essence of nursing knowledge and nursing goals and activities in a manner that is deeply rooted in the beliefs, values, and concepts that are foundational to the nursing model. For the Roy Adaptation Model, this foundation rests on the scientific and philosophic assumptions, and the description of human beings in terms of human adaptive systems.

The nursing process described by Roy relates directly to the view of human beings as adaptive systems. Six steps have been identified in the nursing process according to the Roy Adaptation Model.

1. Assessment of behavior
2. Assessment of stimuli
3. Nursing diagnosis
4. Goal setting
5. Intervention
6. Evaluation

This chapter will explore each of these steps and relate it to Roy's view of human adaptive systems and nursing's responsibility to promote adaptation.

In fulfilling nursing activities, nurses hold a profound regard for human and environment consciousness, meaning, and common destiny. These beliefs are held with respect to individuals and groups receiving care, others participating in the provision of that care, and nurses themselves. As such, nurses promote the right of individuals to define their own health-related goals and seek out health care that reflects their values. The nurse–patient relationship is described further in the document, *Nursing's Social Policy Statement,* "When nursing care is provided to individuals, it is provided within relationships that involve both physical and emotional intimacy . . . The interpersonal closeness that develops between a nurse and patient provides a context for open discussion of the patient's experiences of health and illness" (ANA, 1995, pp. 9–10). Through the array of nursing functions involving physical care, emotional support, anticipatory guidance, health teaching, and counseling, nurses demonstrate compassion, caring, and cognitive and behavioral competencies, in addition to highly developed technical and interpersonal skills. The American social policy statements define nurses as "legally accountable for actions taken in the course of nursing practice as well as actions delegated by nurses to others assisting in the delivery of care" (ANA, 1995, p. 19).

The last chapter focused on the description of human beings as adaptive systems. This chapter highlights the nursing process as it is described within the Roy Adaptation Model. It is important to recognize that, although the steps of the nursing process have been separated and specified for ease of discussion, the process is ongoing and simultaneous. For example, the nurse could be assessing behaviors in one adaptive mode while implementing an intervention in another. This approach is similar to the manner in which Roy's conceptualization of the human adaptive system was presented. Although it was necessary to focus on each aspect as a separate entity, one must bear in mind the belief that human systems function in a holistic manner. Each aspect is related to, and affected by, the others. The image of the kaleidoscope or laser light show, again, exemplifies the whole person or the whole nursing process, both of which can be viewed from different perspectives at different points in time.

► OBJECTIVES

After studying this chapter, the reader will be able to do the following:

1. Given a situation, identify the behaviors demonstrated by a given human system.

2. Apply criteria to evaluate specified behaviors as adaptive or ineffective.

3. In a given situation, identify stimuli influencing designated behaviors.

4. Classify designated stimuli as being focal, contextual, or residual.

5. Identify the specific stimulus of adaptation level as integrated, compensated, or compromised in a given situation.

6. In a given situation, make a nursing diagnosis.

7. Derive complete goal statements when provided with assessment data and nursing diagnoses.

8. In a given situation, identify actions that could serve to appropriately alter a specific stimulus.

9. Propose approaches to strengthen regulator and cognator processes as nursing interventions for given nursing diagnoses.

10. Given goal statements, describe the evidence that would indicate that nursing interventions were effective.

► KEY CONCEPTS DEFINED

Adaptation problems: Broad areas of concern related to adaptation. These describe the difficulties related to the indicators of positive adaptation.

Adaptive behavior: Responses that promote the integrity of the human adaptive system in terms of the goals of survival, growth, reproduction, mastery, and person and environment transformations.

Behavior: Actions or reactions under specified circumstances.

Contextual stimuli: All internal or external stimuli evident in the situation other than the focal stimulus.

Evaluation: Judging the effectiveness of nursing interventions in relation to the behavior of the human adaptive system.

Focal stimulus: The internal or external stimulus most immediately confronting the human adaptive system.

Goal setting: The establishment of clear statements of the behavior outcomes in response to nursing care provided to the human adaptive system.

Ineffective behavior: Responses that disrupt or do not contribute to integrity of the human adaptive system in terms of the goals of survival, growth, reproduction, mastery, and person and environment transformations.

Intervention: Nursing approaches selected to promote adaptation by changing stimuli or strengthening adaptive processes.

Norms: Generally accepted guidelines and expectations used to guide judgment about the effectiveness of behavior.

Nursing diagnosis: A judgment process resulting in a statement conveying the adaptation status of the human adaptive system.

Nursing process: A problem-solving approach for gathering data, identifying the capacities and needs of the human adaptive system, selecting and implementing approaches for nursing care, and evaluating the outcome of care provided.

Residual stimuli: Those stimuli having an undetermined effect on the behavior of the human adaptive system.

▶ STEP 1: ASSESSMENT OF BEHAVIOR

The first step of the nursing process as described in the Roy Adaptation Model is the assessment of behavior. The goal of nursing activities is to promote adaptation. The indicator of how a human adaptive system manages to cope with, or adapt to, changes in health status is behavior. Thus, the first step in the nursing process involves gathering data about the behavior of the human adaptive system and the current state of adaptation. In Figure 3–1, each step of the nursing process as it relates to Roy's description of the human adaptive system is illustrated.

The Roy Adaptation Model views human beings individually and collectively as holistic, adaptive systems. Input, in the form of stimuli from the internal and external environment, activates coping processes that act to maintain adap-

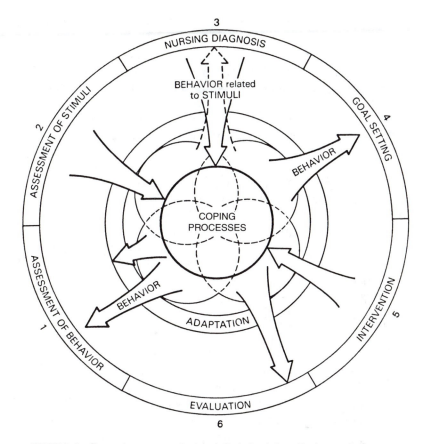

FIGURE 3–1. The nursing process as it relates to Roy's description of the human adaptive system.

tation with respect to the four adaptive modes. The result is behavioral responses, which are identified as either adaptive or ineffective. *Adaptive behavior* promotes the integrity of the human adaptive system in terms of the goals of survival, growth, reproduction, mastery, and person and environment transformation. *Ineffective behavior* disrupts or does not contribute to this integrity.

The responses of the human adaptive system are the focus of the first step of the nursing process, assessment of behavior. Behavior is defined as actions or reactions under specified circumstances. It can be observable or nonobservable. Nonobservable behavior can occur when a person feels anxious, as in the phenomenon commonly described as "butterflies in the stomach." Nonobservable behavior must be reported by the person or be otherwise demonstrated. On the other hand, observable behavior can be discerned by another. A scream from a frightened person would be an observable behavior.

Under usual circumstances, most human adaptive systems cope effectively with the changes that occur in their internal and external environments. However, there may be times, during an illness, for example, when stress is placed on an individual's coping abilities. The stimuli or changes encountered may call for more than the person's usual adaptive strategies. Adaptation levels become vulnerable and integrated life processes may become compensatory or compromised. It is often at these times that the nurse encounters the individual or the group.

In a nursing situation, the primary concern is a certain type of behavior—behavior that requires further adaptive responses as a result of environmental changes straining the coping processes of the human adaptive system. Important aspects of nursing are knowing how to assess these behaviors, compare them to specific criteria in order to evaluate their contribution to the maintenance of integrity, and identify the strengths and strains of the coping processes.

Throughout each step of the nursing process, nurses rely on highly developed technical and interpersonal skills as they assess and initiate interventions involving approaches such as physical care, anticipatory guidance, health teaching, and counseling.

Gathering Behavioral Data

In assessing behavior, the nurse systematically considers responses in each adaptive mode of the individual or group. As noted in Chapter 2, the four adaptive modes for the individual and the collective human system are a classification of ways of coping that manifest coping processes. The adaptive modes include physiologic–physical, self-concept–group identity, role function, and interdependence. It is in relation to these four major categories that responses are carried out and that observable and nonobservable behaviors occur.

All behavior is not directly obvious to another individual. Nonobservable behavior must either be reported by the human adaptive system or demonstrated in some other manner. Observable behaviors typically can be seen, heard, or measured. Thus, in assessing behavior in each adaptive mode, the nurse uses the skills of observation, measurement, and interviewing to obtain behavioral data. The scope of this text permits only a brief look at each of these methods of behavioral assessment. Proficiency in their use is achieved through knowledge and practice of the principles involved.

The nurse, when applying observation skills, uses the senses to obtain data about the behavior of the human adaptive system. In the case of the individual, the nurse may see cyanotic skin color, feel a weakened pulse, smell body odor, or hear unusual chest sounds. There may even be a "sense" of the patient's discomfort, even though the person denies it. In a situation where a nurse is involved with a family where child abuse is suspected, the nurse may observe physical indications such as bruising on a child's arm (an observable behavior) that could indicate trauma.

Behavioral responses can be measured and the measurements compared to preestablished criteria. The nurse may take a blood pressure reading, test a urine specimen, or have a person read an eye chart. In a family situation, the administration of analytic tools can serve to provide further indication of possible abusive behavior to which the child has been subjected. The measured values become the behavioral data.

The nurse uses interviewing skills to listen to and purposefully question to obtain behavioral data. For example, a person's expression of pain should signal the nurse to ask questions regarding the nature of the pain (as discussed further in Chapter 10). The person's verbal response becomes the behavioral data that the nurse identifies and records. When a nurse performs a community assessment, interviewing can be the vehicle through which an understanding is developed of the capacities and needs of that particular human adaptive system. These are behavioral data for the community as a human system.

Effective communication among the nurse, the recipient(s) of care, and the other members of the health care team is important in each aspect of the assessment of behavior, and throughout the nursing process. The emphasis on effective communication and caring (ANA, 1995; Benner & Wrubel, 1989; Watson, 1985), contributes to the effectiveness of all nursing actions.

The process of data collection relative to behavior is systematic. In later chapters, specific behavioral data to be gathered relative to each of the adaptive modes are identified. In addition, the reader is referred to the *Nursing Manual: Assessment Tool According to the Roy Adaptation Model* (Cho, 1998). In initial assessment, the specific data are gathered by means of skillful observation and sensitivity, accurate measurement, and purposeful interview within the nurse–patient relationship. An initial nursing judgment is made as to whether the behavior is adaptive or ineffective. Criteria have been established to assist in this decision.

Tentative Judgment of Behavior

As presented in Chapter 2, adaptive responses are those that promote the integrity or wholeness of the human adaptive system in terms of the goals of survival, growth, reproduction, mastery, and person and environment transformation. Ineffective responses are those that do not contribute to these goals and disrupt integrity.

The individualized adaptive goals of the human adaptive system are a major consideration. Chapter 2 provided an example of the individual in the final developmental stage, preparing for death. At this point, the person's highest goal may not be survival; rather, integrity of the self and interdependent relationships become the priority.

Although the parameters for the designation of adaptive responses are wide, in some areas, normal values are available to guide judgments about the effectiveness of behavior. For example, based on data from large numbers of people, charts have been developed to identify average weights and heights for specific age groups, and we know normal ranges for values of pulse, blood pressure, and temperature. In other areas, *norms,* that is, expectations or generally accepted guidelines, are evident. When behavior does not align with these generally accepted norms, guidelines, or expectations, there is reason to suggest that it may be ineffective. For example, there are some general expectations as to how a new mother behaves toward her baby. These are based on common cultural norms and nursing research. In some cultural groups, babies represent a responsibility for the entire community. In Hutterite communities in Canada, a baby is regarded as the colony's child. The baby's grandmother has a significant role in providing instruction for the new mother. All members of the colony bear some responsibility for the child's nurturing and education. In dominant North American cultures, the baby's mother often assumes the primary role of providing physical care and affection for the child.

In situations where norms are not available, Roy has hypothesized general indications of adaptation difficulty. For individuals, these indications are described as pronounced regulator activity with cognator ineffectiveness. Some signs of pronounced regulator activity are as follows:

1. Increase in heart rate or blood pressure
2. Tension
3. Excitement
4. Loss of appetite
5. Increase in serum cortisol

Signs of cognator ineffectiveness include:

1. Faulty perception and information processing
2. Ineffective learning
3. Poor judgment
4. Inappropriate affect

Similar indications of adaptation difficulty are demonstrated in human systems involving groups of individuals. This is pronounced stabilizer activity with innovator ineffectiveness. In some situations, the loss of a family member could prompt such behavior. Pronounced stabilizer activity would be demonstrated by increased levels of unproductive activity, refusal to acknowledge and accept the death of the family member, and inability to initiate the necessary changes. Signs of innovator ineffectiveness include faulty assessment of environmental factors such as the cause of death, poor judgment regarding changing roles in the family, and inappropriate responses such as delaying burial arrangements. Such behaviors require energy that could be used more effectively to respond to other stimuli. Furthermore, they limit the full potential of the human adaptive system and can ultimately affect integrity.

In making the initial judgment as to whether behavior is adaptive or ineffective, it is important that nurses continually involve those for whom they are caring. Included in the understanding of human adaptive systems is an appreciation of the immense capabilities and responsibilities associated with each person, whether individually or in groups. Nurses define their practice primarily as acceptance, protection, and fostering of human and environment integral relationships. The coping capabilities of humans are used for personal well-being and for creating and enhancing the well-being of the earth and of all creation. In all steps of the nursing process, the nurse holds a deep conviction about the importance of involving the recipients of care in observations and plans related to their health care.

The recipient's perceptions associated with the effectiveness of behavior is an integral consideration in the determination of adaptive or ineffective behavior. For example, a nurse may observe that a patient slept soundly for 8 hours during the night and judge that this behavior was adaptive in meeting the patient's need for rest. However, when asked about the night's sleep, the patient responded, "I only slept 2 hours. I couldn't get to sleep." By validating an observation with the person, the nurse changes the judgment of behavior from adaptive to ineffective.

Through a tentative assessment of behaviors as adaptive or ineffective, the nurse has a basis on which to set priorities of concern. The primary concern would be the behaviors that are disrupting the integrity of the human system and not promoting adaptation. However, the importance of identifying, maintaining, and enhancing adaptive behaviors is acknowledged, as well.

Consider the following example. In a community called Riverside, frequent minor interpersonal disputes are becoming major issues and are increasingly requiring intervention by law enforcement personnel. The behavior from the perspective of the community as an entity would be the increasing number of interpersonal disputes. This behavior is assessed as being ineffective and interfering with the identity integrity of the community. The group members are not able to relate to each other in a manner which effectively and efficiently maintains and enhances the identity of the group and moves it toward its goal achievement.

In this manner, the nurse obtains an indication of whether the human system is coping effectively with changes in the internal and external environment and is able to set priorities with respect to the next level of the nursing process, assessment of stimuli.

▶ STEP 2: ASSESSMENT OF STIMULI

As discussed in Chapter 2, it is change in the internal and external stimuli that places stress on the coping abilities of the human adaptive system. The system's behavior manifests whether or not coping activity is effective in dealing with these changes. Whereas the first level of assessment in the nursing process involves the assessment of behavior and a tentative judgment as to whether it is adaptive or ineffective, the second step of the nursing process involves the identification of internal and external stimuli that are influencing the behaviors.

TABLE 3–1 COMMON STIMULI AFFECTING ADAPTATION

Culture. Socioeconomic status, ethnicity, belief system.

Family/aggregate participants. Structure and tasks.

Developmental stage. Age, sex, tasks, heredity, genetic factors, longevity of aggregate, vision.

Integrity of adaptive modes. Physiologic (including disease pathology); physical (including basic operating resources); self-concept–group identity; role function; interdependence modes.

Adaptation levels. Integrated, compensatory, or compromised life processes.

Cognator–innovator effectiveness. Perception, knowledge, skill.

Environmental considerations. Changes in internal or external environment; medical management; use of drugs, alcohol, tobacco; political or economic stability.

The skills used in assessing stimuli are the same as those used in assessing behaviors, namely, astute and sensitive observation, measurement, and interview. Behavior manifesting a threat to integrity is the initial concern. To assist in setting priorities relative to the behavior of concern, the nurse, in collaboration with the recipient(s) of care and others relevant in the situation, identifies the focal, contextual, and residual stimuli influencing these responses. In addition, the nurse identifies the special stimulus of the adaptation level, and in particular, any compensatory or compromised life processes, as these contribute to adaptive or ineffective behavior. Examples of compensatory and compromised life processes are provided in chapters on the adaptive modes. Additional specific stimuli have been suggested by Roy and colleagues as having an effect on behavior in each adaptive mode. These common stimuli can be focal, contextual, or residual, depending on the situation. They are identified in Table 3–1.

Identifying Focal, Contextual, and Residual Stimuli

A stimulus is defined as that which provokes a response. Stimuli can be internal or external and include all conditions, circumstances, and influences surrounding or affecting the development and behavior of the human adaptive system. A collective term for all internal and external stimuli is environment.

Stimuli are assessed relative to the behaviors identified in the first level of assessment. Behaviors of disrupted integrity, or the ineffective responses, would be of initial concern. Ineffective behaviors are of concern since it is the goal of nursing to promote adaptation. The nurse assists in changing ineffective behaviors to adaptive ones. Adaptive behaviors are also important. They are to be maintained and enhanced. The stimuli are a key to accomplishing this goal. Changes in stimuli challenge the human system's coping abilities. In many instances, stimuli can be altered, thereby enabling the human system to cope more effectively. This idea will be discussed further in subsequent steps of the nursing process. In other situations, the nurse uses knowledge of regulator–cognator and stabilizer–innovator activity so that the coping processes can be dealt with more directly to promote adaptation.

In assessing stimuli, the nurse uses skills of perceptive observation, measurement, and interview. As the stimuli affecting each priority behavior or set of behaviors are identified, they are classified as focal, contextual, and residual. As with step 1, and with each step of the nursing process, consultation with those involved in the situation and validation of observations are extremely important.

The *focal stimulus* is defined as the internal or external stimulus most immediately confronting the human adaptive system. In assessing the focal stimulus, the nurse is looking for the most immediate cause of the identified behavior. Consider an example of a person experiencing a toothache. The focal stimulus in this situation is the fact that the person has just lost a filling from a deep cavity. This loss of filling and subsequent exposure of the nerve is the stimulus or change in environment with which the person is having difficulty coping.

Possible focal stimuli have been identified for given behaviors relative to each adaptive mode. These are identified in the chapters in which specific discussion of each adaptive mode is presented and are summarized in the *Nursing Manual: Assessment Tool According to the Roy Adaptation Model* (Cho, 1998).

It is important to note that behavior in one adaptive mode or system can act as a focal stimulus in another. For example, as a manifestation of anxiety regarding final exams, a teenage girl begins eating while she is studying and subsequently gains weight. This weight gain, a physiologic behavior, may become a stimulus to the self-concept mode causing low self-esteem when she does not meet her own and other's expectations that she remain slim.

From the organizational point of view, consider an organization that is experiencing a threat to its existence. In an effort to resist the threat, the organization launches litigation proceedings over petty issues. This interdependence behavior becomes a stimulus to the physical mode by placing significant pressure on the organization's fiscal resources and actually inflicting another pressure that further compromises the organization's continued existence.

Also reflective of the holism of adaptive systems, one focal stimulus can affect more than one adaptive mode. The loss of a limb not only affects a person's physiologic mode but it may disrupt the self-concept, role function, and interdependence modes. Not only is the individual's mobility affected, self-image, ability to perform roles, and interrelationships with others may be disrupted, as well.

In an aggregate situation, legislation affecting an organization's role will have significant impact on the physical mode, that is, operating resource requirements such as participants, physical facilities, and fiscal resources. Its group identity mode, including group self-image, social milieu, and culture will be affected. Its interdependence mode, for example, interorganizational relations and the group's mission and plans, may also change.

Contextual stimuli are defined as all other internal or external stimuli evident in the situation. They contribute to the behavior triggered by the focal stimulus. Consider, again, the person with the toothache. One contextual stimulus may be a very sticky piece of candy. The candy contributed to the loss of the filling but in the current situation, the sugar on the exposed nerve is aggravating the pain. Contextual stimuli are important because they often are tied to the meaning ascribed to the situation. A person with a toothache who has a family member with cancer of the jaw may react entirely differently from one who does not.

Residual stimuli are the next category of stimuli influencing behavior to be assessed. These stimuli are defined as those having an indeterminate effect on the behavior of the human adaptive system. Their effect has not, or cannot, be validated. Roy identifies two ways in which validation of a stimulus can occur. First, there can be confirmation by those involved that the stimulus is having an effect. Second, the nurse may have theoretical or experiential knowledge to establish confirmation. Residual stimuli become contextual or focal once they have been validated. The rationale for this changed designation is that they are now confirmed present in the situation just as are the focal and contextual stimuli. When residual stimuli are identified as affecting the situation, they are no longer possible influencing stimuli; their effect on the behavior of the human adaptive system has been confirmed.

Residual stimuli affecting the person with the toothache could be the type of toothpaste being used or dental hygiene habits. If one is able to confirm that conscientious care of the teeth has not been taken, the stimulus then becomes contextual. Probable influencing factors can be identified through research and understanding of the human person. Still, based on philosophic assumptions, Roy maintains that parts of human adaptive systems remain a mystery.

It is important to note that changing circumstances can change the significance of the stimuli, as has been noted in using the image of the kaleidoscope or laser lights. What is contextual at one point in time might be focal at another. For example, at the point in time when the filling was actually dislodged, the most immediate cause was the chewing of the piece of candy. This focal stimulus later becomes a contextual factor.

In the previous example relating to the community of Riverside, it was determined that many of the community members were not skilled at resolving conflict when the dispute was minor in nature. As a result, many problems that were readily resolvable early on became major issues when left unattended. Thus, the stimulus in this situation involves the level of capability or skill of the community participants, a factor that is related to resource adequacy in the physical system.

Common Influencing Stimuli

As discussed in Chapter 2, the environment is considered to be all the internal and external stimuli affecting the development and behavior of human adaptive systems. Because of their common influence in the environment, certain stimuli are identified as having an effect on behavior in all of the adaptive modes. Table 3–1 presents an overview of these common influencing stimuli as initially identified by Martinez (1976) and selectively elaborated upon by Sato (1984).

Sato (1984) discussed culture, family, and developmental stage as primary considerations for stimuli affecting human adaptation. Culture is described as involving socioeconomic status, ethnicity, and belief systems. Socioeconomic status provides an indication of the style of living and the material resources upon which the human adaptive system has to draw. Different stimuli are evident in situations of different socioeconomic status. For example, an impoverished community with many inhabitants suffering from malnutrition is affected by entirely different stimuli than those affecting a situation involving a malnourished teenager from an upper-middle-class family.

Ethnicity is viewed as including language, practices, philosophies, and associated values. Ethnic background may influence health practices and responses to illness. Sorrel and Smith (1993) addressed Navajo beliefs and their influence on health practices. For example, consent for a medical procedure or treatment must involve consultation with the family members. It is recognized that ethnicity is a stimulus in a person's response to pain. Generally the experience of pain is believed to be universal. However, perception and behavior regarding pain are influenced by cultural beliefs and practices. Behavior related to pain is taught and socialized within a culture, thus allowing more or less expression of the pain experience by persons of different cultural groups.

Belief systems, as a component of culture, involve spiritual beliefs, practices, and philosophies and may influence all aspects of life for human adaptive systems. As well as being a major support system, belief systems can have a specific influence on health practices and adaptation. For example, attitudes toward death are affected to a great extent by belief systems and the extent to which the beliefs are carried into practice. Religion and spirituality will affect one's deepest beliefs. Often it is important for a Catholic, even one who has not been an active church member, to see a priest when death is imminent.

Another common influencing stimulus pertains to the family or aggregate and its associated structure and tasks. Consider the different stimuli associated with a single-parent family as opposed to a nuclear or extended family. A family in the beginning stages of child-rearing has different duties and responsibilities from a family whose children are grown and have left home.

Consideration of the factors related to the developmental stage of the human adaptive system is important in assessment of contextual stimuli affecting adaptation. Based primarily on the developmental stages and tasks identified by Erikson (1963), it is known that factors such as age, gender, and heredity influence individual behavior, especially relating to the role function mode. For humans in groups, an important consideration includes the longevity of the group. Families and groups proceed through transitional phases much as individuals do, and often the challenges encountered are associated with their particular stage of development.

The interrelationships among the aspects of the human adaptive system cannot be overemphasized. As described earlier in this text, it is important to recognize that a stimulus being assessed may be a behavior in another adaptive mode or system, just as a laser light image may be viewed as a light seen by the person or as a light generated by a computer program operator. Thus, lack of integrity in any area of functioning will, in turn, act as a stimulus for another area. Since the nurse often encounters individuals during treatment for illness, an important consideration relative to adaptation in the physiologic mode is the presence of disease pathology. This lack of integrity in the physiologic mode will act as a stimulus for behavior in each of the other modes and, likewise, lack of integrity of the physical mode will affect the group.

In Chapter 2 it was noted that, at any point in time, adaptation level is a significant internal stimulus. Adaptation levels in individuals and in groups can be described as integrated life processes, or compensatory or compromised life processes. The Roy Adaptation Model has always identified adaptation level as a stimulus. However, until now the concept was only briefly defined and described. Knowledge related to the basic life processes of each component of the adaptive modes is developed in the following chapters, which indicate how these processes will vary at the three levels of integrated, compensatory, and compromised.

Another stimulus demonstrating the interrelated aspects of human adaptive systems relates directly to acquired coping processes, the cognator of the individual and innovator of the group. Coping processes involve the effectiveness with which the particular subsystem is functioning. Inherent in the stimulus of coping processes are the knowledge, perception, and skill to assist in coping with environmental stimuli. Consider an example of a malnourished individual. If the person does not recognize what nutrients constitute a balanced diet, the knowledge necessary to provide for adaptive behavior relative to nutritional health is not present. Therefore, the cognator subsystem cannot perform effectively. Lack of knowledge is a stimulus affecting adaptation level. The previous example with the community illustrates this notion with respect to the innovator coping processes.

The last stimulus to be mentioned relates to the environment. Changes in environment can have a profound effect on the system's state of adaptation. These changes tend to affect the human system's senses and include such stimuli as temperature changes, different noise levels, or unusual diet. The presence of unfamiliar people or absence of familiar ones may be part of an environmental change. Also related to the environment are drugs, alcohol, and tobacco, the use of which has a distinct effect on the person's internal environment. For the collective adaptive system, political and economic stability are important environmental considerations affecting adaptation.

The effect on adaptation of each of the common stimuli identified is a study in itself, as would be the reciprocal effect of the human adaptive system on the environment. The discussion in this chapter is an attempt to identify common stimuli affecting adaptation for human adaptive systems. It is not meant to be exhaustive. Many other stimuli will be evident as each situation is assessed. The stimuli that have been described, however, include those that have been found to be important for primary consideration in the assessment of the stimuli affecting the behavior of human systems relative to each adaptive mode. Such assessment also contributes to the nurse's general understanding of the context and meaningfulness of the world for the human adaptive system.

▶ **STEP 3: NURSING DIAGNOSIS**

Since the nursing process is a problem-solving process, behavioral data must be gathered and interpreted. Data collected thus far in the nursing process take the form of statements about the behavior of the human adaptive system that have been observed, measured, or subjectively reported. Also, data include statements about the focal, contextual, and residual stimuli that are, or may be, influencing these behaviors. The third step of the nursing process involves the formulation of statements that interpret these data. Such a statement is the nursing diagnosis and is depicted in the diagrammatic representation of the Roy Adaptation Model in Figure 3–1. The nursing diagnosis is an interpretive statement about the human adaptive system. This interpretation is accomplished by considering the behaviors, as assessed in the first level of assessment, with the stimuli affecting those behaviors, as assessed in the second level of assessment.

Nursing diagnosis is defined in the Roy Adaptation Model as a judgment process resulting in statements conveying the adaptation status of the human adaptive system. In establishing nursing diagnoses within the framework provided by the model, Roy advocates the development of statements that identify observed behaviors together with the most relevant influencing stimuli. Consider the assessment data associated with the following physiologic adaptation problem. An individual's pulse is rapid and thready, breathing is rapid and shallow, blood pressure tends to rise at first and then fall. The person feels clammy, looks pale, and can be agitated or confused. All of these behaviors are indicative of inadequate circulation and, thus, insufficient oxygenation of body tissue. They can result from a variety of causes, or stimuli, such as loss of blood volume, an infectious process in the body, or a stressful physical or emotional event.

Formulating these data into a nursing diagnosis, the nurse may determine, "blood pressure of 90/60 due to hemorrhage from incision." This would represent one nursing diagnosis related to the problem described. Stated as such, the nursing diagnosis provides specific indication for nursing intervention since, as will be seen later in this chapter, nursing interventions often relate directly to stimuli.

The concept of nursing diagnosis is similarly applicable in situations where the nurse is providing nursing care for humans in groups. Consider the example of a single-parent family with a newborn. The mother is a young girl who has not had access to prenatal care. She has little understanding of the requirements of a newborn and has few material possessions. From the perspective of the family, many of the deficiencies are indicative of physical mode difficulties. A nursing diagnosis that would be relevant in this situation might be "lack of knowledge about baby's requirements due to inadequate prenatal care." The wording of the nursing diagnosis in this fashion becomes important to facilitate the step of goal setting in the nursing process according to the Roy Adaptation Model.

Relating Nursing Diagnosis to Clinical Classifications

Nursing diagnosis is primarily a process of critical thinking or judgment by the nurse. The process results in a statement about the patient status. During the past 25 years, particularly in North America, there has been an effort to develop diagnostic categories to describe the health status of the person, family, or community from a nursing perspective. The categories are not meant to take the place of the nurse's process of reasoning and coming to a conclusion about the patient status observed in the assessment phase of the nursing process. Rather, the various classification systems and taxonomies that have been developed have the specific purpose of aiding the process of nursing diagnosis by providing a common language to communicate the nurse's clinical judgment. The effort has been to provide names for concerns that are within the domain of nursing practice. Many textbooks and clinical agencies currently use the North American Nursing Diagnosis Association (NANDA) Diagnostic Classification System (NANDA, 1994).

Since this is a widely used classification system, and because Roy was involved from 1973 through 1983 in its development, this classification system will be related throughout this text to the clinical classifications based on the Roy Adaptation Model.

Considering the goal of nursing described in the model, namely, to enhance positive life processes and to promote adaptation, Roy (1988) has identified the utility of a typology of indicators of positive adaptation associated with each of the four adaptive modes. This typology is presented in Table 3–2.

Adaptation problems, defined as broad areas of concern related to adaptation, also have been derived to describe deviations from the indicators of positive adaptation. These are presented in Table 3–3. In this manner, the capacities, capabilities, and skills of the human adaptive system are considered in addition to circumstances that may result in a need or problem.

From the typology of commonly recurring adaptation problems listed in Table 3–3, the behavioral assessment information in the postoperative patient example can be clustered and labeled "shock." Shock is a common adaptation problem of the physiologic mode, specifically, the person's need for oxygenation. A nursing diagnosis using this example from the typology of commonly recurring adaptation problems could be "shock due to incisional hemorrhage." The related categories from the NANDA classification are "fluid volume deficit" and "altered tissue perfusion."

TABLE 3–2 TYPOLOGY OF INDICATORS OF POSITIVE ADAPTATION

Physiologic-Physical Mode	
Individuals	*Groups*

Oxygenation

Stable processes of ventilation	Adequate fiscal resources
Stable pattern of gas exchange	Member capability
Adequate transport of gases	Availability of physical facilities
Adequate processes of compensation	

Nutrition

Stable digestive processes

Adequate nutritional pattern for body requirements

Metabolic and other nutritive needs met during
    altered means of ingestion

Elimination

Effective homeostatic bowel processes

Stable pattern of bowel elimination

Effective processes of urine formation

Stable pattern of urine elimination

Effective coping strategies for altered elimination

Activity and Rest

Integrated processes of mobility

Adequate recruitment of compensatory movement
    processes during inactivity

Effective pattern of activity and rest

Effective sleep pattern

Effective environmental changes for altered sleep
    conditions

Protection

Intact skin

Effective healing response

Adequate secondary protection for changes in
    integrity and immune status

Effective processes of immunity

Effective temperature regulation

Senses

Effective processes of sensation

Effective integration of sensory input into information

Stable patterns of perception, interpretation and
    appreciation of input

Effective coping strategies for altered sensation

Fluid, Electrolyte, and Acid–Base Balance

Stable processes of water balance

Stability of electrolytes in body fluids

Balance of acid–base system

Effective chemical buffer regulation

TABLE 3–2 TYPOLOGY OF INDICATORS OF POSITIVE ADAPTATION (CONT.)

Physiologic-Physical Mode

Individuals	Groups

Neurologic Function

Effective processes of arousal and attention; sensation and perception; coding, concept formation, memory, language; planning, motor response

Integrated thinking and feeling processes

Plasticity and functional effectiveness of developing, aging, and altered nervous system

Endocrine Function

Effective hormonal regulation of metabolic and body processes

Effective hormonal regulation of reproductive development

Stable patterns of closed loop negative feedback hormone systems

Stable patterns of cyclical hormone rhythms

Effective coping strategies for stress

Self-concept–Group Identity Mode

Individuals	Groups
Physical Self	
Positive body image	Effective interpersonal relationships
Effective sexual function	Supportive culture
Psychic integrity with physical growth	Positive morale
Adequate compensation for bodily changes	Group acceptance
Effective coping strategies for loss	Principle-based relationships
Effective process of life closure	Value-driven relationships
Personal Self	
Stable pattern of self-consistency	
Effective integration of self-ideal	
Effective processes of moral-ethical-spiritual growth	
Functional self-esteem	
Effective coping strategies for threats to self	

Role Function Mode for Individuals and Groups

Role clarity

Effective processes of role transition

Integration of instrumental and expressive role behaviors

Integration of primary, secondary, and tertiary roles

Effective pattern of role performance

Effective processes for coping with role changes

Role performance accountability

Effective group role integration

Stable pattern of role mastery

TABLE 3–2	TYPOLOGY OF INDICATORS OF POSITIVE ADAPTATION (CONT.)

Interdependence Mode for Individuals and Groups
Affectional adequacy
Stable pattern of giving and receiving
Effective pattern of dependency and independency
Effective coping strategies for separation and loneliness
Developmental adequacy
Resource adequacy

This method of stating nursing diagnoses from established classifications is useful in the complex situations encountered in advanced nursing practice. It is important to be aware that the label stands for a multifaceted clinical situation and points to an established set of cues, signs and symptoms, possible causes or etiologies (Carpenito, 1997), and scientific nursing knowledge that can be used in planning nursing interventions. Diagnostic classifications are useful shorthand ways of communicating with other nurses and with other health care providers, including the federal agencies and private insurance companies which finance health care.

In using the nursing process based on the Roy Adaptation Model, the nurse concludes the first three steps with a clear understanding of patient behavior, the stimuli affecting the behavior, and a diagnostic statement that reflects a nursing judgment about the adaptation status of the person or group.

▶ STEP 4: GOAL SETTING

Goals are established once the nurse has assessed the behavior of the human adaptive system and the stimuli influencing that behavior and has formulated nursing diagnoses from the assessment information. *Goal setting* is defined as the establishment of clear statements of the behavioral outcomes of nursing care.

The general goal of nursing intervention, as defined earlier, is to maintain and enhance adaptive behavior and to change ineffective behavior to adaptive. The behavior of the human adaptive system is the focus of this general statement, and similarly, when establishing specific goals, the behavior of the human adaptive system is the focus.

Throughout the first and second levels of assessment, the human system's behavior and the stimuli influencing it have been identified and recorded. This information was formulated into nursing diagnoses. Step 4 of the nursing process, goal setting, involves the statement of behavioral outcomes of nursing care that will promote adaptation. Figure 3–1 illustrates goal setting as it relates to the other steps of the nursing process.

TABLE 3–3 TYPOLOGY OF COMMONLY RECURRING ADAPTATION PROBLEMS

Physiologic–Physical Mode	
Individuals	*Groups*
Oxygenation	
Hypoxia	Inadequate fiscal resources
Shock	Capability deficits
Ventilatory impairment	Inadequate physical facilities
Inadequate gas exchange	
Inadequate gas transport	
Altered tissue perfusion	
Poor recruitment of compensatory processes for changing oxygen need	
Nutrition	
Weight 20–25% above or below average	
Nutrition more or less than body requirements	
Anorexia	
Nausea and vomiting	
Ineffective coping strategies for altered means of ingestion	
Elimination	
Diarrhea	
Bowel incontinence	
Constipation	
Urinary incontinence	
Urinary retention	
Flatulence	
Ineffective coping strategies for altered elimination	
Activity and Rest	
Immobility	
Activity intolerance	
Inadequate pattern of activity and rest	
Restricted mobility, gait, and/or coordination	
Disuse syndrome	
Sleep deprivation	
Potential for sleep pattern disturbance	
Protection	
Disrupted skin integrity	
Pressure sores	
Itching	
Delayed wound healing	
Infection	
Potential for ineffective coping with allergic reaction	
Ineffective coping with changes in immune status	
Ineffective temperature regulation	
Fever	
Hypothermia	

TABLE 3–3   TYPOLOGY OF COMMONLY RECURRING ADAPTATION PROBLEMS (CONT.)

Physiologic–Physical Mode	
Individuals	*Groups*

Senses
    Impairment of a primary sense
    Potential for injury
    Loss of self-care abilities
    Sensory monotony or distortion
    Sensory overload or deprivation
    Potential for distorted communication
    Acute pain
    Chronic pain
    Perceptual impairment
    Ineffective coping strategies for sensory impairment

Fluid and Electrolytes
    Dehydration
    Edema
    Intracellular water retention
    Shock
    Hyper- or hypo- calcemia, kalemia, or natremia
    Acid–base imbalance
    Ineffective buffer regulation for changing pH

Neurologic Function
    Decreased level of consciousness
    Defective cognitive processing
    Memory deficits
    Instability of behavior and mood
    Ineffective compensation for cognitive deficit
    Potential for secondary brain damage

Endocrine Function
    Ineffective hormone regulation
    Ineffective reproductive development
    Instability of hormone system loops
    Instability of internal cyclical rhythms
    Stress

Self-concept–Group Identity Mode	
Individuals	*Groups*
Physical Self	
Body image disturbance	Ineffective interpersonal relationships
Sexual dysfunction	Oppressive culture
Rape trauma syndrome	Low morale
Unresolved loss	Stigma

TABLE 3–3 TYPOLOGY OF COMMONLY RECURRING ADAPTATION PROBLEMS (CONT.)

Self-concept–Group Identity Mode	
Individuals	*Groups*
Personal Self	
Anxiety	Abusive relationships
Powerlessness	Valueless relationships
Guilt	
Low self-esteem	

Role Function Mode for Individuals and Groups
Ineffective role transition
Prolonged role distance
Role conflict—intrarole and interrole
Role failure
Role ambiguity
Outgroup stereotyping

Interdependence Mode for Individuals and Groups
Ineffective pattern of giving
Ineffective pattern of dependency and independency
Separation anxiety
Loneliness
Ineffective development of relationships
Inadequate resources

Recall from previous discussion the person who, following surgery, was demonstrating a progressive drop in blood pressure caused by hemorrhage from the incision. A nursing diagnosis could be expressed as "blood pressure 90/40 related to hemorrhage." A goal for this person could be stated as follows: "The patient's blood pressure measurement will stabilize in a range of 100/70 to 130/80 within 30 minutes." This is a short-term goal that identifies a behavioral outcome promoting adaptation.

Goals can also be long term. A long-term goal pertaining to the example might be, "The patient will return to his job on a part-time basis within 6 weeks."

The designation of goals as long or short term is relative to the situation involved. For some problems, especially those that are life threatening, short-term goals may be formulated on a minute-to-minute basis, and long-term goals on a day-to-day basis. In other situations, related to self-concept, group identity, or role function, for example, short-term goals may involve the time frame of a week, and long-term goals, months. In situations of community nursing, goals may span much broader time frames. It may take a year or more for a community to make progress in addressing situations of ineffective adaptation.

A goal statement should designate not only the behavior to be observed but the manner in which the behavior will change (as observed, measured, or subjectively reported) and the time frame in which the goal is to be attained. Consider the following.

1. The patient's blood pressure measurement will stabilize *(behavior)* within a range of 110/70 to 130/80 *(change expected)* within 30 minutes *(time frame)*.
2. The patient will be able *(behavior)* to return to his job *(change expected)* on a part-time basis within 6 weeks *(time frame)*.
3. The new mother will demonstrate enhanced ability *(change expected)* to care for her new baby *(behavior)* within 2 days *(time frame)*.
4. Within 1 year *(time frame)* there will be a 25% decrease *(change expected)* in the frequency with which law enforcement personnel will need to be involved in dispute resolution *(behavior)*.

Notice how each of the goals demonstrates the three elements identified above. These elements are important in the evaluation of goal attainment.

In these examples, the goals focus on ineffective behaviors in an attempt to change them to adaptive behaviors. However, it may be just as important to focus on adaptive behaviors in an effort to maintain and enhance them. Consider the following situation: A 5-year-old boy, newly admitted to hospital for surgery, was interacting readily with his new roommate until it was time for his mother to leave, at which point he began to cry and cling to her. In this situation, the goal might focus on the adaptive behavior of interaction with roommate. The goal might be, "Within 5 minutes of mother's departure, child will be playing happily with roommate as evidenced by participation in mutual activity."

In the previous community situation, many members are willing to be involved in learning activities and voluntary programs. This is a physical mode (human resource) adaptive behavior that could be enhanced to help address the problem associated with dispute resolution.

The individuals involved in the situation are actively involved in the formulation of behavioral goals whenever possible. This involvement provides the nurse with the opportunity to explore the rationale behind certain goals and gives the participants, as individuals or a group, the chance to suggest goals and evaluate whether other goals are realistic. Those who are actively involved in the formulation of goals are more likely to be committed to achieving the goal. Consider the following goal: "Within 3 hours after surgery, the patient will stand unsupported by the bed for 5 minutes." Generally, it is considered important for persons undergoing surgery to be mobile as soon as possible following return from the operating room. The patient involved in the formulation of this goal who understands the underlying rationale is more likely to strive to achieve it than someone awakening to, "It's time to get you out of bed," while in pain and still drowsy. It can be noted that individual behavioral goals are aimed at the goals of adaptation, that is, survival, growth, reproduction, mastery, and person and environment transformations. Thus, the nurse helps the human system strive for full human potential.

▶ STEP 5: INTERVENTION

Once the goals have been established relative to behaviors that will promote adaptation, a determination is made as to how best to assist the human system in attaining these goals. This is the fifth step of the nursing process, intervention, as described in the Roy Adaptation Model. *Intervention* is described as the selection of nursing approaches to promote adaptation by changing stimuli or strengthening adaptive processes.

Intervention With Stimuli and Coping Processes

In Roy's description of human adaptive systems, stimuli from the internal and external environment activate the coping process to produce behaviors. When ineffective behavior is identified, there is evidence that the coping processes are not able to adapt effectively to the stimuli affecting them. Interventions can then be focused on both stimuli and coping processes. The first three steps of the nursing process involved the assessment of behaviors and related stimuli and synthesis of this information into a nursing diagnosis. Subsequent goal setting is the statement of the desired behavioral outcomes of nursing care relative to the problem areas identified. Intervention focuses on the manner in which these goals are to be attained. Whereas the focus of goal setting is the behavior of the human system, the focus of intervention is the stimuli influencing the behavior or the ability to cope with the stimuli. Figure 3–1 illustrates this in terms of the Roy Adaptation Model.

As was identified in Chapter 2, the ability of the human system to adapt or respond positively to a change depends on the focal stimulus and adaptation level. The focal stimulus is the degree of change taking place. The adaptation level is the changing condition of the life processes. It is an internal stimulus, which affects the ability of the human system to respond positively in a situation. To promote adaptation, it may be possible to manage the focal or other stimuli present. Management of stimuli involves altering, increasing, decreasing, removing, or maintaining them. Altering the stimuli brings them within the ability of the coping processes of the human system to respond positively. The result is adaptive behavior. In getting the patient out of bed for the first time, the nurse adds positive stimuli to the simple request to get out of bed. This is done in the form of providing specific instructions for each move, for example, to sit on the side of the bed before standing. At the same time, the nurse provides both physical and emotional support.

Nurses are increasing their knowledge about persons in groups as regulatory–stabilizer systems. Likewise, they better understand how thinking and feeling persons promote health for individuals and groups through cognator–innovator systems. Based on this developing knowledge, the nurse increasingly becomes able to design nursing interventions specific to the coping processes. To return to the example of getting the postoperative patient out of bed for the first time, the nurse can affect the cognator by changing perception. Without adequate explanation, the person may perceive the request to stand at the bedside 3 hours after surgery only as an occasion of pain and discomfort. The nurse can provide the opportunity to change this perception by explaining the positive effects of getting out of bed after surgery and increase the perception of this action as beneficial to healing and getting well.

Identification and Analysis of Possible Approaches

The identification of possible approaches to nursing intervention involves the selection of which stimuli to change. Roy incorporates the nursing judgment method as initially presented by McDonald and Harms (1966) in a description of this fifth step of the nursing process. In this method, possible approaches are listed and the approach with the highest probability of attaining the goals is selected. In applying this method to the Roy model, the stimuli affecting specific behaviors are listed and relevant coping processes are identified. Next, the consequences of changing each stimulus, or affecting a coping process, are identified together with the probability of their occurrence. The outcome of the consequence is judged as desirable or undesirable. This is accomplished in collaboration with the individual(s) who is (are) involved in or with the human system.

Consider an example of the person who is unable to sleep in the hospital environment. The second level of assessment yielded the following stimuli as contributing to this sleeplessness.

- Noise level (focal)
- Uncomfortable bed (contextual)
- Hunger (contextual)

Application of the nursing judgment method to these factors is illustrated in Table 3–4.

TABLE 3–4 THE NURSING JUDGMENT METHOD AS APPLIED TO SELECTION OF APPROACHES

Alternative Approach	Consequence	Probability	Value
Alter noise level	Enhance sleep	High	Desirable
	Not enhance sleep	Low	Undesirable
Alter comfort of bed	Enhance sleep	High	Desirable
	Not enhance sleep	Low	Undesirable
	Disrupt intravenous	Low	Undesirable
Alter hunger	Enhance sleep	Moderate	Desirable
	Not enhance sleep	Moderate	Undesirable
	Disrupt plans for surgery in morning	High	Undesirable

The first approach, that of altering the stimulus of noise level, has the best probability of accomplishing the desired goal with undesirable consequences having a low probability. On the other hand, the third approach has a moderate probability of achieving the desired result, but the undesirable consequence of disrupting plans for surgery is highly probable.

Whenever possible, the focal stimulus should be the focus of nursing interventions. However, when this is not possible, contextual stimuli or the coping mechanisms are considered in an effort to change adaptation levels. It also may be appropriate to use several approaches in combination. For example, a person can be suffering severe pain caused by the focal stimulus of a terminal disease process. In this case, it is not possible to deal with the disease itself, and efforts must be directed toward contextual factors enabling the person to handle the pain and be more comfortable. A personal support system may be one of the stimuli that must be increased or maintained. Other factors related to pain management that include strategies for intervening with the regulator and cognator are discussed in Chapter 10.

In the earlier example related to the community with dispute resolution problems, second level assessment indicated that the following stimuli contributed to the problems.

- No resources for dispute resolution other than the law enforcement personnel (contextual).
- Community members not versed in dispute resolution methods (contextual).
- Little positive interaction among neighbors (contextual).

Application of the nursing judgment method in this situation is illustrated in Table 3–5. From this analysis, it appears as if initiating a volunteer mediation program has the highest potential of producing a desirable result, that is, one that would promote the adaptation of the community.

TABLE 3–5 APPLICATION OF NURSING JUDGMENT METHOD TO COMMUNITY SITUATION

Alternative Approaches	Consequence	Probability	Value
Increase law-enforcement capacity	Increased resources to deal with conflict	Low	Undesirable
	Increased cost	Low	Undesirable
Initiate community mediation program	Disputes handled in early stages	High	Desirable
	Community participants develop capabilities	High	Desirable
Prioritize disputes and assist in most serious	Number of unresolved disputes escalates	High	Undesirable

Implementation of Selected Approach

Once the most appropriate approach to nursing intervention has been selected, the nurse works with those involved to determine and initiate the steps that will serve to alter the stimulus and enhance appropriate coping. Having decided that altering the noise level is the best approach to the patient's sleeplessness, the nurse must determine how to do it. Shutting the door to the person's room might help. It may be possible to reduce the volume of the paging system. It may be necessary to move the person away from a disruptive roommate.

To initiate a community mediation program, the nurse works with other agencies and representatives from the community to develop a plan and a process to engage and train volunteer mediators. It is also necessary to provide for the required infrastructure to operate the program. In some cases, law enforcement agencies have offered to fulfill this role in recognition of the extent to which the volunteer mediation program will alleviate their involvement in minor disputes.

Having initiated or accomplished the nursing intervention, the nurse then proceeds with the evaluation of its effectiveness.

▶ STEP 6: EVALUATION

The last step of the nursing process as described in the Roy Adaptation Model is evaluation. *Evaluation* involves judging the effectiveness of the nursing intervention in relation to the behavior of the human system. Was the goal attained that was set in the fourth step of the nursing process? To make this decision, the nurse assesses the behavior of the human system after the interventions have been implemented. As in the initial assessment steps, the skills of sensitive observation, measurement, and interview are used. The nursing intervention would be judged as effective if the system's behavior aligns with the initial goals.

Evaluation as a Reflection of Goals

Understanding the nursing process according to the Roy Adaptation Model thus far, the reader knows that behavior demonstrates the effectiveness with which the coping processes are able to adapt to the stimuli affecting the human adaptive system. Nursing interventions are directed toward altering stimuli in an effort to enhance the ability of the coping mechanisms to respond effectively, or are directed to the coping mechanism activity. When goals are established in step 4 of the nursing process, they are set in terms of the behavior and they aim to maintain and enhance the adaptive behavior and to change ineffective behavior to adaptive. To evaluate the effectiveness of nursing interventions in terms of these goals, the nurse, in collaboration with the individual(s) involved, must look again at the behavior. Have the behavioral goals been achieved? This evaluation is the sixth and final step of the nursing process. Its relationship to the previous steps and to Roy's description of the human adaptive system are illustrated in Figure 3–1.

Skills Used in Evaluation

As in the first assessment steps of the nursing process, the nurse uses the skills of observation, measurement, and interview to evaluate the effectiveness of nursing interventions. Consider the earlier example of the person who was hemorrhaging following surgery. Some of the ineffective behaviors identified were falling blood pressure (measured), a large amount of blood on the dressing (observed), and a decreasing level of consciousness (observed through purposeful questioning). Goals relative to these behaviors would relate to stabilizing blood pressure, cessation of bleeding, and regaining of consciousness, respectively. To evaluate the effectiveness of nursing interventions relative to these goals, the nurse would measure the person's blood pressure, observe the amount of blood on a fresh dressing, and use an established format (see Chap. 12) for determining the level of consciousness, all skills used in making the initial assessment.

In the example of the community with dispute resolution problems, the goal addressed the extent to which law enforcement officers were required to intervene in interpersonal disputes. Evaluation of the attainment of this goal would involve calculation of the frequency with which officers became involved and determining the change 1 year after the initiation of the program. There would most likely be other qualitative measures that could also be employed to measure effectiveness. A survey of those who had used the volunteer mediators to assist with their dispute resolution would constitute a substantive measure of the effectiveness of the program in increasing the ability of group members to relate to each other.

Continuity of the Nursing Process

For the nursing intervention to be judged effective, the behavior of the human adaptive system must reflect the mutually set goals. If the goals are not achieved, the nurse must proceed to discover why the behavior did not change as anticipated. The goals may have been unrealistic or unacceptable to the individual(s) involved, the assessment data may have been inaccurate or incomplete, or the selected interventions may need to be approached in a different manner. The nurse returns to the first step of the nursing process to look closely at behaviors that continue to be ineffective and to work with the individuals involved to further understand the situation.

In the postoperative example, the nurse may evaluate that the person's blood pressure has stabilized and that bleeding has stopped, but there may not be a change in the level of consciousness. Although it is still important to ensure that the stable blood pressure and cessation of bleeding are maintained, the nurse would begin to focus on the person's level of consciousness and proceed through the steps of the nursing process again to identify any other stimuli that might point to the use of an alternative approach to address the ineffective behavior of a decreasing level of consciousness.

Although the steps of the nursing process have been separated and specified for clarity of discussion, it is important to recognize that the nursing process is ongoing. In fact, many of the steps occur simultaneously. The nurse may be assessing behavior in one area while proceeding with a nursing intervention in another area. She may be assessing behavior and stimuli at the same time and discussing goals in another area.

► SUMMARY

The six-step nursing process described in the Roy Adaptation Model has been presented in this chapter. The nurse assesses the behavior of the human adaptive system and the stimuli influencing that behavior and proceeds to formulate nursing diagnoses. Goals establishing behavioral outcomes for the human system are formulated and interventions designed to manage stimuli and enhance coping mechanisms are planned and implemented. Evaluation involves judging the effectiveness of the nursing interventions in relation to the adaptive system's behavior.

Each step of the nursing process is closely aligned with the assumptions and concepts associated with the description of the human adaptive system according to the Roy Adaptation Model. The importance of collaboration with the individuals involved throughout the steps of the nursing process has been emphasized. The effectiveness with which the nurse can assist the human adaptive system in the promotion of adaptation depends on the nurse's understanding of the situation and the effectiveness of collaboration with those involved.

► EXERCISES FOR APPLICATION

1. Suggest a behavioral goal that could apply to you, as the reader of this text, on your completion of this chapter. It should apply to the knowledge gained from reading this chapter.

2. Imagine yourself as a student who has just received a failing grade on an examination. Suggest several stimuli (focal, contextual) that may have influenced the poor performance. Identify and analyze possible approaches to the problem relative to the stimuli or your coping mechanisms. Use the following table as a guideline. Select the approach with the highest possibility of success.

Alternative Approach	Consequence	Probability	Value

3. Assume that, as of last week, you have applied the nursing process to yourself relative to your daily diet and have set the goal that you will begin immediately to eat a nutritionally balanced diet containing all the recommended daily allowances for nutrients. In light of this goal, evaluate your intake of food in the past 24 hours and suggest whether your observations align with the preset goals or are ineffective in moving toward them. Proceed through all the steps of the nursing process relative to your own situation.

▶ ASSESSMENT OF UNDERSTANDING

Questions

1. Underline the behaviors demonstrated by the child in the following situation.

   A mother noticed that her five-year-old son was not actively participating in play with other children. When she questioned him, he stated that he did not feel well and had a sore throat. The mother noticed that he appeared flushed and felt warm to her touch. Looking down his throat, she noticed that it was very reddened and two rather large masses of tissue were protruding from either side.

2. Using the criteria presented in this chapter, label the following underlined behaviors as adaptive (A) or ineffective (I) and provide rationales for your decision.
   (a) _____ A woman of 5 feet <u>weighs 60 pounds</u>.
   (b) _____ The nurse measured the patient's <u>blood pressure at 125/75</u>.
   (c) _____ The patient <u>asked the nurse three times to explain a simple procedure</u>.
   (d) _____ In assessing the family's eating habits, the nurse noted that they <u>never planned meals</u>, they <u>all ate at different times</u>, and that their <u>diet virtually excluded fruits and vegetables</u>.
   (e) _____ Almost <u>50% of children</u> in the elementary school were <u>home from school with flu-like symptoms</u>.

3. In the following situation, suggest stimuli that might be influencing the person's behavior of refusing to taste the food.

   An 80-year-old patient who had been placed on a salt-restricted diet received her first saltless meal. She announced to her nurse that she would rather go hungry than eat such tasteless food. The entire meal was left untouched.

4. In the following situation identify the stimuli that contributed to the student's performance and classify them as being focal, contextual, and residual.

   In preparation for an important exam, an anxious student who was having persistent problems in a course studied all night before the day of the test. During the writing of the exam she found that she was having trouble concentrating on the questions and remembering what she had studied. Handing in her paper, she commented to the instructor, "That exam was really hard; I know I didn't make it." She was right.

5. Formulate a nursing diagnosis statement relative to the behaviors and stimuli underlined in the situation below. Your statement need not include all behaviors and stimuli.

   A 55-year-old woman has <u>lost the use of the right side</u> of her body as a <u>result of a stroke</u>. She is presently in a program of rehabilitation, which is aimed at helping her achieve a degree of independence relative to her activities of daily living. She <u>appears to lack enthusiasm</u> for the program and <u>states that she can see no reason to make an effort</u> to become active again as she has <u>lost her position</u> as an executive secretary. Since she lives alone, she <u>feels she could not manage</u> on her own anyway.

6. Formulate several goal statements for each of the following segments of assessment information and nursing diagnoses.

Behavior	Stimuli	Nursing Diagnosis
a. Sixteen-year-old girl. Weight 85 pounds. Height 5 feet 7 inches. States she does not eat breakfast and only has candy bars for lunch. Feels tired. Appears drawn and pale.	Inadequate caloric and nutritive intake. Always short of time in morning. Peer group does not eat lunch. Parents work; must prepare meals herself. Does not understand principles of good nutrition.	Malnutrition due to inadequate intake of food and lack of knowledge.
b. Elderly male patient. Withdrawn. Uncommunicative. Refuses to do anything for himself. States "No one cares whether I'm dead or alive." States "I'll never leave this place."	Long-term hospitalization. Hospital is long distance from home and family. Has one close relative (a son) who can visit only occasionally.	Loneliness due to absence of support systems.

7. The school nurse in an urban high school has been consulted by the administrative staff and a group of parents to help address a problem of teenage pregnancy among students. The following table represents a segment of information from steps 1 to 4 of the nursing process obtained

when the nurse initiated discussion with a number of girls in the school. Continue with step 5 of the nursing process and identify interventions that could assist in the achievement of the specified goals.

Behavior	Stimuli	Nursing Diagnosis	Goals
Increasing pregnancy rate among high school girls.	Lack of knowledge about consequences	Unwanted pregnancy related to lack of	Within 6 months, the pregnancy rate
All state that they had not intended to become pregnant.	and complications associated with teenage pregnancy.	knowledge about sexual activity and lack of evaluative	among students will have decreased. Within 1 month, all
Many girls state that they acted on impulse and without consideration of long-term outcomes.	Lack of information on which to base decision about sexual activity.	thought prior to decision making. Inadequate knowledge about sexual	students at the school will state confidence in the adequacy of their
Girls stated that their peers expected sexual activity.	Lack of information about birth control.	behavior and potential outcomes.	knowledge related to sexual activity and its ramifi-
Parents of girls are concerned about sexual activity.	Lack of parental involvement in sex education.		cations.

8. For the following goal statements, identify what one would look for in the behavior of the human system that would indicate that nursing interventions had been effective.
   (a) Within 1 week, the patient will have regained full use of his hand as evidenced by his ability to perform a full range of motion.
   (b) Within 6 months, 80% of the staff of the hospital will have received an immunization for hepatitis B.
   (c) Within 1 month, the family will document 1 week's nutritional intake that reflects all of the recommended daily requirements.

Feedback

1. Five-year-old, not actively participating in play, stated that he did not feel well and had a sore throat, appeared flushed, felt warm, (throat) very reddened, large masses of tissue were protruding.

2. (a) I: Normally people of 5 feet weigh much more.
   (b) A: A blood pressure reading of 125/75 is within normal limits.
   (c) I: The patient appears to be demonstrating ineffective learning.
   (d) I: The family is not eating a balanced diet and their nutritional requirements are not being met.
   (e) I: The health status of the school participants indicates that there is a problem affecting half of the school population.

3. Stimuli contributing to the person's refusal to eat: tastelessness of food, inadequate explanation of reason for salt-free diet, diminished acuity of taste sensation associated with aging.

4. Had trouble concentrating and remembering (focal). Studied all night (contextual). Had persistent problems (contextual). Was anxious (contextual). The exam was important (contextual).

5. Examples of nursing diagnosis statements:

   "Appears to lack enthusiasm for rehabilitation and states she sees no reason to make an effort since she has lost her job and feels she will be dependent." This is a statement of behavior connected to the relevant stimuli.

   "Loss of body function due to stroke." The woman has lost the use of the right side of her body as a result of a stroke. She can no longer physically perform her job or care for herself. "Loss" is a common problem associated with the physical self-concept.

6. Examples of goal statements:
   (a) Patient will begin to gain weight as evidenced by a measured gain of 5 pounds in 1 month.

   Patient will eat regular nutritious meals within 1 week as evidenced by a daily diary of food intake that contains all the recommended daily allowances of nutrients.

   Patient's appearance will improve within 6 months as evidenced by weight gain and improved coloring.

   Patient will have more energy within 1 week as evidenced by her statements that she feels less tired and has more energy.

   (b) The patient will begin to interact with other patients and staff by becoming involved actively in an occupational therapy session on a daily basis beginning tomorrow.

   Within 2 days, the patient will begin to assume responsibility for several self-care tasks as demonstrated by shaving himself and cleaning his own teeth.

   Within 2 weeks, the patient will begin to demonstrate optimism about the future by inquiring about potential for discharge to alternative care agency.

7. Examples of interventions:

   In consultation with the students, develop an informational program to address their lack of knowledge.

   Work with the students to enhance their decision-making process by developing several scenarios that illustrate the ramifications and responsibilities of sexual activity.

8. In each case, nursing interventions would be judged effective if the behavior of the human system as identified in the goal statement was attained within the time frame specified.

► REFERENCES

American Nurses Association. (1995). *Nursing's social policy statement.* Kansas City, MO: American Nurses Association.

Benner, P., & Wrubel, J. (1989). *The primacy of caring: Stress and coping in health and illness.* Menlo Park, CA: Addison-Wesley.

Carpenito, L. (1997). *Nursing diagnosis: Application to clinical practice.* Philadelphia: Lippincott.

Cho, J. (1998). *Nursing Manual: Assessment Tool According to the Roy Adaptation Model.* Glendale, CA: Polaris Publishing.

Erikson, E. H. (1963). *Childhood and society* (2nd ed.). New York: Norton.

Martinez, C. (1976). Nursing assessment based on Roy Adaptation Model. In Roy, Sr. C. (Ed.), *Introduction to nursing: An adaptation model* (pp. 379–385). Englewood Cliffs, NJ: Prentice Hall.

McDonald, F. J., & Harms, M. (1966). Theoretical model for an experimental curriculum. *Nursing Outlook, 14(8),* 48–51.

Rantz, M. J., & LeMone, P. (Eds.). (1997). *Classification of nursing diagnosis. Proceedings of the 12th conference NANDA.* Glendale, CA: CINAHL Information Systems.

Sato, M. K. (1984). Major factors influencing adaptation. In Roy, Sr. C. (Ed.), *Introduction to nursing: An adaptation model* (2nd ed., pp. 64–87). Englewood Cliffs, NJ: Prentice Hall.

Sorrel M. S., & Smith, B. A. (1993). Navajo beliefs: Implications for health professionals. *Journal of Health Education, 24(6),* 336–338.

Watson, J. (1985). *Nursing: Human science and human care.* Norwalk, CT: Appleton-Century-Crofts.

► ADDITIONAL REFERENCES

Campbell-Heider, N., & Knapp, T. R. (1993). Toward a hierarchy of adaptation to biomedical technology. *Critical Care Nursing Quarterly, 16(3),* 42–50.

Gordon, M. (1994). *Nursing diagnosis: Process and application* (3rd ed.). St. Louis: Mosby Yearbook.

Mason, G., & Webb, C. (1993). Nursing diagnosis: A review of the literature. *Journal of Clinical Nursing, 2,* 67–74.

Roy, Sr. C. (1984). The Roy model nursing process. In Roy, Sr. C. (Ed.), *Introduction to nursing: An adaptation model* (2nd ed., pp. 42–63). Englewood Cliffs, NJ: Prentice Hall.

II PART

THE ADAPTIVE MODES

Inherent in Roy's description of human beings as individual or collective adaptive systems are four major categories in which coping processes can be observed. These categories are termed the four adaptive modes: the physiologic–physical mode, the self-concept–group identity mode, the role function mode, and the interdependence mode. It is in relation to these four major categories that responses are carried out and that adaptation levels can be observed. Part II of this text is devoted to an exploration of these modes: their integrated processes, compensatory processes, and compromised processes, together with an overview of assessment and planning of nursing care.

In Chapter 4, the authors provide an overview of each of the four modes, with an expanded focus on the physical mode of groups. The major focus in Chapters 5 to 13 is the physiologic mode as it pertains to the individual; however, selective attention is directed to application of the concepts as they apply to human beings in groups or collectives, that is, families, organizations, communities, and society as a whole. The physiologic mode chapters are organized by the five needs and four complex processes of the physiologic mode of the individual. Chapters 14, 15, and 16 present the self-concept–group identity mode, the role function mode, and the interdependence mode, respectively. Each of these chapters includes both individual and collective perspectives. The intent of presenting the physiologic needs and processes first, and then the other modes, is to move from simple to complex, concrete to abstract, and individual to group. Complete discussion of the physiologic mode components provide the basis for understanding application of the adaptation model to more complex nursing practice situations.

4

OVERVIEW OF THE ADAPTIVE MODES

The behaviors of both individuals and collectives that result from coping activity can be observed in four categories, or adaptive modes, developed by Roy to serve as a framework for assessment (Roy, 1984). These four modes are as follows.

1. The physiologic (physical, for collectives)
2. The self-concept (group identity, for collectives)
3. Role function (for individuals and collectives)
4. Interdependence (pertaining to both)

It is through these four modes, or ways of behaving, that responses to and interaction with the environment are carried out. A key aspect of the adaptive person or group is adaptation level, which can be described as integrated processes, compensatory processes, and compromised processes.

These four adaptive modes are discussed in greater detail in Chapters 5 to 16; however, an overview of each is provided in this chapter. Since Chapters 5 to 13 deal with the physiologic mode with focus on the individual human system, concepts associated with the physical mode as pertaining to collective human systems are selectively addressed in expanded detail in this chapter. Presentation of the collective perspective is inherent in the chapters addressing the other three modes.

► OBJECTIVES

After studying this chapter, the reader will be able to do the following:

1. Describe the four adaptive modes as they pertain to both individual human systems and collective human systems.

2. Provide examples of the theoretical basis of each adaptive mode.

3. Identify the five basic needs and their associated life processes inherent in physiologic integrity.

4. Describe the four complex physiologic processes that serve to mediate regulator activity and integrate physiologic functioning.

5. Demonstrate beginning application of the concepts associated with the physical mode as it applies to collective human systems.

▶ KEY CONCEPTS DEFINED

Biobehavioral knowledge: Focus of nursing knowledge that balances understanding of persons as both physiologic beings in a physical world and as thinking and feeling beings with human experience in a cosmic world.

Capacities: The assets that participants involved in collective human adaptive systems bring to the situation including knowledge, skills, abilities, commitments, and associations with others.

Fiscal resources: The component of the physical mode pertaining to the monetary capacity of the collective human adaptive system.

Identity integrity: The basic need of the group identity mode; implies the honesty, soundness, and completeness of identification with the group; involves the process of shared identity and goals.

Operating integrity: The underlying need of the physical adaptive mode; wholeness achieved by adapting to changes in operating resource requirements; encompasses participants, physical facilities, and fiscal resources.

Participants: The component of the physical mode pertaining to those involved in, or members of, the collective human adaptive system.

Personal self: The individual's appraisal of personal characteristics, expectations, values, and worth.

Physical facilities: The component of the physical mode pertaining to the capital and material capacities required for ongoing operation and effective adaptation of the collective human adaptive system.

Physical mode: The manner in which the collective human adaptive system manifests adaptation relative to needs associated with basic operating resources.

Physical self: An individual's appraisal of personal physical being including physical attributes, functioning, sexuality, health-illness states, and appearance.

Physiologic integrity: The underlying need of the physiologic mode; physiologic wholeness achieved by adapting to changes in physiologic needs.

Physiologic mode: One of the four adaptive modes in which a person manifests the physical and chemical processes involved in the function and activities of a living organism.

Physiology: A science dealing with knowledge about the physical and chemical phenomena involved in the function and activities of a living organism.

Process: A series of activities or changes that proceed from one to the next.

Psychic and spiritual integrity: The basic need of the self-concept mode on the individual level; the need to know who one is so that one can be or exist with a sense of unity, meaning, and purposefulness in the universe.

Relational integrity: The underlying need of the interdependence mode; wholeness achieved in terms of the needs for affection, development, and resources.

Role: The functioning unit of society; each role exists in relation to another.

Role clarity: Basic need associated with the role function mode (collective); the need to understand and commit to fulfill expected tasks, so that the group can achieve common goals.

Self-concept: The composite of beliefs and feelings that is held about oneself at a given time, formed from internal perception and perceptions of others' reactions.

Significant others: Persons who are the most important to the individual.

Social integrity: The basic need of the role function mode (individual); the need to know who one is in relation to others so that one can act.

Support systems: Others contributing to meeting interdependence needs.

► EXPANSION OF THE MODES

The adaptive modes, as described in the Roy Adaptation Model, were initially associated with the way in which individual human systems respond to stimuli from the environment. In this book, the modes have been expanded to address collective human systems as well. In describing collectives, Roy specifies terminology for collective human systems—physical, group identity, role function, and interdependence—to correspond with the four adaptive modes associated with the individual.

In situations of advanced nursing practice, nurses often function in roles in which they relate to people in aggregate or group situations. In these circumstances, the collective is regarded as a whole and the nursing process is applied in relation to the whole, just as it is applied to individual circumstances.

In the following section an overview of each of the four modes is provided. As previously mentioned, this chapter contains selective expansion of the concepts associated with the physical mode. This focus is carried into the nursing care example provided later in the chapter.

▶ PHYSIOLOGIC–PHYSICAL MODE

The category of behavior pertaining to physical aspects of human systems is termed the physiologic mode where the individual is concerned and the physical mode for groups and other collectives. Each of these has been developed in further detail to guide the assessment of the effectiveness of adaptation from the physical perspective of individuals and groups. The physiologic and physical modes are addressed separately in this section since Chapters 5 to 13 are devoted to consideration of the individual human system. This separation is not made in the remaining three modes as Chapters 14 to 16 include presentation of individual and collective perspectives in combination.

Physiologic Mode

The *physiologic mode* is associated with the physical and chemical processes involved in the function and activities of living organisms. An understanding of physiologic behavior necessitates a knowledge of the anatomy and physiology of the human body as well as the pathophysiology underlying disease processes. The nurse must be knowledgeable about normal body processes to recognize compensatory processes and compromised processes of physiologic adaptation.

The underlying need of the physiologic mode is *physiologic integrity.* Integrity has been defined as the degree of wholeness achieved by adapting to changes in needs. When a person's physiologic needs are met, physiologic integrity is achieved.

Behavior in this mode is the manifestation of the physiologic activities of all the cells, tissues, organs, and systems comprising the human body. As with each of the adaptive modes, stimuli activate the coping processes, creating adaptive and ineffective behavior. In this case, the coping processes are those associated with physiologic functioning and the resulting responses are physiologic behaviors. It is the person's physiologic behavior that indicates whether the coping processes are able to adapt to the stimuli affecting them.

Five needs are identified in the physiologic mode relative to physiologic integrity: oxygenation, nutrition, elimination, activity and rest, and protection. Each of the physiologic needs involves integrated processes. These needs and associated processes are briefly described here and addressed individually in following chapters.

1. *Oxygenation.* This need involves the body's requirements for oxygen and the basic life processes of ventilation, exchange of gases, and transport of gases (Roy & Andrews, 1991; Vairo, 1984).
2. *Nutrition.* This need involves a series of integrated processes associated with digestion (the ingestion and assimilation of food) and metabolism (provision of energy, building of tissue, and regulation of metabolic processes) (Roy & Andrews, 1991; Servonsky, 1984a).
3. *Elimination.* The need for elimination includes the physiologic processes involved in the excretion of metabolic wastes primarily through the intestines and kidneys (Roy & Andrews, 1991; Servonsky, 1984b).
4. *Activity and rest.* The need for balance in the basic life processes of mobility and sleep provides optimal physiologic functioning of all body components and periods of restoration and repair (Cho, 1984; Roy & Andrews, 1991).
5. *Protection.* The need for protection includes two basic life processes, nonspecific defense processes and specific defense processes.

Also inherent in a discussion of physiologic adaptation are complex processes involving senses; fluid, electrolyte, and acid–base balance; neurologic function; and endocrine function.

1. *Senses.* The sensory processes of sight, hearing, touch, taste, and smell enable people to interact with their environment. The sensation of pain is an important related consideration (Driscoll, 1984; Roy & Andrews, 1991).
2. *Fluid, electrolyte, and acid–base balance.* Complex processes associated with fluid, electrolyte, and acid–base balance are required for cellular, extracellular, and systemic function (Perley, 1984; Roy & Andrews, 1991).
3. *Neurologic function.* Neurologic channels are an integral part of a person's regulator coping mechanisms. They function to control and coordinate body movements, consciousness, and cognitive-emotional processes, as well as to regulate activity of body organs (Robertson, 1984; Roy & Andrews, 1991).
4. *Endocrine function.* Endocrine processes through hormone secretion serve, along with neurologic function, to integrate and coordinate body functioning. Endocrine activity plays a significant role in the stress response and is also part of regulator coping (Howard & Valentine, 1984; Roy & Andrews, 1991).

These four complex processes can be viewed as mediating regulatory activity and encompassing many physiologic functions of the person. The nine components are described within the model as a basis for a nursing assessment of the physiologic mode as it pertains to the individual.

Physical Mode

The *physical mode* for humans in groups and collectives corresponds with the physiologic mode for the individual. It has been described as the manner in which the collective human adaptive system manifests adaptation relative to basic operating resources, participants, physical facilities, and fiscal resources. The basic need associated with the physical mode is *operating integrity,* or the wholeness achieved by adapting to changes in operating resource requirements.

The *participants* component of the physical mode pertains to the people who are involved in the collective human adaptive system. In the case of a family, this includes the relevant family members. Terminology to describe family members includes the nuclear family (two parents and child or children), single-parent family (one parent and child or children), and the extended family (including relatives beyond parent(s) and children). Some families include adults, with or without children, living together, who are bound by legal, kinship, or other relations.

For groups, the participants would consist of members of the group, both formal and informal. In organizations, the participants are those who are involved in or employed by the organization or have some other role to fulfill as part of the organization. Community participants tend to be those who reside in a particular community; however, demographic location may not be a determinant for community membership, as in the case of some ethnic communities where participants reside in numerous locations. Participants in the society as a whole typically are located within the societal boundaries. Whatever the aggregate group, the participants are those who would name themselves as part of the group.

The *capacities* of participants are a major resource for the human adaptive system. Included in the notion of capacities are the capabilities, knowledge, skills, commitments, and health of the individuals within the collective system. The basic need of the physical adaptive mode, operating integrity, cannot be fulfilled unless the participants possess the capacities required to support the collective entity. The refinement and enhancement of the capacities of group participants is a significant requirement to enable the achievement of the goals of adaptation.

Just as the goals of the individual human adaptive system are identified in the Roy Adaptation Model, so are the goals of adaptation for collective human systems. Whether they are families, groups, organizations, communities, or society, effective responses typically pertain to ongoing existence of the collective; its continuing growth; its ability to propagate beliefs, values, and cultural heritage; and the confidence and success in fulfilling its vision and objectives.

Physical facilities are an important component for collective human adaptive systems. This aspect of the physical system includes a physical plant such as shelter for the family, a meeting place for a group, or a physical plant for the organization. Also included in this component are the operational resources required to fulfill the purpose of the group. In a family situation, food and clothing are examples of operational resources. In an organization, supplies and equipment constitute physical resources, for example, books and computers in schools and bed sheets and exercise equipment in a rehabilitation hospital. Some aggregate human systems have need for technologic resources, as well. A community requires communication systems and road maintenance equipment. All of these physical commodities contribute to meeting the need of resource adequacy in the physical system.

Many of these components are dependent on the fiscal adequacy of the collective human adaptive system. Inadequate levels of funding compromise the ability of the system to maintain the integrity of the particular collective entity. In a family situation, if there is not enough food for the members, health of the adults or children can be compromised. If an organization is unable to purchase operating supplies, it will experience difficulty remaining in business.

Capital resources are also an important aspect of fiscal adequacy for most collective human adaptive systems. Capital resources pertain to the significant and infrequent purchases that may be required to support the ongoing integrity of the collective system. In a family situation, this can be a major health care expenditure on behalf of a member or the purchase of a house for the family. For a baseball team, it may be the purchase of uniforms so that the team can be involved in a competition league. Organizations, communities, and societal groups often have major requirements for capital resources to support their ongoing and orderly operation.

If inadequate funding persists over time, the integrity of the entire system is compromised; ineffective behaviors result. This notion will be explored further as the nursing process is applied to the physical mode.

Theoretical Basis

The theoretical background for the physiologic–physical mode lies, for the individual human system, in basic life sciences, particularly anatomy, physiology, pathophysiology, and chemistry. In addition, meeting human needs, either individually or collectively, is influenced by psychologic processes such as motivation and concepts from sociology, anthropology, family studies, organizational behavior, economics, community studies, ecology and cosmology, religious studies, and other disciplines within the humanities. For example, literature can provide understanding of how fictional characters have been drawn to deal with basic themes of life. These fields can be described briefly as follows.

- *Anatomy.* As the study of the structure of the human body, human anatomy provides the structural basis for the physiologic mode.

- *Physiology.* Physiology provides the nurse with knowledge of the processes involved in the functioning and activities of the human body. This knowledge is the basis for the judgment of adaptive and ineffective physiologic behavior.
- *Pathophysiology.* As the study of the abnormal physiologic changes accompanying illness, pathophysiology provides the nurse with a rationale for the identification of ineffective behavioral responses and the stimuli influencing them.
- *Chemistry.* Knowledge from chemistry, dealing with the composition, properties, and reactions of substances, provides the basis for an understanding of body processes such as those involved in fluid and electrolyte activity.
- *Psychology.* The study of the mind and behavior provides a basis for the understanding of psychosocial processes related to self, role, and interdependence, and how the processes relate to illness and ineffective behavior.
- *Sociology.* The study of the development, structure, interaction, and collective behavior of organized groups of people provides a foundation for the nurse's assessment of the self, role, and interdependence modes and their influence on physiologic function in situations of effective and ineffective adaptation.
- *Anthropology.* The study of people in relation to their distribution, origin, classification, and the relationship of races including physical character, environmental and social relationships, and culture contributes to the nurse's ability to identify the impact of these factors on the integrity of the person's adaptive modes.
- *Family studies.* The study of family interactions includes the stages of the family life cycle and consideration of contemporary issues (for example, changing family structures, family violence, addictions).
- *Organizational behavior.* The study of organizations, their environment, strategies, and structures, is basic to understanding groups as adaptive systems.
- *Economics.* The study of the principles of economics provides insight relative to the effects of employment, inflation, monetary policy, and fiscal policy on the provision of health care.
- *Community studies.* The study of community dynamics includes the development, structure, interaction, and collective behavior of community members and is similarly useful to understanding groups as adaptive systems.
- *Ecology and cosmology.* The study of the earth and universe, developmental stages and future, helps nurses understand decisions made by persons concerning the environment.
- *Religious studies and spirituality.* The study of specific religions and approaches to spirituality provides insight into the beliefs and values of individuals and groups. It enables consideration of factors that may be influencing the response to particular environmental influences that are significant in the provision of nursing care.

- *Humanities.* Knowledge from other disciplines focusing on the attributes or qualities of the human person enables the nurse to more effectively consider the individual or group experience and intervene appropriately in situations of need.

These disciplines provide direction for some of the knowledge needed to support understanding of all four modes and the study of nursing itself. At the same time, the view of nursing based on the model indicates what knowledge is relevant and what knowledge needs to be developed. From their experience with persons who are healthy or unhealthy, nurses can determine what knowledge is relevant for nursing care. As with each of the modes, consideration of the physiologic–physical mode involves knowledge from a variety of related disciplines. This knowledge is viewed in the light of nursing's view of the person as an individual or collective system and of the goal of promoting adaptation. Nursing knowledge is *biobehavioral.* Such knowledge balances understanding of persons as both physiologic beings in a physical world and as thinking and feeling beings with human experience in a cosmic world.

▶ SELF-CONCEPT–GROUP IDENTITY MODE

The adaptive mode pertaining to the personal aspect of human systems is termed the self-concept mode for the individual and the group identity mode for collective human systems. These categories have been developed in further detail to guide the assessment of the effectiveness of adaptation from the personal perspective. Chapter 14 expands on the self-concept–group identity adaptive mode.

In the self-concept mode, the personal perspective focuses specifically on the psychological and spiritual aspects of the human system. The basic need underlying the individual self-concept mode has been identified as *psychic and spiritual integrity,* or the need to know who one is so that one can be or exist with a sense of unity, meaning, and purposefulness in the universe. This integrity is basic to health. Adaptation problems in integrity can interfere with the person's ability to heal or to do what is necessary to maintain other aspects of health. It is important for the nurse to have knowledge about the self-concept mode to assess behaviors and stimuli influencing the person's self-concept.

Self-concept is defined as the composite of beliefs and feelings held about oneself at a given time and is formed from internal perceptions and perceptions of others' reactions. The composite sense of self is used to direct one's behavior.

The self-concept mode is viewed as having two components. The *physical self* includes body sensation and body image. The *personal self* is composed of self-consistency, self-ideal, and a moral-ethical-spiritual self. Some examples of these components include the statement, "I look like I haven't slept in a week!"—a behavioral statement related to body image. The statement, "I know I can figure out how to install this new computer program," illustrates self-ideal behavior.

The group identity mode is analogous to the self-concept mode. It reflects how people in groups perceive themselves based on environmental feedback. The group identity mode is comprised of interpersonal relationships, group self-image, social milieu, and culture. The basic need underlying the group identity mode is termed *identity integrity,* the ability of group members to relate to each other with the honesty, soundness, and completeness of identification with the group. Identity integrity involves the process of shared identity and goals.

In a social system such as a school, one can describe an associated culture. There is a social environment experienced by the teachers and students, and a group identity that is reflected by those who are part of the school group. As such, the group identity mode can reflect adaptive or ineffective behaviors associated with the school as a social organization.

Theoretical Basis

The description of the self-concept–group identity mode is based on a number of specific psychologic, biologic, and social theories and principles, synthesized by Driever (1976) and expanded by Roy. These provide direction for the assessment of behavior and stimuli relative to the self-concept or group identity and for each of the other steps of the nursing process. The following is an identification of the theoretical bases of the self-concept–group identity mode described in the Roy Adaptation Model. The works of the identified theorists can enhance knowledge for the use of these theories in the application of the Roy Adaptation Model.

- *Piaget (1954), Erikson (1963), and Neugarten (1969, 1979).* Developmental theories based on physical, social, and cognitive maturational.
- *Mead (1934), Sullivan (1953), Cooley (1964), and Goffman (1959, 1967).* Symbolic interaction theories focusing on social interaction as a basis for developing and maintaining a sense of self.
- *Coombs and Snygg (1959).* Theory of self-perception. Self is seen as a constellation of self-perceptions.
- *Markus (1977).* Self-schema as cognitive generalizations about the self, derived from past experience, that guide the processing of information about the self.
- *Lecky (1945, 1961), Rogers (1951, 1961), Elliott (1986), and Antonovsky (1986).* Theories based on self-consistency, self-organization, and coherence.
- *McMahon (1993).* Introduced term *focusing* to include being in touch with self in a way that surfaces hope, energy, continuity, meaning, purpose, and pride to be on individual self within the whole human community.
- *Campsy (1985), Johnson (1983), Montagu (1986), Johnson and Levanthal (1974), and Amman-Gainotti (1986).* Focus on body sensation, sexuality, and coping, particularly for nursing assessment and intervention.

- *Festinger (1962) and Andrews (1990).* Theory of cognitive dissonance. The individual's behavior reflects an endeavor to minimize perceived discrepancies between the self-concept and other aspects of experience.
- *Rosenberg (1965, 1979) and Driever (1976).* Self-esteem described as stemming from values of self-attributions and as a pervasive aspect of self.
- *Kübler-Ross (1969) and Dobratz (1984).* Described five stages of death and dying, and the process of life closure. Understanding is commonly used in helping people grow through grieving and promoting resolution of the issue of the meaning of one's life and accepting the reality of death.
- *Kimberly (1997).* Describes processes and structures of groups and the bases of cohesiveness as the relationships among liking or attraction, norms and values, and effective pursuit of goals and good working relations.
- *Rabbie and Lodewijks (1996).* A behavioral interaction model for studying groups that includes demands and distance, external social environment, and leadership and responsibility.
- *Zohar (1990) and Swimme and Berry (1992).* The creative self and the human capacity for unity of consciousness and relational wholes. Transaction adds that as persons interact with environment, both are changed and intergration and mutual transformations are possible.
- *Chinn (1995).* Presents a process of transformation, based on experiences of women's groups and represented by the five words, praxis, empowerment, awareness, consensus, and evolvement (PEACE).

This text introduces these theories and describes their relevance to understanding persons and groups as adaptive systems that strive for psychic and spiritual integrity and identity integrity. Nurses will find that continued study and experience can expand upon this knowledge. In this way, they can be enabled to practice nursing with the Roy Adaptation Model at the increasing levels of complexity required in contemporary health care systems.

▶ ROLE FUNCTION MODE

The category of behavior pertaining to roles in human systems is termed the role function mode for both the individual and the group or collective. This category has been developed in further detail to guide assessment of the effectiveness of adaptation as it pertains to the roles that humans occupy relative to each other.

From the perspective of the individual, the role function mode focuses on the roles that the individual occupies in society. A *role,* as the functioning unit of society, is defined as a set of expectations about how a person occupying one position behaves toward a person occupying another position. The basic need underlying the role function mode has been identified as *social integrity,* the need to know who one is in relation to others so that one can act. The role set is the complex of positions that an individual holds.

A classification of role sets as involving primary, secondary, and tertiary roles has been adopted for use in the Roy Adaptation Model. Associated with each role are instrumental behaviors and expressive behaviors, assessment of which provides an indication of social adaptation relative to role function. Each type of behavior can be illustrated with the role of a mother. Caring for a baby's physical needs involves instrumental behaviors; holding and cuddling the baby are expressive behaviors. The manner in which the person fulfills these role expectations is an indication of adequacy of role mastery.

Roles within a group are the vehicle through which the goals of the collective system are actually accomplished. They are the action components associated with group or collective infrastructure. Roles are designed to contribute to the accomplishment of the group's mission or the tasks and functions associated with the group. The role function mode includes the functions of officers and workers, the management of information, and systems for decision making and maintaining order. The basic need associated with the role function mode at the group level is termed *role clarity,* the need to understand and commit to fulfill expected tasks, so that the group can achieve common goals.

In a business, the management function constitutes a role subsystem as do decision-making processes and performance assessment systems. In a family, roles relate to such functions as wage earning, maintenance of a place to live, and child rearing. Interrelated roles are the aggregated role sets of all members and constitute the role function mode for the group.

Theoretical Basis

The description of the role function mode is based on a number of specific theories and principles from sociology, psychology, and nursing. These provide direction for the assessment of behaviors and stimuli relative to the role function mode and, in fact, for each of the other steps of the nursing process. The following is an identification of major theorists and a statement of their important theoretical concepts that are the basis of the role function mode described in the Roy Adaptation Model.

- *Parsons and Shills (1951).* Structural approach to roles. Identification of role requirements and instrumental and expressive behaviors associated with roles.
- *Mead (1934) and Blumer (1969).* Interaction approach to roles. One defines the situation as one "sees it" and acts on the perception.
- *Banton (1965).* Described roles as primary, secondary, and tertiary.
- *Turner (1979).* Role-taking by three standpoints. Described internal and external validation of roles.
- *Merton (1957).* Identifies six processes for integrating role sets.

- *Zohar and Marshall (1994).* Describe a global society where community draws on common culture and collective patterns of thinking, feeling, and acting. The search for meaningful social norms goes beyond individualism or collectivism to creative use of both freedom and ambiguity.
- *Worchel (1996).* Describes six stages of development from observing ongoing groups that are useful in group-based analysis, including nursing assessment.
- *Meleis (1975) and Erickson, Tomlin, and Swain (1988).* Role transitions require incorporation of new knowledge, altering one's behavior, and changing one's definition of self. Role modeling described as a nursing intervention.
- *Roy (1967).* Role cues described and tested as intervention in role transition.
- *Brehm and Kassin (1996).* Describe social perception as involving observations of raw data, analyzing behavior, and attributing characteristics to the other. Stereotyping involves beliefs that associate certain groups of people with certain types of characteristics and then these beliefs influence judgments of individuals.

The theoretical basis for understanding the goals of the role function mode, that is, social integrity and role clarity, includes structural, interaction, and collective pattern approaches. These approaches are compatible with the assumptions outlined in the Roy Adaptation Model. The melding of diverse theories provides a rich perspective of the role function adaptive mode. Again, the reader will find it useful to continue professional development as it relates to theories of roles in society.

▶ INTERDEPENDENCE MODE

The category of behavior pertaining to interdependent relationships of individuals and groups is termed the interdependence mode. This category has been developed in further detail to guide the assessment of the effectiveness of adaptation from the interdependence perspective of individuals and collectives.

The interdependence mode focuses on the close relationships of people (individually and collectively) and their purpose, structure, and development. Each interdependent relationship exists for some purpose and it is through such relationships that people continue to grow as individuals and as contributing members of society.

Interdependent relationships involve the willingness and ability to give to others and accept from them aspects of all that one has to offer such as love, respect, value, nurturing, knowledge, skills, commitments, material possessions, time, and talents. People who have a comfortable balance in interdependent relationships feel valued and supported by others, and can express the same for others. These people have learned to live successfully in a world of others including people, animals, objects, and the environment.

The basic need of this mode, both individually and collectively, is termed *relational integrity,* or the feeling of security in relationships. This basic need consists of three components: affectional adequacy, developmental adequacy, and resource adequacy.

Two specific relationships are the focus of the interdependence mode as it applies to individuals. The first relationship is with *significant others,* persons who are the most important to the individual. The second is with *support systems,* that is, others contributing to meeting interdependence needs (often part of group or collective membership). Specific to these relationships, two major areas of interdependence behavior have been identified (Randell, Tedrow, & VanLandingham, 1982), receptive behavior and contributive behavior. These behaviors apply respectively to the receiving and giving of love, respect, and value in interdependent relationships. For example, a significant other for a child would be the mother. In this interdependent relationship, receptive behavior on the child's part would be allowing the mother to give comfort when the child is hurt. Contributive behavior would be the child's giving the mother a hug and a kiss on leaving for school. The assessment of receptive and contributive behaviors provides an indication of social adaptation relative to the interdependence mode.

The interdependence mode as it applies to collectives has been described in terms of three interrelated components.

1. The context (internal and external influences) in which the collective operates.
2. The infrastructure (procedures, processes, and systems) of the collective.
3. The people who are participants.

Subcomponents of the context of the interdependence mode include governing and political systems, laws, availability of resources, judicial and legal processes, government regulations, ecological concerns, the general economic climate, interorganizational relations, and customer and supplier relationships. The internal context encompasses such aspects as the group's mission, vision, values, and plans.

The infrastructure consists of the procedures, processes, and systems within and by which the collective human system operates. This includes the way in which the members relate to each other, how they communicate, and how they accomplish the requirements for the collective.

The third component, the people, encompasses the knowledge, skills, attitudes, and commitments of all those involved. For the group to be successful in goal attainment, all three components must be in alignment and compatible. Otherwise, disruptive dissonance occurs and adaptation problems are evident.

Many hospitals in the 1990s experienced merger and consolidation with other health care agencies. For the health care organization, these three components (context, infrastructure, and people) become important considerations associated with their interdependent relationships. Of course, economic factors and other external context variables play significant roles in such relationships, as well.

Theoretical Basis

The description of the interdependence mode is based on a number of specific sociological, psychological, nursing, and behavioral theories and principles. These provide direction for the assessment of behaviors and stimuli relative to the interdependence mode and, in fact, for each of the other steps of the nursing process. The following is an identification of the theorists and a statement of their important theoretical concepts that are the basis of the interdependence mode described in the Roy Adaptation Model.

- *Andrews (1994) and Cook (1994).* Interdependence model consisting of three components—context, infrastructure, and people.
- *Berkman (1978).* Development of the social contact index.
- *Cobb (1976).* Described individuals as involved in networks of mutual obligation.
- *Ellison (1976) and Koch and Haugk (1992).* Describe different types of aggression, including physical, nonverbal, verbal, and passive.
- *Erikson (1963).* Eight stages of development and their implication for interdependent relationship.
- *Havighurst (1953).* Developmental tasks for the infant to the mature adult.
- *House, Landis, and Umberson (1988), Cohen (1985), and Gottleib (1981).* Relationship between interdependence and health.
- *Kane (1988) and Caplan (1974).* Conceptual model of family social support with three interaction factors, reciprocity, advice and feedback, and emotional involvement.
- *Klaus and Kennel (1981), Bowlby (1969), Mahler (1979), and Spitz (1945).* Theories related to emotional bonding and attachment and the effects of separation.
- *Maslow (1979).* Hierarchy of needs (physiologic needs, safety needs, need for belongingness, and love–esteem needs) of the individual.
- *Randell, Tedrow, and VanLandingham (1982).* Identification and description of receiving and giving behaviors; development and relinquishing of four adaptive modes.
- *Stanford (1977).* Describes group behaviors during the process of termination and closure.
- *Selman (1980) and McGinnis (1980).* Description of five stages of friendship and activities to deepen friendship.
- *Selman and Andrews (1994).* Committed communication and principles of effective relationships.

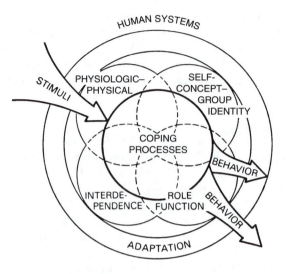

FIGURE 4–1. Diagrammatic representation of human adaptive systems.

Individual and group behavior is viewed in relation to the four adaptive modes. They provide a particular form or manifestation of cognator–regulator and stabilizer–innovator activity within the human adaptive process. Although these modes are frequently viewed separately for teaching and assessment purposes, it must be remembered that they are interrelated.

In Figure 4–1, the four modes are depicted as four overlapping circles, central to which is a circle representing the coping processes as introduced in Chapter 2. As an illustration of interrelationships, it can be noted that the physiologic–physical mode in the diagram is intersected by each of the other three modes. Behavior in the physiologic–physical mode can have an effect on, or act as a stimulus for, one or all of the other modes. In addition, a given stimulus can affect more than one mode, or a particular behavior can be indicative of adaptation in more than one mode. Such complex relationships among modes further demonstrate the holistic nature of humans as individual or collective adaptive systems. The kaleidoscope image or a laser light show illustrates these multifaceted interrelations and how changing the position of one's perspectives changes the patterns perceived.

▶ APPLICATION OF THE NURSING PROCESS

Application of the nursing process to the adaptive modes was illustrated in a general manner in the diagrammatic conceptualization of the model in Figure 3–1. The following section provides an overview of how the six steps of the nursing process described in Chapter 3 are applied in each of these categories.

Nursing assessment according to the Roy Adaptation Model involves two considerations, the assessment of behavior and the assessment of relevant influencing stimuli. Although discussion of these steps is separated for presentation purposes, it is likely that the nurse will identify behaviors and stimuli in a simultaneous fashion while initially interacting with the patient for the purposes of nursing assessment.

Throughout this discussion, an example relating to a collective human adaptive system will be used to illustrate application of the nursing process. Since the following chapters specifically address the nine components of the physiologic mode and the other three modes, the focus of illustration in this chapter will the be physical mode as applied to a collective human system.

Assessment of Behavior

Behavioral assessment of the adaptive modes provides the nurse with an indication of how the human adaptive system is managing to cope with environmental changes affecting the coping processes.

In providing nursing care to individuals, nurses are taught specific ways to conduct physical assessment. These methods must be thorough and efficient. In the Roy Adaptation Model, the approach to assessment of physiologic behavior lies in the five basic needs and the four complex processes of physiologic adaptation. In the study of each of these areas, the nurse learns which behaviors reveal adaptive status in the person. The nurse's background in anatomy, physiology, pathophysiology, and nutrition provides the basis for the decision as to whether the observed behavior in each of the categories is adaptive or ineffective.

Nurses involved with collective human adaptive systems are involved in advanced nursing practice. In preparation for this level of involvement, nurses study areas of knowledge such as family studies, organizational behavior, group psychology, economics, community studies, religious studies, and change theory. In the study of each of these areas, the nurse learns which behaviors reveal adaptive status in the collective system. The nurse's background and interaction with the collective system provide the basis for the decision as to whether the observed behavior in each of the components is adaptive or ineffective.

For each of the behaviors applying to the components of the adaptive modes, there are both general and individual norms against which to judge the behavior of the human adaptive system. The nurse's theoretical background provides the knowledge necessary for this assessment step and for the assessment of stimuli influencing the observed physiologic or physical system behaviors. The nursing model helps to focus that knowledge and provides a lens for looking at the particular mode or system.

Consider the example of a family who, as a result of a motor vehicle accident, is adjusting to a 2-year-old child who is totally paralyzed and ventilator dependent. After a lengthy hospitalization, the child is now stable and plans are being made to move her out of the acute care setting. The family's home is the location under consideration.

In working with the family on these plans, the nurse is involved in assessment related to the associated physical mode. What are the capacities of family members? The child's mother has readily learned the knowledge and skills required to care for an individual on a ventilator. She is committed to assuming care of the child for 8 hours a day, 5 days a week. The father has expressed willingness to learn but has not yet demonstrated competence. There are two other very young siblings who cannot yet be formally involved in care.

With respect to physical facilities, plans are being made to renovate the family's home. A special room close to family activity is being altered to accommodate the mobile bed and equipment. An entrance is being altered to provide wheelchair access. The family has indicated that, financially, they can manage the associated expense.

Each of the above factors represents behaviors in the physical mode associated with the family. The nurse uses theoretical background associated with family roles and responsibilities with respect to caring for a child to label the above behaviors as adaptive with respect to maintenance of the integrity of the family unit.

Assessment of Stimuli

The second aspect of nursing assessment involves the identification of the internal and external stimuli influencing the identified behaviors. In Chapter 3, common stimuli were identified as affecting adaptation in all four modes and as important for primary consideration in the assessment of the stimuli affecting the behavior of the human adaptive system relative to each mode. In addition, stimuli of particular relevance to each of the needs and components have been suggested. These are specified in subsequent chapters. Many of these stimuli relate directly to the common stimuli. Again, the nurse's background knowledge from supporting disciplines provides the insight required for the assessment. The use of a nursing model provides the perspective for integration and making nursing judgments based on that knowledge.

Stimuli are identified, in consultation with the recipient(s) of nursing care, as being focal, contextual, or residual. At this point, it is also possible to determine whether their effect on the human adaptive system is positive or negative. The particular stimuli of adaptive levels are also identified.

Returning to the example cited above, relevant stimuli in the situation involving the paralyzed child may include culture, environmental considerations, and family. From the perspective of culture, the family stems ethnically from an origin generally noted to have very strong commitments to fellow members and a high sense of responsibility regarding family tasks. There is a highly supportive and involved extended family who are willing to be involved in assisting with the child when she comes home.

From a socioeconomic viewpoint, the family is considered to be in the upper quartile with respect to income level and therefore believes they are able to bear the additional financial burden. Environmental considerations related to housing indicate that the family lives in a spacious house with flexibility for renovation to accommodate the particular needs of the handicapped child.

These influencing factors affect the ability of the family to deal adaptively with the focal stimulus, the imminent discharge from hospital of their newly handicapped daughter.

The provision of nursing care to individuals and collective human adaptive systems involves four steps: nursing diagnosis, goal setting, intervention, and evaluation. It is the nursing assessment that provides the direction for these nursing activities.

Nursing Diagnosis

The method of stating a nursing diagnosis according to the Roy Adaptation Model was presented in Chapter 2. This involves relating the observed behavior to the most relevant stimuli. A typology of indicators of positive adaptation and common adaptation problems was presented in Tables 3–2 and 3–3. Specifically, indicators of adaptation and problems were identified as related to the five needs and four complex processes and the collective situation associated with the physiologic–physical mode. With respect to the emphasis on the collective perspective of the physiologic–physical mode as selectively expanded in this chapter and Tables 3–2 and 3–3, three indicators of positive adaptation have been identified: adequate fiscal resources, member capability, and availability of physical facilities. Likewise, there are three common adaptation problems: inadequate fiscal resources, capability deficits, and inadequate physical facilities. Each of these problems represents a cluster of assessment information. Since the typology is an incomplete summary, and since the diagnosis can provide specific direction for nursing intervention, the nurse may prefer to identify individual behaviors and their relevant stimuli. Examples of nursing diagnoses are provided in the following chapters.

An example of a nursing diagnosis related to the previous example could include, "planning to accommodate handicapped child in home supported by adequate fiscal resources, family commitment, and capabilities." Another diagnosis might be, "Inadequate trained personnel to care for child on a 24-hour basis since the mother is the only on-site care giver at this point in time."

Goal Setting

The goal of nursing, when applied to behavior in the adaptive modes, is to maintain and enhance adaptive behavior and to change ineffective behavior to adaptive. Thus, the focus of goal setting is the behavior of the human adaptive system.

The goal statement consists of the three entities identified in Chapter 3, the behavior to be observed, the change expected, and the time frame for achievement of the goal. Examples of goal statements related to the physiologic mode are provided throughout the following chapters.

The second nursing diagnosis example serves as the focus to illustrate a goal statement for the situation described. With respect to the inadequate coverage of care givers, a goal statement may be, "Two weeks prior to discharge (time frame), plans will be in place (change expected) for 24-hour nursing care coverage (behavior)."

Intervention

To promote adaptation, it is necessary to manage the stimuli influencing the behavior under specific consideration. It may be necessary to change the focal stimulus or to broaden the adaptation level by managing other stimuli present or supporting cognator and regulator activity. In selecting approaches, the nurse considers possible alternatives and then selects the approach with the highest probability of achieving the agreed-upon goal.

With respect to the illustrative situation, the stimulus that the nurse will focus on is fiscal resources. The health care plan that provides insurance coverage for the family will provide up to 8 hours of care in the home immediately following discharge from hospital. Since the mother feels that she requires assistance for at least 16 hours a day, it is necessary to pursue additional support above the level provided through the medical insurance plan. It has been determined that, for at least the first month after discharge, 24-hour nursing coverage is required.

In pursuing possible alternatives, the nurse explores with the family the possibility of involvement of members from the extended family. Another possibility is additional funding levels in an exceptional circumstance since the family is willing to take on the care of a person who would otherwise be institutionalized. The health insurance organization will be approached with this request. In planning the alternatives, the nurse collaborates with representatives from several other agencies to develop a workable plan for sufficient nursing care coverage.

Evaluation

The final step of the nursing process, evaluation, involves assessment of the behavioral response in relation to the established behavioral goal. If the goal has been achieved, the intervention was effective; if not, further assessment and reconsideration of goals and intervention is required.

Assessment of the success of the interventions relates to the ability to provide 24-hour nursing care for the child once discharged from hospital. Success in achievement of the goal would be just that. If that goal was not possible to accomplish, the nurse and the family would proceed with further assessment and reconsideration of the goal. Perhaps caring for the child in the home is not realistic. Perhaps there are other sources of funding such as voluntary organizations that could be approached for assistance. Success in achieving the goal would lead to further detailed planning for the child's imminent discharge and the support and achievement of the integrity of the family unit.

▶ SUMMARY

The four adaptive modes as described by the Roy Adaptation Model, and updated for use with groups as well as individuals, have been introduced. Understanding the theoretical basis for and the behaviors to be assessed in each adaptive mode provides the background for applying the Roy Adaptation Model in nursing practice, education, and research. The chapters that follow will build on the general overview of the four adaptive modes to enhance understanding of the modes in both theory and application.

► EXERCISES FOR APPLICATION

1. Select one of the modes and suggest behaviors that would be important to consider. Check your list with those suggested in the relevant following chapters.

2. Compare another framework for physical assessment to that suggested in the Roy Adaptation Model. Look particularly for commonalities. An example of another framework is "head-to-toe assessment."

3. Select a group (family, organization, community) of which you are a part. Identify behaviors and stimuli that are part of the physical mode.

► ASSESSMENT OF UNDERSTANDING

Questions

1. Match the basic need in Column A to the associated adaptive mode in Column B.

   Column A
   Basic Needs

   (a) social integrity
   (b) relational adequacy
   (c) physiologic integrity
   (d) identity integrity
   (e) psychic and spiritual integrity
   (f) resource adequacy

   Column B
   Adaptive Mode

   1. _____ physical mode
   2. _____ group identity mode
   3. _____ self-concept mode
   4. _____ interdependence mode
   5. _____ role function mode
   6. _____ physiologic mode

2. Name five disciplines that form the theoretical basis for the physiologic mode.
   (a) _____
   (b) _____
   (c) _____
   (d) _____
   (e) _____

3. Identify the basic life processes associated with the five basic needs.
   (a) oxygenation (3) _____
   (b) nutrition (2) _____
   (c) elimination (2) _____
   (d) activity and rest (2) _____
   (e) protection (2) _____
4. Name the four complex physiologic processes that mediate regulator activity and integrate physiologic functioning.
   (a) _____
   (b) _____
   (c) _____
   (d) _____

5. Label the following factors as related to one of the three components of the physical mode: participants (P), facilities (F), fiscal resources (R).
   (a) _____ knowledge
   (b) _____ physical plant
   (c) _____ operational resources
   (d) _____ monetary resources
   (e) _____ physical commodities
   (f) _____ commitments
   (g) _____ health

Feedback

1. (a) 5, (b) 4, (c) 6, (d) 2, (e) 3, (f) 1

2. Any five of: anatomy, physiology, pathophysiology, chemistry, psychology, sociology, anthropology, family studies, organizational behavior, economics, community studies, ecology and cosmology, religious studies and spirituality, humanities.

3. (a) Oxygenation: (1) ventilation (2) exchange of gases, (3) transport of gases.
   (b) Nutrition: (1) digestion, (2) metabolism.
   (c) Elimination: (1) intestinal elimination, (2) elimination from kidneys.
   (d) Activity and rest: (1) mobility, (2) sleep.
   (e) Protection: (1) nonspecific defense processes, (2) specific defense processes.

4. (a) senses
   (b) fluid, electrolyte, and acid–base balance
   (c) neurologic function
   (d) endocrine function

5. (a) P, (b) F, (c) F, (d) R, (e) F, (f) P, (g) P

► **REFERENCES**

Amman-Gainotti, M. (1986). Sexual socialization during early adolescence: The menarche. *Adolescence, 21,* 703-710.

Andrews, J. D. W. (1990). Interpersonal self-confirmation and challenge in psychotherapy. *Psychotherapy, 27(4),* 485–504.

Andrews, H. A., Cook, L. M., Davidson, J. M., Schurman, D. P., Taylor, E. W., & Wensel, R. H. (Eds.). (1994). *Organizational transformation in health care: A work in progress.* San Francisco: Jossey-Bass.

Antonovsky, A. (1986). The development of a sense of coherence and its impact to stress situations. *The Journal of Social Psychology, 26(2),* 213–225.

Banton, M. (1965). *Roles: An introduction to the study of social relations.* New York: Basic Books.

Berkman, B. (1978). Mental health and the aging: A review of the literature for clinical social workers. *Clinical Social Work Journal, 6,* 230–245.

Blumer (1969). *Symbolic interactionism: Perspective and method.* Englewood Cliffs, NJ: Prentice Hall.

Bowlby, J. (1969). *Attachment and loss: Attachment* (Vol. 1). New York: Basic Books.

Brehm, S. S., & Kassin, S. M. (1996). *Social psychology* (3rd ed.). Boston: Houghton Mifflin.

Campsey, J. (1985). The sexual dimension of patient care. *Nursing Forum, 22(2),* 69–71.

Caplan, G. (Ed.). (1974). *Support systems and community mental health.* New York: Behavioral Publications.

Chinn, P. L. (1995). *Peace and power: Building communities for the future* (4th ed.). New York: National League for Nursing Press.

Cho, J. S. (1984). Activity and rest. In Roy, Sr. C. (Ed.), *Introduction to nursing: An adaptation model* (2nd ed., pp. 138–158). Englewood Cliffs, NJ: Prentice Hall.

Cobb, S. (1976). Social support as a moderator of life stress. *Psychosomatic Medicine, 38,* 300–312.

Cohen, S. S. L. (1985). *Social support and health.* New York: Academic Press.

Cook, L. M. (1994). Process management: Aligning performance competencies and rewards. In Andrews, H. A., Cook, L. M., Davidson, J. M., Schurman, D. P., Taylor, E. W., & Wensel, R. H. (Eds.), *Organizational transformation in health care* (pp. 139–162). San Francisco: Jossey-Bass.

Cooley, C. H. (1964). *Human nature and the social order.* New York: Schocken.

Coombs, A. W., & Snygg, D. (1959). *Individual behavior: A perceptual approach to behavior.* New York: Harper & Brothers.

Dobratz, M. (1984). Life closure. In Roy, Sr. C. (Ed.), *Introduction to nursing: An adaptation model* (2nd ed., pp. 497–518). Englewood Cliffs, NJ: Prentice Hall.

Driever, M. J. (1976). Theory of self-concept. In Roy, Sr. C. (Ed.), *Introduction to Nursing: An adaptation model* (pp. 255–283). Englewood Cliffs, NJ: Prentice Hall.

Driscoll, S. (1984). The senses. In Roy, Sr. C. (Ed.), *Introduction to nursing: An adaptation model* (2nd ed., pp. 168–188). Englewood Cliffs, NJ: Prentice Hall.

Elliot, G. (1986). Self-esteem and self-consistency: A theoretical and empirical link between two primary motivations. *Social Psychology Quarterly, 49(3),* 207–218.

Ellison, E. (1976). Problem of interdependence: Aggression. In Roy, Sr. C. (Ed.), *Introduction to nursing: An adaptation model* (pp. 330–341). Englewood Cliffs, NJ: Prentice Hall.

Erickson, H., Tomlin, E., & Swain, M. A. (1988). *Modeling and role modeling: A theory and paradigm for nursing.* Lexington, SC: Press of Lexington.

Erikson, E. H. (1963). *Childhood and society* (2nd ed.). New York: Norton.

Festinger, L. (1962). *A theory of cognitive dissonance.* Palo Alto, CA: Stanford University Press.

Goffman, E. (1959). *The presentation of self in everyday life.* New York: Anchor.

Goffman, E. (1967). *Interactional ritual.* New York: Anchor.

Gottlieb, B. H. (Ed.). (1981). *Social networks and social support.* Beverly Hills, CA: Sage.

Havighurst, R. J. (1953). *Human development and education.* New York: Longman.

House, J., Landis, K., & Umberson, D. (1988). Social relationship and health. *Science, 241,* 540–545.

Howard, M., & Valentine, S. (1984). Endocrine function. In Roy, Sr. C. (Ed.), *Introduction to nursing: An adaptation model* (2nd ed., pp. 238–252). Englewood Cliffs, NJ: Prentice Hall.

Johnson, D. (1983). *Body.* Boston: Beacon Press.

Johnson, J. E., & Levanthal, H. (1974). Effects of accurate expectations and behavioral instructions on reactions during a noxious medical examination. *Journal of Personality and Social Psychology, 2,* 55–64.

Kane, C. F. (1988). Family social support: Toward a conceptual model. *Advances in Nursing Science, 10(2),* 188–225.

Kimberly, J. C. (1997). *Group processes and structures: A theoretical integration.* Lanham, MD: University Press of America.

Klaus, M. H., & Kennel, J. H. (1981). *Parent–infant bonding* (2nd ed.). St. Louis: Mosby.

Koch, R. N., & Haugk, K. C. (1992). *Speaking the truth in love.* St. Louis: Stephen Ministries.

Kübler-Ross, E. (1969). *On death and dying.* New York: Macmillan.

Lecky, P. (1945). *Self-consistency: A theory of personality.* New York: Island Press.

Lecky, P. (1969). *Self-consistency: A theory of personality.* New York: Doubleday.

Lecky, P. (1961). In Thorne, C. F. (Ed.), *Self-consistency: A theory of personality.* Hamden, CT: The Shoe String Press.

Mahler, M. S. (1979). *The selected papers of Margaret Mahler: Separation–individuation* (Vol. 2). New York: Jason Aronson.

Markus, H. (1977). Self-schemata and processing information about the self. *Journal of Personality and Social Psychology, 35(2),* 63–78.

Maslow, A. H. (1954). *Motivation and personality.* New York: Harper.

Maslow, A. H. (1968). *Toward a psychology of being.* New York: Van Nostrand.

McMahon, E. M. (1993). *Beyond the myth of dominance: An alternative to a violent society.* Kansas City, MO: Sheed & Ward.

McGinnis, L. (1980). *The friendship factor: How to get close to the people you care for.* Minneapolis, MN: Augsburg Publishing.

Mead, G. (1934). *Mind, self, and society.* Chicago: University of Chicago Press.

Meleis, A. I. (1975). Role insufficiency and role supplementation: A conceptual framework. *Nursing Research, 24(4),* 264–271.

Merton, R. K. (1957). *Social theory and social structure.* New York: Free Press.

Montagu, A. (1986). *Touching: The human significance of the skin* (3rd ed.). New York: Harper & Row.

Neugarten, B. (1969). Continuities and discontinuities of psychological issues in adult life. *Human Development, 12,* 121–130.

Neugarten, B. L. (1979). Time, age, and the life cycle. *The American Journal of Psychiatry, 136(7),* 887–894.

Parsons, T., & Shils, E. (Eds.). (1951). *Toward a general theory of action.* Cambridge, MA: Harvard University Press.

Perley, N. Z. (1984). Fluid and electrolytes. In Roy, Sr. C. (Ed.), *Introduction to nursing: An adaptation model* (2nd ed., pp. 189–210). Englewood Cliffs, NJ: Prentice Hall.

Piaget, J. (1954). *The construction of reality in the child.* Translated by M. Cook. New York: Basic Books.

Rabbie, J. M., & Lodewijks, H. F. M. (1996). A behavioral interactional model: Toward an integrative theoretical framework for studying intra- and intergroup dynamics. In Witte, E., & Davis, J. H. (Eds.), *Understanding group behavior: Small group processes and interpersonal relations.* (Vol. 2, pp. 255–294). Mahwah, NJ: Erlbaum.

Randell, B., Tedrow, M., & VanLandingham, J. (1982). *Adaptation nursing: The Roy conceptual model made practical.* St. Louis: Mosby.

Robertson, M. M. (1984). Neurologic function. In Roy, Sr. C. (Ed.), *Introduction to nursing: An adaptation model* (2nd ed., pp. 211–237). Englewood Cliffs, NJ: Prentice Hall.

Rogers, C. (1951). *Client centered therapy.* Boston: Houghton Mifflin.

Rogers, C. (1961). *On becoming a person.* Boston: Houghton Mifflin.

Rosenberg, M. (1965). *Society and adolescent self-image.* Princeton: Princeton University Press.

Rosenberg, M. (1979). *Conceiving the self.* New York: Basic Books.

Roy, Sr. C. (1967). Role cues and mothers of hospitalized children. *Nursing Research, 16,* 178–182.

Roy, Sr. C. (1984). The Roy Adaptation Model in nursing. In Roy, Sr. C. (Ed.), *Introduction to nursing: An adaptation model* (2nd ed., pp. 27–41). Englewood Cliffs, NJ: Prentice Hall.

Roy, Sr. C., & Andrews, H. (1991). *The Roy Adaptation Model: The definitive statement.* Norwalk, CT: Appleton & Lange.

Selman, R. C. (1980). *The growth of interpersonal understanding: Development and clinical analyses.* New York: Academic Press.

Selman, J. C., & Andrews, H. A. (1994). Effective relationships: Rethinking the fundamentals. In Andrews, H. A., Cook, L. M., Davidson, J. M., Schurman, D. P., Taylor, E. W., & Wensel, R. T. (Eds.), *Organizational transformation in health care: A work in progress* (pp. 53–69). San Francisco: Jossey-Bass.

Servonsky, J. (1984a). Nutrition. In Roy, Sr. C. (Eds.), *Introduction to nursing: An adaptation model* (2nd ed., pp. 110–124). Englewood Cliffs, NJ: Prentice Hall.

Servonsky, J. (1984b). Elimination. In Roy, Sr. C. (Ed.), *Introduction to nursing: An adaptation model* (2nd ed., pp. 125–137). Englewood Cliffs, NJ: Prentice Hall.

Spitz, R. A. (1945). Hospitalism: An inquiry into the genesis of psychiatric conditions in early childhood. In Fenechel, O., Greenacre, P., Hartmann, H., Jackson, E. B., Kris, E., Kubie, L. S., Lewin, B. D., Putnam, M. C., & Spitz, R. A. (Eds.), *The psychoanalytic study of the child* (pp. 53–74). New York: International Universities Press.

Stanford, G. (1977). *Developing effective classroom groups.* New York: Hart.

Sullivan, H. S. (1953). *The interpersonal theory of psychiatry.* New York: Norton.

Swimme, B., & Berry, T. (1992). *The universe story.* San Francisco: Harper.

Turner, R. H. (1979). Role-taking, role standpoint and reference group behavior. In Biddle, B. J., & Thomas, E. J. (Eds.), *Role theory: Concepts and research* (pp. 151–159). New York: Krieger Publishing.

Vairo, S. (1984). Oxygenation. In Roy, Sr. C. (Ed.), *Introduction to nursing: An adaptation model* (2nd ed., pp. 91–109). Englewood Cliffs, NJ: Prentice Hall.

Worchel, S. (1996). Emphasizing the social nature of groups in a developmental framework. In Nye, J. L., & Brower, A. M., (Eds.), *What's social about social cognition? Research on socially shared cognition in small groups* (pp. 261–281). Thousand Oaks, CA: Sage Publishing.

Zohar, D. (1990). *The quantum self: Human nature and consciousness defined by the new physics.* New York: Quill/Morrow.

Zohar, D., & Marshall, I. (1994). *The quantum society: Mind, physics, and a new social vision.* New York: Quill/Morrow.

5

OXYGENATION

Oxygenation is identified in the Roy Adaptation Model as one of five physiologic needs. The basic life processes that provide *oxygenation* include ventilation, gas exchange, and transport of gases. Understanding the physiology of these processes provides the framework for determining adaptation relative to oxygenation. Concepts from pathophysiology are helpful in identifying ineffective behaviors. In this chapter, the three basic life processes of oxygenation are addressed along with identification of parameters for assessment of behaviors and stimuli. Illustrations of innate and learned adaptive responses to compensate for ineffective processes related to oxygenation are described. Examples of compromised processes are discussed. Finally, guidelines for planning nursing care by formulating diagnoses, establishing goals, selecting interventions, and evaluating nursing care are described.

▶ OBJECTIVES

After studying this chapter, the reader will be able to do the following:

1. Describe the three basic life processes associated with the need for oxygenation.

2. Identify important first-level assessment parameters for each of the basic life processes associated with the need for oxygenation.

3. List common stimuli affecting oxygenation.

4. Describe one compensatory process for each of the basic life processes associated with oxygenation.

5. Name and describe two situations of compromised processes of oxygenation.

6. Develop a nursing diagnosis, given an adaptation problem related to oxygenation.

7. Derive goals for an individual with ineffective oxygenation in a given situation.

8. Describe nursing interventions commonly implemented in situations of ineffective oxygenation.

9. Propose approaches to determine the effectiveness of nursing interventions.

▶ KEY CONCEPTS DEFINED

Apnea: The periodic absence of respiration.

Arrhythmia: Irregular pulse rhythm.

Barrel chest: An abnormal condition where the anterior chest diameter is increased and the ribs are more horizontal than the normal downward slant.

Bradycardia: A pulse rate below 60 beats per minute.

Bradypnea: Respiratory rate below 10 breaths per minute.

Cheyne-Stokes Respiration: A pattern of waxing and waning of the respiratory rate and depth.

Dyspnea: The distressful sensation of uncomfortable breathing.

Kussmaul's respirations: Abnormal increase in rate and depth of respirations.

Oxygenation: The processes (ventilation, gas exchange, and transport of gases) by which cellular oxygen supply is maintained in the body.

Pulse rhythm: The time intervals between heart beats.

Respiratory arrest: Prolonged periods of apnea.

Shortness of breath: Observable difficulty with respirations.

Tachycardia: A pulse rate above 100 beats per minute.

Tachypnea: Respiratory rate above 24 breaths per minute.

Tidal volume: The amount of air moved into and out of the lungs during normal respiration.

Ventilation: The complex process of respiration that exchanges air between the lungs and the atmosphere.

▶ BASIC LIFE PROCESS OF OXYGENATION

Oxygenation refers to the processes by which cellular oxygen supply is maintained in the body. The basic life processes responsible for oxygenation are ventilation, alveolar and capillary gas exchange, and transport of gases to and from the tissues. If these processes are functioning effectively, and the environmental oxygen is sufficient, then there is adequate oxygenation of the body tissues. The life of all body tissues depends on maintaining oxygenation, and thus, this need is a high priority in the clinical situation.

▶ VENTILATION: PROCESS AND ASSESSMENT

Ventilation is the complex process of breathing that exchanges air between the lungs and the atmosphere. This process involves both neural control and muscle activity. The neural control is based in a group of neurons referred to as the respiratory center located in the medulla oblongata and lower pons of the brain stem. Afferent and efferent neural pathways transmit signals to the respiratory center to regulate breathing. Further, the peripheral chemoreceptor system, including carotid and aortic bodies, is responsive to changes in oxygen, carbon dioxide, and hydrogen ion concentrations and transmits signals to the main center. This control system operates to serve a fundamental need of all cells, the maintaining of an adequate oxygen supply.

Assessment of Behavior

Given the importance of ventilation to the person's physical and psychological integrity, the nurse assesses oxygenation needs based on the understanding of ventilation as a human life process. Specific assessment factors are examined to determine the adequacy of ventilation and to identify any existing adverse consequences of ventilatory problems.

Ventilatory Patterns

Normal respiratory rate in adults is 12 to 18 breaths per minute when awake. Rates above 24 per minute are termed *tachypnea,* and below 10 per minute, *bradypnea. Apnea* means the periodic absence of respirations. *Respiratory arrest* is the term used for prolonged periods of apnea, a behavior incompatible with life.

Normal respiratory rhythm consists of equal intervals between respiratory cycles with the inspiratory phase shorter than the expiratory phase.

Depth of respirations in terms of *tidal volume,* the amount of air moved into and out of the lungs during normal respiration, is estimated by observing chest movements during inspiration and expiration. Direct measurement of tidal volume, and other respiratory capacities, is done using a spirometer. Spirometry can be done at the bedside, or in an outpatient setting, using simple equipment. At times, spirometry is done in a pulmonary function laboratory with sophisticated equipment and protocols.

Some patterns of altered ventilatory control have specific names. Two patterns most commonly encountered are *Cheyne-Stokes respiration* and *Kussmaul's respiration.* Cheyne-Stokes respiration (CSR) is a pattern of waxing and waning of the respiratory rate and depth. Rate and depth gradually increase and then decrease, followed by a period of apnea, and another cycle of increasing rate and depth. This type of breathing may occur normally in the elderly during sleep, but it may also be seen in patients prior to death or in severe cases of heart failure and drug overdose. Kussmaul's respiration is a term used to describe an abnormal increase in rate and depth of respiration that is seen in cases of metabolic acidosis such as diabetic ketoacidosis. Other types of periodic breathing are described by their characteristics, such as hyperpnea alternating with apnea.

Sleep apnea is a syndrome associated with altered ventilatory control. Persons who are obese are at risk for losing tone in the pharyngeal muscles and consequently having an obstructed airway during sleep. The person exhibits obstructive sleep apnea with episodes of potentially dangerous hypoxemia.

Breath Sounds

Another assessment parameter is breath sounds. Breath sounds are produced by air flow through the airway and are audible through a stethoscope. Normal breath sounds are low pitched with a swishy, breezy quality. Abnormal breath sounds are commonly described as crackles (rales), rhonchi, and pleural friction rub. Nurses learn to distinguish different abnormal breath sounds in studying techniques of physical assessment.

Subjective Experience

The patient's subjective experience of breathing should be perceived as effortless and without conscious thought. *Shortness of breath* is a term indicating observable difficulty with respirations. *Dyspnea* is the distressful sensation of uncomfortable breathing. It is reported by the patient and often is the symptom that limits the person's daily activities. In the case of difficult respirations caused by obstruction, respiratory sounds are audible without the use of a stethoscope. For example, obstruction of the trachea produces a harsh crowing sound (stridor) on inspiration, as seen in a child with acute croup, or laryngotracheitis. Obstruction caused by a foreign body is called aspiration. Severe constriction of the bronchioles, as in asthma, produces a sound known as wheezing that is continuous, high-pitched, and whistling, as air is forced through narrowed respiratory passages.

Assessment of Stimuli

The second level of assessment of oxygenation related to the process of ventilation includes identifying stimuli that influence adaptive and ineffective behaviors. Impairment of structure or function can lead to compromise of the basic breathing processes and affect respiratory rate, rhythm, depth, and ease.

Structural Integrity

Airway patency; musculoskeletal structure of the rib cage; and functioning muscles, neural control centers, and pathways are important for effective ventilation. Assessment of the patency of the patient's airway is a primary responsibility of the nurse. Foreign bodies in the airway; inflammatory reactions from infections, irritants, and allergens; and aspiration of fluids or emesis are all factors that can impede airway clearance.

Pathologic processes can lead to deformity or atrophy of musculoskeletal structures of the rib cage and chest. Skeletal problems of the thoracic cage, such as scoliosis and rib fractures, affect ventilation by decreasing thoracic expansion. *Barrel chest,* as seen in emphysema, is an abnormal condition where the anterior chest diameter is increased and the ribs are more horizontal than the normal downward slant. This change in appearance of the chest results from trapped air due to increased bronchial resistance and the chronic overuse of expiratory muscles. Neuromuscular diseases restricting ventilation include skeletal muscle disorders such as muscular dystrophy; neuromuscular junction disorders such as myasthenia gravis and botulism; and spinal cord disorders such as Guillain-Barré syndrome, poliomyelitis, spinal cord injuries, and tetanus (Dettenmeier, 1992).

Trauma

Head injuries that cause trauma and bleeding in the central nervous system can result in increased intracranial pressure which, in turn, can affect the respiratory center in the brain. Traumatic injuries from motor vehicle accidents, shootings, or stabbings can result in tears of the diaphragm or pleura causing pneumothorax. In this critical condition, air at atmospheric pressure enters the pleural space and causes the lung to collapse. This interferes with both ventilation and tissue perfusion because it also affects gas exchange and transport.

Medications

Depression of the respiratory center can occur with the use of narcotics and anesthetics.

▶ EXCHANGE OF GASES: PROCESS AND ASSESSMENT

In ventilation, atmospheric air reaches the alveoli, where the process of exchange of gases is initiated. Oxygen and carbon dioxide are exchanged across the alveolocapillary membranes. This transfer of gases at the alveolar level is a result of diffusion, which is determined by the partial pressures of the gases on both sides of the alveolocapillary membrane. There is a larger amount of oxygen and a smaller amount of carbon dioxide in the alveoli than in the blood. Thus oxygen diffuses across the membrane and enters the hemoglobin molecules in the blood. Circulation of blood carries oxygen to the body's cells. Carbon dioxide diffuses in a reverse direction across the membrane into the alveoli to be exhaled out of the body. Normal gas exchange depends on the concentration gradients of the gases, on the intact alveolar membrane, and on adequate perfusion of the alveoli.

Assessment of Behavior

Assessment of gas exchange is not made directly since it is not possible to see, hear, or touch the diffusion of gases. However, there are a number of ways to infer the adequacy of gas exchange from noninvasive techniques and from blood samples.

Oxygen Concentration

A variety of technologies are available to noninvasively evaluate arterial oxygen saturation (PaO_2) and partial pressure of serum oxygen and carbon dioxide (PCO_2) in the critically ill patient. These include pulse oximeters and transcutaneous monitoring devices (Von Rueden, 1990). Adequate gas exchange also can be inferred from arterial blood gas levels. If there is a normal concentration of oxygen and carbon dioxide in the blood, it is assumed that there is adequate gas exchange across the alveolar and capillary membranes. Blood gas levels are determined in laboratory testing of blood samples taken from the patient. Often in the intensive care unit, the nurse obtains the arterial blood sample from an indwelling arterial catheter. The most important laboratory finding to determine if there is a problem of oxygen exchange is the level of PaO_2. This reading indicates the partial pressure of oxygen in the arterial blood and generally is about 95 percent, with variations as noted in the discussion of factors influencing gas exchange.

Assessment of Stimuli

In the second level of assessment of gas exchange, one considers the stimuli that influence the exchange of gases. These include concentration of oxygen in the air, adequacy of blood supply to the alveoli, and the thickness and surface area of the alveolar membrane.

Atmospheric Oxygen

Concentration of oxygen in the air varies with such factors as altitude, air quality, and supplemental sources of oxygen.

Disease Pathology

Pathology in the lungs can affect the blood supply to the alveoli. Specific examples are diseases that alter the expandability and elastic recoil of lung tissue such as pnuemonia, tuberculosis, chronic bronchitis, and emphysema.

Pulmonary emboli or thrombi are examples of situations that directly interfere with blood supply to the alveoli. Further, if the alveolar membrane is thick and fibrotic, or if the alveoli are filled with exudate or fluid, as in cystic fibrosis, there will be inadequate gas exchange.

► TRANSPORT OF GASES: PROCESS AND ASSESSMENT

After its diffusion across the alveolo capillary membranes, oxygen is transported to the tissues for uptake. Gas transport includes the processes involved in the movement of oxygen from the alveolocapillary membrane to the mitochondria within the cells and the movement of carbon dioxide from tissue capillaries to the alveolocapillary membrane. Blood transports oxygen in two ways. First, approximately 97 percent of the oxygen is carried in chemical combination with hemoglobin. Second, the remaining 3 percent is carried in physical solution as dissolved oxygen (Sexton, 1990). Under normal conditions, hemoglobin has a high affinity for oxygen, which means it readily absorbs the oxygen transported from the lungs and releases it at the tissue level.

At the tissue level, carbon dioxide is picked up and returned to the lungs for disposal. The blood transports carbon dioxide in three forms: bicarbonate ions; dissolved carbon dioxide in the plasma; and as a compound with other proteins, mainly hemoglobin. Carbon dioxide is 20 times more soluble than oxygen; however, only 7 percent reaches the lungs dissolved in plasma (P_{CO_2}). More importantly, hemoglobin plays a major role in converting carbon dioxide to bicarbonate. Once formed, bicarbonate diffuses out of the red blood cells into the plasma, where it combines with sodium to form sodium bicarbonate. Thus 70 percent of the carbon dioxide is carried back to the lungs in the form of sodium bicarbonate. The remaining 23 percent returns in the form of compounds, mainly attached to hemoglobin proteins.

Assessment of Behavior

The transport of gases is heavily dependent on cardiac output. For this reason, pulses, blood pressure, and heart sounds provide important behavioral indicators in assessing the transport of gases.

Pulses

The apical pulse is felt at the apex of the heart and peripheral pulses are felt in the body's periphery, for example, in the neck, wrist, or foot. In a healthy person, the peripheral pulse is considered equivalent to the heartbeat. Normal adult pulse rates range from 60 to 100 beats per minute. A rate below 60 is called *bradycardia* and above 100 is called *tachycardia*. Pulse rates out of the normal range may not necessarily indicate a pathologic condition. Increased exercise, or any condition that increases the need for tissue oxygenation, will automatically increase the heart rate. When a person is frightened or anxious, stimulation of the sympathetic nervous system will cause temporary tachycardia.

Pulse rhythm is normally regular, that is, the time intervals between beats are of equal duration. Pulse rhythm is recorded as either regular or irregular. An irregular rhythm is referred to as an *arrhythmia* or dysrhythmia. A pulse deficit exists if the apical pulse, on auscultation, is higher than the radial pulse rate, indicating a weakness in the ventricular contractions. Peripheral pulses are assessed for their presence and strength and these are important indicators of the oxygenation status of distal tissues. Patients with cardiac health problems or peripheral vascular disorders may have absent or diminished strength in the peripheral pulses.

In addition to assessing rate and rhythm, the nurse also considers the force of the pulse. The force is an indication of stroke volume and is noted by assessing the pressure exerted to feel the pulse. A full, bounding pulse is difficult to obliterate and is exemplified by the pulse after exercise. Full force of the pulse is also found in a variety of alterations in health, including fever. A weak, thready pulse is easy to obliterate. It may indicate an alteration in health such as hemorrhage. The expected force of a pulse is felt clearly with a reasonable pressure and does not disappear when pressure on the pulse site is slightly adjusted.

Blood Pressure

Blood pressure readings reflect the ebb and flow of blood in waves within the systemic arteries. The systolic pressure occurs at the height of the wave, when the left ventricle contracts, and is recorded as the upper reading. Between the contractions, the heart is at rest and reflects the diastolic pressure, which is recorded as the lower reading. Normal blood pressure readings vary widely in healthy adults. The general norm of 120/80 is used, but it is important to know the patient's blood pressure range to make a sound interpretation of adaptive or ineffective behavior relative to the reading obtained. For example, if a patient's normal range is 150/86 to 138/80, then a sudden change to 106/60 will alert the nurse to possible problems that need further assessment and medical treatment. Useful assessment information is also obtained from taking the blood pressure in several positions, such as lying down, sitting, and standing. Decreased fluid volume can be reflected in changes in blood pressure, which in turn leads to decrease transport of gases. Normally from supine to the standing position, the systolic pressure should not drop more than 15 mm Hg and the diastolic pressure not more than 5 mm Hg. The most common abnormality seen in systolic and diastolic pressure is hypertension.

Further important information about transport of gases is obtained by differentiating and interpreting heart sounds. Discussion of the procedures associated with auscultation of heart sounds can be found in physical assessment resources such as Sims, D'Amico, Stiesmeyer, and Webster (1995).

Diagnostic Tests

Although the nurse cannot assess gas exchange and transport directly, it is increasingly possible to evaluate cellular oxygenation. Nurses can broaden their understanding of expanding technologies such as magnetic resonance imaging (MRI) and positron emission tomography (PET) scanning, which are enhancing the assessment of oxygenation at the cellular level. When cellular impairments are identified, they reflect alterations in the homeostatic relationship between the delivery of oxygen and its cellular utilization (Ahrens, 1993).

Physiologic Indicators

In completing a first-level assessment of oxygenation, the nurse is aware that other components of the physiologic mode can provide useful behavioral indicators. The skin, mucous membranes, and nail beds are often considered for their protective functions; however, pallor and cyanosis of these are seen in situations of decreased tissue perfusion. Decreased cellular oxygenation stimulates the sympathetic nervous system response, which causes the skin to be cool and clammy. A decrease in the level of consciousness can be an early indicator of cerebral hypoxia. With respect to elimination, decreased urinary output can be indicative of a decrease in cardiac output. Monitoring hourly output of urine and detection of production of less that 30 mL/hr signifies ineffective behavior and must be reported to the attending physician for immediate treatment.

Assessment of Stimuli

A thorough first-level assessment of behavioral cues related to transport of gases is accompanied by a complete second-level assessment of factors that influence this process of oxygenation. Key factors in assessment of stimuli relate to cardiac function and the circulating blood volume.

Cardiac Function

Any condition that decreases the pumping ability of the heart will cause oxygenation problems because there will be a deficiency in the number of red blood cells reaching the tissues. Inflammatory conditions of the heart such as bacterial endocarditis, myocardial infarction, and congestive heart failure are disorders which can interfere with the pumping ability of the heart. Hemorrhage and dehydration are common causes of a decrease in cardiac output and circulating blood volume.

Laboratory Results

A decrease in the number of red blood cells or lack of hemoglobin will decrease the oxygen-carrying capabilities of the blood. Under certain circumstances, the ability of hemoglobin to carry oxygen is compromised. Acidosis and increase in body temperature are situations which decrease the uptake of oxygen at the alveolar level. On the other hand, alkalosis and decreased body temperature depress oxygen release at the tissue level.

There are numerous diagnostic studies used specifically to evaluate the effectiveness of the respiratory and cardiovascular systems. As noted in the discussion of all three oxygenation processes, integrity of these systems is basic to meeting needs for oxygen by way of ventilation gas exchange and transport. A detailed discussion of relevant procedures and findings can be found in medical, surgical, or laboratory studies texts. The most common studies are hematocrit, hemoglobin, red cell count, arterial blood gases, chest x-ray, and electrocardiogram. The hematocrit, hemoglobin, and red cell count provide information about oxygen-carrying capabilities of the red blood cells. Arterial blood gas studies, and other noninvasive techniques noted before, reflect the amount of oxygen and carbon dioxide in the blood.

Radiologic Results

Chest x-ray provides information about the gross structures of the lungs and pleural cavity, indicating abnormal growth, inflammation, and fluid within the lungs. Special studies such as angiography, bronchography, barium swallow, and nuclear medicine studies, including MRI and PET scanning, can reveal information not obtained in standard chest x-rays.

Electrocardiography

The electrocardiogram shows the electrical activity of the heart and will reveal abnormal rhythms and other functional changes that affect cardiac output.

Environmental Conditions

Besides the basic physiologic factors affecting oxygenation, noxious environmental stimuli such as tobacco smoke, allergens, and irritating fumes can be considered individually as stimuli affecting oxygenation. They are often part of the pathogenesis of many of the disease conditions mentioned previously. These stimuli and other risk factors can be considered contextual stimuli. While not causing an acute oxygen deficit, they contribute to the situations resulting in compromised oxygenation.

Other Factors

Exercise, stress, changes in altitude, and temperature changes are all stimuli that alter the oxygen demands of the body. Changes of these stimuli are a normal part of the person's external environment. The body, if healthy, adapts to these stimuli with innate regulatory responses. The person can also use learned adaptive responses to enhance processes of oxygenation. Understanding compensatory adaptive responses is important in assessing factors influencing oxygenation.

▶ COMPENSATORY ADAPTIVE PROCESSES

Viewed as an adaptive system (see Chap. 2), the person has innate and acquired ways of responding to the changing environment. Roy conceptualizes these complex adaptive dynamics as the coping processes of the regulator and cognator subsystems. This chapter identifies that the need for oxygenation is met through processes of ventilation, gas exchange, and gas transport. However, when the processes of oxygenation are not stable or adequate, the regulator and cognator activate processes of compensation. Canon (1932), an early physiologist, used the term *the wisdom of the body* to describe the automatic self-regulation of physiologic processes. This phrase is useful when studying Roy's concept of the regulator subsystem. Likewise, the thinking and feeling person, by way of cognator activity, can do much to affect any need of the physiologic mode, oxygenation in particular. Regulator and cognator abilities, then, are important internal stimuli for the person. These subsystems provide compensatory adaptive responses that extend the effectiveness of behavior in reaching the goals of adaptation.

Compensatory abilities that respond to oxygenation requirements include both automatic homeostatic functions of the regulator and voluntary or behavioral activities of the cognator. The nurse must understand as fully as possible the wisdom of the body to identify and interpret changes in the patient's condition. Important to this understanding is the study of physiology and pathophysiology. One particular illustration of a regulator compensatory activity is given to illustrate compensatory adaptation related to oxygenation. A protective mechanism that helps maintain an open airway is mucociliary clearance. The layer of mucus that covers the upper and lower airway traps particles from the inspired air. Cilia then propel the mucus, with entrapped foreign material, toward the pharynx, where it can be swallowed or expectorated. An automatic compensatory response that assists mucociliary clearance is the cough reflex. A cough is initiated by stimulation of irritant receptors in the airway. In particular, these receptors respond to chemical and mechanical stimulation from substances such as high concentrations of dust in the air, noxious fumes, aspiration of foreign material, and mucus accumulation. The complex act of coughing generally involves one deep inspiration, followed by several forced expirations that expel large volumes of air from the lungs. The function of the cough is to clear the upper airways of the irritant. Thus, a cough is a compensatory adaptive response to the need for oxygenation.

An illustration of a compensatory response to oxygen need by way of the cognator is the conscious recruitment of accessory muscles of respiration. Likewise, adequate ventilation depends on respiratory muscles pumping air into and out of the lungs. When oxygen need is challenged, such as in chronic obstructive lung disease, the patient can be taught to recruit additional muscles for the process of ventilation, including sternomastoid, intercostal, and abdominal muscles. Even mandibular, facial, and gluteal muscles can be used (Breslin, Roy, & Robinson, 1992). Similarly, through the cognator, the person can be taught to increase the effectiveness of an automatic regulatory compensating response, such as a cough.

Some environmental changes related to oxygen need, and particularly in a state of illness, can have an overwhelming effect on the individual's ability to adapt. The demands are greater than the compensatory processes can handle, which may lead to compromised processes of oxygenation.

▶ **COMPROMISED PROCESSES OF OXYGENATION**

Adaptation problems can be caused by difficulties in any or all of the processes of oxygenation since ventilation, gas exchange, and gas transport are all interdependent. Two specific examples of compromised processes of oxygenation will be discussed here. Hypoxia is the most pressing concern that reflects a compromised process of oxygenation. Shock is a generalized syndrome that can have many causes; however, a common feature is inadequate tissue perfusion.

Hypoxia

Hypoxia has been classified into four main types: hypoxic, anemic, circulatory, and histotoxic (Berne & Levy, 1992). Hypoxic hypoxia is caused by a decrease in oxygen pressure in the inspired air or in the lungs, or by conditions that prevent or interfere with the diffusion of oxygen across the alveolar membrane. Examples of causes are exposure to high altitudes, obstruction of the airway, asthma, pneumonia, and congenital cardiovascular disease. Anemic hypoxia results from a reduction in the ability of the blood to carry sufficient amounts of oxygen due to a decrease in hemoglobin. Specific examples of such conditions are anemia and carbon monoxide poisoning.

Circulatory hypoxia occurs when there is inadequate circulation of the blood to the tissue cells, even though the oxygen-carrying capacity of the blood may be normal. Specific examples of causes include congestive heart failure or other forms of reduced cardiac output; shock; and arterial spasm or other local obstruction to arterial blood flow. Hystotoxic hypoxia occurs when there is interference with the ability of the cells to utilize oxygen. Causative examples are alcohol, narcotics, and poisons such as cyanide.

Although moderate hypoxia can be compensated for over a period of time, this is not true of acute hypoxia. People have essentially no oxygen reserve and, when exposed to an acute interruption of oxygen, quickly demonstrate signs and symptoms of hypoxia. These vary widely with individuals and their differing abilities to adjust physiologically. However, in general, the higher levels of the brain will show the effects of oxygen deficit very early. Cognitive function is impaired. The person is confused and, because of this, is usually unaware of what is happening. Early signs also include changes in vital signs resulting from the cardiovascular response to hypoxia. There can be tachycardia, and respirations increase in depth and rate. The systolic blood pressure rises slightly as cardiac output increases. As hypoxia increases, a wide variety of central nervous system signs and symptoms may appear including headache, agitation, irritability, depression, drowsiness, apathy, dizziness, decreased concentration, impaired judgment, diminished visual acuity, emotional disturbances, euphoria, poor muscular coordination, fatigue, stupor, and unconsciousness. When the hypoxic state becomes more advanced and the body's compensatory efforts fail, both blood pressure and pulse rate fall precipitously. Hypoxia is also accompanied by changes in the gastrointestinal and renal systems. These changes can occur as a direct result of the hypoxia on the involved tissues or indirectly through the effects of hypoxia on the nervous system. The person can experience anorexia, nausea, and vomiting, as well as oliguria. Since the kidney is very sensitive to hypoxia, frequent measurement of urine output is an important part of the nursing assessment of the patient with acute hypoxia.

The emotional responses of persons who are unable to get their breath are evident. A person may be apprehensive and anxious and compound the problem by hyperventilating. People who are having difficulty breathing will try to sit upright if possible, and if an oxygen mask is being used, may try to push it away because of the sensation that it is stifling them. Respirations become increasingly gasping and as the person's fears increase, so does energy requirement. This places an even greater load on the already overburdened respiratory and cardiac systems, thus increasing the hypoxia.

Specific plans for nursing care for the person with hypoxia will be based on careful individual assessment. However, general interventions can be outlined here. The most important measure in treating hypoxia is oxygen administration. Essential components of oxygen therapy include the following.

- Careful observation of respiratory status, vital signs, and reaction to therapy.
- Use of aseptic technique to assist in preventing infections.
- Thorough explanation to the person of the procedures being used.
- Understanding and correct usage of the equipment being used.

New technology for oxygen flow delivery, such as reservoir-type cannulas, transtracheal cannulas, and intermittent demand flow systems, aim to lower the oxygen flow requirements (Traver, Mitchell, & Flodquist-Priestly, 1991). These methods can be more convenient and comfortable for the patient and have financial benefits as well. Positioning for comfort and correct body alignment are also important for the patient with hypoxia. The position from which the person can usually get maximum ventilation is upright, sometimes leaning slightly forward, such as on an over-bed table. A calm, confident, and supportive manner on the part of the nurse, and a calm physical environment, can help alleviate the stress encountered in breathing difficulties.

Shock

Shock is ordinarily associated with poor tissue perfusion and usually characterized by systemic hypotension. The decrease in blood pressure can be elicited by different mechanisms brought into play by a variety of insults. Thus shock occurs in several forms, including hemorrhagic, septic, myocardial, traumatic, and anaphylactic (Frohlich, 1972). Each of these clinical situations and their treatment are described in medical texts. However, a general nursing assessment and approaches to care can be outlined.

The shock syndrome can be as simple as fainting at the sight of an accident on the highway, or as complex as a medical emergency for the accident victim with internal bleeding. The common feature is inadequate tissue perfusion or lack of oxygen permeation. The circulation becomes progressively inadequate. The behaviors of the person reflect low arterial pressure and increased activity of the sympathetic nervous system in the body's attempt to deal with the emergency. The person in shock appears very pale, and the skin is cool and moist. The pupils are dilated and the person is visibly anxious. Early in the chain of events, a person may be quite restless and agitated, but this progresses to apathy and confusion. Thirst is a common symptom, but usually little water can be tolerated because of nausea. Urinary output is progressively decreased. Breathing is rapid and shallow, and as shock becomes more severe, the pulmonary function progressively deteriorates. Pulse rate is rapid but thready. Arterial blood pressure, particularly systolic pressure, rises early in shock for a brief period and then falls. Further, the pulse pressure tends to be narrow.

Medical therapy of shock aims to restore fluid volume, correct metabolic acidosis, and increase cardiac output. Nursing responsibilities involve careful observation of the patient's appearance, vital signs, and response to treatment, as well as supportive care. The shock syndrome can be divided into three stages. In the initial or compensatory stage, many physiologic reactions are occurring to adapt to the shock state. During the decompensated or progressive stage, the shock state is continuing and the patient's condition is increasingly worse. In some persons, there is a final, refractory stage that can become irreversible. At this point, neither the various compensatory mechanisms nor the treatment is effective in reversing the state of shock and the prognosis is poor.

Positioning of the patient in shock is either lying flat, or in the case of neurogenic shock, horizontal with moderate elevation of the legs. The position of the head lower than the body is not used because the pressure of the abdominal viscera on the lungs impairs ventilation. Supportive care for the respiratory system can include oxygen therapy, suctioning, mechanical ventilation, and pulmonary physiotherapy. Supportive care for the cardiovascular system involves intravenous fluids, either blood or electrolyte solutions, depending on the patient's needs. Cardiac monitoring is continuous and identifying arrhythmia is essential. Renal and gastrointestinal support is provided by accurate monitoring of intake and output, and sometimes hemodialysis and parenteral nutrition as needed. The nursing challenge is to anticipate the development of shock and intervene before the serious progressive changes occur. This challenge involves watchful expectation and vigilance with careful monitoring for early recognition of any changes in the patient's condition (Burrell et al., 1997).

▶ PLANNING NURSING CARE

Oxygenation of body tissues is a priority requirement for the person's physiologic adaptation. In applying the nursing process, the nurse will make a careful assessment of behaviors and stimuli related to the basic life processes of ventilation, gas exchange, and gas transport. In assessing factors influencing oxygenation need, regulator and cognator effectiveness in initiating compensatory processes will be considered. Based on thorough first- and second-level assessment, the nurse makes a nursing diagnosis, sets goals, selects interventions, and evaluates care.

Nursing Diagnosis

As introduced in Chapter 3, nursing diagnosis, according to the Roy Adaptation Model, is a judgment process in which the nurse makes an interpretive statement about the human adaptive system. The statement is formulated by considering the data of the first- and second-level assessment. The statement can include a summary of observed behaviors with the most relevant influencing stimuli. A nursing diagnosis illustrating adaptation and summarizing both behavior and stimuli could be, "Adequate oxygenation of toes of left foot due to good circulation in leg with cast." Also using a summary of behavior and stimuli, the nurse might state an adaptation problem as, "Ventilatory impairment related to copious secretions in the airways."

An alternate way of stating a nursing diagnosis is to use a summary label that best identifies the nurse's judgment of the clinical situation from an established classification system. The Roy model has two classification lists, one for indicators of adaptation and one for commonly recurring adaptation problems. The complete classification lists for the Roy model are included in Chapter 3. In Table 5–1, the Roy model nursing diagnostic categories for the physiologic need of oxygenation are shown in relation to nursing diagnosis labels approved by the North American Nursing Diagnosis Association (Rantz & LeMone, 1997).

An example of use of a summary diagnosis can be considered. Mrs. Jones is an 87-year-old woman who lives alone and has had emphysema for the past 20 years. For many years, she worked outside the home and was a heavy smoker until approximately 12 years ago, when she reportedly quit. The nurse

TABLE 5–1 NURSING DIAGNOSTIC CATEGORIES FOR OXYGENATION

Positive Indicators of Adaptation	Common Adaptation Problems	NANDA Diagnostic Labels
• Stable processes of ventilation	• Hypoxia • Shock • Ventilatory impairment	• Ineffective airway clearance • Risk for aspiration • Risk for suffocation • Inability to sustain spontaneous ventilation
• Stable pattern of gas exchange	• Inadequate gas exchange • Altered tissue perfusion	• Ineffective breathing pattern • Impaired gas exchange
• Adequate transport of gases • Adequate processes of compensation	• Inadequate gas transport • Poor recruitment of compensatory processes for changing oxygen need	• Decreased cardiac output • Dysfunctional ventilatory weaning response

from a neighborhood clinic visits Mrs. Jones and makes a nursing assessment. Mrs. Jones is sitting in a chair and leaning forward on a TV tray. Her rate of respiration is 30 and her lips have a slightly blue tinge. She says she is not really having difficulty breathing, but that she is conscious of every breath. Mrs. Jones has been trying some exercises that the nurse gave her. One is to lift her buttocks and try to use the muscles to help force air out of her lungs. Mrs. Jones indicates that she thinks the exercises are helping but that she is afraid she will forget to do them. Mrs. Jones has asked her friend Sally to help remind her this week. Sally calls Mrs. Jones every day and asks how her exercises are going. The nurse uses a hand-held spirometer to measure Mrs. Jones' ventilatory capacity and notes that it is improved over the last measurement 2 weeks ago. The nurse makes the diagnosis of, "Improving processes of compensation for oxygenation need resulting from respiratory exercise."

The statement of nursing diagnoses, the third step of the nursing process, provides direction for the next step. Based on the nursing diagnosis, the nurse proceeds to the fourth step of the nursing process, known as goal setting.

Goal Setting

Goal setting, according to the Roy Adaptation Model, involves the establishment of clear statements of behavioral outcomes for the person as the result of the nursing care provided. A complete goal statement contains the behavior of focus, the change expected, and the time frame in which the goal should be achieved. Goals may be short-term or long-term and these time frames are relative to the situation.

Consider the example of a patient with a newly applied leg cast. Although the nursing diagnosis indicated that there was adequate oxygenation to the tissue in the toes at that time, the nurse should be aware that swelling often occurs after the application of a new cast, and should monitor the patient's leg. A short-term goal pertaining to this situation could be, "Toes will remain warm and pink within the next hour." The behavior in this goal is, "Toes will be warm and pink." The change expected is no change, that is, oxygenation will remain adequate as evidenced by the toes being warm and pink. The time frame is stated as "within the next hour."

In the case of a patient whose diagnosis is "ventilatory impairment related to copious secretions in the airways," the behavior that the goal will focus on is the ventilatory impairment. The goal is stated, "Within 10 minutes, the patient will be breathing effortlessly." The patient's breathing is the behavior of focus, the criterion is "effortlessly," and the time frame is "within 10 minutes."

In the case of Mrs. Jones, the nurse plans to make the next visit in 1 week. For the diagnosis, "improving processes of compensation for oxygenation need," the nurse sets the goal with the patient that, "Processes of compensation for oxygenation will improve in 1 week." The processes of compensation is the focus of the goal, improvement beyond this week's level is the criterion, and "1 week" is the time frame.

Generally, the nursing goal relative to oxygenation is to ensure an adequate level of oxygen supply to all parts of the body. This goal is operationalized by the identification of the specific goals that address ventilation, gas exchange, transport of gases, and compensatory adaptive responses. The importance of anticipating potential problems associated with oxygenation involves monitoring the person's condition to detect oxygenation problems before they become serious. Thus, many goals established for the patient may be preventive in nature rather than focusing on an already ineffective situation.

In order to assist the patient in the achievement of the established goals, the nurse proceeds to plan nursing interventions.

Intervention

The four previous steps of the nursing process, based on an understanding of oxygenation processes, provide specific direction for the identification of nursing interventions to assist the patient. Whereas the goal focused on specified patient behaviors, the interventions address the stimuli that are effecting the behaviors. The management of stimuli involves either altering, increasing, decreasing, removing, or maintaining the influencing factors.

Some nursing measures used to facilitate ventilation and gas exchange focus on the functioning of the associated structures of respiration, an important factor influencing oxygenation. These include deep breathing and coughing, positioning to encourage maximal breathing capacity, using lung inflation devices, providing oxygen therapy, promoting drainage and removal of tracheobronchial secretion, providing hydration, and providing adequate pulmonary resuscitation in situations of respiratory arrest. The nurse may be responsible for the care of patients on mechanical ventilation and frequently uses suctioning techniques to remove respiratory secretions.

Nursing interventions to enhance gas transport include maintaining adequate circulation through proper positioning and nonrestrictive clothing, providing adequate intake of iron, and promoting effective pumping action of the heart.

In the previous situation involving the patient with the new cast, the stimulus that could interfere with oxygenation of the toes is swelling within the cast and the subsequent interruption of blood flow to the toes. In considering interventions to prevent such an occurrence, the nurse would identify and analyze possible approaches and then select the approach with the highest probability of achieving the goal. Possible interventions could be splitting the cast, elevating the leg on a pillow, or packing the leg in ice to prevent swelling. The last alternative may have a detrimental effect on the plaster cast; the first is not something that would be tried as a preventive measure. Thus the nurse would select the intervention of elevating the leg on a pillow in an attempt to minimize swelling before it becomes a problem. Nursing intervention in situations of oxygenation disruption involves facilitating the processes of ventilation, gas exchange, and gas transport.

In a situation of a patient with ventilatory impairment due to bronchial secretions, the nursing intervention would focus on clearing the secretions from the person's airway. Possible interventions include positioning of the patient, postural drainage, encouraging the person to cough, and suctioning of the patient's airway. The approach selected would depend on the circumstances. A person with an altered level of consciousness may require suctioning while a patient who is aware and can follow instructions may benefit by assistance and encouragement with effective coughing.

Whatever the nursing interventions selected, their effectiveness in attainment of the goals is addressed through evaluation.

Evaluation

As is evident from the initial description of behaviors related to the three basic life processes associated with oxygenation (ventilation, gas exchange, and gas transport), the key to evaluation lies generally in four important behavioral areas: respiratory status, cardiac status, renal status, and mental status. The key to evaluation of the effectiveness of specific nursing interventions lies in determining if the behavior identified in the patient-specific goal changed within the stated time frame. Consider the goal, "Within 10 minutes, the patient will be breathing effortlessly." The behavior of interest in evaluating success in achieving the goal is the person's breathing. If it is effortless within the 10-minute time frame, the goal has been achieved.

Suppose that within 1 hour, the nurse identified that the patient with the cast was demonstrating decreased circulation to his toes in that they were dusky in color and the patient was reporting numbness. This situation would necessitate immediate action on the part of the nurse and prompt, continued reassessment, with further intervention.

With Mrs. Jones and her goal related to improvement in the processes of oxygenation compensation, evaluation of the success of the interventions would relate to compensatory processes and the effectiveness she is experiencing as the result of her exercising. Measurement of ventilatory capacity with the spirometer would provide an indication of this. If no improvement is observed, both the goals and the interventions will need to be reevaluated to determine whether an alternative approach is indicated.

Such situations demonstrate the simultaneous and continuous nature of the nursing process. Although the steps are addressed separately for purposes of teaching and learning, experienced nurses assess behavior and stimuli simultaneously, perhaps while setting goals with the patient and carrying out interventions. The interrelatedness of the steps of the process, based on Roy's conceptualization of the individual human system as a whole, becomes increasingly evident as the nurse becomes more experienced in its application.

► SUMMARY

This chapter focused on the application of the Roy Adaptation Model to the physiologic need of oxygenation. An overview of the basic life processes—ventilation, gas exchange, and gas transport—associated with oxygenation was provided along with the identification of parameters for assessment of behaviors and stimuli. Illustration of innate and learned adaptive compensatory responses related to oxygenation were described and examples of two compromised processes, hypoxia and shock, were provided. Finally, guidelines for planning nursing care through the formulation of nursing diagnoses, goals, and interventions were explored and evaluation of nursing care was described.

▶ **EXERCISES FOR APPLICATION**

1. Develop a tool to assist you with the assessment of oxygenation. Address in the tool important behavioral indicators and stimuli that affect ventilation, gas exchange, and gas transport.

2. Using the tool developed in exercise 1, assess a patient's status relative to oxygenation. Assess the adequacy of your tool by comparing it to an oxygenation assessment guideline in a physical assessment resource.

▶ **ASSESSMENT OF UNDERSTANDING**

Questions

1. Identify the appropriate basic life process of oxygenation in Column A with the associated descriptor(s) in Column B.

Column A	Column B
Basic Life Process	**Descriptor**
Ventilation (V)	(a) _____ depends on concentration gradient of gases
Gas exchange (GE)	
Transport of gases (TG)	(b) _____ inspiratory phase and expiratory phase
	(c) _____ movement of oxygen to the mitochondria within the cells
	(d) _____ involves alveolocapillary membrane
	(e) _____ diffusion of gases
	(f) _____ exchanges air between lungs and atmosphere

2. Label each assessment parameter with the basic life process to which it most closely relates.
   Ventilation (V), Gas exchange (GE), Transport of gases (TG)
   (a) _____ breath sounds
   (b) _____ arterial blood gas levels

(c) _____ tidal volume
(d) _____ pulse rate
(e) _____ pulse oximetry
(f) _____ respiratory rate
(g) _____ pulse rhythm
(h) _____ blood pressure

3. Name two factors that influence each of the basic life processes associated with oxygenation.
   (a) Ventilation: _____ and _____.
   (b) Exchange of gases: _____ and _____.
   (c) Transport of gases: _____ and _____.

4. Provide an example of a compensatory process related to oxygenation that is illustrative of (a) regulator coping mechanism activity and (b) cognator coping mechanism activity.
   (a) _____
   (b) _____

5. Name two serious adaptation problems indicative of compromised processes of oxygenation.
   (a) _____
   (b) _____

6. *Situation:* A young man has been brought into the emergency department from the scene of an automobile accident. He appears very pale. His skin is cool and moist. His pupils are dilated and he is restless and agitated. He complains of thirst and nausea. His pulse is rapid and thready and his blood pressure is lower than normal and is falling. He is being examined for possible internal injury and a ruptured spleen is anticipated but has not yet been confirmed.
   (a) Develop a nursing diagnosis related to the situation described.
   (b) Develop one short-term and one long-term goal relative to the behavior of the falling blood pressure. Each goal should include the behavior of concern, the change expected, and the time fame involved.

7. List five nursing interventions commonly used in situations of hypoxia.
   (a) _____
   (b) _____
   (c) _____
   (d) _____
   (e) _____

8. Which of the following evaluative methods would be appropriate for assessing the effectiveness of the nursing interventions aimed at enhancing tissue perfusion in the patient demonstrating shock?

(a) cardiac status
(b) renal status
(c) respiratory status
(d) mental status
(e) all the above

Feedback

1. (a) GE, (b) V, (c) TG, (d) GE, (e) GE, (f) V

2. (a) V, (b) GE, (c) V, (d) TG, (e) GE, (f) V, (g) TG, (h) TG

3. (a) Examples: impairment of structure or function, increased intracranial pressure, trauma to diaphragm or pleura.
   (b) Examples: oxygen concentration in air, adequacy of blood supply to alveoli, thickness and surface area of alveolar membrane.
   (c) Examples: cardiac function, circulating blood volume, hemorrhage, dehydration.

4. (a) Regulator coping mechanism activity: coughing, sneezing, yawning, increased heart rate upon exertion.
   (b) Cognator coping mechanism activity: use of additional muscles to facilitate air exchange, use of positioning with head elevated on extra pillows, mouth breathing in situations of high spinal cord injury.

5. (a) hypoxia
   (b) shock

6. (a) Example of nursing diagnosis: Altered tissue perfusion due to decrease in circulating blood volume; or shock due to possible internal hemorrhaging.
   (b) Example of a short-term goal: Within 5 minutes, the patient's blood pressure will have stabilized.
   Example of a long-term goal: Within 1 hour, the patient's blood pressure will demonstrate an upward trend.

7. (a) oxygen administration
   (b) comfortable and aligned positioning
   (c) calm and supportive physical environment
   (d) correct usage of oxygen equipment
   (e) thorough explanation of procedures being used

8. e

▶ **REFERENCES**

Ahrens, T. (1993). Changing perspectives in assessment of oxygenation. *Critical Care Nurse, 13(7),* 78–83.

Berne, R., & Levy, M. (1992). *Physiology.* St. Louis: Mosby.

Burrell, L. O., Gerlach, M. J. M., & Pless, B. S. (1997). *Adult nursing: Acute and community care* (2nd ed.). Stamford, CT: Appleton & Lange.

Breslin, E., Roy, C., & Robinson, C. (1992). Physiological nursing research in dyspnea: A paradigm shift and a metaparadigm exemplar. *Scholarly Inquiry for Nursing Practice, 6(2),* 81–104.

Canon, W. (1932). *The wisdom of the body.* New York: Norton.

Dettenmeier, P. (1992). *Pulmonary nursing care.* St. Louis: Mosby Year Book.

Frohlich, E. (1972). *Pathophysiology: Altered regulatory mechanisms in disease.* Philadelphia: Lippincott.

Rantz, M. J., & LeMone, P. (Eds.). (1997). *Classification of nursing diagnosis. Proceedings of the 12th conference NANDA.* Glendale, CA: CINAHL Information Systems.

Sexton, D. (1990). *Nursing care of the respiratory patient.* Norwalk, CT: Appleton & Lange.

Sims, L., D'Amico, D., Stiesmeyer, J., & Webster, J. (1995). *Health assessment in nursing.* Redwood City, CA: Addison-Wesley.

Traver, G., Mitchell, J., & Flodquist-Priestley, G. (1991). *Respiratory care: A clinical approach.* Gaithersburg, MD: Aspen.

Von Rueden, K. (1990). Noninvasive assessment of gas exchange in the critically ill patient. *AACN Clinical Issues in Critical Care Nursing, 1,* 239–247.

▶ **ADDITIONAL REFERENCES**

Bates, B. (1995). *A guide to physical examination and history taking* (6th ed.). Philadelphia: Lippincott.

Grimes, J., & Burns, E. (1992). *Health assessment in nursing practice.* Boston: Jones and Bartlett.

Marieb, E. N. (1994). *Essentials of human anatomy and physiology* (4th ed.). Redwood City, CA: Benjamin/Cummings.

Porth, C. (1994). *Pathophysiology: Concepts of altered health states* (4th ed.). Philadelphia: Lippincott.

Vander, A., Sherman, R., & Luciano, D. (1993). *Human physiology: The mechanisms of body function.* New York: McGraw Hill.

6

NUTRITION

Nutrition, identified in the Roy Adaptation Model as one of five physiologic needs, relates to the series of processes by which the person takes in and assimilates food necessary for maintenance of human functioning, promotion of growth, and replacement of injured tissues. Marieb (1989) described nutrition as "one of the most overlooked areas in clinical medicine" (p. 851) and Linton, Matteson, and Maebius (1995) have called it "the cornerstone of the healing process" (p. 125). These observations have important implications for nurses in their goal of promoting health. Level of nutrition influences every phase of metabolism and plays a major role in each person's overall health. Consideration of the individual's state of nutrition and promotion of an optimal nutritional level are important nursing activities in the holistic role that nurses occupy in the promotion of adaptation and health.

Basic life processes of nutrition as described within the Roy Adaptation Model include digestion and metabolism. Understanding the physiology of these processes provides the framework for determining adaptation relative to nutrition. Concepts from pathophysiology are helpful in identifying ineffective behaviors. In this chapter, the two basic life processes of nutrition are addressed along with identification of the parameters for assessment of behaviors and stimuli. Illustrations of compensatory and compromised processes related to nutrition are described. Finally, guidelines for planning nursing care by formulating diagnoses, establishing goals, selecting interventions, and evaluating nursing care are considered.

▶ OBJECTIVES

After studying this chapter, the reader will be able to do the following:

1. Describe the two basic life processes associated with the need for nutrition.

2. Identify important first-level assessment parameters for each of the basic life processes associated with the need for nutrition.

3. List common stimuli affecting each basic life process associated with nutrition.

4. Describe one compensatory process related to each of the basic life processes associated with nutrition.

5. Name and describe two situations of compromised processes of nutrition.

6. Given a situation related to nutrition, develop a nursing diagnosis.

7. In a given situation, derive goals for an individual with ineffective nutrition.

8. Describe nursing interventions commonly implemented in situations of ineffective nutrition.

9. Propose approaches to determine the effectiveness of nursing interventions.

▶ KEY CONCEPTS DEFINED

Absorption: The movement of digested substances into the blood or lymph for transport to body cells.

Appetite: A pleasant sensation involving the person's desire for and anticipation of food and fluids.

Chemical digestion: The breaking down of food into molecules small enough to be absorbed.

Defecation: The elimination of undigested substances.

Digestion: A series of mechanical and chemical processes by which food is taken into the body and prepared for absorption into the blood and lymph for transport to the body cells.

Hunger: A physiologically aroused sensation related to the body's need for food.

Ingestion: The process of taking food and liquids into the digestive tract.

Mechanical digestion: The breaking down of food components into smaller parts by chewing, mixing, and churning in preparation for chemical digestion.

Nausea: An unpleasant sensation reported as a feeling of sickness with the urge to vomit.

Nutrition: The series of processes by which a person takes in nutrients and assimilates and uses them to maintain body tissue, promote growth, and provide energy.

Propulsion: The movement of food through the alimentary canal by peristalsis.

Thirst: A desire for fluid or the dry sensation resulting from a lack of or need for water.

Vomiting: The forceful ejection of stomach contents through the mouth.

► BASIC LIFE PROCESS OF NUTRITION

Nutrition concerns the food people eat and how their bodies use it (Williams, 1995). It is defined as the series of processes by which the person takes in nutrients and assimilates and uses them to maintain body tissue, promote growth, and provide energy. Second only to the need for oxygen, nutrition provides the foundation for life and health. For purposes of this overview of nutrition, two major processes are identified: digestion and metabolism.

Although it is difficult to separate consideration of assessment related to digestion and metabolism, for purposes of discussion here, the assessment of digestion pertains to the physiologic processes associated with foods and fluids that are ingested. Assessment of metabolism, on the other hand, addresses factors associated with the adequacy of nutrient intake relative to the body's requirements.

► DIGESTION: PROCESS AND ASSESSMENT

Digestion can be described in general terms as a series of mechanical and chemical processes by which food is taken into the body and prepared for absorption into the blood and lymph for transport to the body cells. The organs of the digestive system function to keep the body supplied with the nutrients required by the body tissues and organs. Digestive organs can be categorized into two main groups. The gastrointestinal tract, or alimentary canal, consists of the mouth, pharynx, esophagus, stomach, small and large intestines, and the anus (the terminal opening). Within the alimentary canal, food is digested, digested fragments are absorbed, and undigested substances are eliminated. The accessory digestive organs include the teeth, tongue, gallbladder, salivary glands, liver, and pancreas. These assist in the process of digestive breakdown of foods.

Marieb (1994, p. 412) described digestion in terms of the following five major processes.

1. *Ingestion.* The process of taking food and liquids into the digestive tract.
2. *Food breakdown.* The breakdown of food into its building blocks through *mechanical digestion* and *chemical digestion*. Mechanical digestion is the breaking down of food components into smaller parts by chewing, mixing, and churning in preparation for chemical digestion. Chemical digestion is the breaking down of food into molecules small enough to be absorbed. This is accomplished by secretion of digestive juices, acid, mucus, bile, and other materials in various parts of the alimentary canal.
3. *Propulsion.* The movement of food through the alimentary canal by peristalsis, or wavelike contractions by which the smooth muscles of the digestive system propel the contents through the tract.
4. *Absorption.* The movement of digested substances into the blood or lymph for transport to body cells.
5. *Defecation.* The elimination of indigestible substances.

Assessment of Behaviors

When assessing behaviors related to the process of digestion (first-level assessment) as described in the Roy Adaptation Model, the nurse observes several categories of behavior. These include eating patterns, sense of taste and smell, food allergies, pain, and altered ingestion.

Eating Patterns

The nurse obtains a diet history listing the quantities of all food and fluids ingested during a 24-hour period. Of particular interest with respect to digestion are types of foods ingested, times of food intake, the situations associated with mealtimes and eating, and the person's bodily response in terms of the digestive process. Many of these factors are specified further in the following discussion.

Sense of Taste and Smell

The taste and smell of food to the individual have a significant influence on the person's response to it. The normal person determines taste on the anterior two thirds of the tongue. Four basic sensations are experienced. They are sweet, sour, bitter, and salt. The sensory receptors for taste are the glossopharyngeal nerve (cranial nerve IX) and the facial nerve (cranial nerve VII). Nasal passages should be patent. Testing each nostril separately, the person should be able to identify such odors as coffee or tobacco.

Food Allergies

The nurse assesses whether the person has a known food allergy or sensitivity. An allergic reaction to a certain food or food group is the result of an inappropriate antibody–antigen reaction in the body. Foods causing problems are identified and the behaviors (skin rash, swelling of the face or mouth, or gastrointestinal reaction) that occur if the food is ingested are noted.

Pain

The nurse assesses for any pain related to the ingestion of food or fluids. Pain can be noted as a behavior by listing the person's statements regarding discomfort and pain following ingestion of food. For example, a person may identify a burning sensation, or "heartburn," after the ingestion of foods such as onions. All verbal and nonverbal behaviors are recorded. Pain is further specified in terms of severity; duration; onset (gradual or abrupt, before or after meals); location, spread, and radiation; precipitating factors; frequency; and quality (sharp, dull, burning, pressure, stabbing). In addition, treatment measures (diet, rest, position, medications), aggravating factors, associated symptoms, and the patient's attitude toward the pain are explored.

Altered Ingestion

If the person is unable to eat and drink normally, the altered means of nutritional intake are assessed. For example, a person may be nourished through a nasogastric or gastrostomy tube. The amount and substance ingested should be noted. If the person is receiving intravenous fluids and electrolytes or a hyperalimentation solution, the solutions and rate of delivery are recorded. The knowledge and skills related to these particular altered means of ingestion are continually developing. The nurse is challenged to maintain the knowledge and skill necessary to provide nursing care in these situations through reading, clinical practice, and continuing education.

Assessment of Stimuli

Assessment of stimuli involves the identification of the factors that appear to be influencing the person's behavior relative to digestion. Common stimuli affecting the process of digestion include the physical structures and physiologic functions of digestion, medication, conditions of eating, and cues for eating.

Integrity of Structure and Function

The alimentary canal consists of the upper, middle, and lower regions and is responsible for the digestion and absorption of nutrients. When food is ingested, a series of physical and chemical changes occur, which prepare the nutrients for absorption and utilization by the cells. The alimentary canal is regulated by the neural, chemical, and endocrine processes that Roy describes as the regulator subsystem (see Chap. 2). Residue remaining after digestion and absorption is then excreted from the body.

Through physical assessment of the structures associated with the process of digestion, the nurse identifies whether or not a disease state is present that affects the normal processes of the digestive system. Such examination would involve inspection of the oral cavity, abdomen (inspection, auscultation, percussion, and palpitation), and a rectal examination, in addition to inquiring about the person's experiences surrounding ingestion and elimination. Examples of disease states influencing digestive function would include such conditions as obstructive lesions of the esophagus and malabsorption, which are explained in general textbooks of pathology. Also, the nurse assesses for conditions that prohibit the person from eating, such as recent surgery, and for restricted or special diets, such as that for a person with a medical diagnosis of diabetes.

Medication

The nurse identifies whether or not the person takes any medication that can influence the intake of food or the digestive process. For example, drugs that can decrease the appetite may be taken if the person is attempting to lose weight. It is important to ascertain whether supplemental vitamins and minerals are used, as well.

Conditions of Eating

The nurse identifies who purchases and prepares the food the person eats. In the family setting, the health beliefs of the food purchaser and preparer regarding nutrition will greatly influence the ingestion behaviors of all members. The nurse determines whether or not the family meal planning provides a well-balanced diet and notes what social and moral values are placed on eating. For example, is eating a highly social event, and is food used as a punishment or reward? The nurse further identifies the level of family or peer group influence regarding eating and considers if the person or family sets aside a special time for mealtime. For example, are the meals taken alone, with a group, at home, at fast-food services, or in a restaurant? Another important consideration is the person's familiarity with different types of food.

Cues for Eating

Finally, when assessing factors influencing the person's food intake and the process of digestion, it is important to identify the internal and external cues to which the individual responds. A healthy, functioning hypothalamus sends the person internal cues which signal that enough food has been ingested. In cases of overeating, the nurse helps the person which identify what external cues they are responding to when eating. Generally, other cues are being used when the person is failing to respond to internal cues relating to satiety and hunger control. For example, some people might overeat as a means of coping with the stresses of daily living. The nurse identifies if the person's eating and drinking behaviors are influenced by emotions, social pressures, habits, or the good taste and palatability of food, rather than the internal cues that control appetite. Cues from the external environment, such as a pleasant environment and freedom from pain and stress, also influence ingestion.

► METABOLISM: PROCESS AND ASSESSMENT

Williams (1995, p. 7) described metabolism as the sum of all body processes that accomplish three basic life-sustaining tasks: the provision of energy sources, building of tissue, and regulation of metabolic processes. Through the process of metabolism, nutrients are synthesized to fulfill these tasks.

Nutrients are described as substances that provide nourishment to the body and are used by the body to promote normal growth, maintenance, and repair. Three major and two minor nutrients have been categorized by Marieb (1994, p. 422). The major nutrients include carbohydrates, lipids, and proteins, while the body requires smaller amounts of minor nutrients, known as vitamins and minerals. Carbohydrates, some lipids, and some proteins are converted into chemical energy (metabolic products), electrical energy (brain and nerve activity), mechanical energy (muscle activity), and thermal energy (warmth). Proteins and other nutrients including minerals, vitamins, and fatty acids contribute to building cells, to replacing worn structures, or to synthesis of functional molecules. Other nutrients contribute to regulation and control within body systems.

Assessment of Behavior

The role of nursing in the person's need for nutrition and in relation to the process of metabolism, in particular, relates to ensuring that the individual's diet is meeting body requirements. In particular, in assessing behaviors related to the process of metabolism and the associated nutrient intake, the nurse is interested in the person's physical appearance relative to height and weight, appetite and thirst, nutrient profile, condition of the oral cavity, and any relevant laboratory indicators.

Height and Weight

In a behavioral assessment of the process of metabolism, the nurse measures and records the height and the weight of the person. Height measurements are taken without shoes and the weight, preferably, is taken without clothing.

A daily weight is also useful when assessing a person's fluid balance. In this case, it is particularly important that the weight be taken at the same time of day and on the same scale. When a person is underweight or overweight, measurements taken over a period of time are more useful than a single measurement. Tables specifying appropriate height and weight for male and female adults have been established and serve as a guideline when making judgments regarding adaptive weight according to a person's height, gender, and body frame. These tables are found in textbooks on nutrition. In general, the nurse may use the following criterion. Females should weigh 100 pounds for 5 feet, with 5 pounds added for each additional inch of height. For males, an extra 5 pounds per inch is suggested. Standard and reference growth charts for infants, children, and adolescents have also been established, and these guidelines are found in any growth and development or pediatric textbook.

Appetite and Thirst

Appetite is a pleasant sensation involving the person's desire for and anticipation of food and fluids. Frequently, the appetite is affected by such specific stimuli as the sight, smell, and thought of food. It is psychological and is dependent on memory and associations. An example of an adaptive appetite behavior would be the statement, "I have a good appetite in the morning and eat a well-balanced breakfast," whereas an ineffective appetite behavior would be, "Although I ate a large lunch, the smell of freshly baked cinnamon buns tempted me into eating two large ones. I now feel very uncomfortable."

Thirst is a desire for fluid or the dry sensation resulting from a lack of or need for water. Often this sensation of dryness is felt in the mouth and the back part of the throat. Thirst is usually a reliable guide to the body's need for water. The normal adult should consume an average of 1 to $1^1/_2$ liters of water or other liquids daily to provide a sufficient amount of water for all physiologic processes. Water is available to the body through other sources, such as beverages, solid foods, and a small amount through the oxidation of essential nutrients. The maintenance of water balance is explored further in Chapter 11.

Nutrient Profile

The factors to be considered when evaluating a diet for optimal nutrition are described by Williams (1995, pp. 321–323). To promote health, the diet should provide all essential nutrients in adequate amounts for the daily needs of the body. Accepted standards for recommended daily allowances of nutrients have been developed by the National Academy of Sciences. The optimal diet provides a caloric level that will meet the energy needs of the body. Foods containing fiber will be ingested since the fiber provides bulk, which stimulates intestinal elimination. The food eaten should promote health and provide a measure of prevention in protecting the person from illness throughout all stages of the life cycle.

The established nutrient profile must be acceptable to the person or family. Acceptability includes establishing a diet that includes culturally defined differences such as those noted later in this chapter. Taking into account such differences can be accomplished with ease since there are many kinds and combinations of foods that constitute a well-balanced diet. Finally, the diet chosen should promote a good supply of energy for optimum performance of the person's activities of daily living and total human functioning.

The Department of Agriculture in the United States (1992) and Health Canada (1992) developed a daily food guide for the purpose of promoting good nutrition. This guide provides a flexible framework to help people achieve nutrient needs as outlined in the recommended daily dietary allowances. The daily food guide combines foods with similar nutritional values into four main groups—milk, meat, vegetable and fruit, and grain—commonly referred to as the basic four. In planning a diet, the person should choose a variety of foods from each group that they like and can afford. (Refer to nutrition textbooks for further information about nutritional requirements and dietary planning.)

Condition of the Oral Cavity

Appraisal of the oral cavity, that is the lips, teeth, gums, and tongue, is useful in determining the person's nutritional health and in identifying deficiencies. The lips of the healthy adult are smooth and free from lesions. The skin is thin with many vascular structures, which give the lips their reddish appearance. The oral mucosa is normally smooth, moist, and pink-red in color, with expected variations based on ethnic differences. The adult has 32 permanent teeth. They are examined for conditions that decrease their grinding action, such as loose or missing teeth, cavities, or wear. If dentures are used, they are removed to allow complete inspection of the mouth. Normal gums are solid in turgor and free of inflammation or bleeding. The tongue is pink in color. The dorsal surface is rough and the ventral surface is smooth.

Laboratory Indicators

Many laboratory tests provide indicators of the body's nutrition status. Plasma protein measures assist in the detection of protein and iron deficiencies. Twenty-four hour urine tests measure products of protein metabolism. Elevated levels may indicate excess body tissue breakdown. In advanced nursing practice roles, nurses may be involved in ordering such laboratory procedures as further behavioral indicators of the patient's nutrition and metabolic status.

Assessment of Stimuli

Stimuli related to the process of metabolism are assessed relative to the factors that may be affecting metabolic status and nutrition adaptation. These factors include nutrient requirements, cognator effectiveness, availability of food, culture, and weight consciousness.

Nutrient Requirements

Factors affecting nutrient requirements are age, gender, size, activity, temperature, diet, race, climate, pregnancy, and endocrine functioning. For example, an infant, because of a high rate of metabolism and relatively large body surface area, requires more calories per kilogram of body weight than an adult. A person exposed to severely cold weather expends additional calories to maintain body temperature. In periods of rapid growth during infancy, adolescence, and pregnancy, there is an increased caloric need. Males, who usually have a greater body size and greater proportion of lean body tissue, have a greater caloric requirement than do females. Additionally, there is a steady decline in caloric need starting with the early adult years. Inactive people require fewer calories than those with greater levels of activity (Phipps, Long, & Woods, 1991, p. 1210). Exercise patterns of the person are assessed when they will also influence caloric requirements.

Cognator Effectiveness

The person's level of knowledge regarding nutrition and perception of what constitutes a healthy and nutritious diet is a major stimulus. The nurse assesses this knowledge and perception since it greatly influences what the person is ingesting or what the person desires to eat, and thus results in either adaptive or ineffective patterns of nutrition. Based on the patient's level of knowledge about sound nutrition, diet counseling may be required. The nurse explores the person's beliefs regarding types of food eaten. Some people, for religious, economic, health, ethical, or ecologic reasons, are vegetarians. Such beliefs are taken into account in diet counseling.

Availability of Food

The nurse considers the availability of food to the person including financial and other resources. For example, an elderly person may find it difficult to travel to the store and may have limited financial resources with which to purchase food.

Culture

The nurse inquires about the person's cultural, social, and religious patterns that influence eating and drinking. Food habits and preferences based on cultural experience begin early in life. Cultural patterns affect both the kinds of foods used and the way they are prepared. As examples, two cultural perspectives described by Williams (1995) are cited here.

Basic dietary laws for Jewish people are identified in the Rules of Kashruth. These apply to the slaughter, preparation, and serving of meat; the combining of meat and milk; types of fish eaten; and eggs. Some food is restricted. Pork is not used, no combining of meat and milk is allowed, and only fish with fins and scales are to be eaten. Eggs with blood spots may not be eaten. Orthodox Jewish people strictly observe these laws, conservative Jewish people are less strict, and there is minimal general use by reform Jewish people. It is important for the nurse to understand and observe the person's preference in this regard.

A second example pertains to Asian food patterns. The dietary habits of Asian people include the use of meat, fish, eggs, cereals, and a variety of vegetables. Rice is used instead of bread. Meat is eaten in small amounts and is usually served with vegetables. Food is cut or chopped into small pieces and cooked quickly in small amounts of liquids or fats.

It is thus of utmost importance that culture be assessed as a factor potentially influencing intake of nutrients and the process of metabolism.

Weight Consciousness

Finally, the nurse identifies the person's desire to gain, lose, or maintain body weight. This weight consciousness influences the person's present and future eating patterns.

▶ COMPENSATORY ADAPTIVE PROCESSES

Viewed as an adaptive system (see Chap. 2), the person has innate and acquired ways of responding to the changing environment. Further, Roy conceptualizes these complex adaptive dynamics as the coping processes of the regulator and cognator subsystems. As described in this chapter, the need for nutrition is met through processes of digestion and metabolism. However, when the processes of nutrition are not integrated, then the regulator and cognator activate processes of compensation. Further, the thinking and feeling person, by way of cognator activity, can do much to affect any need of the physiologic mode, nutrition in particular. Regulator and cognator abilities then, are important internal stimuli for the person. These subsystems provide compensatory adaptive responses that extend the effectiveness of behavior in meeting the goals of adaptation and person and environment transformations.

Compensatory abilities that respond to nutrition needs include both automatic homeostatic functions of the regulator and voluntary, or behavioral, activities of the cognator. The nurse needs to understand as fully as possible the "wisdom of the body" to identify and interpret changes in the patient's condition. Study of physiology and pathophysiology are important to this understanding. One particular illustration of a regulator compensatory activity is given to illustrate compensatory adaptation related to nutrition.

The hypothalamus contains the hunger and satiety centers of the body and is the principal organ involved in the physiologic regulation of eating. A functioning hypothalamus is responsible for initiating internal cues that signal the person to eat to supply the body with needed energy. *Hunger* is the physiologically aroused sensation related to the body's need for food. The hypothalamus again signals through the satiety center to tell the person to stop eating. A healthy individual who responds to these internal cues that regulate energy balance is able to maintain a normal weight and control appetite.

At particular times of rapid, specialized growth throughout the life cycle, the body's nutritional demand is heightened. This is particularly true during pregnancy and lactation, in the first year of life, and at the onset of puberty. It is the regulator mechanisms within the body that stimulate enhanced appetite at these crucial times.

Another example of regulator compensatory response pertains to situations in which large portions of small intestine have been surgically removed as in some patients with Crohn's disease, an inflammatory bowel disease. With less intestinal absorptive surface available in the digestive system, it is apparent that the body responds through hypertrophy of the remaining villi to offset the loss of length of bowel and enhance the total absorptive surface in the bowel.

An illustration of a compensatory response to nutritional need by way of the cognator is a person with a medical diagnosis of diabetes mellitus, a metabolic disorder of energy balance involving the body's production of or response to the hormone insulin. Many people with this disorder have learned to effectively manage their diabetes by balancing food intake, exercise, and insulin requirements. In some cases, this means self-administration of insulin; in other situations, dietary control is effective. The keystone of effective management is sound diet therapy, and many people with the disorder become very skilled at determining dietary and insulin requirements based on self-assessment of blood sugar levels and exercise requirements. They are compensating for a physiologic problem through their cognator coping mechanisms (perceptual and information processing, learning, judgment, and emotion).

Some environment changes related to nutrition, particularly in a state of illness, can have an overwhelming effect on the individual's ability to adapt. The demands are greater than what compensatory processes can handle and the result can be compromised processes of nutrition.

▶ COMPROMISED PROCESSES OF NUTRITION

Adaptation problems can be caused by difficulties in any or all of the processes of nutrition since digestion and metabolism are interdependent. Two specific examples of compromised processes of nutrition will be discussed here. Obesity is a common nutritional problem in North American society, affecting an estimated 30 to 40 percent of the adult population (Burrell, Gerlach, & Pless, 1997, p. 285). Anorexia, or the loss or lack of appetite for food, is another common problem. It is particularly prevalent among adolescent females.

Obesity

Obesity is a clinical term for excess body weight generally applied to those who are 20 percent or more above a desired weight for height. Burrell et al. (1997, p. 1381) classify the condition as an eating disorder indicative of substance abuse. The substance of concern in this case is food. This is one of the most common adaptation problems related to nutrition in contemporary North America. Excessive accumulation of fat in the body increases the weight beyond the recommended measures with regard to bone structure, height, and age. The male is termed as having an intake exceeding metabolic needs when his weight exceeds 20 percent of the average weight found in standard height and weight tables. For the female, excess weight is 25 percent above the listed standard.

Although many individual differences exist in the factors contributing to obesity, the most common cause is an imbalance between the amount of food ingested and the amount of energy expended. In Burrell et al. (1997, p. 1381), influencing factors are described further:

> Partly to blame for obesity is the abundance of food and a sedentary lifestyle with little exercise except in leisure activities. Individual metabolism also plays a

part in the rate at which calories are burned. Misinformation about nutrition and dieting also contribute to the problem. Similar to other substance abusers, overeaters may indulge as a reaction to stress, to allay anxiety or depression, or to supplement a sedentary, boring lifestyle.

Unfortunately, there are no shortcuts to successful weight control. As Williams (1995) clearly states, "it requires hard work and strong individual motivation" (p. 284). An effective program of weight management must be personalized for the individual. It must focus on healthy lifestyle eating and exercise behaviors, and include stress management with supportive interpersonal relationships.

The nurse's primary role in supporting people with a weight management problem is to teach and encourage healthy dietary patterns. In many situations, referral to a health professional involved exclusively in dietetics and nutrition may be required. In situations where further physiologic problems are suspected, referral to a physician specializing in metabolic disorders may be required.

Anorexia

Williams (1995) noted, "America's obsession with thinness carries social and physiologic costs," and further explained that, "sometimes family and personal tensions as well as social pressures for thinness cause adolescent girls, even as young as grade-school age, to develop serious body image and eating problems that may become psychiatric disorders" (p. 276).

Anorexia nervosa, as described by Burrell et al. (1997), is, "generally considered to be a psychosomatic eating disorder of young adults with self-induced severe weight loss, starvation, malnutrition, and emaciation, which can progress to death without treatment" (p. 1381). Williams (1995, p. 291) described the typical situation surrounding the disorder.

> The young girl, usually a high achiever who pushes herself constantly toward perfection, sees food and her body as ways in which she can be in control. Her distorted body image—she sees herself as fat even when she is really emaciated—keeps her in a state of near panic. She plans her days around ways of avoiding food. It becomes a full-time obsession, and she grows more and more depressed, irritable, and anxious.

Obviously, serious problems including lowered resistance to infection, poor general health, and reduced strength can result from being seriously underweight. Without help, the disorder can lead to fatality.

Treatment of a serious psychological disorder such as anorexia nervosa requires the therapy of a skilled team of professionals—physicians, psychologists, and nutritionists. The nurse's role is one of teaching and supporting the individual with respect to healthy lifestyle, balanced diet, and support for a realistic perception of expectations and accomplishments. Ongoing monitoring and the support of treatment regimen may be required.

▶ **PLANNING NURSING CARE**

Adequate nutritional status is a priority requirement of the person's physiologic adaptation. In applying the nursing process, the nurse will make a careful assessment of the behaviors and stimuli related to the basic life processes of digestion and metabolism. In assessing factors influencing nutrition need, regulator and cognator effectiveness in initiating compensatory processes will be considered. Based on these thorough first- and second-level assessments, the nurse makes a nursing diagnosis, sets goals, selects interventions, and evaluates care.

Nursing Diagnosis

As has been described previously in this text, the assessment information related to behaviors and stimuli are interpreted in the form of a nursing diagnosis. The statement is formulated by considering the data of the first- and second-level assessment. The statement can include a summary of observed behaviors with the most relevant influencing stimuli. An example of a nursing diagnosis illustrating adaptation and summarizing behavior and stimuli is, "Evidence of adequate nutritional pattern related to a balanced diet for body requirements containing appropriate foods from all four food groups."

In situations where problems exist relative to the need for adequate nutrition, it is important that the nursing diagnosis convey the essence of the problem such that direction is provided for the subsequent steps of the nursing process. This is facilitated by the recommended structure of a nursing diagnosis: a statement of observed behaviors with most relevant influencing stimuli.

Consider an example of a 75-year-old man who has recently become a widower. Although he has been in good health, he has been losing weight gradually since his wife's death. When asked about his eating patterns, he states that he does not bother cooking for himself. Rather, he eats primarily cereals and bread, never cooks meat or vegetables, but occasionally enjoys baked food that his neighbor prepares. A nursing diagnosis relevant to this situation might be, "Weight loss due to inadequate intake of required nutrients."

A summary label is an alternate way of stating a nursing diagnosis. The nurse's judgment of the clinical situation may be expressed by using a statement from an established classification system. The Roy model has two classification lists, one for indicators of adaptation and one for commonly recurring adaptation problems. The complete classification lists for the Roy model are included in Chapter 3. In Table 6–1, the Roy model nursing diagnostic categories for the physiologic need of nutrition are shown in relation to nursing diagnosis labels approved by the North American Nursing Diagnosis Association (Rantz & LeMone, 1997).

Labels that summarize a behavioral pattern when more than one mode is being affected by the same stimuli are often very meaningful to experienced nurses. They convey much information in a single term. An example of such a label would be the term *anorexia,* that is, the loss or lack of appetite

TABLE 6–1   NURSING DIAGNOSTIC CATEGORIES FOR NUTRITION

Positive Indicators of Adaptation	Common Adaptation Problems	NANDA Diagnostic Labels
• Stable digestive processes	• Nausea and vomiting	• Risk for aspiration • Altered oral mucous membrane • Impaired swallowing
• Adequate nutritional pattern for body requirements	• Nutrition more or less than body requirements • Weight 20–25% above or below average • Anorexia	• Altered nutrition: more than body requirements • Altered nutrition: potential for more than body requirements • Altered nutrition: less than body requirements
• Metabolic and other nutritive needs met during altered means of ingestion	• Ineffective coping strategies for altered means of ingestion	• Feeding self-care deficit • Ineffective breast-feeding • Interrupted breast-feeding • Effective breast-feeding • Ineffective infant feeding pattern

for food. As described earlier, stimuli contributing to this disorder are often very complex and are associated with modes in addition to the physiologic mode. For example, the self-concept and interdependence modes may be involved. The person may feel attractive only at a weight of less than 100 pounds. Significant others may reinforce this belief by commenting adversely whenever additional weight becomes evident. A nursing diagnosis illustrating this could be, "Anorexia related to peer pressure and low self-esteem."

Another nursing diagnosis related to altered nutrition, "More or potentially more than body requirements due to excessive intake," defines the state in which a person experiences or is at risk of experiencing an intake of nutrients that exceeds metabolic needs.

The behaviors and stimuli related to these diagnoses are individual and may include such assessment factors as sedentary activity level or responding inappropriately to internal and external cues for eating. It is important to consider metabolic and endocrine factors that may be contributing to the problem. If these physiologically based factors do not exist, other stimuli should be explored.

A diagnosis of "altered nutrition, less than body requirements due to poverty" is defined as the state in which a person experiences an intake of nutrients insufficient to meet metabolic needs. Stimuli related to this diagnosis may include the person's ability to ingest or digest food or absorb nutrients because of psychological, biologic, or economic factors. The person is referred to as having an intake of nutrients insufficient to meet metabolic needs when the body weight is 20 percent or more under the ideal weight for bone structure, height, and age. The behaviors and stimuli related to this diagnosis are varied and can include such assessment factors as lack of interest in food; decreased availability of food; or painful, inflamed condition of the mouth.

Nausea and vomiting are other common adaptation problems related to nutrition. These problems are frequently associated but can be experienced separately. *Nausea* is an unpleasant sensation reported as a feeling of sickness with the urge to vomit. *Vomiting* is the forceful ejection of stomach contents through the mouth. The vomiting reflex can be stimulated by a number of intrinsic and extrinsic factors, for example, unpleasant odors, tastes, sights; sensations such as severe pain; chemical agents used in the treatment of disease; and radiation therapy. Identification of the stimuli contributing to the problem is an important factor in its solution.

Once the nursing diagnosis related to nutrition has been established, the nurse proceeds to formulate goals that address each of the identified problems or support areas in which adaptation has been observed.

Goal Setting

In the fourth step of the nursing process as described in the Roy Adaptation Model, the nurse establishes goals in collaboration with the person receiving care, namely, statements of clear behavioral outcomes of nursing care planned with the person. The goal should address the behavior, the change expected, and the time frame in which the goal is to be achieved. Goals may be long-term or short-term and these time frames are relative to the situation involved.

When setting a goal for the person experiencing an intake of nutrients exceeding metabolic needs, it is realistic and healthy to establish a goal providing for gradual weight loss of 1 to 2 pounds per week while eating a well-balanced diet. An appropriately worded goal could be, "The patient will lose 2 pounds each week for the next 4 weeks." In this objective, the person's weight is the behavior of focus, the change expected is the loss of 2 pounds each week, and the time frame is 4 weeks.

An appropriate goal for the situation described previously of the elderly man experiencing altered nutrition with less than body requirements would be the ingestion of a well-balanced, high-caloric diet so as to initially stabilize the weight and then increase weight gradually. A short-term goal may relate to the daily intake, "Today Mr. Smith will ingest an evening meal which is balanced in nutrients and of sufficient caloric content to meet his energy requirements." A longer term goal could be related to his status in 1 month: "By this date next month, Mr. Smith will have gained 5 pounds and documented a balanced intake containing all recommended nutrients."

For the person experiencing the adaptation problems of nausea and vomiting, the goal should directly reflect a decrease in the stated assessed behavior or an increased ability to cope with it. As has been identified before, goals pertain directly to the person's behavior and are stated in behavioral terms from the patient's perspective.

The focus for the next step of the nursing process, intervention, is the change of the stimuli identified as contributing to the observed behaviors and strengthening compensatory processes, in particular.

Intervention

Once the goals have been established relative to behaviors that will promote adaptation, the nurse determines the interventions that will assist the person in attaining the stated goals. Nursing interventions for promotion of nutrition depend on the stimuli and, particularly, the coping processes identified. The nurse manages the stimuli by either promoting or reinforcing them, or by taking action to change or eliminate them. For example, if the stimulus related to overeating is a response to internal cues of feeling stressed has been identified, the nurse can assist the person in establishing coping strategies to adapt to the stresses of daily living. Additionally, if a decreased exercise pattern is identified as a stimulus, the nurse can assist the individual with measures to increase activity level. New coping strategies may be learned, such as taking a walk to handle stress.

If a person wants to change a situation of being overweight, it is important to establish the motivation for the desired weight-loss regimen. One reason for wanting to lose weight may include an improved health status in order to avoid many of the chronic disorders linked to obesity. Other motivators may be a desire for improvement in personal appearance and peer pressures from family and friends to lose weight.

An intervention that has been used successfully for changing a person's response pattern of eating because of external cues is behavior modification (Burrell et al., 1997). It is often helpful for the person to write down specific feelings before eating to identify whether the eating is in response to emotions such as anxiety, boredom, or loneliness. The person is then instructed to try to substitute other activities in place of eating at these times. Other techniques in this approach include slowing down and making the act of eating a conscious acknowledged action. A meal should last at least 20 minutes so that the hypothalamus can send out satiation signals. In the process of slowing down, doing only one activity at a time may be helpful, that is, preparing each bit of food separately, putting the utensils down between bites, taking a sip of beverage between bites, and using the napkin frequently while concentrating on slowing down all actions.

In the previous situation of the elderly man, the short-term goal focused on one balanced meal. In addressing the stimuli involved in the situation, it was evident that Mr. Smith had never received instruction related to the four basic food groups, or had the opportunity to do any cooking. By reviewing the dietary requirements associated with a balanced meal and discussing preparation methods with him, Mr. Smith made a commitment to make a list and go to the grocery store to buy the required supplies, then cook himself a meal. He invited his neighbor to observe the cooking session, intervene in case of a problem, and share the meal with him.

General interventions for nausea and vomiting will focus, where possible, on the stimuli causing the problem. For example, unpleasant, strong odors in the environment should be eliminated; or the person's environment should be kept quiet and sudden movements prevented. If pain is causing the problem, it may be that something can be done to alleviate it. Other conservative treatments for nausea and vomiting include limiting the person's food and fluid intake until the problem subsides. If fluids are tolerated, offering carbonated beverages may be comforting. Ice chips may be tolerated and oral hygiene is refreshing for the patient. Positioning the patient with the head raised and turned to the side may assist and will be necessary if vomiting is occurring. If none of these interventions is successful, it may be necessary to administer an antiemetic medication as ordered by the physician. When the problem subsides and the diet is resumed, offering foods that are bland, such as dry toast or soda crackers, is often appropriate. If nausea and vomiting persist, the use of intravenous fluids to prevent fluid and electrolyte imbalance may be warranted.

The nurse's intervention in relation to nutrition planning may be to provide for referral to a health professional involved exclusively in dietetics and nutrition.

Evaluation

Evaluation involves judging the effectiveness of nursing interventions in relation to the person's behavior and in terms of the preset goals. The nursing interventions would be identified as effective if the person's behavior is in accordance with the stated goal. For example, in a previous illustration, the goal was, "The patient will lose 2 pounds each week for the next 4 weeks." The goal would be achieved if the person loses 2 pounds each week for 4 weeks. Achievement of this goal could be measured by weekly assessment of weight.

For Mr. Smith, evaluation would be accomplished as he reported on his success with his first meal and, in the longer term, his ability to continue to consume a balanced diet and his subsequent weight stabilization and gain. If this optimistic scenario did not materialize, other approaches to the problem would be sought. If the goal has not been achieved, the nurse identifies alternative interventions or approaches by reassessing the behavior and stimuli, particularly the use of compensating strategies, and continuing with the other steps of the nursing process.

► SUMMARY

This chapter has focused on the application of the Roy Adaptation Model to the physiologic need of nutrition. An overview of the basic life processes—digestion and metabolism—associated with nutrition was provided along with the identification of parameters for assessment of behaviors and stimuli. Illustrations of innate and learned adaptive compensatory processes related to nutrition were described and examples of two compromised processes (obesity and anorexia) were provided. Finally, guidelines for planning nursing care through the formulation of nursing diagnoses, goals, and interventions were explored and evaluation of nursing care was described.

▶ EXERCISES FOR APPLICATION

1. Assess your own eating patterns by recording a diet history for a 24-hour period. Determine if the quantity and quality of the nutrients ingested are adaptive or ineffective.

2. Identify a person with good eating habits and preferences based on cultural experience that is different from your own. Determine the cultural, social, and religious patterns that influence that person's ingestion of food and fluids.

▶ ASSESSMENT OF UNDERSTANDING

Questions

1. List the five major processes (and subprocesses where applicable) associated with the basic life process of digestion.
   (a) _____
   (b) _____
   (c) _____
   (d) _____
   (e) _____

2. List three categories of behavior associated with each of the basic life processes of nutrition.
   (a) Digestion: _____, _____, _____.
   (b) Metabolism: _____, _____, _____.

3. The following is the list of common influencing factors that were identified in Chapter 3. Identify the factors which are of concern with respect to the need for nutrition.
   (a) Culture
   (b) Family and aggregate participants
   (c) Developmental stage
   (d) Integrity of modes and systems
   (e) Cognator and innovator effectiveness
   (f) Environmental considerations

4. Label the following examples of compensatory responses as associated with regulator (R) or cognator (C) mechanisms.
   (a) _____ In situations of illness, the person often loses his or her appetite for food.
   (b) _____ When blood glucose levels are too low, the liver breaks down stored glycogen and releases glucose into the blood.

(c) _____To lose weight, the person alters intake of fats and increases his or her exercise pattern.

(d) _____When caloric intake is inadequate for the body's level of activity, fat and even tissue proteins begin to break down to satisfy the body's requirements.

(e) _____The diabetic person calculates daily requirement for insulin and self-administers the required amount.

5. An altered means of ingestion can be the outcome of compromise relative to a particular process involved in nutrition. In the situation of a person being fed through a gastrostomy tube, identify two processes that could be compromised to warrant such an alternative.

Situation

Nancy James is a 40-year-old career person who works as an executive for a publishing company. She commutes 2 hours each day, leaving early and arriving home late. She rarely has time for breakfast and does not bother preparing dinner for herself. She frequently has business luncheons and does not feel hungry until later in the evening. Whenever she does feel hungry, she snacks on soda pop, chocolate bars, and chips since the dispensing machine is located close to her office. Nancy wants to lose some weight. She is 5 feet 2 inches tall and weighs 160 pounds. She states, "I can't understand why I keep putting on weight. I usually eat only one meal a day!"

6. Formulate a nursing diagnosis for the described situation.

   _____

   _____

7. State a goal to address weight loss in the described situation. Identify the behavior, the change expected, and the associated time frame.
   Goal: _____
   Behavior: _____
   Expected change: _____
   Time frame: _____

8. List two interventions that might assist Nancy in the achievement of the goal stated. What stimuli are being managed?

Interventions	**Stimuli**
_____	_____
_____	_____

9. What behavior would provide evidence that the identified goal had been achieved?

   _____

Feedback

1. (a) ingestion
   (b) food breakdown (mechanical digestion and chemical digestion)
   (c) propulsion
   (d) absorption
   (e) defecation

2. (a) Any three of: eating patterns, sense of taste and smell, food allergies, pain, altered ingestion.
   (b) Any three of: physical appearance relative to height and weight, appetite and thirst, nutrient profile, condition of oral cavity, laboratory indicators.

3. All of the factors are of relevance to the need for nutrition.

4. (a) R, (b) R, (c) C, (d) R, (e) C

5. Ingestion: The person may be unable to swallow. Movement of food: It may not be possible for food to move down the esophagus.

6. Nursing diagnosis example: Body weight greater than 20 percent above average due to diet in excess of body requirements.

7. Goal example: Within 4 weeks, Nancy will have lost 10 pounds.
   Behavior: weight
   Change expected: loss of 10 pounds
   Time frame: within 4 weeks

8. | **Interventions** | **Stimuli** |
   |---|---|
   | Documentation of intake | Cognator effectiveness: Nancy's perception of how much she eats is erroneous. |
   | Adherence to 1,000-calorie diet | Caloric requirements: Nancy's required intake for weight loss will relate to her needs. |

9. Within 4 weeks, Nancy will have lost 10 pounds.

▶ REFERENCES

Burrell, L. O., Gerlach, M. J. M., & Pless, B. S. (1997). *Adult nursing: Acute and community care* (2nd ed.). Stamford, CT: Appleton & Lange.

Health and Welfare Canada. (1992). *Canada's food guide*. Ottawa, Canada: Minister of Supply and Services.

Linton, A. D., Matteson, M. A., & Maebius, N. K. (1995). *Introductory nursing care of adults.* Philadelphia: Saunders.

Marieb, E. N. (1989). *Human anatomy and physiology.* Redwood City, CA: Benjamin/Cummings.

Marieb, E. N. (1994). *Essentials of human anatomy and physiology* (4th ed.). Redwood City, CA: Benjamin/Cummings.

Phipps, W., Long, B., & Woods, N. (1991). *Medical-surgical nursing: Concepts and clinical practice.* St. Louis: Mosby.

Rantz, M. J., & LeMone, P. (Eds.). (1979). *Classification of nursing diagnosis. Proceedings of the 12th conference NANDA.* Glendale, CA: CINAHL Information Systems.

U.S. Department of Agriculture. (1992). *The food guide pyramid, Home and Garden Bulletin,* No. 252. Washington, DC: Government Printing Office.

Williams, S. R. (1995). *Essentials of nutrition and diet therapy* (6th ed.). St. Louis: Mosby.

▶ **ADDITIONAL REFERENCES**

Guyton, A. C. (1992). *Human physiology and mechanisms of disease* (5th ed.). Philadelphia: Saunders.

Servonsky, J., & Opas, S. (Eds.). (1987). *Nursing management of children.* Monterey, CA: Jones and Bartlett.

7

ELIMINATION

Elimination is a basic life process essential to adaptation. Just as nutrients are provided for survival and maintenance of physiologic balance by digestion and metabolism processes, so do metabolic waste products need to be eliminated. These waste materials are expelled to maintain homeostasis. Wastes are excreted from the intestines, by the kidneys, and by the skin and lungs. Chapter 5 addresses excretion by the lungs through gas exchange with the environment, and Chapter 9 deals with excretion by the skin through perspiration.

In this chapter, the basic life processes of intestinal elimination and urinary elimination are addressed along with the identification of parameters for assessment of behaviors and stimuli. As well, illustrations of compensatory and compromised processes related to elimination are described. Examples of compromised processes are provided. Finally, guidelines for planning nursing care by formulating diagnoses, establishing goals, selecting interventions, and evaluating nursing care are described.

▶ OBJECTIVES

After studying this chapter, the reader will be able to do the following:

1. Describe two basic life processes associated with the need for elimination as presented in this chapter.

2. Identify important first-level assessment parameters (behaviors) for each of the basic life processes associated with the need for elimination.

3. List second-level assessment parameters (common stimuli) that affect elimination.

4. Describe one compensatory process related to each of the basic life processes associated with elimination.

5. Name and describe two situations of compromised processes of elimination.

6. Develop a nursing diagnosis, given a situation related to elimination.

7. Derive goals for an individual with ineffective elimination in a given situation.

8. Describe nursing interventions commonly implemented in situations of ineffective elimination.

9. Propose approaches to determine the effectiveness of nursing interventions.

► KEY CONCEPTS DEFINED

Anuria: The complete suppression of urine formation by the kidneys.

Bowel incontinence: The involuntary passage of stool.

Constipation: A condition in which the fecal matter in the bowel is too hard to pass with ease, or a state in which the bowel movements are so infrequent that uncomfortable symptoms occur. It is clinically defined as less than three bowel movements per week.

Diarrhea: The rapid movement of the fecal material through the intestines, resulting in poor absorption of water, essential nutrients, and electrolytes, and an abnormally frequent passage of watery stool.

Flatulence: Gas or air in the gastrointestinal tract that can result in pain or feelings of abdominal fullness.

Intestinal elimination: The expulsion from the body of undigested substance via the anus in the form of feces.

Micturition: The process by which the bladder is emptied.

Oliguria: Diminished urine secretion in relation to fluid intake.

Peristalsis: Movements of the intestinal tract that both mix and propel the mixture of food and enzymes that come from the digestive process in the stomach.

Urinary elimination: The elimination of fluid wastes and excess ions as a result of the filtering process in which the kidneys maintain the purity and constancy of internal fluids.

Urinary incontinence: The involuntary passage of urine from the bladder.

Urinary retention: The inability to void, with the resultant accumulation of urine within the bladder.

▶ BASIC LIFE PROCESSES OF ELIMATION

Although many basic life processes participate in the elimination of waste products from the body, the focus of this chapter is intestinal elimination and urinary elimination. *Intestinal elimination* is the expulsion from the body of undigested substances via the anus in the form of feces. *Urinary elimination* pertains to the elimination of fluid wastes and excess ions as a result of the filtering process in which the kidneys maintain the purity and constancy of internal fluids. As mentioned previously, other elimination processes are addressed in other chapters of this text.

▶ INTESTINAL ELIMINATION: PROCESS AND ASSESSMENT

Maintenance of adequate intestinal elimination requires a functioning gastrointestinal tract. As noted in Chapter 6, it is the primary function the gastrointestinal, or alimentary, tract as a whole to provide water, electrolytes, and nutrients to sustain life. Basic structures of the upper gastrointestinal tract consist of the mouth, esophagus, stomach, and duodenum. The lower gastrointestinal tract is made up of the small intestines, jejunum, and ileum; the large intestine, which includes the ascending, transverse, descending, and sigmoid colon; and the rectum and the anus. This tract carries out three functions: the movement of food through the tract; secretion of digestive juices; and absorption of the digested nutrients, water, and electrolytes. The upper gastrointestinal tract deals with ingestion and digestion of food. The small intestine involves both digestion and absorption of nutrients. The function of the large intestine is primarily the absorption of water and electrolytes, and the elimination of the waste products of digestion through the anus.

Movements of both the small and large intestine are key to the process of elimination. *Peristalsis* is the term used to describe movements of the intestinal tract that both mix and propel the mixture of food and enzymes that comes from the digestive process in the stomach. Such movements are divided into two types, mixing and propulsive movements. In the small intestine, rapid segmental contractions chop the solid food particles to promote mixing with digestive secretions. The peristaltic waves are weak and die out quickly; thus chyme (mixture of food with stomach secretions as it passes through the tract) moves slowly, taking 3 to 5 hours to pass from the stomach to the large intestine.

The proximal half of the colon is concerned primarily with absorption, and the distal half with storage. Less intense mixing movements are required for these functions. Thus, in the colon, the fecal material is gradually turned over and exposed to the surface of the large intestine, where fluid is progressively absorbed. In this way, about 1500 mL of chyme enters the large intestines each day but only 80 to 150 mL are excreted as feces.

The propulsive movements of small and large intestines also differ. In the latter case, instead of peristaltic waves, mass movements primarily occur in the large intestine. The movements involve the constriction of a ring occurring at a distended or irritated point, followed rapidly by the constriction of a long segment (20 cm or more) of colon contracting almost as a unit. This action forces the fecal material as a mass down the colon. These movements usually occur only a few times a day, most frequently for about 15 minutes during the first hour or so after eating breakfast. On the other hand, the peristaltic waves of the small intestine occur throughout the day, but are greatly increased after a meal.

Defecation is the action whereby feces is emptied from the rectum. A weak sphincter approximately 20 cm from the anus, at the juncture between the sigmoid colon and the rectum, keeps the rectum empty of feces most of the time. Normally, when a mass movement forces feces into the rectum, the process of defecation is initiated. This process includes the defecation reflex and conscious sphincter control. Control of fecal evacuation involves tonic constriction of two sphincters. The internal sphincter is a circular mass of smooth muscle that constricts immediately inside the anus. The external anal sphincter is composed of striated voluntary muscle and surrounds the internal sphincter, slightly distal to it.

The defecation reflex initiates the process that ordinarily results in defecation. Sensory nerve fibers in the rectum are stimulated by stretch and carry their signals to the spinal cord, then reflexively, back to the lower gastrointestinal tract by way of the parasympathetic system. These signals set up strong peristaltic waves that can effectively empty the entire large bowel. Other effects that are part of the reflex response are taking a deep breath, closing the glottis, and contracting the abdominal muscles and the pelvic floor muscles. In infants and people without conscious control, this process proceeds naturally to defecation. However, in others, despite the defecation reflex, voluntary efforts are used in expelling feces.

In addition to several other reflex systems, the gastrointestinal tract has an intrinsic nervous system of its own called the enteric nervous system (Guyton, 1992). It begins at the esophagus and extends all the way to the anus. This system particularly controls gastrointestinal movements and secretions. However, the degree of activity of the enteric nervous system can be altered strongly by both parasympathetic and sympathetic nervous system signals from the brain (see Chapter 12). The influence of both branches of the autonomic nervous system, parasympathetic and sympathetic, are particularly active at the upper end of the gastrointestinal system, down to the stomach, and at the distal end, from the midcolon region to the anus. The neurons of the parasympathetic system generally enhance activity of most gastrointestinal functions, whereas stimulation of the sympathetic branch inhibits activity of the tract. Strong stimulation of this branch can totally block the movement of food. Understanding these connections, and the relationship of these processes within the thinking and feeling person, can be useful in assessing problems of elimination and in planning nursing care.

Assessment of Behavior

The formation of a positive nurse–client relationship is essential to collect data about a person's elimination patterns. Since the topic of bodily secretions is considered personal by many, the nurse is aware of the privacy needs of the person, and one's own reaction when inquiring about another's elimination pattern. In addressing elimination, the nurse establishes privacy and an intrusion-free environment. The nurse's interaction with the patient considers the person's language level and communication skills, as influenced by one's cultural and educational background. Main aspects of assessment include characteristics of stool, bowel sounds, and laboratory findings.

Characteristics of Stool

When assessing intestinal elimination, the nurse observes the following behaviors. Stool is described by stating the amount, color, consistency, frequency, odor, and effort. Normally, the stool that is evacuated is soft, formed, and brown in color for adults. The frequency of a bowel movement varies with each individual, although one bowel movement a day is average.

In healthy people, variations can range from stool evacuated twice a day to stool evacuated every 2 to 3 days. When making a judgment as to whether the frequency is adaptive or ineffective, the nurse assesses if the observed behavior represents a change from the person's normal pattern.

Stool is to be passed with ease without straining or discomfort when the defecation reflex is first felt. Stool containing any unusual matter such as blood, mucus, pus, or intestinal worms is also noted. A careful, exact description of the stool is essential when blood is present. Observe whether the blood appears on the surface of the stool or if it is mixed throughout. If the female is menstruating, this may be the source of bright red blood on the surface of stool. Normal stool has a characteristic odor caused by bacterial action on the foods that are eaten. Any unusual odor should be noted, for it can have clinical significance.

Bowel Sounds

Bowel sounds indicate the movements within the small and large bowel. In assessing these, the nurse notes the presence, frequency, or absence of bowel sounds. The abdomen is auscultated in all four quadrants proceeding in a clockwise fashion. Using the diaphragm part of the stethoscope, listen in each quadrant, changing the auscultatory site 2 or 3 inches with each move. It is important to remove the stethoscope completely from the abdomen when changing locations, for pulling the stethoscope across the abdomen will produce interfering sound, can cause involuntary muscle spasms, and can be uncomfortable for the person.

Normal bowel sounds will be high-pitched, gurgling noises usually occurring five or more times a minute. Ineffective bowel sounds include extremely weak or infrequent sounds, or a complete absence of sounds, which can indicate bowel hypomobility or immobility. Before a determination of bowel sounds can be made, the abdomen is auscultated for at least 3 minutes. Bowel sounds indicating possible hypermotility of the bowel will be heard as frequent rushes of loud, high-pitched sounds. Passage of gas is a good indication that peristaltic movement is occurring.

Pain

Pain related to bowel elimination is included as assessment of behavior by listing the person's statements regarding discomfort and pain on evacuation of the bowel or the excessive accumulation of flatus or gas in the intestines. All verbal and nonverbal behaviors and the location, severity, duration, and onset of the pain are noted.

Laboratory Findings

In completing the behavioral assessment of the bowel elimination component of the physiologic adaptive mode, laboratory results related to stool are checked, if available. Specimens of the feces may be tested for occult blood when intestinal bleeding is suspected, but gross blood is visible on inspection. (Laboratory values and procedures for assisting with these tests are available from resource texts such as Burrell, Gerlach, & Pless, 1997.)

Assessment of Stimuli

With the assessment of stimuli, the nurse gathers data about factors influencing the behaviors identified in the first assessment phase of the adaptation nursing process. This includes the important factor of the body's adaptive ability to maintain integrated processes of elimination, as well as the coping strategies the person uses to maintain or change behaviors.

Intact Homeostatic Processes

Homeostasis comprises the steady physiologic states which enable people to counteract changes both in external conditions and in internal bodily functions. The intact homeostatic process in the bowel is primarily responsible for adaptive intestinal elimination behaviors. As noted earlier, the digestion of food is completed in the small intestine as it absorbs nutrients from the ingested substances. Peristaltic waves push the substance through the ileocecal valve into the large intestine, which absorbs a high percentage of the liquid as well as salts from the wastes. Intestinal contents are then propelled toward the rectum for evacuation.

Presence of Disease

A major stimulus disrupting intestinal elimination is the presence of a disease state that affects the normal processes of the gastrointestinal system. Examples include such conditions as ulcerative colitis and intestinal obstruction, which are explained in general textbooks on pathology.

Diet

The type and amount of diet are important influences in bowel elimination. The nurse notes the person's present daily nutritional intake and evaluates whether or not these foods provide roughage and bulk, such as high-residue foods or fresh fruits and vegetables; contain natural laxative effects that promote normal stool consistency, such as prunes and brans; influence the production of excessive intestinal gas, such as cabbage and beans; and influence the color or consistency of stool. For example, the high milk intake of an infant can cause light-colored stool, and intolerance to certain foods can promote diarrhea.

Fluid Intake

Assessment of stimuli influencing bowel elimination includes fluid intake. The nurse notes the amount of fluid the person is taking, both orally and intravenously. Decreased fluid intake can promote stool that is dry and hard.

Immediate Environment

The immediate environment contributes to adaptation in this mode component as it does in others. This would include whether or not the person has maintenance or lack of privacy for evacuation. The nurse assesses the availability of the toilet to the person or if the use of a bedpan is required. The person immobilized in traction who uses a bedpan while in the reclining position may have difficulty adapting usual bowel evacuation to this changed environment. The temperature and comfort of the room is assessed since this also may influence the situation.

Medications and Treatments

Other factors in the immediate situation that influence bowel elimination are medications, treatments, or tests. The nurse notes specific medications that the person may be taking that influence stools. For example, iron can cause dark, hard stools; codeine can cause behavior indicative of constipation; and sensitivities to certain other drugs, particularly antibiotics, can cause diarrhea. Any treatments or tests influencing bowel elimination behaviors, such as barium enemas, gastrointestinal x-ray series, or soapsuds enemas, are identified as well. Of specific significance is any altered means of elimination, such as an ileostomy or a colostomy.

Painful Conditions

The nurse validates with the person the cause of any pain related to bowel elimination. Possible causes include the presence of disruptive processes, such as hemorrhoids, anal fissure, or abdominal cramping caused by excessive intestinal gas. The coping strategies the person uses for this pain are assessed. For example, with hemorrhoids, the person may use sitz baths, ointments, or special skin care for the irritated skin around the anus.

Elimination Habits

The nurse also assesses the normal pattern of bowel habits as influencing the current behavior observed. She notes factors that maintain or increase peristalsis, such as the person's daily activity level or pattern of exercise. Factors that decrease peristalsis include bed rest, immobility, or recent anesthesia. The coping strategies that the person uses to maintain elimination are identified. These could include drinking a hot liquid or fruit juice, or the use of laxatives, mineral oil, enemas, or suppositories. The nurse assesses if the person has a routine schedule or time set aside each day for evacuation. Whether the person thinks the strategies used are effective or ineffective is important to note.

Stress

Because of the connection of bowel motility and the defecation reflex with the autonomic nervous system, stress may be an important factor influencing ongoing habits and current behaviors noted by the nurse. Awareness of signs of physical and psychological stress, such as illness or anxiety, is part of the nursing assessment as these factors influence elimination behaviors.

Family or Cultural Beliefs

Family or cultural beliefs concerning elimination often begin early in childhood and can involve specific views about the need and schedule to eliminate wastes from the bowel. The expected schedule of elimination may be related to beliefs about health. These background factors are relevant information regarding assessment of bowel elimination.

Developmental Stage

Age is another contextual stimulus that the person brings to the situation. The age of the person is noted, since this will influence intestinal elimination. For example, the older person may show a decline in the motility of the gastrointestinal tract, which occurs with advancing years, or the young child may have difficulties with toilet training.

▶ URINARY ELIMINATION: PROCESS AND ASSESSMENT

The structures of urinary elimination include the kidneys, ureters, bladder, and urethra. One function of this system, to balance body fluids and electrolytes, is discussed in Chapter 11. The second function of these structures is the excretion of most of the end-products of bodily metabolism. The intact operation of both of these functions contributes to internal homeostasis and to the regulation of body processes.

The functional nephron is the basis for understanding renal function. The two kidneys together contain more than two million nephrons, each of which is capable of forming urine by itself. The nephron cleans, or clears, the blood plasma of unwanted substances as it passes through the kidney.

The nephron's filtering process prevents waste substances from being reabsorbed. These unwanted substances, such as urea, creatinine, uric acid, and urates, are end-products of metabolism. Wanted substances such as water and electrolytes are reabsorbed into the plasma. In addition, the nephron clears the plasma of excesses of other substances—such as sodium ions, potassium ions, chloride ions, and hydrogen ions—that tend to accumulate in the body. The unwanted portions of the fluid from the nephron filtration process are passed into the urine. This system has two special feedback mechanisms that act together with the arterial blood pressure to bring about the necessary degree of filtration autoregulation. The principles of urine formation and the mechanisms of metabolism in the kidney are discussed further in basic physiology texts.

As urine collects in the kidneys, pressure increases and initiates a peristaltic contraction of the ureter. The ureters are small smooth muscle tubes that pass downward from the kidneys to the bladder. The ureters have both sympathetic and parasympathetic nerves, as well as other nerve fibers, along their entire lengths. The urinary bladder is composed of smooth muscle and has two principal parts: the body, where the urine collects; and the neck, a funnel-shaped extension of the body. The muscle of the bladder neck is referred to as the internal sphincter. It acts to keep the bladder neck empty of urine. Beyond the bladder neck, the urethra passes through a layer of muscle called the external sphincter of the bladder. This is a voluntary skeletal muscle. As with the gastrointestinal tract, this voluntary sphincter is under the control of the central nervous system and can be used consciously to prevent urination.

Micturition is the process by which the urinary bladder is emptied. A micturition reflex is a cycle involving three stages: progressive and rapid increase in pressure in the bladder, a period of sustained pressure, and return of the pressure to a baseline level. After such a reflex cycle that has not ended in emptying the bladder, the nervous system structures remain inhibited for at least a few minutes, to as long as an hour, before another micturition reflex occurs. With an increasingly distended bladder, the micturition reflexes occur more frequently and powerfully. Eventually they will force the bladder neck to open, leading to further reflexes.

Assessment of Behavior

When assessing urinary elimination the nurse observes amount and characteristics of urine, frequency, urgency, pain, and laboratory findings.

Amount and Characteristics of Urine

The amount of urine per voiding and the total for 24 hours is stated. The color and transparency, odor, frequency, urgency felt, and effort are noted as well. Normally, the amount of urine voided by the average adult will vary from 1000 to 2000 mL in a 24-hour period. Urine is normally pale yellow or amber in color because of the presence of the yellow pigment urochrome. In healthy individuals, urine that is pale and almost colorless is probably very dilute with a low specific gravity, while urine that is darker in color may have a higher specific gravity. Freshly voided urine has a clear transparency, and cloudy urine or urine containing a sediment can represent a disease state. This change in transparency could be caused by a reactional change of the urine if left standing for a period of time, as the pH changes from acidic to alkaline. The odor of fresh-voided urine is aromatic. When left standing, urine may develop an ammonia smell caused by the decomposition of urea by bacteria.

Presence of Frequency or Urgency

The frequency of urination, urgency felt, and effort in starting and stopping the flow of urine can depend on many factors. In general, the musculature of the bladder is capable of distending to the approximate capacity of 300 mL before the urge to void is felt. This begins the process of the micturition reflex described earlier. The stretch receptors in the bladder being stimulated, together with involuntary and voluntary control of the sphincters located at the opening of the bladder into the urethra, permit the flow of urine.

Pain

The nurse assesses any pain related to urinary elimination. This includes pain or burning sensations prior to, during, or after urination. Normally, the person will void with ease, without pain or discomfort.

Laboratory Findings

Laboratory data are useful, especially in comparing the findings in a routine urinalysis and findings of other specific tests with normal values.

The adaptive response of the urinary system, which is discussed later in this chapter, plays a major role in homeostasis or physiologically steady states by the removal of waste products from the bloodstream, and regulation of fluid and electrolyte balance, acid–base balance, and osmotic pressures within the body. Nursing assessment of factors influencing urinary elimination begins with an understanding of the intact homeostatic processes that result in the production and elimination of urine. (These processes are described earlier in this chapter and in other basic physiology and nursing science texts.)

Assessment of Stimuli

As the basic life processes operate, bladder elimination is influenced by many of the same categories of stimuli that influence intestinal elimination. Specifically, the following are factors to be considered in the assessment of stimuli for urinary elimination.

Presence of Disease

The nurse identifies whether what has taken place is a disease process or condition, a surgical procedure, or trauma, which affects the normal structure, function, or regulation of the urinary system. Examples include urinary tract infections; disturbances of the central nervous system pathways, causing loss of voluntary control; tissue damage to the sphincters; relaxation of the perineal structures from childbirth; pressure on the bladder during pregnancy; poorly regulated diabetes mellitus; and chronic renal failure.

Fluid Balance

Of particular significance as a stimulus for urinary output is the amount of fluid intake. The nurse notes both oral and intravenous intake of fluids within the most recent 24 hours. Intake naturally influences the amount of urine excreted. Insensible loss of water through the skin and lungs are considered in relation to urinary output. Basically, when evaluating intake and output for 24 hours, these values will be approximately equal, allowing for some margin of difference. In instances that are critical to the maintenance of health, a basic measurement of fluid loss or gain is taken by weighing the person at the same time each day. Related to fluid balance, the person is assessed for conditions that can affect the fluid and electrolyte balance of the body. Examples are losses of fluids via other routes such as liquid stools, nasogastric tube drainage, emesis, or insensible loss occurring with high body temperature. Fluid, electrolytes, and acid–base balance are discussed in greater detail in Chapter 11.

Immediate Environment

In assessing the immediate environmental stimuli, the nurse observes for factors that can influence the person's ability to void, such as the maintenance or lack of privacy to void; temperature and comfort of the room; availability of the toilet, bedpan, or urinal; and the position the person requires to void. For example, the male who is unable to stand to void may have difficulty adapting his usual pattern within this environmental change.

Medications

Another immediate influence to consider is medications the person may be taking that can influence the color or amount of urine. For example, certain vitamins and Pyridium can cause dark orange urine, and diuretics increase the amount of urine excreted.

Pain and Coping

When the person has pain or discomfort with urination, the nurse assesses both the factors influencing the pain and the coping strategies the person uses to deal with the pain. For example, one stimulus influencing pain could be mucosal irritation caused by recent removal of a urinary catheter or by a cystoscopy examination. The presence of a urinary tract infection can also be a source of pain. The nurse also considers the person's ability to cope with ineffective behaviors such as burning or pain with urination.

How these behaviors have affected the voiding pattern and how they are coped with are assessed. For example, the person may use sitz baths, or avoid voiding. For behaviors indicating retention, incontinence, difficulty starting or stopping the stream of urine, or dribbling, the effect of these alterations on the person's activities of daily living and social relations is assessed. Predisposing factors that make the urinary behaviors better or worse are noted. For example, urinary incontinence may be precipitated by laughing, coughing, stress, activity, and so forth. The nurse assesses what coping strategies are being used presently and if the person feels that they are effective or ineffective.

Usual Elimination Pattern

A key assessment factor is the person's usual daily urinary elimination pattern. The usual pattern is noted and its effect on and comparison with the behaviors observed are assessed. A change in the present pattern from the person's normal patterns is particularly important. In assessing usual patterns, the nurse is aware of any altered means of elimination such as a urinary catheter or ureterostomy.

Stress

Stress may be present as a focal or contextual stimulus in the daily pattern or for a currently observed behavior. The nurse thus assesses for physical or psychological states that can stimulate or hinder urination. For example, under anxious or stressful situations, a person may notice a feeling of urgency to void, although the bladder has just been emptied. Another example is fear of a recurring painful experience from urinating. In this case, the person develops muscular tension, which inhibits relaxation of the perineal muscles that promote urination.

Family and Culture

As with bowel elimination, there may be family and cultural beliefs concerning the need, schedule, and particular circumstances for emptying the bladder. The nurse identifies these beliefs as contextual stimuli.

Developmental Stage

The age of the person is also an important contextual stimulus affecting urinary elimination. For example, the young child may lack sphincter control or not yet be toilet trained. With the natural aging process, there are generalized circulatory changes, and blood flow to the kidneys can be diminished due to a decrease in cardiac output. Therefore, renal function may decrease. With aging, the pelvic floor muscles become weakened and the supporting connective tissue alters, causing the bladder to become funnel shaped. This change can result in bladder wall irritability. There can also be decreased bladder capacity due to its inability to elongate.

Therefore, the aging person may present behaviors of frequency, incontinence, retention, and dysuria (Phipps, Long, & Woods, 1991). Another example would be an elderly male who has frequency of voiding accompanied by problems in initiating and ending the stream of urine. This can be due to prostatic enlargement with resultant urinary retention. Also, the elderly female with relaxation of the perineal muscles may present behaviors of stress incontinence.

► COMPENSATORY ADAPTIVE RESPONSES

Viewed as an adaptive system (see Chap. 2), the person has innate and acquired ways of responding to the changing environment. Further, Roy conceptualizes these complex adaptive dynamics as the coping processes of the regulator and cognator subsystems. The basic life processes described in this chapter are intestinal elimination and urinary elimination. However, when the processes of elimination are not integrated, then the regulator and cognator control mechanisms activate processes of compensation. Here we return to Canon (1932), the physiologist who used the term "the wisdom of the body" to describe the automatic self-regulation of physiologic processes. This is a useful phrase when studying Roy's concept of the regulator subsystem.

Further, the thinking and feeling person, by way of cognator activity, can do much to affect any need of the physiologic mode, elimination included. Regulator and cognator abilities, then, are important internal stimuli for the person. These subsystems initiate compensatory adaptive responses that extend the effectiveness of behavior in reaching the goals of adaptation, including higher adaptation levels.

Compensatory abilities that respond to elimination needs include both automatic homeostatic functions of the regulator and voluntary, or conscious, activities of the cognator. The nurse needs to understand as fully as possible the wisdom of the body to identify and interpret changes in the patient's condition. Study of physiology and pathophysiology are important to this understanding. One particular illustration of a regulator activity was described by Marieb (1994, p. 419). When a person's diet is lacking in bulk, the colon narrows and its circular muscles contract more powerfully to effectively move the contents along the length of the colon.

The micturition reflex is a completely automatic spinal cord reflex. It is the basic initiator of urination, but the higher brain centers normally exert final control. According to Guyton (1992), these include strong facilitatory and inhibitory centers in the brain stem, probably located in the pons and several centers located in the cerebral cortex, which are mainly inhibitory but can, at times, become excitatory. The higher centers keep the micturition reflex inhibited when micturition is not desired. They can also facilitate it when desired, and can inhibit the closure of the external urinary sphincter so that urination can occur.

An illustration of a compensatory response to elimination by way of the cognator is the conscious cognitive process through which a person voluntarily controls intestinal elimination. We are familiar with the processes undertaken to toilet train young children. In a toddler, the nervous system develops to the point that the child learns to control both urinary and intestinal elimination. For example, in bowel training, the child learns to inhibit contraction of the external anal sphincter and thereby allow defecation to occur or to contract the sphincter if the time is not socially acceptable for defecation to occur. If the sphincter is kept contracted, the defecation reflex can die out after a few minutes. Usually it does not return until an additional amount of feces enters the rectum, possibly several hours later.

In some situations where persons have lost control over their elimination processes, through either disease or injury, it is possible to implement bowel training (often in combination with bladder training). Here, individuals learn to regulate their elimination by understanding their normal pattern of defecation, regulating the amount of fiber and fluid in their diet, and using perineal exercises. Many have been able to regulate their elimination patterns through cognitive mechanisms even though they have lost the ability to neurologically control these processes.

► COMPROMISED PROCESSES OF ELIMINATION

Changes in adaptation levels and adaptation problems can be caused by difficulties in any or all of the processes of elimination since intestinal and urinary elimination, and other means of elimination of wastes from the body, are all interdependent. Two specific examples of compromised processes of elimination, constipation and urinary retention, will be discussed.

Constipation

One of the most common adaptation problems of elimination is *constipation*. However, as Burrell et al. (1997, p. 1368) indicate, the concept has a variety of meanings. Although generally understood as a change in bowel habits involving either a decrease in frequency or stools that are harder in consistency and difficult to expel, constipation, by definition, refers to a stool frequency of less than three per week.

Constipation can result from a number of factors including dietary change, decreased fluid intake, lack of dietary fiber, lack of physical activity, or ignoring the urge to defecate. As Burrell et al. (1997) described, "when the urge to defecate is ignored, the rectal contents are returned to the sigmoid colon. Prolonged retention of feces in the colon can lead to drying of the stool through reabsorption of the water content. Gradually, the normal response to rectal filling becomes dulled, and chronic constipation can occur as the gastrocolic reflex weakens" (p. 1369).

The intervention for constipation is determined by the underlying cause. Dietary fiber, fluid, and exercise all influence the consistency of stool and the stimulation of peristalsis. Adequate levels of each of these factors assist in decreasing the incidence of constipation for many individuals. If an organic disorder is present, medical management of the primary problem may be required. Laxatives, suppositories, and enemas can be used to treat the symptoms but it is important that the underlying cause be identified and addressed.

Urinary Retention

The inability to void, with resultant accumulation of urine within the bladder, is known as *urinary retention*. The absence of voided urine due to retention is to be distinguished from *anuria*, complete suppression of urine formation by the kidneys, or *oliguria,* diminished urine secretion in relation to fluid intake. Possible causes of urinary retention include obstruction at or below the bladder outlet, spinal or general anesthesia, muscular tension, emotional anxiety, and medications such as sedatives, opiates, psychotropic drugs, and antispasmodics, which interfere with the normal neurologic function of the voiding reflex.

Besides the absence of voided urine, in retention, the nurse may assess a distended bladder. As the bladder fills with urine, it rises above the level of the symphysis pubis and can be displaced to either side of the midline. The person may report increasing discomfort and pain, which can be accompanied by increased blood pressure. Patients who are unable to communicate or are confused may become restless. When the cause is neurologic dysfunction, the person may not sense the fullness of the bladder.

Nursing activities related to urinary retention are focused on prevention and reduction of risk, particularly as related to postoperative patients. Measures including encouraging postoperative physical activity, positioning, allowing adequate time, relaxation exercises, running water, positive reassurance, or warm water poured over the perineum may promote urination and prevent retention. When preventive nursing measures are unsuccessful, one-time catheterization may be required to prevent subsequent complications.

▶ PLANNING NURSING CARE

Intestinal and urinary elimination are priority requirements for the person's physiologic adaptation. In applying the nursing process, the nurse will make a careful assessment of behaviors and stimuli related to these basic life processes. In assessing factors influencing intestinal and urinary elimination, regulator and cognator effectiveness in initiating compensatory processes will be considered. Based on this thorough first- and second-level assessment, the nurse makes a nursing diagnosis, sets goals, selects interventions, and evaluates care.

Nursing Diagnosis

Assessment data of behaviors and related stimuli are interpreted and used in establishing a nursing diagnosis. The nurse prepared to use the Roy Adaptation Model of nursing can state diagnoses as specific behaviors with the stimuli that are most relevant. Some examples have already been given, such as the example of involuntary release of urine related to relaxed muscles in an elderly person.

Roy has developed a typology of indicators of positive adaptation related to intestinal and urinary elimination (see Table 3–2). Included in the typology are effective homeostatic bowel processes, stable pattern of bowel elimination, effective processes of urine formation, stable pattern of urine elimination, and effective coping strategies for altered elimination. Chapter 3 demonstrated the importance of recognizing situations of effective adaptation so that these can be maintained or enhanced. A nursing diagnosis addressing an indicator of positive adaptation could be, "Stable pattern of urine elimination following surgery due to early ambulation and relaxed surroundings."

Commonly recurring adaptation problems as defined within the Roy Adaptation Model include diarrhea, bowel or urinary incontinence, constipation, urinary retention, flatulence, and ineffective coping strategies for altered elimination. *Diarrhea* is defined as a state in which the person experiences a change in normal bowel habits characterized by the frequent passage of loose, fluid, unformed stools. When the person presents with behaviors of diarrhea, abdominal cramping and tenesmus (ineffectual and painful straining) may also occur. Frequently, diagnostic procedures or laboratory tests may be necessary to determine the exact cause and other related influencing factors.

Bowel and *bladder incontinence* refers to the involuntary passage of stool or urine. Excessive gas in the stomach and intestines is termed *flatulence* and may be accompanied by abdominal distention. Certain foods contribute to the formation of excessive gas and should be reduced or eliminated from the diet.

The use of a summary label to develop a nursing diagnosis when more than one mode is being affected by the same stimulus is often an effective way of communicating a cluster of behaviors to experienced nurses. For example, "urinary incontinence related to spinal cord damage" might be such a diagnosis because the nurse would be immediately aware that the person's physical self-concept, role function, and interdependence modes would also be involved. After extensive, successful rehabilitation, a person with such injuries might have the diagnosis of, "effective coping strategies for altered elimination due to successful bladder and bowel training." In Table 7–1, the Roy

TABLE 7–1 NURSING DIAGNOSTIC CATEGORIES FOR ELIMINATION

Positive Indicators of Adaptation	Common Adaptation Problems	NANDA Diagnostic Labels
• Effective homeostatic bowel process	• Diarrhea	• Diarrhea
	• Flatulence	
• Stable pattern of bowel elimination	• Bowel incontinence	• Bowel incontinence
	• Constipation	• Colonic constipation
		• Perceived constipation
		• Constipation
• Effective processes of urine formation		
• Stable pattern of urine elimination	• Urinary incontinence	• Stress incontinence
		• Functional incontinence
		• Reflex incontinence
		• Urge incontinence
		• Total incontinence
	• Urinary retention	• Urinary retention
• Effective coping strategies for altered elimination	• Ineffective coping strategies for altered elimination	• Altered urinary elimination pattern
		• Toileting self-care deficit

model nursing diagnostic categories for the physiologic need of elimination are shown in relation to nursing diagnosis labels approved by the North American Nursing Diagnosis Association (Rantz & LeMone, 1997).

Consider the following example. Mr. Beard is a 72-year-old man with a medical diagnosis of benign prostatic hypertrophy, a noncancerous enlargement of the prostate gland that has necessitated surgical intervention of a transurethral prostatectomy. Following the surgical procedure, he had an indwelling Foley catheter that was in place for 48 hours and has been removed in preparation for discharge. It has been 6 hours since the catheter removal and he has not yet voided. He is expressing anxiety about the situation and is experiencing some pain, and his bladder is now palpable above the symphysis pubis. A nursing diagnosis in this situation could be, "Urinary retention following catheter removal possibly due to urethral edema."

Goal Setting

Based on thorough assessment and understanding of adaptation problems related to elimination, the nurse sets goals in terms of outcomes for the person. A complete goal statement includes the behavior of focus, the change expected, and the time frame in which the goal is to be achieved. For example, for the person experiencing the adaptation problem of constipation related to poor normal bowel habits, the long-term goal may be, "within 2 weeks, the person will establish a regular pattern of bowel movements." An initial short-term goal could be that during the next week, the person would identify the best time of day for bowel elimination. This would take into consideration personal patterns of mass movements of the large bowel and the individual's life activities. An attempt for the person to reach this goal effectively may include drinking either hot liquid or fruit juice to facilitate normal evacuation on 3 days of the week.

In the previous example of Mr. Beard, the goal would focus on the behavior of urinary retention. A short-term goal may be, "In the next 30 minutes, Mr. Beard will have passed at least 30 mL of urine." The behavior in this goal is passing urine, the change relates to the amount (30 mL as opposed to none), and the time frame is within 30 minutes.

Intervention

The intervention step of the nursing process according to the Roy Adaptation Model depends on the identified stimuli as the nurse either promotes or reinforces the stimuli or takes action to change or delete them. In some instances, direct intervention by way of the regulator and cognator processes is possible. Interventions for the common adaptation problems related to elimination will be discussed in this section.

For the problem of constipation, general interventions include increasing fluid intake to ensure adequate hydration; exercise; providing a diet that is adequate in residue, including increasing the intake of fruits, juices, bulk-producing vegetables, and bran cereals; and responding to the urge to defecate to prevent additional reabsorption of water from the stool, thus avoiding hard, dry stools.

Setting time aside to evacuate the bowel (for example, 30 minutes after the morning meal) or drinking a warm beverage or water early in the morning can help to initiate a bowel movement for some people. In learning healthy habits, chronic laxative use is avoided, for this abuse can lead to atonic bowel syndrome. However, if other conservative measures fail, the occasional use of a laxative to stimulate peristalsis and bowel evacuation may be indicated.

Interventions should be directed toward those identified causes when intervening for the problem of diarrhea. Other interventions include avoidance or elimination of allergic dietary substances or drugs that promote loose, watery stools. Many persons are aware of the foods that cause diarrhea, for example, alcoholic beverages, highly caffeinated liquids such as coffee, or rich pastries high in sugar content.

With mild cases of diarrhea, nothing but clear liquids, such as water, tea, carbonated beverages, bouillon broth, and sweet fruit juices, is taken during the first 12 hours. Citrus juices are avoided, as well as cold liquids and concentrated sweets, which are poorly tolerated. During the next 12 hours, more foods, such as toast, soda crackers, and uncreamed soups may be added. After the stool begins to firm, other bland foods can be added, with gradual advancement to the person's regular diet.

With more severe cases of diarrhea, fluid and electrolyte replacement may be necessary, or the person may need administration of medication to decrease peristalsis and relieve abdominal cramping. Medical treatment of diarrhea is discussed in texts concerned with pathophysiology. The person with diarrhea is provided with an atmosphere conducive to relaxation and rest. The anal region is cleansed with mild soap and water after each movement to reduce local irritation and discomfort.

When anal incontinence (the inability of the anal sphincter to control the passage of stool) is present, a bowel training program may be initiated. It is important to set aside a consistent time for evacuation. Hot fluids may be given, followed by a glycerine suppository, or for some, the insertion of a gloved finger into the rectum will provide enough stimulation. The person should then attempt evacuation and allow adequate time.

In addition, the person should be encouraged to follow many of the interventions outlined in the section addressing constipation, such as adequate fluid intake, a diet high in roughage, and the intake of fruit juices.

Incontinent persons may be embarrassed and have emotional distress. Special nursing care includes support and understanding, as well as measures to reduce possible skin irritation, odor, and the soiling of clothing and linen.

For urinary retention, as in Mr. Beard's situation, interventions include early ambulation following surgery, acquiring a sitting position or a standing posture in the male, providing the person with privacy, listening to the sound of running water, dangling the hands in warm water, pouring warm water over the perineum or sitting in a warm bath to promote perineal muscle relaxation, or any other measure that might promote relaxation. If these measures fail, medications can be employed to promote the ease of voiding. Ultimately, bladder catheterization may be required.

A complete diagnostic workup is done to identify the causative and contributing stimuli for the adaptation problem of incontinence. If stress incontinence is present, the person tries to avoid excessive straining or conditions such as chronic coughing. Weight reduction and pelvic exercises are helpful in regaining bladder control. Kegel exercises increase the tone of the perineal muscles. Instruct the person to contract the perineal muscles as though trying to stop the flow of urine. This should be done 10 to 15 times per session at least four times a day. Also, the person should try to start and stop the stream of urine when voiding.

A bladder training program may be required, which includes an adequate intake of fluids, strengthening exercises for the perineal muscles, and a definite schedule set aside for voiding. The intake of fluids should be carefully spaced throughout the day and limited before sleep to promote adequate rest. The person is encouraged to void every 30 minutes to 2 hours, and as the program progresses, the urine is held for longer periods of time. As with anal incontinence, nursing care should include supportive measures to decrease emotional stress and possible skin irritation. (Additional information on nursing management of incontinence is found in basic nursing texts and in textbooks on neuroscience nursing and care of the elderly.)

Evaluation

Evaluation involves judging the effectiveness of the nursing interventions in relation to the person's adaptive behavior. Whether or not the patient has attained the behavior stated in the goal is identified. The nursing interventions would be identified as effective if the person's behavior is in accordance with the stated goal. If the goal has not been achieved, the nurse identifies alternative interventions or approaches by reassessing the behavior and stimuli and continuing with the other steps of the nursing process.

Consider the example given earlier of a short-term goal set with the person with constipation. In 1 week, the person has identified that prior to breakfast is the best time of day for bowel elimination. He consumed a cup of hot decaffeinated coffee after he awoke and had prune juice with breakfast. During the week, he had four bowel evacuations in the morning that were hard but expelled without undue difficulty. At this point, another short-term goal would be set. This would be to add other contextual factors to create good bowel habits, such as drinking more fluids, getting more exercise, and a consuming diet higher in residue.

In Mr. Beard's situation, evaluation of the success of interventions would be focused on his ability to void within the 30-minute time period. If he has been able to produce at least 30 mL of urine, the goal would have been achieved and a new goal established to continue to monitor the situation. If he was not able to void, another intervention may be initiated such as a one-time catheterization.

► SUMMARY

This chapter focused on the application of the Roy Adaptation Model to the physiologic need of elimination with particular attention to intestinal and urinary elimination. An overview of these basic life processes was provided along with the identification of parameters for assessment of behaviors and stimuli. Illustration of adaptive compensatory processes related to elimination were described and examples of two compromised processes (constipation and urinary retention) were provided. Finally, guidelines for planning nursing care through the formulation of nursing diagnoses, goals, and interventions were explored and evaluation of nursing care was described.

► EXERCISES FOR APPLICATION

1. Assess the bowel elimination behaviors of a child, adolescent, adult, and elderly person. Relate the stimuli of age for each person to the assessed behaviors.

2. Develop a teaching plan to help a person utilize strategies to cope with the adaptation problem of urinary incontinence.

► ASSESSMENT OF UNDERSTANDING

Questions

1. Designate each of the following statements as related to either intestinal elimination (I) or urinary elimination (U).
   (a) _____ elimination of fluid wastes and excess ions
   (b) _____ defecation reflex and conscious sphincter control
   (c) _____ works to balance body fluids and electrolytes
   (d) _____ expulsion of undigestible substances
   (e) _____ excretion of the end products of body metabolism

2. List three first level assessment parameters (behaviors) that are related to intestinal elimination and three related to urinary elimination.
   (a) _____   (d) _____
   (b) _____   (e) _____
   (c) _____   (f) _____

3. Discuss stimuli that can influence peristalsis and relate these to your understanding of the processes involved in movements of the intestines.

4. Label the following compensatory processes as indicative of regulator (R) or cognator (C) activity.
   (a) _____ narrowing of colon in response to diet lacking in bulk
   (b) _____ voluntary control of micturition

(c) _____ powerful contraction of circular muscles of the colon
(d) _____ bowel training after spinal cord injury
(e) _____ regulation of elimination patterns through diet and exercise

5. Name and describe one situation of compromised elimination.

6. State a potential nursing diagnosis related to urinary elimination for a patient after surgery.

7. Identify two interventions that help a person cope with increased flatulence.
(a) _____
(b) _____

8. If a suggested nursing intervention has not been effective in meeting the goal established with the patient to meet elimination needs, discuss how the nurse will proceed based on the Adaptation Model nursing process.

Feedback

1. (a) U, (b) I, (c) U, (d) I, (e) U

2. Intestinal elimination behaviors: (a) amount and characteristics of stool, (b) bowel sounds, (c) pain.
   Urinary elimination behaviors: (d) amount and characteristics of urine, (e) frequency and urgency, (f) pain.

3. Factors that maintain or increase peristalsis include the person's daily activity level or pattern of exercise. Factors that decrease peristalsis include bed rest, immobility, or recent anesthesia. Movements of the intestines are both mixing and propulsive types. Mixing movements aid in absorption functions and propulsive movements move waste products toward elimination. General increase of muscle activity and related neurologic activity promotes such movement, thus facilitating bowel elimination.

4. (a) R, (b) C, (c) R, (d) C, (e) C

5. One example of compromised elimination is urinary retention. This means that the person is unable to void urine that has been collected in the bladder. Possible causes include obstruction at or below the bladder outlet, spinal or general anesthesia, muscular tension, emotional anxiety, and medications.

6. Example of a nursing diagnosis: Urinary retention related to recent anesthesia.

7. Any of the following: reduce or eliminate foods that contribute to flatus formation such as beans, cabbage, onions, cauliflower, and milk products; avoid carbonated beverages; avoid swallowing excessive air; and increase activity level.

8. The nurse will return to the earlier steps of the process to see if the assessment is accurate and complete, the diagnosis is appropriate, the goal is realistic, and the interventions are adequate.

▶ **REFERENCES**

Burrell, L. O., Gerlach, M. J. M., & Pless, B. S. (1997). *Adult nursing: Acute and community care* (2nd ed.). Stamford, CT: Appleton & Lange.

Canon, W. (1932). *The wisdom of the body.* New York: Norton.

Guyton, A. (1992). *Human physiology and mechanisms of disease* (5th ed.). Philadelphia: Saunders.

Marieb, E. N. (1994). *Essentials of human anatomy and physiology* (4th ed.). Redwood City, CA: Benjamin/Cummings.

Phipps, W., Long, B., & Woods, N. (1998). *Medical-surgical nursing: Concepts and clinical practice* (5th ed.). St. Louis: Mosby.

Rantz, M. J., & LeMone, P. (Eds.). (1997). *Classification of nursing diagnoses. Proceedings of the 12th conference NANDA.* Glendale, CA: CINAHL Information Systems.

▶ **ADDITIONAL REFERENCES**

Ellickson, E. (1988). Bowel management plan for homebound elderly. *Geronontology Nursing, 14(1),* 16–19.

Linton, A. D., Matteson, M. A., & Maebius, N. K. (1995). *Introductory nursing care of adults.* Philadelphia: Saunders.

Maresca, T. (1986). Assessment and management of acute diarrhea illness in adults. *Nurse Practitioner, 11(11),* 15–16.

McShane, R., & McLane, A. (1988). Constipation: Impact of etiological factors. *Journal of Gerontology Nursing, 14(4),* 31–34.

Resnick, B. (1985). Constipation: Common but preventable. *Geriatric Nurse, 6(4),* 213–215.

Sparks, S. M., & Taylor, C. M. (1995). *Nursing diagnosis reference manual* (3rd ed.). Springhouse, PA: Springhouse.

8

ACTIVITY AND REST

Activity and rest are basic needs in the physiologic mode. Through activity, persons go about daily living and present who they are within the environment. Activity also provides the physical stresses on body structures that promote normal growth and development. Rest, on the other hand, provides periods of restoration, repair, renewal of energies, and effectiveness of life processes.

Two basic life processes that act to maintain an appropriate balance in both activity and rest are mobility and sleep. These two processes are the focus of this chapter. Assessment of behaviors and stimuli related to the needs of activity and rest are outlined based on an understanding of the two life processes. Innate and learned compensating strategies that act to maintain adaptation and health are discussed. Examples of compromised processes of activity and rest are identified, with particular focus on the effects of immobility and sleep deprivation. Finally, guidelines for planning nursing care based on nursing diagnoses, goals, and nursing interventions are described. Emphasis is placed on the overall goal of preventing problems with activity and rest and promoting health in this physiologic mode component.

▶ OBJECTIVES

After studying this chapter, the reader will be able to do the following:

1. Describe the basic life processes associated with activity and rest.

2. Identify important first-level assessment parameters (behaviors) for the needs of activity and rest.

3. List second-level assessment parameters (common stimuli) affecting activity and rest.

4. Describe one compensatory process related to the needs of activity and rest.

5. Name and describe two situations of compromised processes of activity and rest.

6. Develop a nursing diagnosis, given a situation related to activity and rest.

7. Derive goals for an individual with ineffective activity and rest in a given situation.

8. Describe nursing interventions commonly implemented in situations of ineffective activity and rest.

9. Propose approaches to determine the effectiveness of nursing interventions.

► KEY CONCEPTS DEFINED

Activity: Body movement that serves various purposes such as carrying out daily living chores and protecting self or others from injury.

Activity intolerance: A state in which an individual has insufficient physiologic or psychological energy to endure or complete required or desired daily activities.

Disuse consequences: Changes in major body functions that result from a period of physical inactivity.

Disuse syndrome: The potential negative effects of curtailed physical activity, particularly when imposed by medical restrictions.

Gait: The manner of walking; the basic means of moving around from place to place.

Limbic system: Brain structures which govern basic biologic drives and emotional behavior by controlling neuroendocrine and autonomic systems through the hypothalmus.

Mobility: The basic life process for activity whereby one moves or is moved.

Nonlimbic structures: The sensory and motor cortex and associative systems.

Posture: Anatomic arrangement of body parts in a given position.

Recreation: A change in activity in which one becomes renewed for other activities.

Rehabilitation: A process through which a person achieves optimal physical, emotional, psychological, social, and vocational potential.

Rest: Changes in activity in which energy requirements are minimal; more generally, refreshing relaxation.

Sleep: The basic life process for rest in which most of the body's physiologic activities slow down to allow renewal of energy for future activity.

Sleep apnea: The periodic cessation of breathing during sleep.

Sleep pattern disturbance: A commonly occurring compromised process associated with the need for rest.

▶ BASIC LIFE PROCESSES OF ACTIVITY AND REST

Activity and rest are both key to human survival; their associated basic life processes are mobility and sleep. *Activity* refers to body movement and serves various purposes such as carrying out daily living chores and protecting self or others from bodily injuries. Mobility is the basic life process for activity. *Recreation* is a change in activity in which one becomes renewed for other activities. *Rest,* on the other hand, involves changes in activity in which energy requirements are minimal. During rest, energy is conserved and restored. *Sleep* is the basic life process for rest in which most of the body's physiologic activities slow down to allow for renewal of energy for future activity.

As more of the institutionalized patient population, as well as people receiving health care at home, is made up of elderly or seriously ill persons, inadequate processes of mobility and their effect become an important focus for nursing care. At the same time, there are increasing numbers of individuals in society whose daily activity leads to stresses that interfere with getting adequate sleep and rest. Because of increasing difficulties in meeting the needs for activity and rest in today's society, the nurse is concerned with assisting persons in meeting these needs, particularly by promoting effective mobility and sleep processes.

▶ MOBILITY: PROCESS AND ASSESSMENT

Mobility is the process whereby one moves or is moved. To move is to change location or position. The body structures of normal movement are the voluntary and autonomic neuromuscular and skeletal systems. About 50 percent of body mass is composed of muscle and 25 percent of bone and connecting structures (Burrell, Gerlach, & Pless, 1997). Muscles act through tension applied at the points of attachment to bones; bones serve as levers. Muscles and bones combine with neurologic inputs to provide locomotion and activity. Nurses note that in addition to intact body systems, mobility also involves the motivation to move and a free, nonrestrictive environment in which to move (Hodges & Callihan, 1988).

In terms of brain function, limbic and nonlimbic structures are involved (see Fig. 8–1). The *limbic system* governs basic biologic drives and emotional behavior by controlling the neuroendocrine and autonomic systems through the hypothalmus, as noted in Chapter 6 in relation to nutrition. A need for motion is generated, and influenced, by the sensorimotor part of the brain. The *nonlimbic structures* consist of sensory and motor cortex and their associative systems.

Brooks (1986) describes a command hierarchy for the control of postures and movements. The highest level operates in the association areas of the cerebral cortex and elaborates perceptions and overall motor plans or strategies. As part of this process, the limbic system denotes what is relevant to the perceived needs of the body. The middle level of the command hierarchy is where strategies are converted into motor programs or tactics. This level involves the sensorimotor cortex, cerebellum, basal ganglia, and brain stem. These programs correlate body equilibrium, movement directions,

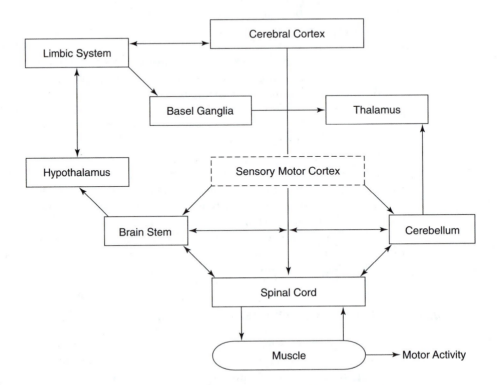

FIGURE 8–1. Central nervous system structures involved in motor activity.

force, and speed, as well as mechanical stiffness of the joints, that is, whether the joints move or are held in one position. Natural movements of everyday life involve several joints and are composed of a series of simple movements that affect only one joint. The lowest level of control is the spinal cord, which translates commands into muscular activity. The spinal cord also regulates movement through stretch reflexes. (Chapters 10 and 12 further describe related sensory and neurologic processes and relevant reviews are found in basic anatomy and physiology texts.) The result of all these structures working in coordination is motor activity.

All of these processes are integrated so intricately that human movement has not yet been duplicated in efforts to built robots. An article in a popular science journal (Dworetzky, 1987) noted:

> It's no wonder movie makers still use people dressed up in robot suits instead of using the real thing. Today's commercial robots don't walk like men [*sic*], actually balancing their bulk, but stay on their feet statically, like tables on wheels. They're incapable of counter-balancing, of shifting their center of gravity to make lifting or pushing more efficient, so they must be over-engineered into glorified forklifts in order to work without toppling over (p. 18).

This type of robot movement was evident to the world in the wide media coverage of the mechanical success of the rover Sojourner, even as it carried out the extraordinary mission of exploring Mars.

For the person, the stress caused by physical movement is essential in maintaining all major body functions. Bones themselves are dynamic tissues that undergo continuous remodeling. Where bone experiences stress, it will increase osteoblastic activities to increase ossification. Bone that is not stressed will have increased osteoclastic activity and bone resorption. Therefore, the musculoskeletal system maintains its bone strength, as well as muscle tone, only if adequate stresses are imposed regularly.

Physical movement also promotes the normal oxygenation process by stimulating cardiovascular circulation and proper lung expansion with mobilization of its secretions. Skeletal movement promotes the normal urinary tract flow and stimulates the gastric mobility that is essential for proper digestion of foods. It also has a positive effect on bowel elimination. Maintenance of normal metabolic rate requires adequate physical stresses to maintain proper equilibrium between catabolic and anabolic activities.

The human dimensions of what it means to a person to plan and carry out movement is noted in a neurologist's account of witnessing patients become suddenly mobile, after years of virtual immobility, after receiving a new treatment for parkinsonian symptoms induced by encephalitis. Sacks (1983) called what he saw in patients "awakenings," and he commented that we are critically dependent on a continual flow of impulses and information to and from all the sensory and motor organs of the body. More poignantly he states, "We must be active or we cease to exist: activity and actuality are one and the same" (p. 302).

Assessment of Behavior

Given the importance of mobility to the person's physical and psychological integrity, the nurse assesses activity needs based on understanding mobility as a human life process. Specific assessment factors are examined to determine the adequacy of mobility level and to identify any existing adverse consequences of immobility. Two major categories of assessment are considered. The first category is the frequency, intensity, and duration of daily physical activity carried out by the person. The second is the assessment of the person's motor function status, which depends on muscle and joint mobility, posture and gait, and coordination.

Physical Activity

The benefits of physical activity for fitness have been widely recognized since the 1950s, when President Eisenhower called attention to this need. Regular exercise by adults has increased in this country since that time. Federal policy and programs on health promotion have continued to emphasize physical exercise. However, current studies show that the majority of people, particularly women, children, low-income populations, and minorities, still do not get enough regular exercise.

Obtaining information on the person's patterns of daily physical activity is important in planning care to avoid the consequences of inadequate activity and to promote health, fitness, and well-being. By observing, discussing, and recording the frequency, intensity, and duration of physical activity, the nurse can judge the adequacy of activity level in relation to the person's total physical condition.

Motor Function

Through assessment of motor function, the nurse determines the type of physical activity the person is capable of performing and identifies consequences of inactivity.

Functional Assessments. The types of physical activity that the person can perform are evaluated by functional assessments. Specific instruments developed for functional assessment are divided into three basic categories: global instruments for comprehensive assessments; activities of daily living scales; and functional profiles, which assess limitations due to a specific condition or evaluate a single function such as use of a hand or the ability to climb stairs (Hollerbach, 1988). Of particular significance is whether or not a person is capable of performing self-care activities. Assessment of muscle mass and tone and joint mobility is accomplished through active or passive demonstration of the range of motion. All active movements, such as lifting, pushing, and pulling, require muscle contractions.

Muscles Mass and Tone. Muscle mass (size) and tone (firmness) are assessed by grasping the center of the muscle and feeling that it is firm, supple, and full-bellied. In the older person, it is expected that there is less shape and contour of major muscles. In the child, muscles are softer and have less mass.

Muscle Strength. Muscle strength varies widely according to age and training. Strength is tested by asking the person to move using certain muscles, using resistance, or holding an instrument still while the examiner tries to move it. An example is testing flexion and extension at the elbow by having the patient pull and push against the examiner's hand. Levels of strength are commonly scaled from 0 (no muscular contraction either seen or felt) to 5 (normal muscle strength). Table 8–1 describes commonly used levels of strength. Generally, a muscle strength rated below 3 is considered indicative of disability.

Joint Mobility. Joint mobility is assessed by an active or passive demonstration of each joint's range of motion. The range of motion is the direction and degree a joint is capable of moving. This varies for different joints, for example, the ankle moves by flexing about 50 degrees and extending about 20 degrees, whereas the hip can flex as much as 135 degrees, extend 28 degrees, abduct 50 degrees, and adduct about 30 degrees as well as rotate (see Fig. 8–2). Some expected limitation of joint mobility occurs with aging. When there is good mobility, bones move freely and smoothly without pain (Mourad, 1986).

Posture. The anatomic arrangement of body parts in a given position is called *posture*. Correct posture is a factor in physical safety since inappropriately aligned muscles and joints during activity can result in injury or deformity. Good posture is body alignment that permits optimal weight balance and operation of motor function. In the upright standing position, the head, shoulders, and pelvis are aligned; the arms hang freely from the shoulders; and the feet are aligned with toes pointing straight ahead (see Fig. 8–3). A person's preferred posture is a significant behavioral indicator since deviations from good posture may be indicative of some dysfunction. For example, a person with obstructive lung disease tends to lean forward with arms braced.

Gait. *Gait* is the manner of walking and provides the basic means of moving around from place to place. The nurse assesses whether or not the person walks

TABLE 8–1   LEVELS OF MUSCLE STRENGTH

Grade	Strength
5	Free range of motion against normal resistance and gravity
4	Full range of motion against moderate resistance and gravity
3	Full range of motion against gravity only
2	Full range of motion with gravity eliminated
1	Slight muscle contraction palpable, but no movement noted
0	No visible or palpable contraction; paralysis of limb

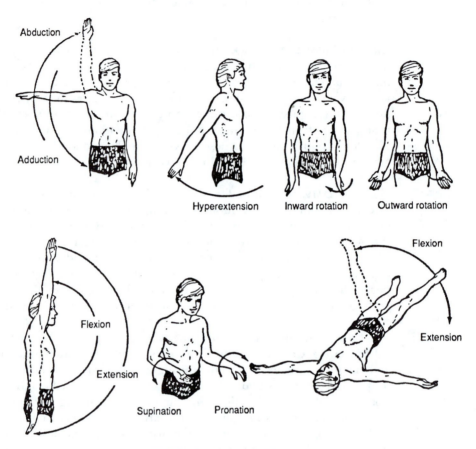

FIGURE 8–2. Range of motion movements.

easily and comfortably, with self-assurance, good balance, and symmetry of movement. Is there the presence of a limp, pain or discomfort, fear of falling, loss of balance, difference in movement from one side to the other, or unusual movements? A deviation in gait can impose undue stress on certain musculoskeletal parts and, in time, lead to deformity. For example, when a patient is using a "swing through" gait on crutches, the movement is not the same as normal walking; it will eventually result in weakening of the lower extremities. A proper gait with good posture will allow a safe and optimal level of mobility.

Motor Coordination. Good motor coordination requires both intact neurologic and musculoskeletal function and will have an effect on the person's activity status, particularly self-care activities. Coordination is easily tested by having the person perform rapidly alternating movements such as placing one foot on the opposite knee and sliding it down that shin to the big toe or moving a finger from the examiner's finger to one's own nose. A child as young as

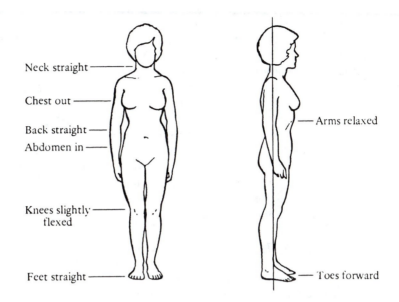

Neck straight

Chest out

Back straight

Abdomen in

Knees slightly
flexed

Feet straight

Arms relaxed

Toes forward

FIGURE 8–3. Correct standing position.

6 years can easily do these tasks. (Further details on assessing each of these aspects of motor function can be found in texts on physical assessment.)

Assessment of Stimuli

Along with the behavioral assessment of activity needs, the nurse assesses the stimuli affecting these needs and how they are being met. Some of the categories of possible stimuli are physical condition, current psychological condition, the surroundings, and personal habits related to activity. These factors act together and are assessed as the pattern of stimuli affecting the person.

Physical Condition

For activity needs, disruptions in the structure and function of the musculoskeletal system are physical conditions that act as key focal stimuli affecting the person. Such disruptions can occur by either direct physical injuries to muscles and bones or by central nervous system disorders. Regardless of the underlying causative factor, a dysfunctioning musculoskeletal system will cause a direct and immediate effect on motor function. A fractured bone will inevitably necessitate a limitation of physical activity due not only to the loss of function, but also to the discomfort and pain experienced. A person with an illness, depending on the nature and severity of the condition, will limit physical mobility either voluntarily or because of medically imposed restrictions. Bed rest is often an integral part of therapeutic treatment because rest provides a period of restoration and repair. Particular concerns for planning nursing care when the person is on bed rest will be addressed later in this chapter.

Psychological Condition

Besides intact physical abilities, it was noted earlier that activity involves the motivation to move. Motivation is a psychological condition and includes knowledge about activity and its beneficial effects for health. A situation in which misinformation is a focal stimulus for inactivity is that of a new mother on a postpartum unit who does not get out of bed to take a shower. With further assessment, the nurse might learn that the mother's cultural background taught her not to move out of bed for several days following giving birth. Psychologically depressed persons tend to reduce their physical activity to a bare minimum. The catatonic state of a psychotic individual exemplifies this case to the extreme. In a catatonic state, the individual is not able to initiate body movements, even though physical and physiologic dysfunction cannot be demonstrated.

Surroundings

A free, nonrestrictive environment in which to move is required for physical activity. A suitable environment for activity includes availability of space and adequate physical and personal assistance. Unsuitable factors, such as adverse environmental temperature and surroundings, will act to restrict the person's activity. For example, encouraging daily walks for a person after a heart attack, or for health promotion and fitness for a working professional person, will be ineffective if the person is contending with severe winter weather conditions and has no indoor alternative, or if the neighborhood seems to be an unsafe place to walk. Lack of privacy can also be a focal or contextual stimulus. A person may be reluctant to do exercises on a mat or in a swimming pool of a busy physical therapy department. A child placed in a playpen will have a restricted range of physical activity which, over time, could affect the child's normal growth and development.

Personal Habits

Any motivational or conditional factors that last over a period of time can affect the individual's personal habits related to activity. The effect of a habit, or accustomed pattern of behavior, can be a strong influence in a given situation. If a health care worker has the habit of doing physical aerobic exercise every day, finding a way to exercise when away from home for business or a holiday will be a high priority. Helping others to overcome poor habits related to levels of activity is an important health promotion effort for the nurse.

▶ SLEEP: PROCESS AND ASSESSMENT

Rest needs are as important as the need for activity, and sleep is an important life process for obtaining rest. *Rest* generally means changes in activity in which energy requirements are minimal. It is the prelude to sleep. However, rest can also be thought of in a broader context of refreshing relaxation. In the latter meaning, rest is not defined as mere physical inactivity. Rest includes the quality of relaxation that comes with freedom from physical discomfort and psychological stresses such as anxiety. Most notably, rest is an individualized matter. What leads to relaxation and restoration of energy will vary from person to person. Rest may be changing activity, such as taking a walk during a lunch break at work. Vacation and other kinds of recreation also provide rest. For some individuals, rest is best attained while doing nothing—sitting outside watching the ocean, beside a fireplace indoors in winter, or watching raindrops on the window in spring.

During rest, physiologic processes slow down to allow renewal of energy. Physiologically, heart rate recovery is greatest at the beginning of a rest period. Thus, it is suggested that several short rest periods rather than one long, extended period are more effective. Industrial studies suggest that 15 percent of work time be given to rest, with increases of 20 to 30 percent in evenly distributed times for strenuous work loads.

Most rest is accomplished through the basic life process of sleep, with human beings spending an average of one third of their lives sleeping. Behaviorally, rest becomes sleep when the ability to respond to minute environmental stimuli is diminished. Sleep is a rhythmic and active life process with defined stages. Physiologically, sleep is defined by polygraph criteria that include cortical activity scored from electroencephalogram (EEG) waveforms, muscle activity noted on the electromyogram (EMG), and eye movements recorded by electro-oculogram (EOG). Standardized terminology, techniques, and a scoring system are used to define the stages of sleep in the adult (Rechtschaffen & Kales, 1973) and in the child (Anders & Parmelee, 1971). During a typical night of 7 to 8 hours of sleep, the person goes through several cycles of sleep in an orderly sequence of stages approximately every 60 to 90 minutes. Stages 1 through 4 are called the NREM (nonrapid eye movement) phase, and stage 5 is called the REM phase because of the rapid eye movements characteristic of this stage. This pattern of sleep, including occurrence, timing, and duration of stages, is called the architecture of sleep.

Generally, the night's sleep begins with the lights out and less than 20 minutes of awake time. A period of drowsiness, stage 1, follows and will reoccur at intervals throughout the night, especially to begin a new sleep cycle. Stage 1 makes up less than 1 to 5 percent of the night. A person is easily aroused during this stage and if awakened, will state that they were not asleep. In stage 2 there is increased muscular relaxation and several cortical changes, including low-voltage activity and bursts of sleep spindles. The person's ability to respond spontaneously to stimuli is further diminished. Stages 3 and 4 are the deeper levels of sleep, also known as delta sleep, or slow wave sleep (SWS). The percentage of particular waveforms differentiates the two stages. The fourth stage is actually deep sleep in which one may be able to respond only to strong stimuli. Bed wetting in children usually takes place during this stage because of an inability to respond to internal stimuli as well as external stimuli. Following the fourth stage, the cycle usually reverses, returning to stage 2 before entering stage 5, the REM phase of sleep. On the EEG, REM sleep looks much the same as the awake state. However, the characteristic eye movements are both phasic and tonic (high number of movements and periods of fewer movements). These movements can be observed through the closed eyelids as well as on the EOG.

During sleep, the person's physiology differs significantly from that when awake (Robinson, 1993). The cardiovascular, respiratory, and gastrointestinal systems are most affected. Other alterations include cerebral blood flow, metabolism, temperature regulation, and endocrine and renal function. These effects differ in the various stages of sleep and are based on the characteristics of sleep. For example, with the loss of wakefulness, neural control of respiration changes as the cortical component is lost and metabolic control predominates. The result may be normal variations, such as rapid or irregular breathing, or abnormal responses such as snoring or obstructive apnea.

Beginning in stage 1, there is decreased activity in vital bodily functions such as heart rate, temperature, respiration, and basal metabolic rate. During the deep sleep that starts with stage 3, the basic metabolic rate is decreased by 10 to 20 percent. This is demonstrated by a drop in body temperature, heart rate, and blood pressure. Muscle tone becomes atonic. The skin may become flushed and warm, with mild diaphoresis. Blood pressure decreases during stages 3 and 4. It is believed that during stage 4, growth hormone is released and there is a decreased concentration of corticosteroids. These changes seem to promote protein synthesis, which assists in restoration and repair of biologic structures and functions (Oswald, 1976).

Thus, sleep researchers postulate that NREM sleep is an anabolic state and responsible primarily for physiologic restoration. This possibility is supported by the fact that NREM sleep takes precedence over REM sleep when a person is recovering from sleep deprivation. Still, more is known about the description and mechanisms of sleep than about its functions or how it acts to renew the person for another day's activities.

Variability of both blood pressure and heart rate is increased during REM sleep, possibly due to other changes such as decreased cardiac output. During this stage, there is an overall but transient increase in physiologic activities in the body. This may result from marked but brief cutaneous vasoconstriction, a reduction in urine volume, and possibly, an increased level of plasma catacholamines. Body temperature, heart rate, and blood pressure are all increased, sometimes even to above the level of the person's waking state. An increase in cerebral activity is indicated by increased cerebral blood flow. When awakened during this stage, many persons report vivid dreams. Nocturnal attacks of conditions such as anginal pain, gastric pain, and asthma can be triggered during this stage. Although REM sleep is included within each cycle, the cycles occurring later in the sleep period, that is, closer to normal awakening, have more REM sleep; thus there is greater vulnerability to these attacks around 5 or 6 AM.

In relation to the processes whereby sleep occurs, researchers have identified the neurotransmitter-active neurons and the anatomic sites on which they act for each stage of sleep (Robinson, 1993). One model attempts to provide a global view of the action and interaction of three neurochemical systems of the brain that are the mechanisms for the cycles of waking and sleeping (Hobson, 1974). As the processes continue to be better understood, functions can be identified more clearly. This knowledge—what causes sleep and what sleep does for people—is important to nursing practice in helping persons meet the need for rest.

Assessment of Behavior

Sleep and rest are important to the person's physical and psychological integrity. Behavioral observations of adequacy of meeting sleep and rest needs, and background knowledge in this area, provide the basis for planning nursing care. The nurse examines specific assessment factors based on understanding the processes related to these needs. For rest and sleep, the following are assessed: quantity and quality of daily rest, sleep pattern, and signs of sleep deprivation.

Quantity and Quality of Daily Rest

Behavior related to rest can be assessed simply by observing and recording rest periods throughout the day. The need for daily rest periods other than nightly sleep depends on a person's physical and psychological condition in a given situation. However, for most hospitalized patients, deliberately planned rest periods may be a necessary part of total care. Continuous tossing and turning while resting in bed or fidgeting of hands may indicate restlessness. The mere absence of physical activity may not provide effective rest for a person who is under mental stress. Persons with activity intolerance may show one or more of the following behaviors: exertional discomfort, difficulty completing activities, and verbal report of being easily fatigued (American Nurses Association and American Association of Neuroscience Nurses, 1985). The person's assessment of being "well rested" or "tired" is the most important indicator (behavior).

Sleep Pattern

A person's sleep pattern is assessed by recording observations or reports of how long it takes to fall asleep, restlessness during sleep, number of arousals during each sleep period, early awakening, and sleepiness during the day. Behavioral cues of sleep deprivation include reddened eyes, puffy eyelids, dark circles around the eyes, and frequent yawning. Understanding the person's usual pattern of sleep in relation to any recent change is important in the assessment. Characteristics of a sleep pattern disturbance include the following additional behaviors: reduction in one's role performance (work, school, or home), increasing irritability, restlessness, disorientation (progressive), listlessness, slight hand tremors, expressionless face, and thick speech with mispronounced and wrong choice of words (Schreier, 1986).

Signs of Sleep Deprivation

Humans, unlike animals, can deliberately postpone the initiation of sleep. The record for sleep postponement is about 10 days (Friedman, 1993). The effects of sleep on physiologic and psychological integrity have been studied by observing and recording behavioral changes that occur following a period of sleep deprivation (Pasnau, Naitoh, Stier, & Kollar, 1968; Opstad, Bugge, & Magnus, 1979; Sassin, 1970). These studies indicate that loss of sleep brings changes in brain function and causes alteration in biochemical processes in the body. Sleep loss causes not only physical fatigue and poor neuromuscular coordination, but also signs of psychological dysfunction which are manifest as general irritability, inability to concentrate, disorientation, and confusion. The severity of these effects depends on the degree and length of deprivation and the individual's predeprivation condition.

More extensive assessment tools for clinically evaluating sleep and rest have been developed. An example is the Sleep Questionnaire and Assessment of Wakefulness (SQAW), from the Stanford Sleep Disorders Clinic (Miles, 1979). These tools depend on self-report and subjective feelings about being well rested. The person's sense of having enough sleep is the important behavior to assess regardless of additional data from observation.

Assessment of Stimuli

The nurse also assesses stimuli affecting these rest and sleep needs. Sleep occurs in a circadian, or 24-hour, rhythm maintained by internal hormonal factors and neurologic activity.

Environmental Factors
The timing for normal sleep is regulated further by external factors such as sunrise, sunset, and length of day; ambient temperature; physical activity and rest; timing and type of meals; and timing of social cues such as increased morning noise from traffic or farm animals.

Physical Stress
Rest and sleep also are influenced by the physical stresses experienced at a given time. The extent of illness is assessed as affecting rest and sleep. The more serious the illness, the more time a person will need to spend in rest and sleep. Levels of daily physical activity also are assessed. Whereas vigorous physical activity tends to lengthen the deep sleep cycle, a lack of physical activity will cause a feeling of unsatisfied sleep caused by lack of deep sleep. Physical discomfort and pain are other common causes that reduce the level of satisfactory rest and sleep. Travel by jet airplane across time zones or working shifts that rotate can alter the body's rhythmic sleep–wake cycle.

Developmental Stage
Another contextual stimulus for sleep is age. Generally, younger persons sleep longer, until the individual reaches young adulthood. The average time spent for sleep in different age groups can be summarized as 22 hours for the neonate, 14 to 16 hours for infants, 10 to 12 hours for toddlers and preschoolers, and 8 to 10 hours for school children. Young adults, those in middle years,

and elderly individuals spend an average of 7 to 8 hours daily for sleep. Recent studies have demonstrated that elderly men and women have multiple miniature arousals to stage 1 or awake during the normal night's sleep.

Psychological Condition

Psychological condition in a given situation and at a given time has an effect on both activity and rest. Since sorting and consolidating daily living experiences seems to be done by the brain during sleep, a person who is under psychological stress has increased need for rest and sleep. However, the increased cortical activity of stress and worry can also disrupt the person's normal sleep pattern, inducing a feeling of unsatisfied sleep need. It is not uncommon for a psychologically stressed person to wake up with dreams and complain of unsatisfactory rest and sleep even after spending many hours in bed.

Immediate Environment

The immediate environment affects rest and sleep. Since human beings require an average of one third of their total lifetime for sleep, each individual develops unique habits and patterns related to the immediate environment for sleep. Through the years, these individualized patterns take on the character of ritualistic habits. It is not uncommon for an individual to experience difficulties in falling asleep, or staying asleep, if the usual sleep habits cannot be followed, or if the bedtime schedule of activity is altered. An unfamiliar or unsuitable environment also disrupts rest and sleep. Such stimuli as unpleasant noise, light, odor, and room temperature can be disturbing factors. This was likely a factor in a study which recorded the EEGs of intensive care patients for 48 hours. In these patients, only 50 to 60 percent of total sleep during a 24-hour period occurred at night. The remaining 40 to 50 percent occurred during the day. Patients also had less total sleep time than they would have usually had at home (Hilton, 1976).

Substance Use

A person's use of drugs and alcohol acts as a focal or contextual stimulus for sleep and rest. A person who is sedated with medications, or consuming large amounts of alcoholic beverages, will not be ready, either physically or psychologically, to be involved in physical activity. In turn, changes in activity levels then influence the quality of sleep. Alcoholic beverages and drugs such as barbiturates and opiate derivatives may be effective for initiating sleep and rest on a temporary basis. However, over time, they actually induce sleep deprivation because of their tendency to suppress REM sleep. These substances are habit forming, and as a person develops a tolerance, they become ineffective with prolonged use.

The person's bed partner can also be a source of assessment information and be able to describe sleep behavior and possible psychological influences, such as stress at home or on the job.

► COMPENSATORY ADAPTIVE PROCESSES

Many compensating strategies for activity and rest are embedded in an understanding of mobility and sleep and rest processes. Some of these are innate, some are learned, and some are a combination of both. Combining innate responses with learning is an important approach for nurses in promoting patient adaptation. Two examples of combined compensating strategies are the use of feedback in movement and the learned relaxation response to promote rest and sleep.

Use of Feedback in Movement

The command hierarchy for movement described earlier makes it possible for the person to complete simple tasks, such as casually throwing a piece of paper into the wastebasket and very complex tasks such as feeding oneself. In the first action, the person uses a ballistic control system. Prior to movements, a precise sequence of motor commands is worked out to produce the correct pattern of muscular contractions that are needed to achieve the goal of hitting the basket. It is clear that, once the paper leaves the hand, no amount of sensory feedback about its trajectory is going to enable a person to modify the flight. In the example, the individual begins with the desired result, and translates this into an appropriate pattern of commands, drawing on a library of motor programs suitable for different acts. These commands produce the actual result through their effect on the body's muscles. If the program is a good one, the actual result is the same as the desired result, that is, the paper lands in the basket.

This type of movement, however, is not efficient in most human action because a person cannot have an infinite number of motor programs to draw upon. Also, noise or unpredictable circumstances are always present. The system needs to cope with the problem of noise, such as the slightest breeze blowing from an air conditioner. It also must make complex computations in advance including the nature of the load to be moved and a host of internal factors such as body temperature, the degree of fatigue, and the amount of energy available. Feedback control systems are the answer. These operate on the same general principles as the adaptation level described for the person as an adaptive system.

In a motor control system, the possibility of using feedback greatly improves the functioning of the system. A simple feedback control system starts with the desired result and, at every moment, compares this with the actual result. This comparison is made by sensory information feedback, and the difference between the two is a measurement of error. The smaller the error, or the difference between actual and desired result, the more nearly the person succeeds in accomplishing the task. The error signal is used to generate motor commands to reduce the difference between the desired and actual results. The computation of correcting commands is a much simpler process than the calculations needed in a ballistic system.

An additional capability of the human motor feedback control system is that of learning. When this feature is added, the system is a sort of compromise between a guided and a ballistic system. The main forward pathway is the same as in a ballistic system in that the desired result is again converted into a suitable pattern of output commands by means of stored programs. What is new about this system is that it also incorporates feedback about the actual result, which is compared with the desired result to provide an error signal. However, this error signal, instead of being used to generate commands directly in the course of the movement, is used instead to modify the parameters of the program for movement. The system learns by experience and faulty programs are altered for future successful motor activity.

This behavior is highly characteristic of human motor systems learning to execute complex actions. A person throwing darts at a target for the first time may use a preexisting program from throwing a ball, or initially from tossing toys on the floor from a highchair. As the person practices, the feedback from each throw is used to reduce error and gradually evolve an accurate program for dart throwing.

Another positive feature of the motor feedback control system is that, when it is difficult to obtain feedback about actual results quickly enough for them to be of use during an action (like throwing the dart), it may be possible to use internal feedback to predict the result of a particular motor command before the actual result is known. From a general sensory knowledge of the mechanical properties of the hand and arm, and information about the kinds of loads that are present, an individual can form an estimate of what position the limb is going to adopt in response to any particular pattern of motor commands. This estimate is formed entirely within the brain; it is available long before any feedback from the actual movement has returned from the peripheral sensory motor system. In the internal feedback control system, the desired result is not compared with the actual result, but with the predicted result. The prediction is derived by sending a copy of the motor commands to a neural model of the mechanical properties of the body, which is used to predict the probable result. Again, actual results are compared with the predicted result. Errors are used to correct the model itself, thus improving the accuracy of the predictions. In a very real sense, learning motor skills becomes a matter of learning to predict the behavior of the body. The compensating strategy of using feedback in making mobility more effective is particularly important in rehabilitation.

Learned Relaxation Response

It has been noted that life stresses and worry can interfere with restful sleep. The relaxation response can be a learned compensatory process that enhances an innate, autonomic response to promote rest and sleep. In this response, the person is alert, but the body processes slow down as sympathetic nervous system arousal is decreased and the person feels a sense of calmness.

The relaxation response has been studied extensively by Benson (1975) and colleagues. It is used as complementary treatment of serious health conditions such as cardiac disease and cancer. There are many possible approaches to elicit the relaxation response. A simple approach that nurses can use in many clinical situations is progressive muscle relaxation. The rationale for the effectiveness of this approach is that the stress response cannot exist when the muscles of the body are relaxed. The purpose of teaching progressive muscle relaxation is to provide a sense of control and to minimize the effects of stress, rather than to directly affect stress and illness.

The relaxation response benefits the person by decreasing the anxiety associated with strange environments and stressful or painful situations; increasing the effect of pain medications and helping the patient to dissociate from pain; decreasing fatigue by interrupting protective muscle tensing; increasing relaxed breathing to replace shallow breaths that result from anxiety and fear; providing periods of rest that are as beneficial as a nap and are preparation for restful sleep; decreasing heart rate, blood pressure, and respirations; and improving effectiveness of the endocrine and immune systems (Dossey, Buzzetta, & Kenner, 1992).

In teaching progressive muscle relaxation, the nurse keeps in mind four basic components of relaxation techniques.

- A quiet environment that deletes all possible noise and distractions.
- A comfortable position, such as sitting or lying without undue muscle tension.
- Focusing on muscle groups as a mental device to shift the mind from logical, externally oriented thoughts.
- Use of the principle that a muscle will relax when it is let go after being tensed.

Progressive relaxation consists of tensing and relaxing muscle groups and focusing on the feelings of relaxation (Cassmeyer, Long, & Wykle, 1993).

After discussing the approach with the patient, the nurse leads the person to develop the relaxation response by instructions to assume a comfortable position and to begin by focusing on breathing easily. For each muscle group, the muscles are tensed for 5 to 7 seconds, then relaxed completely. The person then focuses for about 10 seconds on the sensations of the relaxed muscles, such as warmth, tingling, and lightness. Sequential tensing of the following muscle groups has been found to be effective.

1. Hands, arms, and shoulders. Clench fists, extend the arms in a slightly raised position and pull the shoulders tight.
2. Outer face. Raise eyebrows to hairline and protrude the lower jaw.
3. Inner face. Squeeze eyes tightly closed, wrinkle nose, purse lips.
4. Neck. Rest ear on right shoulder then left shoulder.

5. Shoulders, chest, and abdomen. Push shoulders back and chest forward, with abdomen pulled in.
6. Trunk, legs, and feet. Pinch buttocks together raising slightly, extend legs and point toes upward.

The nurse coaches the person through this sequence and observes for effectiveness of the teaching.

Nurses can practice progressive muscle relaxation exercises and teach them to colleagues. Cues that the relaxation response has been learned include: changes in breathing, that is, slower, deeper breaths progressing to slow, somewhat more shallow breathing as relaxation deepens, and more audible breathing; fluttering of the eyelids; easing of jaw tightness, sometimes to the extent that the lips part and the jaw drops slightly; lack of muscle holding. Lack of holding is demonstrated by lifting the arm gently by the wrist without detectable resistance. In addition, the arm moves as easily as an object of similar weight (Dossey et al., 1992).

As an aid to rest and sleep, the nurse can suggest that, once learned, the relaxation response can be practiced twice a day for 20 minutes. Time spent in sensing the feelings of relaxation are an integral part of the exercise and receive about twice the amount of time as the muscle tensing. Between focusing on different muscle groups, the person is directed to return to being aware of breathing easily. Abbreviated forms of the muscle relaxation exercises can be repeated in any stressful situation and can be done before preparing to go to bed for sleep.

► COMPROMISED PROCESSES OF ACTIVITY AND REST

There are many situations in both health and illness when a person's needs for activity and rest are not being met and when compensatory processes are not adequate for adaptation. The result can be compromised processes of mobility and sleep.

Adaptation problems can result when any of the processes related to activity and rest are disrupted. Two specific examples of compromised adaptive processes related to activity and rest are discussed in this section. *Disuse syndrome* is the term used for the potential negative effects of curtailed physical activity, particularly when imposed by medical restrictions. *Sleep pattern disturbance* is a commonly occurring compromised process associated with the need for rest.

Disuse Syndrome

A major issue of physical immobility is disuse syndrome. The North American Nursing Diagnosis Association defines "high risk for disuse syndrome" (Rantz & LeMone, 1997, p. 494) as a state in which an individual is at risk for deterioration of body systems as the result of prescribed or unavoidable inactivity.

There are many neuromuscular, skeletal, and other conditions that lead to inactivity. A fractured bone may require a period of immobile therapeutic alignment preoperatively to prevent further damage to the fractured bone or the surrounding soft tissues. Postoperatively, immobility promotes proper healing of the repaired fracture.

In the case of a patient who is suffering acute cardiac insufficiency, absolute bed rest is one of the most important aspects of the therapeutic regime. This measure is to conserve the oxygen and energy consumption required by nonpriority physical activity, minimizing the cardiac load for the damaged heart muscle.

The same principle applies when the nurse places a patient with a fever on bed rest. An elevation of 1° in body temperature will require a 7 percent increase in basic metabolic rate, or energy needed. The nurse uses bed rest to prevent further exhaustion of the already stressed body. At the same time, the risks of immobility must be addressed by recognizing the potential for disuse syndrome.

Some specific consequences of physical inactivity are listed in Table 8–2. The first two columns are organized by major body functions and the underlying changes that result from a period of physical inactivity. The behavioral effect of these changes, termed *disuse consequences,* is summarized in column 3 (Cho, 1984; Long et al., 1993; Rubin, 1988a, b).

Changes from inactivity can further affect adaptation related to the physiologic need for activity and rest. For example, a deficit in muscle mass, tone, and strength indicates muscle atrophy, which is a part of the disuse syndrome. In turn, the atrophied muscle is less effective in performing physical activity. The older person is especially prone to disuse syndrome when immobile.

From the perspective of the Roy Adaptation Model, physical inactivity affects the psychosocial aspects of the person as well. The nurse uses knowledge of the other adaptive modes to recognize that the inability to move about and interact with people and the environment in one's usual pattern greatly affects the person's self-concept, role function, and interdependence (see Chaps. 14, 15, and 16). The effect on the other modes takes place through the sensory perceptual processes that involve, in particular, anxiety, change of body image, and egocentricity. All four adaptive modes are affected by the stimulus of inactivity. Disuse syndrome is a diagnostic term broad enough to include these effects, particularly when viewed from the perspective of a specific nursing model such as the Roy Adaptation Model and from an understanding of the scientific work related to this concept.

Sleep Pattern Disturbance

It is estimated that more than one half of all adults cite difficulties with sleeping at some time in their lives. Sleep problems are often overlooked in health care settings because other symptoms are given higher priority. However, inadequate sleep leads to an increased risk for accidents, inefficiency at work, irritability in social relations, and exacerbation of other health problems. The nurse is frequently the person with whom the patient talks about sleep distur-

TABLE 8–2   CONSEQUENCES OF PHYSICAL INACTIVITY–DISUSE SYNDROME

Body Function	Underlying Changes	Disuse Consequences	Preventive Interventions
Musculoskeletal	*Muscles:* Autolysis of unused muscles	Muscular atrophy with weakness and decreased endurance	Muscle conditioning exercises: isometric, isotonic, resistive
	Bones: Increased osteo-clastic process due to lack of physical stresses of weight bearing on the bones leads to increased urinary excretion of calcium	Osteoporosis and vulner-ability to pathologic fracture	Physical activities that would produce the stresses of weight bearing: standing and walking, pushing and pulling
	Joints: Decreased pliability and increased density of the collagen meshwork leads to fibrous forma-tion and shortening of the muscle fibers	Joint contractures with permanent loss of joint mobility	ROM (range-of-motion) exercises: active, assisted, passive
	Nerves: Denervation due to prolonged compression of nerve fibers and decreased circulation	Paralysis, foot drop, and wrist drop	Frequent change of position; use of foot board
Circulatory	Cardiac overload due to central pooling of the circulatory volume	Deconditioning leads to poor exercise tolerance	Frequent change of position; including sitting up and standing positions, if possible
	Loss of regulatory mechan-ism to maintain central BP (normally with position change to sitting up, the splenic and peripheral vessels constrict to maintain the central blood volume)	Postural hypotension, dizziness, and fainting in upright position	
	Sluggish venous return due to lack of pumping mechanism generated by muscular contractions of physical activity	Dependent (local) edema, especially of the lower extremities	Muscle exercises to stimulate the circulation
	Hypercoagulability of blood (due to injury or surgery) combined with physical inactivity	Thrombus formation leads to pulmonary embolism	Well-fitting antiembolic stockings
Pulmonary	Limited expansion of lungs due to arms crowding chest and diaphragm not dropping	Hypoventilation	Positions of maximum chest expansion
	Medium for infection due to stasis of secretions in lungs and poor pulmon-ary circulation	Hypostatic pneumonia	Frequent change of positions, and deep-breathing and coughing exercises

TABLE 8–2   CONSEQUENCES OF PHYSICAL INACTIVITY–DISUSE SYNDROME (CONT.)

Body Function	Underlying Changes	Disuse Consequences	Preventive Interventions
Metabolic	Increased catabolic processes lead to increased excretion of nitrogen via gastrointestinal and urinary tract combined with poor protein intake due to poor appetite	Negative nitrogen balance leads to poor tissue healing	Ensure adequate intake of dietary protein
Eliminative	Urinary stagnation due to lack of natural position of gravity in recumbent position and loss of proprioception	Urinary retention Urinary tract infection	Frequent encouragement to void, providing adequate toilet facility and position of comfort; ideal position for male client is standing up, while sitting up is for female client
	Increased calcium content in the urine	Nephrolithiasis	Ensure adequate fluid intake with cranberry juice to acidify the urine pH level
	Decreased gastrointestinal mobility combined with dependency on others to obtain toilet facility, lack of privacy, lack of bulk in the diet, and poor abdominal and pelvic muscle tones	Constipation Fecal impaction	Avoid unnecessary use of CNS depressants; muscle toning exercise for abdominal and pelvic muscles; ensure adequate fluid and bulk intake
Integumentary	Inability to carry out daily personal hygiene measures and prolonged compression of tissues, resulting in decreased circulation	Pressure sores and decubiti ulceration formation with secondary infection	Frequent change of position; use of protective devices (pillow, padding); frequent massaging of all bony prominences
Sensory-perceptual	Decreased environmental stimuli lead to decreased sensory stimulation; changed perceptual axis with recumbent position; inability to manipulate own environment	Anxiety, disorientation, loss of proprioception–change in body image; boredom; egocentricity	Environment structuring to provide meaningful stimuli; use of calendar, radio, TV, and wall clock can be helpful Provide opportunity to carry out meaningful conversations with others Visits from family and friends are very important

From Cho, J. S. (1984). Activity and rest. In S. C. Roy, Introduction to nursing: An adaptation model (pp. 141–143). Englewood Cliffs, NJ: Prentice Hall.

bance. Careful assessment of the problem can be useful in helping the person get the help that is needed.

The Association for Sleep Disorders Centers (Sleep Disorders Classification Committee, 1979) published a diagnostic classification of sleep and arousal disorders. The classification system has four major categories: disorders of initiating and maintaining sleep, such as insomnia; disorders of excessive daytime somnolence, for example, narcolepsy; disorders of sleep–wake schedule, as experienced with rapid travel across time zones; and parasomnias, such as sleepwalking and sleep terror. Literature in the field provides information on each major type of disorder and subcategory of specific conditions with their associated patterns of signs and symptoms.

Increasingly, major medical centers have sleep disorder clinics where patients can be referred to receive diagnostic evaluation and treatment. Nurses can also help the person establish good sleep habits and possibly prevent sleep pattern disturbance. Adequate time, an appropriate environment, and freedom from worry all contribute to good sleep habits.

▶ PLANNING NURSING CARE

Meeting activity and rest needs is important for the physiologic adaptation of the person, as well as for integrity of the other adaptive modes. With an understanding of mobility and sleep processes, and related compensatory processes, as well as the factors that influence these, the nurse can complete a holistic first- and second-level assessment for a person's activity and rest needs. Based on judgment about nursing care needs, the next step of the nursing process is the nursing diagnosis. The assessment and diagnoses are then used to set goals with the patient, to select interventions, and to evaluate the outcomes of care.

Nursing Diagnosis

As noted in Chapter 3, the data from the nursing assessment of behaviors and stimuli are interpreted in the statement of a nursing diagnosis. The statement includes a clustering of the observed behaviors with the most relevant influencing stimuli. A nursing diagnosis related to adequate activity may be stated, "Good muscle tone and 4+ muscle strength in major muscle groups of all four extremities due to knowledge of health benefits of fitness and commitment to regular exercise program."

In situations where there are problems related to needs for activity and rest, the nursing diagnosis will convey the essence of the problem in a way that will direct the subsequent steps of the nursing process. This clarity of communication is facilitated by using the approach recommended by the Roy Adaptation Model for stating the diagnosis, that is, a statement of observed behaviors with the most relevant influencing stimuli.

For example, the nurse may see a young professional woman in an outpatient department who says that she must have a virus because she is not feeling well. In assessing activity and rest needs, the nurse notes the following data.

The person reports difficulty falling asleep and frequent arousals from sleep during the night. Her eyes are reddened with puffy eyelids, dark circles under the eyes; and she states she knows she is not sleeping well. She also mentions concerns about the responsibilities associated with a job promotion.

The diagnosis can be stated as, "Reports of poor sleep pattern, with eyes showing evidence of sleep deprivation, due to a recent change in job responsibilities."

Another way of stating a nursing diagnosis is to use a summary label from an established classification system that best identifies the nurse's judgment of the clinical situation. In earlier discussion of the Roy model, two classification lists were described, one for indicators of adaptation and one for commonly recurring adaptation problems (see Chap. 3). In Table 8–3 the Roy model nursing diagnosis categories for the physiologic mode need of activity and rest are shown in relation to nursing diagnosis labels approved by the North American Nursing Diagnosis Association (Rantz & LeMone, 1997).

For experienced nurses, a summary diagnostic label can convey a behavioral pattern when more than one mode is being affected by the same stimulus. Consider the following illustration. A 28-year-old male was involved in a car accident with resultant paraplegia (loss of voluntary muscle control and sensation of the lower extremities). He is involved in aggressive physical and occupational therapy to learn to care for himself while in a wheelchair. Nurses on the 24-hour-care unit, where the patient stays, use knowledge of movement processes to make the following diagnosis, "High potential for disuse syndrome related to prolonged immobility and paralysis." As noted ear-

TABLE 8–3   NURSING DIAGNOSTIC CATEGORIES FOR ACTIVITY AND REST

Positive Indicators of Adaptation	Common Adaptation Problems	NANDA Diagnostic Labels
• Integrated processes of mobility	• Immobility • Activity intolerance • Restricted mobility, gait, and/or coordination	• Impaired physical mobility • Activity intolerance • Risk for activity intolerance
• Adequate recruitment of compensatory movement processes during inactivity	• Disuse syndrome	• Bathing/hygiene self-care deficit • Dressing/grooming self-care deficit • Risk for disuse syndrome
• Effective pattern of activity and rest • Effective sleep pattern	• Inadequate pattern of activity and rest • Sleep deprivation	• Diversional activity deficit • Fatigue • Sleep pattern disturbance
• Effective environmental changes for altered sleep conditions	• Potential for sleep pattern disturbance	• Energy field disturbance

lier, immobility has a profound effect on the physiologic needs of the body. At the same time, the person's feelings about self and what he is able to do with respect to social roles is greatly affected. The nursing diagnosis with the summary diagnostic label "disuse syndrome" conveys this complex interrelationship.

Activity intolerance has been defined by NANDA as a state in which an individual has insufficient physiologic or psychological energy to endure or complete required or desired daily activities. This diagnosis can be related to such factors as anxiety, acute and chronic pain, weakness and fatigue, sedentary lifestyle, deconditioned status, and pathology (such as cardiac arrhythmias, circulatory or respiratory problems) resulting in imbalance between oxygen supply and demand. This condition can be recognized by behaviors of complaints of fatigue and weakness, abnormal heart rate or blood pressure in response to activity, and exertional discomfort or dyspnea.

Sleep apnea is the periodic cessation of breathing during sleep. Further, neurologic, respiratory, and cardiovascular systems are also involved. Because sleep apnea results in frequent awakenings, irritability and daytime drowsiness can result. For this reason, sleep apnea can be a dangerous sleep disorder for the community as well as for the individual (automobile accidents can occur when the person experiences daytime sleepiness). The nurse can be helpful in identifying persons who need immediate diagnosis and treatment. Often the first manifestation of a problem is a complaint from a spouse, family, or significant other about loud, irregular snoring. Obese males are particularly prone to this disorder because fat deposition in tissues can reduce the diameter of the oropharynx and diminish upper airway exchange.

Following a careful assessment of activity and rest needs and the derivation of nursing diagnoses, the fourth step of the nursing process—goal setting—is undertaken.

Goal Setting

In using the Roy Adaptation Model, goal setting is the stating of clear outcomes for the person as a result of nursing care. As noted earlier, a complete goal statement contains the behavior of focus, the change that the nurse and patient together expect, and the time frame in which the goal can be achieved. Depending on the situation, the goal may be long-term or short-term.

Consider the person with the diagnosis of "good muscle tone and 4+ muscle strength in major muscle groups of all four extremities due to knowledge of health benefits of fitness and commitment to regular exercise program." If this person suddenly is hospitalized with a fractured pelvis suffered in an automobile accident, an appropriate goal in the new situation of immobility is, "Upper extremity muscle tone will be maintained at a good level and strength will be increased from 4+ to 5+ during the 4 weeks of acute care." This goal is influenced by the need to prepare the person for use of the arms to bear weight on crutches during rehabilitation.

In the case of the person who reports a poor sleep pattern, with eyes that show evidence of sleep deprivation, due to a recent change in job responsibilities, a short-term goal is, "In the next week, the person will identify in writing early in the day the two major responsibilities that are of most concern, and for the concern that is most distressing, consider several alternate ways of dealing with it."

Within the activity and rest component of the physiologic mode, the general overall goal is to promote adequate activity and rest for normal growth and development and for restoration, repair, and renewal of energies and effectiveness of life processes. Balance is the goal. Activity is balanced with the need for activity, and rest is balanced with the need for rest. These goals are made specific in the many situations that nurses encounter that can interfere with meeting these needs for activity and rest. For example, the person's rest needs may be adequately met in terms of length and quality of sleep, but if the individual's ongoing physical stress level is beyond the available energy level, a negative energy balance indicates the need to set a goal related to increasing the quality and quantity of rest. Similarly, in earlier examples of the individuals with heart disease or a fever, the need for rest increases; providing more rest becomes part of the goal of nursing care to achieve balance of this need. Since nurses often see patients during times of change that affect their activity and rest, they are in a position to develop preventive goals rather than allow consequences of imbalances in activity and rest to occur.

Based on knowledge related to movement and sleep processes, and the specific goals for the person, the nurse plans appropriate nursing interventions.

Intervention

Each step of the nursing process provides direction for the intervention stage. The goal focuses on the behavioral description of the patient situation. The interventions address the context of the behaviors, that is, the focal, contextual, and residual stimuli, and the person's ability to cope with these (regulator and cognator coping processes). Understanding this combined effect on individuals and their abilities is the basis for assisting the person to handle the experience in the direction of positive adaptation.

► ACTIVITY AND MOBILITY

Nursing measures used to promote adequate activity include health teaching to promote physical activity that maintains physical fitness, removing any discomfort or restriction that is unnecessarily limiting movement, providing timely feedback in reestablishing neurologic control of movement, and careful planning of preventive measures for those who must be immobilized. Two interventions will be discussed in detail because of their significance in promoting health for individuals and the community as a whole.

Health Teaching

Health teaching to promote exercise for physical fitness involves both information and motivational factors. It has been noted that, although exercise is recognized as enhancing health, many people in North America do not include enough physical activity in their daily lives. At one end of the continuum, only 22 percent of adults in the United States engage in leisure time physical activity at recommended levels, and at the other end, an estimated 24 percent of Americans are totally sedentary and never engage in beneficial physical exercise (U.S. Centers for Disease Control and Prevention and the American College of Sports Medicine, 1993). In health teaching, the nurse acknowledges with the person the difficulties of establishing and maintaining an adequate exercise program and identifies with the person the particular barriers and positive influences. The benefits of exercise are stressed and accurate information is provided about exercise recommendations.

Just as immobility affects all body systems and the four adaptive modes, so, too, does physical activity benefit the person as a whole. Positive effects have been shown on the functioning of the cardiovascular, respiratory, and musculoskeletal systems, as well as improved metabolism, nutrition, and bowel elimination. In addition, exercise positively affects self-esteem, intellectual activity, and social and emotional status. Evidence shows that a primary benefit of regular physical activity is protection against coronary artery disease. Likewise, regular exercise appears to provide some protection against such chronic conditions as hypertension, adult-onset diabetes, some cancers, osteoporosis, and mental health changes such as depression (Sims, D'Amico, Stiesmeyer, & Webster, 1995).

The nurse can teach the person to assess physical fitness in relation to needs for activity using five criteria: cardiovascular endurance, muscle strength and endurance, joint flexibility, body weight and composition, and motor performance skill. The nurse helps the person to use insight into personal needs, to problem solve, and to plan within the given social context to create a healthy lifestyle. The following recommendations for exercise have received backing from the U.S. Centers for Disease Control and Prevention and the American College of Sports Medicine.

1. Individuals should engage in a total of 30 minutes of moderate-intensity exercise over the course of most days of the week. The individual is not required to do all 30 minutes during one session, but can accumulate this total throughout the day. Walking, gardening, dancing, and walking up stairs (rather than taking the elevator) are all ways to incorporate more physical activity into daily life. People can also fulfill this recommendation through planned exercise or recreation such as tennis, swimming, or cycling.

2. People who do no exercise should begin by incorporating even a few minutes of exercise into their daily routine with the goal of eventu-

ally reaching 30 minutes per day. Activities to increase joint flexibility and muscle strength should also be included.

Preventive Measures

Preventive measures for those who must be immobilized are discussed in detail because of their importance in care of hospitalized people, as well as for the elderly or debilitated at home or in long-term care facilities. Intervention for disuse syndrome has general and specific aspects. The general aspect includes those preventive measures that promote maintenance of normal movement functions. By promoting a person's movement, the nurse facilitates accomplishment of daily living tasks and also helps provide the body with the physical stresses that are essential in maintaining the internal physiologic functions.

In planning preventive nursing interventions, the nurse takes the nature and extent of medically imposed restrictions into consideration. As noted earlier, at times, a period of complete bed rest or other limited movement is medically indicated; therefore, the nurse cannot manage the focal stimulus, that is, the enforced physical inactivity. However, other factors are managed through well-planned preventive measures so that disuse syndrome is avoided and the effects of immobility are minimized without impeding the purpose of the needed temporary immobilization. A similar situation exists when pathology of the neuromuscular skeletal system limits mobility, as in the case of paraplegia.

General preventive nursing interventions include the following four major principles: maintenance of good body alignment, frequent change of positions, maintenance of joint mobility, and conditioning of muscles. These interventions are summarized in column 4 of Table 8–3.

Good Body Alignment

Good body alignment is a body posture in which the body parts are arranged in an anatomically functional position and the weight distribution is well balanced in a stable manner. The normal functional standing position is shown in Figure 8–3. Good body alignment is assumed in all body positions. For example, in the supine, or lying position, the body is in full extension, resembling the upright position. Incorrect body alignment or posture will impose undue stresses on muscles, ligaments, and joints. Poor body alignment that is frequent or prolonged can leave permanent defects such as flexion contracture of the neck or foot drop. These outcomes are not uncommon among bedridden patients.

Positioning

Disuse syndrome is a direct result of static body positions for prolonged periods of time. Changing the patient's position is another way to manage the major stimulus for these consequences. The supine position is the most common position assumed by ill individuals. For some patients, this static position becomes prolonged without spontaneous body movements, for example, in situations of paralysis or unconsciousness. Frequent changes of position with proper body alignment are provided to prevent nerve damage in the pressure areas, joint contractures, pressure sores, and loss of the postural adjustment mechanism for the maintenance of central blood pressure in the upright position.

Within mobility restrictions, body position can include many different positions including prone, or lying on the stomach. Frequent changes of position not only relieve the pressure of body weight, promoting general circulation, but the movement of changing positions also facilitates dislodging of bodily discharges, such as mucus secretions of the respiratory tract. An active change of position to a sitting-up position is effective in maintenance of the postural adjustment mechanism and consequently prevents the symptoms of postural hypotension (lowered blood pressure upon standing).

At times, it is easy to think that sitting up in a chair is too big a task for a particular patient. However, the nurse knows that, although the process of struggling to get out of the bed and moving to a chair takes a lot of effort on the parts of both the patient and the nurse, the benefits of such movement, when within therapeutically indicated limits, are paramount. This activity provides almost all of the physical exercises that contribute to the prevention of disuse syndrome.

Mobilization

To maintain joint mobility either active or passive exercises must be done. In active range-of-motion (ROM) exercise, the patient initiates and completes the full range of motion (see Fig. 8–2). For a person who is too weak or is partially paralyzed, assisted or passive ROM exercising is accomplished. In assisted ROM exercise, the person initiates the movement but requires assistance to complete the full range of motion. For a paralyzed or unconscious person, passive ROM exercises are done, that is, initiating and completing the full range of motion is accomplished by the nurse. The involved limb is supported at all times during the motion to prevent straining the muscles and ligaments. Passive limb movement does not involve muscle contractions as in active motion. Therefore, it does not achieve muscle conditioning but it is effective in preventing joint contractures. Joint motion exercise is never carried out beyond the point of pain or resistance.

Muscle Conditioning

There are several types of exercises that contribute to muscle conditioning. The primary purpose of muscle conditioning exercise is to prevent muscular atrophy and weakening. However, because muscle exercise provides physical stress on other structures, it aids, to some extent, in promotion of general circulation and prevention of osteoporosis.

All active body movements, such as lifting and moving objects, induce isotonic exercise. In isotonic exercise, the muscle fibers shorten during the muscle contraction and the joint moves. This is distinguished from isometric exercise, which is performed to maintain muscle tone without moving the joint. A setting exercise is an example of an isometric exercise. Muscle setting is accomplished simply by purposefully contracting or hardening of a group of muscles for 10 seconds and then releasing to relax. This type of exercise is effective in conditioning the abdominal, gluteal, and quadriceps muscles. The use of isometric exercise requires a certain degree of caution. During the muscle-setting period, intrathoracic pressure increases due to the trapping of air against the closed epiglottis, a phenomenon called the Valsalva maneuver. The Valsalva maneuver can precipitate cardiac arrest in a person who has a damaged heart. This untoward reaction occurs because the increased intrathoracic pressure prevents normal cardiac input, and subsequently decreases cardiac output and the coronary circulation. In any case, if this type of exercise is instituted, the person is taught to exhale during the muscle-setting period.

Resistive exercise is another form of muscle conditioning. This exercise is done by pulling or pushing against a stationary object. Because of its pumping effect on the venous system, this type of exercise is effective not only for muscle conditioning, but also in stimulating venous return. Simple activity such as pushing the feet against a foot board is effective for conditioning the gastrocnemius and quadriceps muscles. Pulling on the trapeze bar is effective for conditioning the upper arms and shoulder muscles. Basic nursing skills textbooks provide detailed steps for instituting these exercises. Further, the nurse works with other members of the health care team including physiotherapists or occupational therapists who have special expertise in this area.

► **REHABILITATION**

Nurses are involved in rehabilitation, an intervention involving the whole person, but particularly focusing on activity needs. *Rehabilitation* is an active and dynamic process through which a person achieves optimal physical, emotional, psychological, social, and vocational potential. Basic premises include maintaining dignity and personal wholeness in a life that is as independent and self-fulfilling as possible. The Association of Rehabilitation Nurses defines their practice as facilitating individuals, through optimum adaptation, to reengage in the mainstream of living whereby each person functions maximally within the environment.

An individual's goals for rehabilitation may range from employment or reemployment for the handicapped person to the more limited achievement of developing self-care abilities. Restoration to former capacity may be possible in some situations such as a mild head injury or a slight stroke. However, in other situations, such as severe head injury, paralyzing spinal cord injury, or stroke, complete recovery of function may not be possible and permanent disability is likely. In this case, the person and the family are helped to accept, adjust to, and compensate for the existing deficit and to establish an optimal level of function.

The principles of rehabilitation are an integral component of nursing practice and include the major elements of prevention, maintenance, and restoration (Hickey, 1992). Nursing protocols directed at preventing disability include skin care, positioning and alignment, frequent turning, and range-of-motion exercises. The nurse helps to maintain intact skills and functions by encouraging the patient to be as independent as possible in activities of daily living. The nurse's participation is key in exercise programs aimed at restoring functions, particularly mobility. Details of prevention, maintenance, and restoration protocols can be found in textbooks on rehabilitation.

Rehabilitation programs include many health care providers working in collaboration with the patient and family. However, the nurse spends the most time with the patient on a daily basis and can help coordinate a schedule so that optimum benefit is derived from rehabilitation activities. The patient needs a high energy and motivation level for demanding activity such as learning ambulation. Nursing knowledge of mobility processes and of feedback as a compensatory process in learning efficient movement can be helpful throughout the rehabilitation process. An example of use of this knowledge may be with a patient who has neuromuscular deficits that affect mobility of one side. This may be the result of a stroke on the side of the brain that controls motor programs for the opposite side of the body. The patient may be receiving occupational therapy to learn to eat independently. In helping the patient with an evening meal, the nurse is aware of the need for added feedback to relearn motor movements. The patient is directed to visually scan the tray and verbal cues are provided as the patient reaches for items on the tray. Past-pointing errors are common after certain types of brain damage, but can be overcome with coaching to relearn the motor program involved.

Application of Interventions for Activity Needs

An illustration of specific planning of nursing interventions to meet activity needs is provided for a person who suddenly is hospitalized with a broken pelvis suffered in an automobile accident. Two nursing diagnoses for this person are: (1) good muscle tone and 4+ muscle strength in major muscle groups of all four extremities due to knowledge of health benefits of fitness and commitment to regular exercise program; and (2) potential for disuse consequences related to sudden, therapeutically enforced immobility and age of 62 years. A number of long- and short-term goals are indicated, each with interventions that identify stimuli that can be managed to reach the goal.

For the first goal, the nurse plans a series of interventions. The patient is involved in self-care activities as soon as possible after admission. Simple activities such as participating in bathing, combing the hair, shaving, or putting on makeup in bed allows the pulling and weight bearing of active movement. This is effective in muscle conditioning, as well as stimulating general circulation and promoting mobility of joints.

Recognizing strengths within the person such as knowledge of health benefits and commitment to regular exercise, the nurse explains that, even though the exercises done in the hospital will be different from the person's usual pattern of exercise, they are even more important at this time. The nurse describes the exercises and their specific purpose. Then, the patient is involved in setting up a schedule of muscle strengthening exercises for the upper extremities that includes lifting on a trapeze bar, increasing the number of times and the frequency gradually. Since pushing and pulling against a stationary object is important, the nurse can use ingenuity to provide such an object, such as stabilizing the over-bed table.

To maintain an effective exercise program, the nurse focuses on the person's knowledge and commitment, the scheduled use of muscles that are the primary target, providing the equipment to complete the exercises, and providing an environment that does not restrict the program (a conflicting schedule of therapies, for example). For this particular patient, a chart of progress of muscle strength can be made. The patient and the nurse will recognize that some unavoidable muscle weakness can occur early in the program. However, keeping the long-term goal in mind is useful. Knowing that, even if this goal is not achieved, the person will be better ready to undertake the next stage of rehabilitation than if the muscle strengthening program had not been instituted and carefully carried out is encouraging for both patient and nurse.

▶ REST AND SLEEP

Some general measures for promoting quality rest and sleep by managing the major stimuli identified earlier include the following: provision of physical comfort, alleviation of psychological stresses, structuring daily activity schedule, structuring a restful environment, and controlled use of hypnotic drugs and alcohol.

Physical Comfort

Since physical pain and discomfort are among the most common causes for disruption in rest and sleep, providing physical comfort is a method of relief from the disruption. Good personal hygiene aids physical comfort and improves the quality of rest and sleep. A warm bath can be relaxing. For some persons, spicy food may interfere with sleep. This possibility, as well as whether or not the person is hungry, is discussed with the person and remedied as appropriate. Soothing backrubs can be comforting and effective in inducing sleep. As noted earlier, mere physical inactivity does not provide good quality rest.

In some situations, administration of an analgesic medication is indicated for relief of pain to enhance comfort. Appropriate timing of analgesic administration is important. For patients in pain, the nurse is not concerned with long-term drug dependency (see Chap. 10); however, the choice of drug is made carefully so that the person does not experience the consequences of REM sleep deprivation.

Alleviation of Psychological Stress

Alleviation of psychological stress may be necessary to allow for rest and sleep. The nurse provides the person with opportunities to ventilate feelings of fear, anxiety, and frustration. In a hospital setting, lack of knowledge or understanding of what is happening often generates feelings of powerlessness. These feelings can trigger anxiety (see Chap. 14). Sometimes it is a misperception or incorrect understanding that causes unnecessary anxiety. The nurse is in a position to check out the patient's understanding of the situation and its particular personal meaning. She is sensitive to the person's subtle, as well as obvious, behaviors indicating distress and interfering with restful sleep. From the person's perspective, then, the nurse can help in dealing appropriately with these factors, focal or contextual, that are interfering with rest and sleep.

For persons in the hospital or at home, anxiety about not sleeping can be the psychological stress that is focal in disturbing sleep. Researchers have noted that trying too hard to sleep aggravates the problem. When struggling with the need for sleep and the inability to fall asleep, feelings of anxiety, frustration, and anger can trigger arousal and tension. Practical interventions to deal with these situations have been suggested (Sloan et al., 1993). They include going to bed only when sleepy and using the bed only for sexual activity and sleeping (not reading or watching television). If a person is unable to fall asleep in about 20 minutes, getting up and going to another room until sleepy, or turning the clock toward the wall may assist. With wakefulness during the night, likewise, it is suggested that the individual get up and return to bed only when sleepy. Finally, it is useful to awake at the same time every day and not to take daytime naps. Eventually, going to bed is associated with rapid falling asleep.

Physical Activity

As noted earlier, physical activity induces NREM sleep; therefore, adequate amounts of physical activity, within the individual's restrictions, are worked into the daily schedule. However, any vigorous physical activity or events that trigger strong emotional responses are avoided near bedtime. Every effort is made to ensure that the sleep cycles can take their full course so that the person will not suffer from REM sleep deprivation. Treatment procedures and other activities are grouped together in such a way that the number of interruptions is kept to a minimum. Each sleep cycle takes 60 to 120 minutes. Therefore, scheduling the interruptions at longer than 2-hour intervals will allow each sleep cycle to take its full course. A large amount of food and fluid taken in the late evening will require unnecessarily frequent arousals caused by increased gastrointestinal and bladder stimulations. Any drugs that have a diuretic effect are not administered at bedtime. For healthy persons, moderate exercise used consistently can lengthen and deepen sleep.

Restful Environment

In structuring a restful environment, the nurse takes into consideration the individual's personal habits and bedtime routine. The environment in general is to be free of all kinds of noxious stimuli. Room temperature, light, noise, and odor are checked out for suitability. Unavoidable, but unpleasant, noise can be disguised by pleasant music. People will differ in the degree of quiet needed for restful sleep. Some need absolute quiet and others prefer some background noise. Increasingly, it is possible to arrange the environment differently for each patient as more hospital rooms are private accommodations. The effects of a strange environment on a person's sleep usually does not last more than 3 or 4 days. This information can help the person control anxiety about changes in sleep pattern in the hospital.

Special care units present problems in establishing a restful environment by reason of their equipment and activities. Nonetheless, the nurse strives to make this environment as conducive to rest and sleep as possible. The nurse can emphasize a sense of security in the constant watchfulness of the person's condition throughout the night. The careful scheduling of activities as noted is particularly relevant in these settings. In this case, however, activity for one patient may affect another patient more readily because of the physical setup of many units. Sometimes it is staff conversation, a stimulus easily managed by the nurse, that is most disturbing to the patient.

Hypnotic Drugs

Lastly, hypnotic drugs are controlled carefully and used in selected situations for sleep since they have been identified as related to quality of sleep and rest. The same is true of alcohol, particularly when it is used habitually for sleep. The nurse explains that such substances are effective on a short-term basis only and that they tend to suppress restful or REM sleep. The person is encouraged to restrict their use. The nurse then assists the person to find alternate means to promote sleep. Given the scope and variety of settings and situations that call for individually designed nursing interventions to assist persons with activity and rest needs, careful evaluation of the effectiveness of these interventions is particularly important.

Evaluation

As in each of the modes of adaptation, with the physiologic need for activity and rest, the evaluation phase of the nursing process reflects the behavioral assessment. In the example given earlier, a person who reported poor sleep pattern, with eyes showing evidence of sleep deprivation, due to a recent change in job responsibilities, returns to the clinic with the same behaviors that the nurse noted 1 week earlier. That is, the person reports difficulty falling asleep and frequent arousals from sleep during the night, as well as having reddened eyes, puffy eyelids, dark circles under the eyes, and feelings of poor sleep. This person also reports continuing concerns about the responsibilities associated with the job promotion. As related by the patient, these concerns have been intensified by difficulty in identifying in writing the two major responsibilities that are of concern and frustration in trying to develop strategies to handle this part of the job. The person is also more anxious about the sleep disturbance and struggles with efforts to go to sleep and with concern about meeting the short-term goal set for beginning to handle the difficulty. The nurse notes evidence of unclear and slightly confused thinking (see Chap. 12), possibly related to on going sleep disturbance.

Since the behaviors of interest have not changed and the nurse is concerned about the increasing behavioral signs of the problem worsening, she provides the person with specific instructions for moderate active exercises at noontime and relaxation exercises to use at bedtime. She also decides to have the patient evaluated for the prescription of a short-term hypnotic. The nurse then asks the person to come back for a morning appointment in 3 days, after getting some sleep, so that they can work together on the problem. The goals of identifying in writing the two major job responsibilities that are of most concern and developing several alternate ways of dealing with the most distressing concern will again be attempted. The nurse will provide guidance in the use of a problem-solving process. This example shows a revision in the intervention plan based on evaluation of an ineffective intervention and assessment of additional behaviors.

► SUMMARY

In this chapter, the Roy Adaptation Model was used as a perspective from which to view activity and rest needs. A theoretical basis related to this need was developed which includes the processes of mobility and sleep. Related compensatory adaptive processes were identified, as well as examples of compromised processes. Each step of the nursing process was discussed and demonstrated with examples of behavior and stimuli, of nursing diagnoses, goals, and interventions, as well as evaluation of the effectiveness of nursing care.

► EXERCISES FOR APPLICATION

1. Identify the factors that influenced (focal and contextual stimuli) the amount of physical activity you engaged in on a particular day in the past week.

2. Develop a tool that can be used in the assessment of rest and sleep. In your tool consider both the usual pattern and current condition.

3. Using the tool developed in item 2, assess the rest and sleep needs of one person under 25 and one person over 60 years of age.

► ASSESSMENT OF UNDERSTANDING

Questions

1. The basic life process associated with activity is (a)_____ and with rest is (b)_____. Describe each of these concepts.

2. Label the following first-level assessment parameters as to whether they are associated with the need for activity (A), rest (R), or both (B).
   (a) _____ 24-hour pattern of activities
   (b) _____ self-report of status
   (c) _____ muscle mass and tone
   (d) _____ joint mobility
   (e) _____ lifestyle
   (f) _____ gait
   (g) _____ irritability and restlessness

3. Name three contextual factors (stimuli) that affect activity and three that affect rest.

4. Describe a compensatory process associated with the need for activity and rest that was not included in the discussion in the chapter.

Situation:

Mrs. L. is a 73-year-old widow with a social history of no known relatives or close friends who can visit her during her hospital stay. While waiting for a major surgical procedure for a fractured left femur, she is placed on the activity restriction of complete bed rest. Without a properly planned preventive nursing intervention, Mrs. L. likely will develop some of the very serious disuse consequences.

5. For Mrs. L., identify the disuse consequences that can occur in three of the following bodily functions: metabolic, musculoskeletal, circulatory, pulmonary, eliminative, integumentary, and sensory perceptual.

6. Formulate a nursing diagnosis for Mrs. L.

7. Develop a short-term and a long-term goal statement for Mrs. L.

8. Understanding that repair and restoration take place during rest and sleep, you are trying to improve the quality of sleep for Mrs. L. List at least two major nursing interventions to accomplish this.

9. What would be the behavior that would indicate that Mrs. L. had achieved the goals developed in your answer to (c)?

Feedback

1. (a) Mobility: the process whereby one moves or is moved.
   (b) Sleep: the process whereby most of the body's physiologic activities slow down to accomplish renewal of energy for future activity.

2. (a) B, (b) B, (c) A, (d) A, (e) B, (f) A, (g) R

3. Activity: physical condition, psychological condition, surroundings, or personal habits.
   Rest: physical stresses, environmental factors, age, psychological condition, or consumption of substances such as hypnotic drugs or alcohol.

4. Examples:
   At times, it is important to stay awake rather than fall asleep, for example, when driving. Some people use caffeine, loud music, or conversation to help them avoid sleep when occasionally required.

   Some people find a repetitive activity (counting "sheep") is helpful to divert their mind and induce sleep.

   When the ability to move about is limited, for example, when nurses in the operating room are "scrubbed" on a case or for choir members during a lengthy performance, circulation in the leg muscles is maintained by continually moving the toes.

5. Metabolic: negative nitrogen balance.
   Musculoskeletal: osteoporosis, joint contractures, denervations.
   Circulatory: postural hypotension, dependent edema, thrombosis.
   Pulmonary: hypoventilation.
   Eliminative: urinary rentention, kidney stones, constipation.
   Integumentary: pressure ulcers.
   Sensory perceptual: disorientation, confusion, anxiety.

6. Example of nursing diagnosis: Potential for disuse consequences related to the activity restrictions associated with complete bed rest.

7. Example of short-term goal: Prior to surgery, Mrs. L. will be actively participating in range-of-motion exercises for unaffected muscle groups.
   Example of long-term goal: Within 6 hours of surgery, Mrs. L. will sit in a chair for 10 minutes, or within 1 week following surgery, Mrs. L. will achieve sufficient mobility to enable her to return home with assistance provided as required.

8. Any two of the following:
   Maintain physical comfort and freedom from pain.
   Maintain an adequate amount of physical activity in order to induce deep sleep.
   Limit nighttime interruptions to a minimum to allow full cycles of sleep to take place.
   Alleviate psychological stress, which may increase need for REM sleep.

9. Examples: Mrs. L. would demonstrate and report doing the range-of-motion exercises for unaffected muscle groups at regular intervals.

Mrs. L. would understand the importance of early mobilization following surgery and would accomplish sitting in a chair for 10 minutes within the first 6 hours after surgery.

Mrs. L. would be confident with her ability to get around and, with required assistance provided in her home, be discharged from the hospital.

▶ **REFERENCES**

American Nurses Association and American Association of Neuroscience Nurses. (1985). *Neuroscience nursing practice: Process and outcome standards for selecting diagnoses.* Kansas City, MD: American Nurses Association.

Anders, E., & Parmelee, E. (Eds.). (1971). *A manual of standardized terminology and criteria for scoring states of sleep and wakefulness in newborn infants.* Los Angeles: University of California.

Benson, H. (1975). *The relaxation response.* New York: Morrow.

Brooks, V. (1986). *The neural basis of motor control.* New York: Oxford University Press.

Burrell, L. O., Gerlach, M. J. M., & Pless, B. S. (1997). *Adult nursing: Acute and community care* (2nd ed.). Stamford, CT: Appleton & Lange.

Cassmeyer, V., Long, B., & Wykle, M. (1993). Stressors, stress, and stress management. In Long, B., Phipps, W., & Cassmeyer, V. (Eds.), *Medical-surgical nursing: A nursing process approach* (pp. 88–107). St. Louis: Mosby.

Cho, J. (1984). Activity and rest. In Roy, Sr. C. (Ed.), *Introduction to nursing: An adaptation model* (2nd ed., pp. 138–158). Englewood Cliffs, NJ: Prentice-Hall.

Dossey, B., Buzzetta, C., & Kenner, C. (1992). *Critical care nursing: Body-mind-spirit.* Philadelphia: Lippincott.

Dworetzky, T. D. (1987, October). The willowy six-footer that bends at the waist. *Discover,* p. 18.

Friedman, D. (1993). Sleep disorders. In Long, B., Phipps, W., & Cassmeyer, V. (Eds.), *Medical-surgical nursing: A nursing process approach* (pp. 228–243). St. Louis: Mosby.

Hickey, J. (1992). *The clinical practice of neurological and neurosurgical nursing.* Philadelphia: Lippincott.

Hilton, J. (1976). Quantity and quality of patients' sleep: Disturbing factors in respiratory intensive care unit. *Journal of Advanced Nursing, 1,* 453–468.

Hobson, J. (1974). The cellular basis of sleep cycle control. *Advances in Sleep Research, 1,* 217–250.

Hodges, L. C., & Callihan, C. (1988). Human mobility: An overview. In Mitchell, P. H., Hodges, L. C., Muwaswes, M., & Walleck, C. A. (Eds.), *American Association of Neuro-*

science Nurses' Neuroscience Nursing: Phenomena and practice (pp. 269–281). Norwalk, CT: Appleton & Lange.

Hollerbach, A. (1988). Assessment of human mobility. In Mitchell, P. H., Hodges, L. C., Muwaswes, M., & Walleck, C. A. (Eds.), *American Association of Neuroscience Nurses' Neuroscience Nursing: Phenomena and practice* (pp. 283–302). Norwalk, CT: Appleton & Lange.

Long, B., Phipps, W., & Cassmeyer, V. (Eds.). (1993). *Medical-surgical nursing: A nursing process approach.* St. Louis: Mosby.

Miles, L. (1979). Sleep Questionnaire and Assessment of Wakefulness (SQAW). Stanford: Stanford Sleep Disorders and Sleep Research Program. As reprinted in Guilleminault, C. (1979). Sleeping and waking disorders: Indications and techniques (pp. 383–413). Menlo Park, CA: Addison-Wesley.

Mourad, L. (1986). Musculoskeletal system. In Thompson, J. (Ed.), *Clinical nursing* (pp. 427–541). St. Louis: Mosby.

Opstad, P., Bugge, J., & Magnus, P. (1979). Performance, mood, and clinical symptoms in men exposed to prolonged, severe physical work and sleep deprivation. *Aviation, Space and Environmental Medicine, 49,* 1065–1073.

Oswald, I. (1976). Why do we sleep? *Nursing Mirror, 138,* 71.

Pasnau, R., Naitoh, P., Stier, S., & Kollar, E. (1968). The psychological effects of 205 hours of sleep deprivation. *Archives of General Psychiatry, 18,* 496–505.

Rantz, M. J., & LeMone, P. (Eds.). (1997). *Classification of nursing diagnoses. Proceedings of the 12th conference NANDA.* Glendale, CA: CINAHL Information Systems.

Rechtschaffen, A., & Kales, A. (Eds.). (1973). *A manual for standardized terminology, techniques and scoring system for sleep stages of human subjects.* Los Angeles: Brain Research Institute, UCLA.

Robinson, C. (1993). Impaired sleep. In Carrieri-Kohlman, V., Lindsey, A., & West, C. (Eds.), *Pathophysiological phenomena in nursing* (pp. 490–528). Philadelphia: Saunders.

Rubin, M. (1988a). The physiology of bedrest. *American Journal of Nursing, 88,* 50.

Rubin, M. (1988b). How bedrest changes perception. *American Journal of Nursing, 88,* 55.

Sacks, O. (1983). *Awakenings.* New York: Dutton.

Sassin, J. (1970). Neurological findings following short-term sleep deprivation. *Archives of Neurology, 39,* 187–190.

Schreier, A. (1986). Nursing diagnoses pattern 13, Activity and rest: Sleep pattern disturbance. In Thompson, J. (Eds.), *Clinical nursing* (pp. 2099–2104). St. Louis: Mosby.

Sims, L., D'Amico, D., Stiesmeyer, J., & Webster, J. (1995). *Health assessment in nursing.* Redwood City, CA: Addison-Wesley.

Sleep Disorders Classification Committee, Association of Sleep Disorders Centers. (1979). Diagnostic classification of sleep and arousal disorders. *Sleep, 2,* 137.

Sloan, E., Hauri, P., Bootzin, R., Morin, C., Stevenson, M., & Shapiro, C. (1993). The nuts and bolts of behavioral therapy for insomnia. *Journal of Psychosomatic Research, 37 (1),* 19–37.

United States Centers for Disease Control and Prevention and American College of Sports Medicine. (1993). Summary statement: Workshop on physical activity and health. *Sports Medicine Bulletin, 28(2),* 7.

► ADDITIONAL REFERENCES

Bootzin, R., & Perlis, M. (1992). Nonpharmacologic treatments of insomnia. *Journal of Clinical Psychiatry, 53 Suppl.,* 37–41.

Canavan, T. (1984). The psychobiology of sleep. *Nursing, 84,* 682.

Dement, W. (1960). The effect of dream deprivation. *Science, 131,* 1705–1707.

Downs, F. (1974). Bestrest and sensory disturbances. *American Journal of Nursing, 74,* 434–438.

Dunn, M. (1987). Guideline for an effective personal fitness prescription. *Nurse Practice, 12(9),* 9–10.

Ferrandez, A. M., & Teasdale, N. (Eds.). (1996). *Changes in sensory motor behavior in aging.* Amsterdam: Elsevier.

Hoch, C., & Reynolds, C., III. (1986). Sleep disturbances and what to do about them. *Geriatric Nursing, 7,* 24.

Kerr, E. H. (1988). Exercise and health related fitness. *Physiotherapy. 74,* 411–420.

Kryger, M., Roth, T., & Dement, W. (1989). *Principles and practice of sleep medicine.* Philadelphia: Saunders.

Mitchell, P. H., Hodges, L. C., Muwaswes, M., & Walleck, C. A. (Eds.). (1988). *American Association of Neuroscience Nurses' Neuroscience nursing: Phenomena and practice* (pp. 501–515). Norwalk, CT: Appleton & Lange.

Perlis, M., Giles, D., Mendelson, W., Bootzin, R., & Wyatt, J. (1997). Psychophysiological insomnia: The behavioral model and a neurocognitive perspective. *Journal of Sleep Research, 6(3),* 179–188.

Roy, C. (1988). Altered cognition: An information processing approach. In Mitchell, P. H., Hodges, L. C., Muwaswes, M., & Walleck, C. A. (Eds.), *American Association of Neuroscience Nurses' Neuroscience Nursing: Phenomena and practice* (pp. 185–211). Norwalk, CT: Appleton & Lange.

Shannon, M. L. (1984). Five famous fallacies about pressure sores. *Nursing, 84,* 13–34.

Walsenben, J. (1965). Sleep disorders. *American Journal of Nursing, 150,* 971.

9

PROTECTION

Protection is the fifth basic need identified in the Roy Adaptation Model as essential to adaptation. Through both nonspecific and specific life processes of defense, the body is protected against disease and integrity of the human adaptive system is maintained. Whereas the nonspecific defense mechanisms include both surface membrane barriers and cellular and chemical defenses, it is the immune system that constitutes the specific defense processes of the body. Working hand in hand, these complex functional systems serve a vital role in meeting the need for protection by providing lines of defense against the invasion of disease-causing substances, thus promoting adaptation.

In this chapter, the basic life processes associated with protection—non-specific defense processes and specific defense processes—are addressed, along with the identification of parameters for assessment of behaviors and stimuli. Illustrations of compensatory and compromised processes related to protection are described. Finally, guidelines for planning nursing care by formulating diagnoses, establishing goals, selecting interventions, and evaluating nursing care are described.

▶ OBJECTIVES

After studying this chapter, the reader will be able to do the following:

1. Describe two basic life processes associated with the need for protection as presented in the chapter.

2. Identify important first-level assessment parameters (behaviors) for each of the basic life processes associated with the need for protection.

3. List second-level assessment parameters (common stimuli) that affect protection.

4. Describe one compensatory processes related to each of the basic life process associated with protection.

5. Name and describe two situations of compromised processes of protection.

6. Develop a nursing diagnosis, given a situation related to protection.

7. Derive goals for an individual with ineffective protection in a given situation.

8. Describe nursing interventions commonly implemented in situations of ineffective protection.

9. Propose approaches to determine the effectiveness of nursing interventions.

► KEY CONCEPTS DEFINED

Antigens: Substances such as proteins, nucleic acids, large carbohydrates, and some lipids that trigger the immune system.

Antimicrobial chemicals: Nonspecific defense chemicals that include interferons, complement, and urine.

Cellular (cell-mediated) immunity: Specific defense processes involving lymphocytes and macrophages.

Complement: A group of about 20 plasma proteins that causes destructive lesions in foreign cells and amplifies the inflammatory response.

Fever: Abnormally high systemic body temperature that inhibits multiplication of bacteria and increases metabolic rate to enhance repair processes.

Humoral (antibody-mediated) immunity: Specific defense processes involving antibodies in the body's fluids.

Immune system: A functional system that recognizes foreign molecules (antigens) and acts to inactivate or destroy them (Marieb, 1994, p. 351).

Immunity: The ability of the body to resist disease-causing agents. **Active immunity** is produced by an encounter with an antigen. **Passive immunity** is short-lived immunity resulting from antibodies obtained from another human or animal donor; no immunologic memory is established.

Immunocompetent: The ability of lymphocytes to respond to a specific antigen.

Inflammatory response: The body's second line of defense; initiated when cells are injured. Inflammatory chemicals cause blood vessels to dilate, capillaries to leak, and neutrophils and monocytes to be attracted to the area.

Interferons: Antimicrobial chemicals released by virus-infected cells to protect uninfected cells from the virus and interfere with the ability of the virus to multiply within the infected cells.

Natural killer cells: Cells that attack and destroy virus-infected or cancerous body cells.

Nonspecific defense processes: Surface membrane barriers and cellular and chemical defenses which function to hinder pathogen entry, prevent the spread of disease-causing microorganisms, and strengthen the immune response.

Phagocytes: Defense cells (nonspecific) that engulf and digest pathogens that enter the body through the mechanical barriers.

Pressure ulcers: Any lesions resulting from unrelieved pressure that causes damage to underlying tissue.

Pus: A mixture of dead or dying cells and living and dead pathogens; often a product of the inflammatory response.

Specific defense processes: Defense processes that are targeted against specific antigens.

Surface membrane barriers: Intact skin and mucous membranes; the body's first line of defense.

▶ BASIC LIFE PROCESSES OF PROTECTION

The physiologic need of protection is viewed as consisting of two basic life processes: nonspecific defense processes and specific defense processes. Together these two functional defense systems work to protect the body from "foreign" substances such as bacteria, viruses, transplanted tissues, and abnormal body cells.

▶ NONSPECIFIC DEFENSES: PROCESSES AND ASSESSMENT

Nonspecific defense processes are associated with two categories of protective mechanisms including surface membrane barriers involving the skin and mucous membranes; and cellular and chemical defenses, namely phagocytes, natural killer cells, the inflammatory response, antimicrobial chemicals, and fever. According to Marieb (1994), nonspecific defenses function "to hinder pathogen entry, to prevent the spread of disease-causing microorganisms, and to strengthen the immune response" (p. 345).

Surface Membrane Barriers

Surface membrane barriers, consisting of intact skin and mucous membranes, are the body's first line of defense. Unbroken skin forms a mechanical barrier against pathogens and other harmful substances. Its acidic epithelial surface inhibits bacterial growth. Sebum, the oily secretion of sebaceous glands, contains bacteria-killing chemicals. Keratin, a tough, insoluble protein in the hair, nails, and epidermis, resists acids, alkalis, and bacterial enzymes. The skin functions to protect deeper tissues from mechanical, chemical, and bacterial damage; ultraviolet radiation and thermal damage; and desiccation (drying out).

Sweat glands in the skin aid the body in heat loss and heat retention, and, through the process of perspiration, aid in the excretion of urea and uric acid. In addition, hairs and hair follicles provide minor protective functions while the nails protect fingers and toes. Consider this quotation from Marieb (1994, p. 98): "Would you be enticed by an advertisement for a coat that is waterproof, stretchable, washable, and permanent press, that invisibly repairs small cuts, rips, and burns, and that is guaranteed to last a lifetime with reasonable care?" Such are the properties of our first line of defense— the skin. It is a functional system that is often taken for granted, yet without which we could not maintain physiologic integrity.

Mucous membranes, the second component of the body's first line of defense, also function as a physical barrier against pathogens for the body. Mucus in respiratory and digestive tracts traps microorganisms. Nasal hairs filter and trap microorganisms, and cilia in the lower respiratory passages propel debris-laden mucus toward the upper respiratory tract. Secretions in the stomach, vagina, oral cavity, and eyes either destroy pathogens or inhibit the growth of bacteria and fungi.

Cellular and Chemical Defenses

Nonspecific cellular and chemical defenses include phagocytes, natural killer cells, the inflammatory response, antimicrobial chemicals, and fever. *Phagocytes* confront pathogens that manage to enter the body through the mechanical barriers by engulfing the pathogen and then digesting it. *Natural killer cells* directly attack and destroy any virus-infected or cancerous body cells.

The *inflammatory response* is considered to be the body's second line of defense. It is initiated when cells are injured, releasing inflammatory chemicals. These substances cause blood vessels to dilate, capillaries to leak, and neutrophils and monocytes to be attracted to the area. The four signs of inflammation are redness, heat, swelling, and pain. As Marieb (1994) identified, the inflammatory response "(1) prevents the spread of damaging agents to nearby tissues, (2) disposes of cell debris and pathogens, and (3) sets the stage for repair" (p. 348). A product of the inflammatory response may be *pus,* a mixture of dead or dying cells and living and dead pathogens.

Antimicrobial chemicals include interferons, complement, and urine. *Interferons* are released by virus-infected cells. They protect uninfected tissue cells by interfering with the ability of the virus to multiply within the cell. *Complement,* a group of about 20 plasma proteins, causes destructive lesions in foreign cells and amplifies the inflammatory response. Interferon molecules protect unaffected cells from viral takeover. The acidic nature of urine serves to inhibit bacterial growth and flush the lower urinary tract on an ongoing basis.

The final component of the nonspecific defense mechanisms of the body is fever. *Fever* involves an abnormally high systemic body temperature. The high body temperature inhibits multiplication of bacteria and increases metabolic rate in general, enhancing repair processes.

Assessment of Behavior

The first level of assessment as it relates to the nonspecific defense processes provides the nurse with an indication of how the person is managing to cope with factors affecting the surface membrane barriers and the cellular and chemical defenses associated with the need for protection. The nurse's background in anatomy, physiology, and pathophysiology provides the basis for decisions as to whether the observed behavior is adaptive or ineffective. As with assessment of other components of the physiologic mode, assessment related to the nonspecific defense processes involves observation, measurement, and subjective reporting.

History

The nurse initially obtains an understanding of the person's history related to the nonspecific defense mechanisms, past medical history, family history, and psychosocial history including lifestyle.

Skin

Inspection of the skin is a primary aspect to be addressed in the initial phase of assessment. This includes a description of the skin's appearance in terms of color. For example, erythema (redness of the skin), cyanosis (dusky blue color), jaundice (yellowness of skin), and pallor (paleness of face, conjunctiva, and mucous membranes) are some terms that may be applicable. Any changes in the normal pigmentation should be noted. Nurses are knowledgeable of variations in skin appearance for racial groups commonly encountered in their specific area of practice.

Initial assessment of the skin also includes a description of skin lesions that may be present, noting color, distribution, shape and arrangement, and whether lesions appear to be primary (direct result of a causative factor) or secondary (resulting from changes in a primary lesion).

Vascularity of the skin is the third aspect to be addressed. Vascular lesions resulting from the dilation of small blood vessels may be apparent. Birthmarks, nevi, and scars should also be noted and recorded as to their location, their dimensions, and, in the case of scars, how they were acquired.

Palpation of the skin provides further important information related to temperature, moisture, texture, mobility, turgor (elasticity of the skin), and skin thickness. Normal skin is warm to touch. Its texture is typically smooth and soft. Normal skin moves easily over most areas and when pinched, should immediately return to its normal shape (turgor).

Skin lesions related to sexually transmitted diseases such as herpes genitalis are of significance to nurses and the public because of their rising incidence. Herpes genitalis initially appears as a blister or pimple progressing to an ulcerated state. It is generally located on the vagina, cervix, and female or male external genitalia.

Pain and Skin Condition Related to an Operative Incision

The nurse carefully assesses postoperative pain and skin condition as it relates to an incisional area. People who have had surgery are expected to experience pain as a protective response following an incision. The duration of the pain depends on the nature of the surgery and on the person's tolerance of pain. The presence of pain is identified through the observation of activities such as crying, tense positioning, tightening of facial muscles, and through patient statements. In describing the pain experience, the nurse must note the type, duration, and location of the pain. Further discussion of pain is found in Chapter 10.

The nurse assesses skin integrity at the operative site by observing the color of the skin, whether the sutures or adhesive strips are intact, and the presence or absence of drainage. If drainage is present, the nurse must note the color, amount, and odor. The patient's phagocytic immune response and humoral-mediated immune response operate as protective functions, which cause the drainage and odor. With early discharge of surgical patients, the nurse provides education to the patient and family about assessing wound healing.

Hair and Nails

Examination of the hair should address distribution, quantity, texture, and condition of the scalp. The scalp should be smooth, moist, and clean. The presence of cysts, dandruff, or scabs would be considered unexpected or ineffective behaviors.

The distribution of the person's hair is assessed, bearing in mind that there are many normal variations. Variations that warrant further assessment are alopecia, unexpected general or local hair loss; a noticeable change in the character of the hair; excessive hair growth in women; and the disappearance of body hair from an area where it normally is present. Observations are made about the cleanliness of the hair. The expected adaptive behavior is the presence of clean hair in normal distribution and consistency on the head, extremities, trunk, pubic area, and face.

Nails should be examined closely because they are useful in assessing the person's general state of health. The nurse should note the color, shape, thickness, adherence to the nail bed, and presence lesions. Normal nails are transparent with a translucent, white end. Observe by asking whether the nails are soft, hard, brittle, peeling, pitted, or splitting. What is their color? Is the surface ridged and are there transverse lines indicative of injury or other pathologic processes? Clubbing of the fingers is indicative of decreased oxygenation and is an important indicator of cardiopulmonary disease.

Perspiration and Body Temperature

The nurse assesses the quantity, color, and location of perspiration on the body. Perspiration has a protective function to control the amount of heat loss from the body. When a person has an elevated temperature, the quantity of perspiration increases in an attempt to cool the body. The adaptive behavior for perspiration is a musty, salty, or sour odor. Perspiration is termed "malodorous" if it is particularly offensive, a situation caused by the breakdown of bacterial products found on the skin.

Measurement of body temperature is an important indicator of the final component of the nonspecific defense processes, fever. Alterations of body temperature above 98.6°F (37°C) are generally indicative of fever. Hypothermia is a term used to describe body temperature below normal.

Mucous Membranes

First-level assessment of mucous membranes includes the person's description of, or signs of, pain or discomfort in oral and nasal mucous membranes, the eyes, or the vaginal mucous membranes. Aspects to be noted include excess or decrease in secretions, edema, color of membranes, and lesions. Assessment of the oral cavity should describe the presence of stomatitis, oral plaque, carious teeth, coated tongue, or dry mouth.

Inflammatory Response

As previously mentioned, the inflammatory response is considered to be the body's second line of defense. The four signs of inflammation are redness, heat, swelling, and pain. If the inflammatory response is noted, there must be a careful description in terms of location, appearance, and presence of discharge.

Laboratory Examination

Laboratory examination of blood, urine, and secretions provides important information about microscopic defense activities which are underway in the human body. The presence of bacteria, plasma proteins, or foreign cells and molecules contributes to the determination of specific factors that are contributing to behaviors associated with the cellular and chemical defense processes.

Sensitivity to Pain and Temperature

Assessment of a person's level of sensitivity to pain and temperature is important for persons who lack this protective function since the defense mechanism of withdrawal from danger is decreased. This withdrawal behavior can be elicited for the assessment process by testing the person's perception of warm and cold objects applied to an area or by touching the person with a pin and seeing if the sensation was experienced. The expected behavior is skin that is sensitive to a pin and temperature.

Assessment of Stimuli

In the second level of assessment, assessment of stimuli, the nurse gathers data about internal and external factors influencing the behaviors identified in the first assessment phase of the adaptation nursing process. This includes the body's adaptive ability to maintain the structure, function, and regulation of the protection component, as well as the coping strategies the person uses to maintain or change behaviors.

Environmental Factors

Many of the factors that influence the nonspecific defense processes originate in the environment. For example, environmental stimuli that influence perspiration include room temperature, the amount of circulating air, and humidity. Factors that influence perspiration include the thickness of clothing worn and personal hygiene measures, such as frequency of bathing and the use of soaps and deodorants. Increased exercise or activity and stressful or anxiety-producing situations also contribute to increased perspiration.

Factors that influence the color of the skin include variation in emotions, extremes of temperature, and products that the person may be using such as cosmetics, lotions, and powders, or the presence of tattoos. Erythema may be a reflection of body temperature, environmental temperature, or the inflammatory process. Cyanosis results from deoxygenated hemoglobin, a situation that could arise from a variety of causes. Chemical and mechanical irritants can also interfere with the integrity of the surface membrane barriers and cellular and chemical defenses.

Cold weather as an environmental stimulus contributes to dry skin, whereas exposure to the sun can burn the skin. Poison ivy, urine, feces, soap, and some medications can irritate the skin and this can lead to the development of a rash.

Scars often are the result of injuries or previous surgical interventions. The factors causing scars often point the nurse in the direction of other physiologic problems that may or may not be of immediate concern. Skin piercing is a practice accepted by some groups of people. The practice is assessed as a factor interrupting skin integrity.

Integrity of the Modes

Disruptions to other components of the physiologic mode, or self-concept, role function, and interdependence modes, may be manifest in the nonspecific defense processes. Generalized rise in body temperature may be an indication of an increased metabolic rate associated with medical conditions such as hyperthyroidism; or it may be the manifestation of fever, strenuous exercise, or sunburn. Localized rise in skin temperature may be indicative of injury or infection. Situations where skin temperatures are cooler than normal may be indicative of shock or arterial disease.

Skin becomes drier as a person ages. Dryness can also be associated with physiologic conditions such as dehydration, myxedema, and chronic renal disease.

Texture of the skin, which is normally smooth and soft, can be influenced by local irritation, trauma, or a systemic problem. Mobility of the skin is decreased in situations of edema or with certain pathologic conditions such as scleroderma, an autoimmune disease that results in fibrosing of tissue. Turgor is also affected in situations of dehydration and with aging. Thickness of the skin is affected by disease conditions or frequent injection. The skin is also thinner in the elderly.

Alterations in the condition of hair and nails may be indicative of disease processes such as hormonal imbalance and endocrine problems, or indicative of a side effect of drugs. Although gray hair is normally associated with aging, it can result from local nerve injury.

Alterations in nails may also be indicative of injury or disease processes. Clubbing of the fingers is associated with cardiopulmonary disease, for example.

It is also suggested that stress is a factor that can lead to cutaneous disorders such as puritus, urticaria, psoriases, dermatitis, and acne.

Nutritional status affects the overall condition of the skin, hair, and nails. Pale-appearing skin may be due to anemia caused by a diet low in iron. Hair loss is evident in those suffering from some nutritional disturbances. Psychological disturbances are sometimes manifest through skin disruptions such as rashes, itching, and acne.

The role of malnutrition in the development of pressure ulcers is increasingly understood. It is important that the person's diet include nutrients required to support healing.

Cognator Effectiveness

Other factors that influence the condition of the skin and mucous membranes include hygiene practices. Maintaining clean, dry skin is important in the avoidance of infection. Effective oral hygiene maintains healthy mucous membranes and teeth. A well-balanced diet and adequate fluid intake are necessary for optimal general health, and for the health and functioning of the skin and mucous membranes in particular. There is increasing awareness of the importance of protection from sunlight. Exposure to chemical and physical agents is also an important consideration.

Developmental Stage

Aging is another factor that contributes to changes in the skin. Infants are prone to skin disorders because their skin structures are functionally immature. The infant dehydrates easily because the epidermis is very permeable. Milia and cradle cap are common protective behaviors caused by the increased activity of the sebaceous glands during late fetal life and early infancy. Temperature regulation is more labile in the neonate since the skin has an immature ability to shiver in response to cold or perspire in response to heat.

During the adolescent period, the sebaceous glands become extremely active and increase in size. The condition of the skin can be disrupted by the development of acne.

The behavioral manifestations of skin integrity for an elderly person are affected by the aging process. Skin pigmentation becomes uneven due to the clustering of melanocytes. The elasticity of the skin is decreased and the skin is more delicate as a result of decreased hydration and vascularity of the dermis. Lines and wrinkles appear as a result of the loss of subcutaneous fat. The hair becomes thicker in the nose and ears, while the scalp hair grays and thins. The nails become hard and brittle. Steps can be taken to prevent many of these changes. Protection from undue exposure, safety, and nutrition play important roles in the avoidance of injury to the skin.

▶ SPECIFIC DEFENSES: PROCESSES AND ASSESSMENT

The body's third line of defense is considered to be the immune system, the body's *specific defense processes.* Marieb (1994) described the *immune system* as "a functional system that recognizes foreign molecules (antigens) and acts to inactivate or destroy them" (p. 351). The action of the immune system is "targeted" against specific antigens. It protects the body against a wide variety of pathogens and abnormal body cells by recognizing foreign substances and mounting a systemic and targeted attack against them.

Two interrelated aspects of the immune system have been described: first, *humoral immunity* or *antibody-mediated immunity;* and second, *cellular* or *cell-mediated immunity.* In the first case, the protective factors are the antibodies in the body's fluids. In the second, the protective factors are living body cells—the lymphocytes and macrophages. The reader is referred to textbooks on anatomy and physiology for a more in-depth description of the cells involved in humoral immunity and cellular immunity. These cells act upon cellular targets either by directly lysing the foreign cells or by releasing chemicals that enhance the inflammatory response and activate other lymphocytes or macrophages.

Substances that trigger the immune system are called *antigens.* These can include foreign proteins, nucleic acids, many large carbohydrates, and some lipids. Any substance that consists of such foreign molecules is antigenic. At times, small molecules link up with body proteins and this results in a combination that is recognized as an antigen by the immune system. Initial exposure to an antigen primes the body to react more vigorously thereafter.

As previously mentioned, the cells of the immune system are lymphocytes (T cells and B cells) and macrophages. Lymphocytes originate in the red bone marrow. Only as they mature do they become *immunocompetent,* that is, capable of responding to a specific antigen. Immunocompetence happens for lymphocytes before they encounter the antigen and it is therefore understood that genes determine resistance to specific foreign substances. T cells are nonantibody-producing lymphocytes and B cells are associated with humoral (antibody-mediated) immunity.

Macrophages are distributed throughout lymphoid organs and connective tissues and tend to remain fixed in these areas. Their role in the immune response is to engulf foreign particles and to assist in the development of T lymphocytes.

Marieb (1994, p. 351) identified three important aspects of the immune response. One aspect is antigen specific, that is, it recognizes and acts against particular foreign substances. Another is systemic, not restricted to the initial site of infection. The third aspect of immune response is that it has memory, recognizing previously encountered pathogens and mounting even stronger attacks thereafter.

Humoral immunity can be acquired naturally or artificially and can be active or passive in nature. Naturally acquired active immunity occurs through contact with a pathogen or infection, while artificially acquired active immunity is generated artificially by the introduction of dead or attenuated pathogens. Passive immunity is acquired naturally when antibodies pass from the mother to the child either via the placenta before birth or through breast milk after delivery. Passive immunity is provided to a person with the injection of immune serum (gamma globulin) containing antibodies capable of binding with a specific antigen.

Antibodies are proteins produced by sensitized B cells in response to an antigen and are capable of binding to that antigen. This process involves fixation, neutralization, precipitation, and agglutination.

The information provided in this chapter about nonspecific and specific defense processes related to the need for protection is designed as an overview. The reader is encouraged to seek more detailed information about these important human processes from anatomy and physiology resources. At this point, however, discussion turns to the assessment of behaviors related to the specific defense processes.

Assessment of Behavior

The first level of assessment regarding immunologic status also involves the skills associated with observation, measurement, and subjective reporting.

Indications of the Immune Response

The nurse observes the person for indications that the immune response is occurring. Low-grade fever is often indicative of the initial viral attack and the release of interferon by the damaged cells. Second, there may be localized swelling of lymph nodes progressing to local inflammatory signs, generalized inflammatory response, malaise, aches and pains, and further progression to nausea, vomiting, and diarrhea.

Immunologic Status

In assessment of an individual's status relative to communicable diseases, several areas of behavior are of concern. It is important to know which communicable diseases the person has had or has been immunized against. In some chronic and degenerative diseases such as leukemia and acquired immunodeficiency syndrome (AIDS), the individual's immunologic protection is compromised. The complications prompting the person's need for care are a result of ineffective or absent immune responses of the body. The nurse anticipates that persons with such diagnoses will demonstrate many ineffective behaviors related to the need for protection. For example, there may be evidence of infectious processes within the body such as symptoms associated with pneumonia.

Laboratory Examination

Clinical indications of the immune response are also evident in laboratory findings related to blood cell counts, immunoglobulin levels, and serum complement level, for example.

As the nurse identifies the person's behaviors relative to the need for protection, an initial evaluation is made as to whether these behaviors are adaptive or ineffective. To guide this evaluation, the nurse uses knowledge related to normal physiologic functioning, established normal values, and the person's report of what is personally "normal" or adaptive. In consultation with the patient or family, the nurse establishes the tentative identification of adaptive and ineffective behaviors. With the initial priorities being the ineffective behaviors, the nurse then proceeds to identify the related stimuli.

Assessment of Stimuli

Many of the stimuli potentially affecting the specific defense processes of the immune system relate to the integrity of the modes, developmental stage, environmental considerations, and cognator effectiveness.

Integrity of the Modes

According to Burrell (1992, p. 164), stress is understood to make an individual more vulnerable to organisms in the immediate environment. Nutrition status also affects cell-mediated immunity; malnutrition and protein deficiency cause atrophy of the thymus and other lymphoid tissue.

Developmental Stage

As with the nonspecific defense processes, the specific defense mechanisms of the immune system are also affected with aging. The older person encounters a greater number of infections, which are more severe in nature, and this may be the result of the body's inability to trigger an effective immune response. It appears that the production and function of the T- and B-cell lymphocytes are affected in some manner as the aging process proceeds.

Environmental Factors

Environmental considerations include the use of tobacco, alcohol, and other drugs. Cigarette smoke suppresses T cell formation and alcohol destroys lymphocytes. Antibiotics, cytotoxic drugs, and nonsteroidal anti-inflammatory drugs suppress the immune response, while corticosteroids cause the lysis of T cells and inhibit protein synthesis in lymphocytes and phagocytes.

Radiation also affects the immune process by killing lymphocytes and diminishing the number of cells able to replenish them. Surgical removal of the thymus, lymph nodes, or spleen can also seriously impair immune system functioning.

Cognator Effectiveness

The person's perception, knowledge, and skill are often factors that interfere with adaptation as related to protection. Good nutrition is necessary for a properly functioning immune system. According to Lehmann (1991), protein-calorie malnutrition is considered to be one of the most frequent causes of immunosuppression. Malnutrition can affect the functioning of the T cells, B cells, and macrophages. When the amount of protein is diminished, it causes a depressed antibody response, decreased numbers of T cells, and ineffective phagocytic activity.

Research in the field of psychoneuroimmunology is exploring connections among psychological factors such as emotions and attitudes, the nervous system, and the immune system (Santrock, 1989). Relationships between emotional status and the immune system are being demonstrated. For example, depression is thought to adversely affect and suppress the immune system.

Associated with cognator effectiveness is the person's knowledge about prevention and early detection of disease processes. Increasingly, prevention and health promotion are becoming a major focus of health care systems throughout the world. Immunization programs provide people with the opportunity to avoid many communicable diseases that in times past claimed many lives. For example, flu immunizations are available in many areas to prevent particular strains of influenza from infecting susceptible individuals in the population.

Knowledge about communicability, diagnosis, and treatment of sexually transmitted diseases is becoming increasingly important. In many areas, programs are being mounted to assist in the education of the public relative to prevention of and protection against this widespread health problem.

Education of the public is important in the prevention and early detection of sexually transmitted diseases. It is important for the nurse to assess the person's understanding and practice of preventive and health promotion activities related to the need for protection.

► **COMPENSATORY ADAPTIVE PROCESSES**

Viewed as an adaptive system (see Chap. 2), the person has innate and acquired ways of responding to the changing environment. Further, Roy conceptualizes these complex adaptive dynamics as coping mechanisms of the regulator and cognator subsystems.

As described in this chapter, the need for protection is met through nonspecific defense processes and specific defense processes. However, when the processes of protection are not stable or adequate, the regulator and cognator coping processes activate compensation. Further, the thinking and feeling person, by way of cognator activity, can do much to affect any adaptation levels within the physiologic mode. Cognator and regulator subsystems provide compensatory adaptive responses that extend the effectiveness of behavior in meeting the goals of adaptation. Adaptation levels, as an internal stimulus, can be integrated, compensatory, or compromised.

Compensatory adaptation for protection includes, in many respects, what the nonspecific and specific defense processes are all about, that is, providing lines of defense against the invasion of disease-causing substances. Under normal situations, the defense processes carry out their work without human consciousness of the cellular activity that is occurring in and around the body. It is at times of particular challenge to these processes that awareness of their functioning takes place.

The inflammatory response was described earlier in this chapter. Considered to be the body's second line of defense, the inflammatory response is initiated when cells are injured. The four signs of inflammation are redness, heat, swelling, and pain.

Fever, an abnormally high systemic body temperature, is a compensatory process that inhibits multiplication of bacteria and increases metabolic rate, thus enhancing repair. There are situations, however, in which an abnormally high fever, particularly in young children, is deemed to be ineffective and, ultimately, a threat to the integrity of the individual. There are ways to control abnormally high fever (through learning as a cognator compensatory mechanism). These actions include the intake of large amounts of fluids, tepid sponges, and the administration of salicylic acid (aspirin).

Another example of a compensatory adaptation level relates to individuals traveling in a foreign country, particularly one in which the food and water supply is of questionable purity. Travelers have learned that it is important to carefully assess the food to be eaten for the possibility of contamination and to rely on a dependable supply of bottled water or other processed beverages for fluids.

The development and application of immunization programs represents an organized and massive undertaking to provide a compensatory adaptation level for entire populations. As described earlier, scientists have learned that it is possible to assist immune systems to develop protection against specific communicable diseases. Through immunization programs, many infectious diseases have been virtually irradicated. The immunization process for the individual and programs for the community can be regarded as a learned (cognator) activity indicative of compensatory adaptation.

▶ COMPROMISED PROCESSES OF PROTECTION

When adaptation levels are neither integrated nor compensatory, compromise leads to adaptation problems. Adaptation problems can be caused by difficulties in any or all of the processes of protection. With respect to the need for protection, eight compromised processes are identified. They are disrupted skin integrity, pressure ulcers, itching, delayed wound healing, infection, potential for ineffective coping with allergic reaction, ineffective coping with changes in immune status, and ineffective temperature regulation. Two specific examples of compromised processes of protection are further explored: pressure ulcers and ineffective coping with changes in immune status.

Pressure Ulcers

Pressure ulcers are any lesions resulting from unrelieved pressure, which causes damage to underlying tissue. It is estimated that approximately 9 percent of all hospitalized patients and 23 percent of all personal care home residents are affected by pressure ulcers (Agency for Health Care Policy and Research, 1994). According to Sparks (1993), three factors have been identified as the best discriminators for pressure ulcer risk: friction, dependence in self-care, and confinement to bed or chair. Prolonged localized pressure on bony prominences or from external devices (casts, traction, catheters, or tubes, for example) causes tissue necrosis, which results in ulceration. As Burrell (1992) points out, "the incidence of a single pressure ulcer will prolong the patient's hospitalization and increase health team care and costs. In addition, there is the added discomfort to the patient that, in most cases, could have been avoided or prevented" (p. 2013). Preventive measures will be addressed later in this chapter.

Immunodeficiency

Ineffective coping with changes in immune status is particularly evident in immunodeficiency disorders. Defective function of one or more mechanisms of the immune system results in inadequate protection for the body against microbial infections or other antigens. These disorders are classified as either primary, when there is improper development of the immune system, or secondary, if it results from depression of the immune system from environmental factors or infection.

Of particular significance in the 1990s is acquired immunodeficiency syndrome (AIDS), described by the U.S. Secretary of Health and Human Services (Marieb, 1994, p. 366) as the "plague of the twentieth century." One report by the Interagency Coalition on AIDS (1996/97) noted, "Each day, 1,000 new HIV infections occur in children worldwide. The World Health Organization estimates that by the year 2000, between five and ten million children will be infected with HIV." As Marieb described in 1994:

> AIDS is characterized by severe weight loss, night sweats, swollen lymph nodes, and increasingly frequent infections, including a rare type of pneumonia . . . and a bizarre malignancy Kaposi's sarcoma, a cancer-like condition of blood vessels evidenced by purple lesions of the skin. Some AIDS victims develop slurred speech and severe dementia. The course of AIDS is grim, and thus far inescapable, finally ending in complete debilitation and death from cancer or overwhelming infection (p. 366).

Recent research advances in improving health and prolonging life for people with HIV infection and AIDS have occurred in the area of drug therapies, for example, protease inhibitors and vaccines. However, as effectiveness of antiviral therapies increases, disease complexities increase as well. With the accumulation of new information about HIV infection and disease progression, the Office of AIDS Research of the National Institutes of Health (NIH) sponsored a panel to define principles of therapy of HIV infection in clinical practice. The panel defined 11 principles to provide the scientific basis for specific guidelines for the treatment of HIV-infected persons. The principles are being widely disseminated to health care providers in an attempt to keep treatment current with research (National Institutes of Health, 1998).

Other compromised processes of protection involve such situations as allergic reactions, infection, itching, rashes, and delays in wound healing. The reader is directed to pathophysiology resources for complete discussion of these situations.

Once the stimuli associated with the ineffective and adaptive behaviors have been identified, the nurse, in consultation with the patient, establishes their focal, contextual, or residual influence on the person. This classification assists the nurse in setting priorities in the subsequent steps of the nursing process.

▶ PLANNING NURSING CARE

Protection is a priority requirement for the person's physiologic adaptation. In applying the nursing process, the nurse makes a careful assessment of behaviors and stimuli related to the basic life processes of nonspecific and specific defense processes. In assessing factors influencing the need for protection, regulator and cognator effectiveness in initiating compensatory processes is also considered. Based on this thorough first- and second-level assessment, the nurse makes a nursing diagnosis, sets goals, selects interventions, and evaluates care.

Nursing Diagnosis

The assessment information related to behaviors and stimuli are interpreted in the form of a nursing diagnosis. The statement of the diagnosis is formulated by considering the data of the first and second levels of assessment. The diagnosis includes a statement of observed behaviors with the most relevant influencing stimuli.

Indicators of effective adaptation relative to the need for protection would be evident in nursing diagnosis statements such as "intact skin free of excoriation and lesions due to nutritious diet and conscientious hygiene," or "profuse perspiration due to outside temperature of 102°F." In the latter situation, perspiration is the body's method of adapting to warm temperatures in the external environment.

An alternate way of stating a nursing diagnosis is to use a summary label that best identifies the nurse's judgment of the clinical situation from an established classification system. The Roy model has two classification lists, one for indicators of adaptation and one for commonly recurring adaptation problems. The complete classification lists for the Roy model are included in Chapter 3. In Table 9–1, the Roy model nursing diagnostic categories for the physiologic need of protection are shown in relation to nursing diagnosis labels approved by the North American Nursing Diagnosis Association (Rantz & LeMone, 1997).

Common adaptation problems, or broad areas of concern, within the component of protection include pressure ulcers (decubitus ulcers) and itching (puritis). Pressure ulcers occur frequently in the elderly and those who are immobilized; they result from disrupted circulation to the affected tissue. (Issues related to immobility are discussed in Chap. 8.) A relevant nursing diagnosis for this adaptation problem could be "pressure ulcer on left lateral ankle due to prolonged pressure and immobility." Indicators of positive

TABLE 9–1   NURSING DIAGNOSTIC CATEGORIES FOR PROTECTION

Positive Indicators of Adaptation	Common Adaptation Problems	NANDA Diagnostic Labels
• Intact skin	• Disrupted skin integrity • Pressure ulcer • Itching	• Impaired tissue or skin integrity • Risk for impaired skin integrity • Altered protection • Pressure ulcer (specific stage)
• Effective healing response	• Delayed wound healing • Infection	• Risk for infection • Risk for trauma • Risk for poisoning • Risk for injury • Risk for perioperative injury
• Adequate secondary protection for changes in skin integrity and immune status	• Potential for ineffective coping with allergic reaction	
• Effective processes of immunity	• Ineffective coping with changes in immune status	• Altered protection
• Effective temperature regulation	• Ineffective temperature regulation • Fever • Hypothermia	• Ineffective thermoregulation • Hypothermia • Hyperthermia • Risk for altered body temperature

adaptation related to the problem of pressure ulcers would include skin integrity with the absence of skin infection.

Alteration in comfort related to skin lesions is often termed "itching." The focal stimulus for itching may be a skin disorder resulting from a systemic disease or pregnancy. An allergic reaction (immune response), local lesion, dry skin, and emotional upset are other influencing factors. The time of day is a contextual stimulus since itching is often worse at night when there are fewer activities on which to focus. A warm environment also increases itching. A nursing diagnosis reflecting this adaptation problem is "itching related to contact with poison ivy."

Once the nursing diagnoses have been established, the nurse proceeds to the next step of the nursing process, goal setting. The priority nursing diagnoses, those relating to the ineffective behaviors and the focal stimulus, would be given initial consideration although the importance of maintaining adaptive behavior is acknowledged.

Goal Setting

In the fourth step of the nursing process as described in the Roy Adaptation Model, the nurse, in collaboration with the person receiving care, establishes goals, that is, statements of clear behavioral outcomes of nursing care for the person. The goal should address the behavior, the change expected, and the time frame in which the goal is to be achieved. Goals may be long-term or short-term and these time frames are relative to the situation involved.

In the example of the nursing diagnosis, "pressure ulcer on left lateral ankle due to prolonged pressure and immobility," a relevant goal would focus on the pressure ulcer. A short-term goal could be, "Within 3 weeks, the pressure ulcer on the left ankle will decrease in diameter from 1 inch to $1/2$ inch." In this goal, the behavior relates to the size of the pressure ulcer and the healing that is expected to occur, the time frame is "within 1 week" and the change is the decrease in the diameter of the ulcer.

Another example of goal setting illustrates the importance of focusing on the maintenance of effective adaptation. The situation pertains to the postoperative status of an incision, a disruption in skin integrity that could lead to ineffective adaptation should an infection develop. The nursing diagnosis indicates that the patient has an incision with a dressing resulting from surgery to the abdomen. A goal statement focuses on the status of the incision: "Within 2 days, incisional edges will be approximated with evidence of normal healing and the absence of infection." Here, the behavior focuses on the healing of the incision; the time frame is within 2 days; and the change expected is the evidence of normal healing, the approximation of the wound edges, and the absence of infection.

Although the goals illustrated pertain to situations in which skin integrity has been disrupted, it is important for the nurse to derive goals aimed at preservation of the protective functions of the body. Within this context are many preventive and health promoting goals relating to protection. As was mentioned in Chapter 2, in response to an increasing incidence of HIV infection and AIDS in native Canadians, the Atlantic First Nations AIDS Task Force has undertaken a program to teach native people about HIV and AIDS and the effect it could have on their communities and their people as a whole. Native communities across Canada have become involved in an effort to decrease behaviors that contribute to the spread of the disease. A population goal related to this particular initiative could be: "Within 3 years, the new cases of HIV infection will be reduced from the 1997 levels by 50 percent." Here, the time frame is 3 years, the measured behavior for the population is "new cases of HIV infection," and the change expected is a 50 percent reduction.

Within the context of protection are many preventive and health promoting goals. A nurse in a community agency may establish a goal for an infant that pertains to immunization status at a particular age. For example, "At 4 years of age, the child will demonstrate active immunity against common communicable childhood diseases." The behavior associated with this goal is "immunity."

Once the behavioral goals have been established, the nurse proceeds to identify the nursing interventions most likely to assist in the achievement of the desired outcomes.

Intervention

Once the goals have been established relative to behaviors that will promote adaptation, the nurse determines the interventions that will assist the person in attaining the stated goals. Nursing interventions for the promotion of protection depend on the stimuli identified. The nurse manages the stimuli by either promoting or reinforcing them or by taking action to change or eliminate the stimuli. In addition, the nurse can affect the internal stimulus of adaptation level by interventions that focus on the cognator or regulator processes.

In the situation relating to pressure ulcers, frequent positioning of the immobilized patient assists in promoting circulation by ensuring that bony prominences are cushioned against pressure. From a different perspective and situation, the body's internal protective response is facilitated through programs of immunization in the community agencies. Many health promotion programs have been designed to assist individuals in protecting and promoting their own health by early detection of disease processes. Each of these examples can be viewed as attempts to manage stimuli that compromise an individual's protective processes.

Many of the nursing interventions associated with aseptic technique are directed at the control of microorganisms and the minimization of inflammatory and infectious responses of the body. For example, preoperative skin cleansing is an attempt to manage the opportunity for foreign substances to enter the incisional site.

Specific interventions are directed at factors contributing to the observed adaptation problems related to protection. Interventions to control itching include soothing baths, trimming the nails, and the use of firm pressure instead of scratching. For localized itching, the application of cool, wet compresses may be used. Temperature control and the use of diversionary activities such as watching television are other suggested interventions.

The nurse routinely observes the skin color of the person and notes localized areas of red, blue, or mottled skin, which indicate decreased circulation. Rubbing around these areas helps to restore circulation. If the skin integrity becomes disrupted, as in the case of a pressure ulcer, then other interventions are necessary.

There are many nursing interventions applicable to the care of persons with pressure ulcers. Once again, these interventions are directed at the stimuli identified in the second level of assessment.

1. Nutritional status must be addressed. Adequate dietary intake or supplementation is necessary if the person is malnourished. This may require supplementation with vitamins or minerals if deficiencies are confirmed.
2. Tissue load (the distribution of pressure, friction, and shear on the tissue) must be managed. Positioning techniques include staying off the ulcer and using appropriate positioning devices. Pressure-relieving overlays, mattresses, and beds can be helpful adjuncts to turning every 2 hours.
3. Support surfaces including standard mattresses, foam, static flotation, alternating air, low-air loss, and air-fluidized mattresses should be considered, but cost and availability may be prohibitive.
4. Care of the ulcer itself can involve debridement, wound cleansing, and application of dressing or other therapy. Debridement of necrotic tissue is necessary before healing will occur. Wet-to-dry dressings are one method to accomplish this, as is enzymatic debridement.
5. Wound cleansing should be gentle and use of antiseptics should be avoided as these agents are cytotoxic and retard the healing process. Normal saline is the preferred choice.
6. Dressings should protect the wound, be biocompatible, and provide hydration.
7. Bacterial colonization and infection must be managed. Topical antibiotics may be indicated.
8. Patient education can enable people to become partners in the healing process, where possible. Information should include risk factors, pathology, principles of wound healing and nutrition, product selection, and assessment of healing.

Nursing interventions must be directed at the prevention of pressure sores. The identification of patients at risk can assist in this prevention. Sparks (1993) identified three factors that are suggested to be the best discriminators for pressure ulcer risk: friction, being dependent in self-care, and being confined to bed or chair. To decrease the stimulus of moisture on the skin, the patient and bed need to be clean and dry. Lifting when repositioning, instead of pulling, as well as keeping the bed wrinkle free, decreases the problem of friction. A diet high in protein and vitamins is essential to the repair of tissue. The application of lotion helps to keep the skin soft and intact.

Protection is a component of the physiologic mode where nursing interventions often focus on the maintenance of adaptive behaviors in an effort to prevent adaptation problems. Thus, many interventions are protective and preventive in nature. Specifically, nurses are conscientious in their efforts to minimize the opportunity for infectious processes to enter the body. For example, herpes genitalis is a sexually transmitted disease and much can be done in the form of prevention. Nurses are often functioning in positions where they can help to prevent the spread of such infections through a program of counseling and education. It is important that nurses maintain current knowledge regarding sexually transmitted diseases and their treatment.

Protective and preventive interventions are particularly important as they pertain to the increasing incidence of AIDS. Nursing measures associated with the prevention of the spread of AIDS and the care of the increasing numbers of hospitalized persons in the final stages of the disease are vitally important and have widespread implications for nurses functioning in all aspects of practice. As Rogers (1989, p. 254) pointed out, "prevention is the only approach to dealing with this epidemic [AIDS]." This intervention includes information regarding protection from and prevention of the disease, particularly in relation to self, other patients, and staff. Standard precautions set forth by the Centers for Disease Control and Prevention include a two-tiered approach to infection control that is used in many settings for all patients and includes bloodborne, airborne, and epidemiologically important pathogens (West & Cohen, 1997).

The success of the interventions such as those described in assisting the person to achieve the preset behavioral goals is determined through evaluation. This is the sixth step of Roy's nursing process.

Evaluation

Evaluation involves determining the effectiveness of nursing interventions in relation to the person's behavior and in terms of the preset goals. Was the goal that was set in the fourth step of the nursing process attained? To make this decision, the nurse assesses the behavior of the person after the interventions have been implemented. As in the initial assessment steps, observation, measurement, and subjective reporting are used. The nursing intervention would be considered effective if the person's behavior aligns with the preset goals.

Looking back to the goal related to the pressure ulcer, it was identified that the diameter of the lesion should reduce from 1 inch to $1/2$ inch within 1 week. If the nursing interventions described were assisting with the healing process, it would be noted by the nurse that the size of the lesion had decreased. If no change was noted, the nurse would proceed through the nursing process again, perhaps establishing that the goal was unrealistic, that not all stimuli have been identified, or that there are other interventions that may be appropriate to attain the goal.

Expected outcomes for the protection component would be the maintenance of integrity of the nonspecific and specific defense processes. The person's skin should be intact and free of discomforts such as itching. It may be helpful for the person to acquire knowledge regarding skin care and its importance in the area of protection. Indicators of positive adaptation related to the problem of itching would include patient statements indicating relief of discomfort, a skin free from scratch marks and abrasions, and an intact skin surface. Indicators of positive adaptation related to the problem of pressure ulcers would be the maintenance of skin integrity with the absence of skin infections.

Once the effectiveness of the nursing intervention has been determined, the nurse returns to the first step of the nursing process to look more closely at behaviors that continue to be ineffective. It is important to recognize that the nursing process is ongoing and simultaneous. Although it is necessary to discuss each aspect of the nursing process as a separate entity, one must bear in mind that each aspect is related to and affected by the other.

▶ SUMMARY

This chapter has focused on the application of the Roy Adaptation Model to the physiologic need of protection. An overview of the basic life processes, nonspecific body defense processes and specific body defense processes, associated with protection was provided along with the identification of parameters for assessment of behaviors and stimuli. Illustration of innate and learned adaptive compensatory responses related to protection were described and examples of two compromised processes (pressure ulcers and ineffective coping changes in immune status) were provided. Finally, guidelines for planning nursing care through the formulation of nursing diagnoses, goals, and interventions were explored and evaluation of nursing care was described. In providing for the person's need for protection by promoting and maintaining nonspecific and specific defense processes, the nurse contributes to the overall integrity of the person.

▶ EXERCISES FOR APPLICATION

1. Identify activities that you engage in, as a healthy adult, that are directed at your adaptation relative to the need for protection.

2. If you were a resident in a nursing home as a result of the progression of multiple sclerosis and immobilized in a wheelchair, what nursing interventions would you require to assist you in the maintenance of adaptation relative to protection?

3. You have an acquaintance who has offered to provide hospice care in her home for a friend with AIDS. What advice would you offer as to how she should protect herself and her family?

▶ ASSESSMENT OF UNDERSTANDING

Questions

1. Classify the following components of protection as associated with non-specific defense processes (N) or specific defense processes (S).
   (a) _____ antibodies
   (b) _____ phagocytes
   (c) _____ mucous membranes
   (d) _____ lymphocytes
   (e) _____ skin
   (f) _____ natural killer cells
   (g) _____ macrophages
   (h) _____ inflammatory response
   (i) _____ fever

2. In behavioral assessment of an operative site, which of the following factors would be important to note and measure?
   (a) approximation of wound edges
   (b) temperature of skin at wound edge
   (c) color of skin at wound edge
   (d) presence of discharge
   (e) pain in the incisional area

3. Developmental stage is an important stimulus affecting protection behaviors. Label the following behaviors according to the developmental stage to which they pertain: infant (I), adolescent (A), or older adult (O).
   (a) _____ uneven skin pigmentation
   (b) _____ epidermis very permeable
   (c) _____ nails become hard and brittle
   (d) _____ sebaceous glands active and increase in size
   (e) _____ temperature regulation labile

4. Label the following compensatory adaptation level as indicative of regulator (R) or cognator (C) activity.
   (a) _____ wound healing process following incision
   (b) _____ universal precautions practiced by health care workers
   (c) _____ covering one's mouth when coughing
   (d) _____ swelling of tissue following an insect bite
   (e) _____ cold symptoms
   (f) _____ preoperative skin cleansing

5. Name and describe one compromised adaptation process of protection related to (a) nonspecific defense processes and one related to (b) specific defense processes.

   (a) _____

   _____

   (b) _____

   _____

Situation:

A 45-year-old woman with multiple sclerosis has been admitted to a continuing care facility as a result of progression of the disease. Although she has limited movement of one arm, the rest of her body is paralyzed. Contractures have developed in her legs and arms and careful positioning is required. She has very limited ability to fulfill any of the activities of daily living and is catheterized intermittently for bladder control. She has developed a reddened area on her coccyx that is at risk for breaking down without careful attention.

6. Construct a nursing diagnosis focusing on the need for protection, with particular attention to the potential for disrupted skin integrity.

7. Develop a goal relative to the behavior of "reddened skin over coccyx." The goal should include the behavior of concern, the change expected, and the time frame involved.

8. Nursing interventions are focused on the stimuli causing the behavior of concern, in this situation, reddened skin over the coccyx. For each of the stimuli identified below, suggest a nursing intervention that could assist in dealing with the problem.

Stimuli	**Nursing Intervention**
(a) Continual pressure on coccyx from supine positioning	_____ _____
(b) Friction on skin when moving up in wheelchair	_____ _____
(c) Incontinence between catheterizations	_____ _____
(d) Nutritional status less than body requirements	_____ _____

9. Which of the following behaviors would indicate that the nursing intervention had been effective in goal achievement?

   (a) breakdown of skin over coccyx

   (b) increase in size of reddened area

(c) disappearance of redness over coccyx

(d) patient's report of pain and discomfort

Feedback

1. (a) S, (b) N, (c) N, (d) S, (e) N, (f) N, (g) S, (h) N, (i) N

2. a, c, d, and e

3. (a) O, (b) I, (c) O, (d) A, (e) I

4. (a) R, (b) C, (c) C, (d) R, (e) R, (f) C

5. (a) A burn (disrupted skin integrity) is a situation in which the skin has been damaged by heat, friction, or chemicals. This results in disruption of the surface membrane barrier of the body.
    (b) A reaction to mismatched blood (ineffective coping with allergic reaction) is a situation in which the immune system mounts an attack on infused blood cells that are not appropriately matched to those of the individual.

6. Example of nursing diagnosis: "Potential for disrupted skin integrity (pressure ulcer) due to immobilization and pressure on coccyx."
7. Example of goal: "Within 2 days, the skin over the coccyx will be free of redness and irritation."
8. (a) management of tissue load to relieve pressure on the area at all times; repositioning every 2 hours.
    (b) assistance with repositioning to avoid friction on the area
    (c) keep area clean and dry and exposed to air as much as possible
    (d) consultation with dietitian to ensure adequate intake and nutritious diet
9. c

▶ REFERENCES

Agency for Health Care Policy and Research. (1994). *Quick reference guide for clinicians: Pressure ulcer treatment.* U.S. Department of Health and Human Services. Washington, DC: (AHCPR Publication No. 95–1653).

Burrell, L. O. (1992). *Adult nursing in hospital and community settings.* Norwalk, CT: Appleton & Lange.

Interagency Coalition on AIDS. (1996/97). New international network calls for urgent action on children and AIDS. *Canadian AIDS News, IX(3),* 2.

Lehmann, S. (1991). Immune function and nutrition: The clinical role of the intravenous nurse. *Journal of Intravenous Nursing, 14(6),* 406–420.

Marieb, E. N. (1994). *Essentials of human anatomy and physiology* (4th ed.). Redwood City, CA: Benjamin/Cummings.

National Institute of Health. (1998). Report of the NIH panel to define principles of therapy of HIV infection. *Annals of Internal Medicine, 128,* 1057–1078.

Rantz, M. J., & LeMone, P. (Eds.). (1997). *Classification of nursing diagnoses. Proceedings of the 12th conference NANDA.* Glendale, CA: CINAHL Information Systems.

Rogers, B. (1989). AIDS and ethics in the workplace. *Nursing Outlook, 37(6),* 254–256.

Santrock, J. W. (1989). *Life-span development* (3rd ed.). Dubuque, IA: Brown.

Sparks, S. M. (1993). Clinical validation of pressure ulcer risk factors. *Ostomy Wound-Management, 39(4),* 40–41, 43–46, 48.

West, K., & Cohen, M. (1997). Standard precautions—a new approach to reducing infection transmission in the hospital setting. *Journal of Intravenous Nursing, 20(6 Suppl.),* 7–10.

▶ **ADDITIONAL REFERENCES**

Bruner, L. S., & Snygg, C. (1989). *Textbook of medical-surgical nursing.* Philadelphia: Lippincott.

Gordon, M. (1995). *Manual of Nursing Diagnosis 1995–96.* St. Louis: Mosby.

Manrex Limited. (1996). Treatment of pressure ulcers. *The Art of Geronursing* (Pamphlet). Winnipeg, Manitoba, Canada: Author.

10

SENSES

The senses play an important role in adaptation. They are channels of input necessary for the person to interact with the changing environment. The model of integrated cognitive processing presented in Chapter 12 indicates that immediate sensory experience is the focal stimulus to be processed. Sensations, and the resulting perceptions, are influenced greatly by who the person is and their context, that is, environmental, cultural, and other background experiences. In the Roy Adaptation Model, these influences are contextual and residual stimuli, as is adaptation in the other modes. In turn, one's life functioning depends on intact sensory function and adapting to the effect of temporary or permanent disabilities related to sensation.

The life processes related to primary senses of seeing, hearing, and feeling are explored in this chapter. Examples of compensatory adaptive strategies and compromised processes related to sensory processes are described. There is particular focus on the compromised sensory experiences of pain and hyperactivity, which nurses encounter frequently in clinical practice. The nursing process is explored as it relates to promoting adaptation related to the senses.

► OBJECTIVES

After studying this chapter, the reader will be able to do the following:

1. Describe three primary senses associated with the complex process by which a person receives and exchanges information as presented in this chapter.

2. Identify important first-level assessment parameters (behaviors) for each of the primary senses.

3. List second-level assessment parameters (common stimuli) that affect primary senses.

4. Describe one compensatory process related to each of the primary senses.

5. Name and describe two situations of compromised processes of the primary senses.

6. Develop a nursing diagnosis, given a situation related to the primary senses.

7. Derive goals for an individual with adaptation problems associated with the primary senses in a given situation.

8. Describe nursing interventions commonly implemented in situations of adaptation problems associated with the primary senses.

9. Propose approaches to determine the effectiveness of nursing interventions.

▶ KEY CONCEPTS DEFINED

Detectors: Sensory receptors that act to detect the presence or absence of some component of the environment.

Feeling: A complex process involving the somatosensory system whereby touch and pressure, position sense, heat and cold, and pain are detected, transmitted, and interpreted.

Hearing: A complex process involving the peripheral structure of the ear, auditory neural pathways, and the auditory areas of the brain whereby sound waves are detected, transmitted, and interpreted.

Hyperactivity: The general term given to a group of behaviors such as constant movement, short attention span, distractability, and poor impulse control; also referred to by terms such as attention deficit disorder, hyperkinesis, or minimal brain dysfunction.

Kinesthesia: Position sense resulting from mechanical changes in the muscles and joints, both the sense of static limb position and the sensation of limb movement.

Pain: A biobehavioral, subjective, and personal experience of noxious stimuli, considered to be whatever the patient says it is and occurring whenever the patient says it does. **Acute pain** is short in duration, has an identifiable cause, and follows an expected time course depending on the cause. **Chronic pain** is persistent and does not have a predictable time limit.

Perception: The interpretation of a sensory stimulus and the conscious appreciation of it.

Sensation: Processes whereby energy (light, sound, heat, mechanical vibration, and pressure, for example) is transduced into neural activity that becomes perception.

Suffering: Endurance of a difficult state, physiologic, phychological, or both; a severe state of distress associated with loss or threat of loss of the integrity of the person.

Transducers: Sensory receptors that act to sample a portion of the energy associated with a component of the environment and convert the sampled energy into an electrical signal containing information.

Vision: A complex process involving the peripheral structure of the eye, visual neural pathways, and the visual area of the cerebral cortex in the occipital lobe of the brain whereby light energy is detected, transmitted, and interpreted.

▶ BASIC LIFE PROCESSES OF SENSATION

Sensation includes processes whereby energy, such as light, sound, heat, mechanical vibration, and pressure, is transduced into neural activity that becomes perception. A particular characteristic of sensation is that it can cause an immediate reaction or its memory can be stored in the brain for minutes, weeks, or years and then can help to determine the person's reactions at some future date.

As noted in Chapter 12, Guyton (1992) considered the sensory division as one of the four complex networks whereby neurologic function is fulfilled. The neurologic basis for sensory processes provides some common principles for understanding these processes. These can be summarized briefly as follows.

1. Specialized receptors, whereby sensory energy is transduced into neural activity in the form of graded potentials or action potentials.
2. Receptive fields, which allow stimuli to be located in space or on the body surface.
3. Localization and detection, determined by receptor density and overlap.
4. Neural relays of three or four neurons, connected in sequence from receptor cells to cortex.
5. Information transmission, involving the coding of action potentials from all sensory systems and carrying that information along nerves, then tracts of the brain and spinal cord.

6. Sensory subsystems that include multiple pathways such as different pathways to the cerebral cortex for color perception and for tracking moving objects.
7. Multiple representation, whereby there are both primary and secondary representations of each sensory field on the cortex (Kolb & Whishaw, 1985).

Reducing an enormous array of environmental factors and influences to the single common language of the nervous system is a first and very important step in enabling an individual to cope with a highly complex world (Meiss & Tanner, 1982). There are a large variety of sensory receptors in the human body and a continuous stream of stimulation to these receptors. Sensory receptors act as both *detectors* and *transducers*. They detect the presence or absence of some component of the environment. Then as transducers, they sample a portion of the energy associated with the particular component and convert the sampled energy into an electrical signal containing information such as the intensity of sound.

Sensation gives rise to perception, another complex process that involves the central nervous system. *Perception* is a process of the cognator subsystem identified in the Roy model (see Chap. 2) and is defined as the interpretation of a sensory stimulus and the conscious appreciation of it. It has been noted that sensation is a result of activity of receptors and their associated pathways and corresponding cortical sensory areas. Perception, in comparison, is the result of activity of cells in the cortex beyond the first synapse in the sensory cortex. From the perspective of the Roy Model and a nursing view of information processing (Roy, in press), one considers that the immediate sensory experience is transformed into a perception in association with such factors as education and experience; that is, the focal stimulus is processed in the light of contextual and residual stimuli. Perception includes providing meaning to what is sensed. For example, knowing that one's house is located within the area where airplanes descend for landing at a nearby airport, a person will attach a nonthreatening meaning to the roar of a low flying aircraft at night. As noted earlier, previous sense experiences can be stored as part of the interpretation of a present sense experience.

The primary senses of seeing, hearing, and feeling are processes by which a person receives and exchanges information needed for life's activities, including relating to others. The sensory network initiates most neural activity with stimuli acting on the visual, auditory, tactile (on the surface of the body), or other kinds of receptors.

▶ VISION: PROCESS AND ASSESSMENT

Vision is a complex process involving the peripheral structure of the eye, visual neural pathways, and the visual area of the cerebral cortex in the occipital lobe of the brain. The retina of the eye is the visual receptor. Light enters the eye and is bent slightly by the cornea. It is then bent further by the lens so that images are focused on the receptors at the back of the eye. The human retina has two types of photoreceptor cells, the rods, which are sensitive to dim light and used for night vision, and the cones, which transduce bright light for daytime and color vision. The axons of ganglion cells (the third type of cells) leave the retina to form the optic nerve. Axons from the inner half of each eye cross over in the optic chiasm and terminate in the opposite occipital lobe. A number of separate pathways are formed, some for visual perception and some for reflex activity. This is how different parts of the visual field are represented in different parts of the brain. Thus, a person may have varying visual disturbances after brain damage, for example, from a stroke, depending on areas of the brain affected. If the stroke affects the left side of the brain, the person may not be able to see in the right visual field.

To understand how the brain cells representing vision act, researchers have used microelectrodes to record the activity of these cells in cats and monkeys under local anesthesia. Visual stimuli are presented on a screen placed in the animals' visual fields. Results from studies indicate that the cells seem to differ in two ways (Kolb & Whishaw, 1985). The receptive fields (areas of responding cells) seem to be larger at each succeeding level of cortex. Thus complexity increases at higher brain levels. Second, cells in different levels of the visual system respond to different properties of visual stimulation. For example, there are cells that respond to the corners of objects and others that respond to moving objects.

Assessment of Behaviors

Behavioral assessment of vision, as with other physiologic mode components, involves physical assessment skills using both observation and measurement. In addition, the nurse uses sensitive interviewing and perceptiveness.

Visual Tests

At times the nurse may conduct baseline assessments, for example, performing vision screening tests for schoolchildren. At other times, these assessments may be more precise and complete, for example, when visual field tests are done by a nurse practitioner in the annual physical examination of a person who is a pilot.

Functional Examination. The external, or functional, examination of the eye includes its ability to move in its orbit and the reaction of the pupil to light and accommodation. Visual acuity refers to the ability of the eye to form an image in the finest detail. Visual acuity is measured for both distance or far vision and for reading or near vision. Far vision can be tested by use of a Snellen chart, with which the person is asked to identify letters or objects of varying sizes. The acuity of each eye is measured separately while the other eye is covered with an opaque card. The expected response is that the person can identify letters of the 20 line at 20 feet when asked to read the chart. The term 20/20 is used for normal vision. Test cards for near vision are made for the person with normal vision to read at 14 inches.

Legal blindness usually involves visual acuity between 20/200 and 20/400. Reading is possible with this level of visual acuity, but high-powered magnifiers are needed and speed and endurance are limited. Gross orientation and mobility are usually adequate, but traffic signs are difficult to see. Near blindness means that the person can count figures at 4 feet. Vision is reliable only under ideal circumstances and nonvisual aids are used. Total blindness means that the person has no light perception and must rely entirely on other senses (Burrell, Gerlach, & Pless, 1997).

Usually there is greater importance placed on clarity of central vision. However, losses of peripheral or color vision can also be incapacitating. A perimeter is the instrument used to test peripheral vision. This indicates how far to the side the person can see without moving the eye. The test is conducted with the person's vision fixed with test objects moved in from the far periphery. Sometimes this can be done electronically with lights on a 360 degree field on the wall. Other times, the moving object is a piece of chalk on a string so that a mark is made on the spot where the person first reports seeing the object in the line of vision. Normally, the person can report visualizing objects in each of the four visual quadrants. To test color vision, the person is asked to identify colored figures or test plates having a background of colored dots with a superimposed figure or number that can be discriminated only if the person has the ability to identify colors. Referral to an ophthalmologist is indicated if the person notices vision problems, there is unexplained or unnoticed vision loss of 20/30 or more, or upon examination the person has losses in given visual fields or fails the test for color vision (Burrell, Gerlach, & Pless, 1997).

Internal Examination. Internal examination of the structure of the eye is done in several ways. A tonometer is used to measure the intraocular pressure, which normally is 11 to 22 mm Hg. The interior of the eye can be seen with an ophthalmoscope, which directs a small beam of light through the pupil. Refraction tests ascertain the ability of the lens and cornea to focus on the retina. Again, a referral to a physician is made if the nursing assessment reveals evidence of eye pathology.

Assessment of Stimuli

Besides physical assessment skills, interview questions are useful in assessing factors influencing visual and other sensory processes. The introduction to sensory processing has highlighted the fact that sense experience becomes perception in the context of an individual's total life experience. As with each mode of the Roy Adaptation Model, in addition to assessing the behaviors, the nurse looks carefully at the context, or total life experience, relative to adaptation of the senses.

Neurologic Pathology
Neurologic pathology is often the focal stimulus for altered sensation. Understanding such pathology is one way the nurse uses knowledge from pathophysiology in clinical practice.

TABLE 10–1 QUESTIONS FOR NURSING ASSESSMENT OF SENSORY IMPAIRMENT

1. Is sense impairment temporary or permanent?
2. Is impairment recent or of long standing?
3. Is more than one impairment present?
4. How does the person view the loss of function?
5. How is the person affected in the current environment?
6. What is the person's level of knowledge, the knowledge needed, and readiness for teaching?

Basic Sensory Questions. Guidelines for assessing focal, contextual, and residual stimuli for all sensory processes are summarized in six basic questions (see Table 10–1) by which the nurse can assess the person's life experience. These questions are discussed in this chapter in assessing the context of sensory impairment of seeing, hearing, and feeling.

► HEARING: PROCESS AND ASSESSMENT

Hearing is defined as the complex process whereby sound waves are detected, transmitted, and interpreted. The anatomy of the ear provides the basis for understanding the process whereby the ear transduces sound waves into action potentials. The eardrum vibrates when sound waves strike it. Transmission of the vibrations is by way of three small bones in the middle ear to the fluid of the inner ear. One of the bones, the stirrup, drives the fluid back and forth in the rhythm of the sound waves. The movements of the fluid cause a thin membrane, the basilar membrane, to resonate. It is this movement of the basilar membrane that causes movements of the auditory receptors. These receptors are the hair cells in the organ of Corti, whose cell membrane potentials are altered, resulting in neural activity. Different frequencies of sound are coded by way of the structure of the spiral-shaped cochlea, which holds the basilar membrane and organ of Corti.

Axons of the hair cells leave the cochlea to form the major part of the auditory nerve, the eighth cranial nerve. After projecting to the level of the medulla in the lower brainstem, synapses are formed and two distinct pathways emerge. One pathway projects to the primary auditory cortex and the other to the secondary regions. Representation of each cochlea in both sides of the brain is one way these pathways differ from the visual pathways. Less is known about the auditory cortex than about either the visual or the somatosensory. In general, it appears that in each subfield that has been mapped, low tones are represented farther back, with high tones more forward. Single neurons in the auditory system code the frequency or pitch of sounds with different neurons having their greatest sensitivity to different sound frequencies. Below the level of the cortex, generally, cells are responsive to a broader band of frequencies than are cells higher in the central nervous system.

Assessment of Behavior

Testing to ascertain the degree and type of auditory processing or hearing loss can be carried out by an audiologist, a physician, a nurse, or other appropriately trained health care personnel.

Audiometry

The basic instrument for the measurement of hearing is called the audiometer. Two types of stimuli (pure tones and actual words) are presented to measure the sensitivity (acuteness of hearing) and discrimination (how clearly the ear distinguishes different sounds) of the person's hearing. The expected response for adequate discrimination is hearing selected spoken words correctly over 50 percent of the time. Indications of hearing difficulty involving discrimination are such comments as "You are speaking too softly; I don't understand you," or, "They just mumble; the words are loud enough but I can't make out what they are saying."

Selecting an auditory screening test depends on the age of the person. Hearing tests for the infant (1 to 3 months) require the infant to respond to some sound, for example, shaking a rattle out of sight. Behaviors indicating that the sound has been heard may be subtle, such as moving or stopping a movement or widening the eyes. From 3 months to 1 year, the child is expected to respond to localized sound; from 6 months on the child should be vocalizing; and from 2 years on, speech should be present (Servonsky & Opas, 1987). The parents' reports of how the child responds to ordinary sounds are particularly important. Audiometer screening tests may be performed for children as young as 3 years of age and are generally used for 5-year-old children and older. Play audiometry also can be used between ages $1^1/_2$ and 5 years (Hill, 1987). The child first learns a specific task such as putting rings on a peg, then is instructed to do this whenever a sound is heard through the earphones.

Other Diagnostic Tests

Some health care centers are now equipped to measure electrical changes in the auditory system following sound stimulation and these tests are replacing the traditional audiometry tests. Electrocochleography (ECochG) measures electrical responses arising from the cochlea and auditory nerve. Auditory brainstem evoked response (ABR, BER, or BSER) measures the electrical responses arising from the auditory neural pathway. Both tests use electrodes applied to the scalp and a series of clicks emitted at a rapid rate through earphones. The electrical activity detected by the electrodes following stimulation is delivered to a computer that extracts the acoustic response from ongoing neural activity. The acoustic response is then transferred to paper, as in an EEG or EKG, and the resultant waveforms can be studied. These tests are useful to identify hearing threshold and to distinguish between cochlear and retrocochlear pathology.

There are two additional tests related to hearing function. The Rinne test is used to compare bone conduction with air conduction of sound. The tone produced by the tuning fork is generally heard approximately twice as long by air as by bone conduction. Weber's test is used to compare hearing in the two ears. In this test, the tone produced by the tuning fork is heard with equal loudness by both ears.

In addition to the behaviors noted on testing, the nurse is also alert to other behaviors that may indicate difficulty hearing such as faulty speech, inattentiveness, unresponsiveness, strained or intense facial expression, and a tendency toward withdrawal in social situations.

Assessment of Stimuli

In a situation of an impairment of hearing processes, the nurse assesses the context in which the person is experiencing the loss using the questions listed in Table 10–1 and discussed in the next section.

► FEELING: PROCESS AND ASSESSMENT

Feeling is the common term given to the complex processes whereby sensation from the somatosensory system is detected, transmitted, and interpreted. The somatosensory system includes the nervous system mechanisms that receive information from the body. It is a multiple sensory system composed of the following submodalities.

1. Touch and pressure, which is elicited by mechanical movement of body tissue.
2. Position sense or *kinesthesia,* resulting from mechanical changes in the muscles and joints, including both the sense of static limb position and the sensation of limb movement.
3. Heat and cold, showing neural discharges related to skin temperature changes.
4. Pain that is activated mainly by factors that damage tissue.

In describing the somatosensory pathways, the complexities involved are simplified by considering that there are two subsystems. The first is for fine touch, pressure, and kinesthesis, and the other is for pain and temperature (Kolb & Whishaw, 1985). The first system has fibers that leave the receptors and ascend the dorsal columns of the spinal cord to synapse in the lower brainstem. These fibers cross over and terminate in the thalamus and from there projections go to several areas of the cortex.

The second subsystem follows a different pattern. The fibers related to pain and temperature leave the receptors to synapse in the dorsal horn of the spinal cord. These cells then cross over to the other side of the cord and form a new tract. This tract terminates primarily in two areas of the thalamus. Finally, projections go to various areas of the cortex, as is the case with the other sensory systems.

The results of the work of numerous researchers have suggested that at least five basic sensations are coded in the somatosensory system: light touch to the skin, deep pressure to the fascia below the skin, joint movement, pain, and temperature. Specific cells in the thalamus respond to only one mode of stimulation. At the level of the cortex, there is response also to a specific stimulus, but a given cell is responsive to a smaller region, making it possible to locate the stimulus on the skin. Other cells, even at the skin surface, have more complex properties, such as those of the hand, which respond to movement and precise orientation of stimuli. These properties make it possible to explore tactilely shape and three dimensions.

Assessment of Behavior

Assessment of somatosensory processing has many facets. These relate to the five basic sensations previously identified and are assessed for intact sensation and symmetry of feeling.

Sensation

Light touch is tested by touching the skin with a wisp of cotton. With eyes closed, the person states when and where he or she is being touched. Joint movement is tested by having the person identify the position of fingers as up or down as the examiner moves them. The sense of pain is estimated by pin prick, occasionally substituting the blunt end of a saftey pin. The person reports whether the stimulus is sharp or dull. Two test tubes filled with hot and cold water can be used to test temperature. As the person reports temperature changes, the examiner charts any areas of loss with oblique lines, one way for heat and the other direction for cold.

Symmetry

The ability to perceive the stimulus is the basic behavior assessed in sensory processing within each of the modalities of seeing, hearing, and feeling. Bates (1991) makes some general suggestions about assessment of feeling and sensory processing. The first is to compare the symmetry of sensation on the two sides of the body. With pain, temperature, and touch, compare distal and proximal areas of the extremities. If vibration and position are normal in the fingers and toes, then it can be safely assumed that the more proximal areas will also be normal. The examiner scatters the stimuli and varies the pace of testing so that most major peripheral nerves are covered and so that the patient does not merely respond to a repetitive pattern of testing. If an area of sensory loss or hypersensitivity is detected, the examiner maps out the boundaries in detail. Textbooks on physical assessment and general clinical nursing practice are available to provide additional details on assessment of feeling.

Assessment of Stimuli

A major focus of the nursing assessment related to sensations is the context that affects the person's experience of altered sensation. The questions listed in Table 10–1 are used to assess the stimuli affecting adaptation to sensory impairment.

Impairment Temporary or Permanent

An important factor influencing the person's adaptation is whether the impairment is temporary or permanent, or if this is an unanswerable question at the current time. An example is a nurse's encounter with three people newly admitted to a hospital neurologic unit. They all have paralysis and loss of sensation in their right arms and hands. In reviewing the medical reports and in interviewing these people, the nurse determines by first- and second-level assessment (see Chap. 3) that one of them probably has a correctable situation. He has been admitted for a workup before brain tumor surgery, which is thought to have good possibilities for correcting the loss of arm sensation. The second person sustained the loss of sensation in a skydiving accident 5 years ago, and the loss appears permanent. The third person had a cerebral vascular accident 3 days ago, and it is uncertain at this time whether or not sensation will return to the right limb. It is clear that without incorporating this kind of information in assessment data, it would be difficult to complete the remaining steps of the nursing process with these people.

Impairment Recent or Long Standing

The second question closely follows the first, as it is fundamental to assessment. Is the impairment recent or long standing? When an 80-year-old man casually comments that he has not been able to hear anything with his left ear since he was young, the nurse may register this information with a sense of significance different from the response to another person's complaint of sudden loss of hearing after a period of unconsciousness caused by a malfunction of scubadiving equipment.

More than One Impairment

The third question raises the concern of whether or not more than one impairment is present. Perhaps a person with diabetes is learning to adjust to paresthesia (loss of feeling) affecting both feet, but is also experiencing retinal degeneration causing pronounced loss of vision.

Person's View of Loss of Function

Throughout the assessment, the nurse is incorporating information regarding the fourth question, how does the person view the loss of function? There is a wide range of reactions regarding both old and new problems involving the major senses, and these reactions are based on all the contextual and residual factors that make the person unique. For example, the slightest danger of a potential loss of hearing could be very threatening to a musician, whereas a person who works around jet aircraft might take it in stride as an expected component of the job. Nurses assess how individuals feel about newly developed losses, and also try to understand how people are coping with long-standing incapacities. Does the blind person confront the loss of vision with continued anger, forced resignation, or matter-of-factness? Some people, for example, may still require a great deal of help in reaching a level of adaptation many years after becoming blind, while others may be at a stage of knowing they have met such a challenge with the best possible adaptation.

Effect in Current Environment

The nurse deals with the fifth question and considers it of immediate relevance in all nursing encounters. It is, how is the person affected in the current environment of home, work, school, clinic, or hospital and moving from one place to another? The person's comfort in these settings is very important, but even more fundamental are safety factors. The nurse is very careful to assess any loss of sensation with a view to potential safety problems. To what degree does the person not see, hear, or feel, and what hazards does this present? Can the schoolchild with retinitis pigmentosa safely play sports in the bright sunlight, or would school gym sports such as tumbling and swimming be better choices? Does the hard-of-hearing hospitalized person tend to smile and nod even when addressed by a name other than his own? Does the patient with cataracts see well enough to ambulate safely around obstacles in the long-term care facility? The nurse learns quickly that nursing according to the Roy Adaptation Model fosters and encourages physical independence. However, responsibility in assessing the sensory processes is rooted in a sharp awareness of potential situations that could result in harm to the person. In particular, the combination of a new environment, as when a person is admitted to the hospital or has to travel to visit a clinic, and the stress of illness may change the context so as to reduce the safety level for a usually adapted person.

Level of and Need for Knowledge and Readiness for Teaching

The sixth assessment question follows naturally from the other five, and helps the nurse finalize the assessment. It asks what is the person's level of knowledge, the knowledge needed, and readiness for teaching. Is teaching for long-range purposes needed, as, for example, the proper method for inserting contact lenses, or how the newly diagnosed glaucoma patient will instill eye drops daily? Is the concern short-term specific bits of information, such as safety precautions while one eye is bandaged? Is it appropriate for one nurse to conduct the teaching, or do notes need to be made on charts, care plans, or home care flowcharts so that more than one nurse can contribute to teaching information, reinforcing the learning that has been accomplished and reassessing learning needs? Are persons significant to the patient also involved in health teaching? How much can the person be expected to absorb, and on which senses can one rely? The nearly blind person will learn little from a teaching film, and the person who is in the process of adapting to a hearing aid will profit little from a small-group discussion.

From the data that are generated by these questions, the nurse can identify which factors are most immediately influencing the person, that is, what is focal and what is contextual or contributing to adaptation of sensory processes, and any alterations in their functioning. Finally, the nurse can note stimuli that need further assessment because they may be affecting the person's ability to respond positively to the situation, but they have not yet been verified by the nurse or the patient. Basically, many of the problems of altered sensation are medical problems with associated medical interventions to treat the many possible disruptions to the underlying neurologic pathways. The nurse's total assessment of the person's behavior and context provides the understanding of the person's life experience from which the nursing diagnoses are derived and plans for nursing care implemented.

► COMPENSATORY ADAPTIVE PROCESSES

According to the Roy Adaptation Model, compensatory adaptive processes are activated by way of the regulator and cognator subsystems. The processes of sensation provide many examples of compensatory adaptive processes. An example of an innate regulatory process related to vision is light and dark adaptation. It is a common experience that when entering a darkened area, such as a movie theater, or going outside after sunset without lighting, it takes time for the eyes to adapt. Dark adaptation, or a decline in visual threshold, is at a maximum within 20 minutes in the dark environment. Light adaptation, when returning to a light environment, however, takes the eyes only about 5 minutes. While adapting visually in a dark environment, the person may lose balance and have trouble moving around effectively. During light adaptation, the person feels an uncomfortable brightness that makes vision less effective. Both the rods and cones of the eye structures are involved in light and dark adaptation. However, the sensitivity to darkness is much greater in the rods than the cones. Adaptation to the dark takes place in two stages. Unknown changes in the cones occur in the first 7 minutes in the dark environment, accounting for a small increase in visual acuity. This is followed by a less rapid, but quantitatively greater rod adaptation. In the second stage, the rhodopsin stores are rebuilt in the rods (Bullock & Rosendahl, 1992).

Dark adaptation can be maintained by using a learned behavior in conjunction with the innate compensatory process of the regulator. When visual acuity in the dark is necessary, for example viewing fluoroscopy, red goggles are worn on returning to bright light. The wavelengths in the red part of the spectrum allow cone vision to continue while stimulating rods only to a small degree. Thus, the person can avoid having to wait 20 minutes to repeat the whole process of dark adaptation.

► COMPROMISED PROCESSES OF THE SENSES

Adaptation problems can be caused by difficulties in any of the sensory processes. Two examples of compromised processes related to sensation will be discussed here. A specific compromised process of sensation is the adaptation problem of pain. Varying degrees of discomfort usually accompany the conditions for which people seek health care. The nurse constantly encounters people in pain. Although pain is increasingly understood, all the advances of science have not eliminated the experience of pain. Further, although many treatment options are available, undertreatment of pain remains a significant problem in health care (Marks & Sachar, 1973; Thorpe, 1990).

Hyperactivity of a child is another instance of compromised sensation. This problem also has broad relevance for nursing practice. It is estimated that 5 to 20 percent of the population is affected. Although hyperactivity is not fully understood, families face the challenge of helping the child to effectively integrate sensory input and to modulate a response appropriate to environmental information.

Pain

Pain involves input to certain sense receptors and deserves special consideration because the phenomenon of pain is one of the most significant areas of nursing practice. Constantly meeting people in pain, both from disease and from treatments, can be distressing for the nurse. However, the novice quickly realizes that the ability of the nurse to provide comfort and alleviate suffering is a fundamental component of nursing responsibility. The experienced nurse never forgets this responsibility and strives throughout a career to improve abilities to provide comfort-giving measures.

Writings by McCaffery (1979, 1997; McCaffery & Beebe, 1989) have been influencial in providing a practical and comprehensive statement about pain. Basically *pain* is a biobehavioral, subjective, and personal experience of noxious stimuli, considered to be whatever the patient says it is and occurs whenever the patient says it does. This definition emphasizes the subjective and personal nature of the pain experience. Numerous publications provide evidence of research that opens new perspectives on understanding the experience of pain. The reader is referred to McCaffery's seminal work that appeared in 1979 and more recent publications. These and other sources provide an in-depth discussion of topics related to pain.

Theoretical Basis

In its simplest form, pain acts as a protective mechanism to warn the person of actual and potential sources of tissue damage. An example is withdrawing a hand quickly from a hot stove. This example illustrates the elements of sensation from specialized receptors, transduced into neural activity, then neural relays through the spinal cord, and finally, the involvement of specialized brain centers in interpretation of the pain stimulus. However, because of its complex biobehavioral nature, and the difficulty of contexts in which it occurs, pain more often loses its compensatory function and becomes a compromised process of sensation. The nurse learns to help the person deal with pain that continues long after its adaptive purpose has been achieved.

Pain research has been widely influenced by the gate control theory of pain proposed by Melzack and Wall (1965, 1970, 1989). The theory also receives wide attention in practice because the concepts have been useful in treating pain. In this theory, both the peripheral and central nervous systems are involved. Understanding the biobehavioral nature of pain, and contextual factors influencing this experience, provides a basis for effective nursing intervention.

The receptors that transmit noxious stimuli (pain) are called nociceptors. These nerve endings are undifferentiated or free nerve endings and are found in nearly every tissue of the body. The nociceptors respond to thermal, chemical, and mechanical stimulation such as pressure. Scientists believe that certain neurotransmitters, such as bradykinin, histamine, serotonin, and substance P, may be important in sensitizing the nerve endings and enhancing transmission of pain (Thorpe, 1997). Different types of nerve fibers and special spinal tracts form a complex network for relaying the pain sensation. Different types of sensory nerve fibers are distributed in different ways throughout the body. The extensive supply of A-delta myelinated (fast) fibers, larger C unmyelinated (slow) fibers, and large A fibers on the skin result in the ability to localize pain when a finger is cut with a sharp object, for example. This combination of fibers also accounts for the initial stinging, sharp pain, and the slightly delayed throbbing and more diverse pain. In contrast, the viscera has fewer A-delta fibers and large A fibers. Thus, it is difficult to localize intraabdominal pain.

The primary processing area, or gate for pain, is located in the dorsal horn of the spinal cord. Groups of nerve cells lie in layers of the central portion of the gray matter of the spinal cord. Each group of nerves has a different function in relaying pain sensation messages. For example, one group is called lamina V and seems to be the key area for transmission of nociceptive stimuli from the dorsal horn to the opposite side of the spinal cord, where an ascending pathway transmits the sensation to the thalamus. The specialized ascending spinal tract is supplied with A-delta fibers and has only two synapses. Pain sensation by this route is sharp, well-localized, and relayed rapidly. Another ascending tract originates in the dorsal horn of the spinal cord and transmits impulses to the thalamus and limbic system. It travels close to the other ascending tract, but differs in that it has many synapses and mainly C fibers. Consequently, transmission of nerve impulses by this route is slower and more diffuse. Another tract, the dorsal column, also originates in the dorsal horn, but ascends dorsally and does not cross until the medulla and then synapses at the thalamus. Sensations received by way of this column specifically help the person locate an injury.

The ascending spinal tracts carry the varying pain sensations to the thalamus, from which other neurons send the impulses to the cortex. The central mechanisms of pain involve the brain structures of the thalamus, limbic system, and reticular formation. The thalamus is a relay station, but also seems to play an important role in translating the sensation to a perception. Interactions of the ascending spinal tracts with the limbic system can be the source of fear, anxiety, and attention to pain in the person experiencing pain. Within this system, the hippocampus and amygdala seem to be structures for translating short-term memory into long-term memory. This is an important factor in the management of pain. The reticular formation, and in particular the reticular activating system (RAS), influences the person's level of arousal, including anxiety and distractibility. Further, the role of the cerebral cortex in memory and learning is significant for purposes of managing pain.

While various categories of pain are recognized, the focus here is on pain felt as a physiologic process that affects the other three adaptive modes, self-concept, role function, and interdependence. Pain can be acute or chronic, and the assessments and interventions are different. *Acute pain* is short in duration, has an identifiable cause, and follows an expected time course depending on the cause. Acute pain goes away as healing occurs. Acute pain serves a useful purpose when it alerts a person to an illness or injury. The symptom of pain may aid the health care personnel to determine the nature of the problem. Short-term pain can also accompany many therapies and diagnostic procedures. Perhaps the most common example of this is postoperative surgical incision pain.

Chronic pain is persistent and does not have a predictable time limit. Sometimes chronic pain is referred to as pain lasting longer than 6 months. However, rather than using an arbitrary time limit, the nurse focuses on the characteristics of chronic pain. When pain is chronic, it serves no useful purpose and may or may not have an identifiable cause that can be dealt with directly. The persistence of chronic pain is a constant source of suffering for the patient, and a challenge for the nurse in helping the patient with pain management.

Understanding some common terms used in relation to the pain experience—pain levels, threshold, tolerance, and suffering—can be useful in nursing practice. However, using the subjective definition given by McCaffrey (1979) and the premises of holistic and individualized nursing care, assures that the terms are used correctly and avoids negative judgment on any person's individual experience and interpretation of it.

Pain levels simply means that various stimuli provoke varying amounts or degrees of pain. For example, a small area of burned tissue does not hurt as much as more extensive burn trauma, and although a surgical incision can always be uncomfortable, a chest wall incision that is aggravated by breathing and coughing can produce a more intense level of pain than an abdominal incision. *Pain threshold* is the level of intensity of the stimulus that causes the sensation or feeling of pain. Given the same intensity of a noxious stimulus, the awareness of the beginning of the pain experience varies from person to person.

Finally, *pain tolerance* is the amount of pain a person can endure at a given time. Two people may experience pain at the same threshold, but the higher pain-tolerant person may more readily incorporate the pain into overall sensations at the time without it becoming a major focus of attention. Further, for a given person, pain tolerance will vary in different situations. An example is the patient with a severe headache who told the nurse, "I can stand a lot of pain, except if it is in my belly; my mother died of ovarian cancer." Suffering relates to endurance of a difficult state, physiologic, psychological, or both. *Suffering* has been defined as a severe state of distress associated with loss or threat of loss of the integrity of the person (Cassell, 1989). Although pain and suffering are not the same human experience, they are frequently linked. Given the individual nature of the pain, the nurse who compares the pain experience of various people, or uses a personal standard of expected responses to pain stimuli, does patients an injustice. Rather, the nurse will want to accept the challenge of learning more about the complexity of pain and the individual person's experience of it.

Assessment of Behavior

Some basic guidelines for assessment of pain can be followed even though the phenomenon is complex and presents itself in multiple forms. Whether the situation involves a school nurse and a 10-year-old child complaining of a stomach ache, a hospital nurse responding to a patient in the postanesthesia room, or a home care nurse visiting a person with chronic rheumatoid arthritis or terminal cancer, certain information is useful to plan for promoting adaptation. As in assessment of the senses in general, the nurse obtains a behavioral description of the person's pain experience and the factors influencing it.

Rapport. Initially in assessing pain, the nurse establishes rapport with the patient and believes the report of pain, recognizing that the patient as the only authority on the pain being felt. The patient's report of pain is accepted in a caring manner. The nurse listens without interrupting and uses accepting nonverbal communication, such as making eye contact and touching the patient. Repeating and clarifying information show concern and are helpful in making an accurate assessment.

Description of Pain. The next step in pain assessment is to describe the pain: location, quality, intensity, onset, and duration. Although the location of pain may seem apparent, such as that derived from an obvious problem such as a fracture or deep cut, the fact is that nurses sometimes erroneously assume that they know the source of a person's pain complaint. For example, a 65-year-old man recovering from laminectomy surgery complained of being miserable and was grimacing. The nurse assumed that he was experiencing pain related to the surgical incision site and administered the potent intramuscular analgesic that was prescribed. After the injection, the patient commented "At home I just take a couple of aspirin when I have a headache like this."

It is also common for a person to have pain in more than one location at the same time. It is important that the nurse confirm the source of the person's pain during each assessment of the situation. Whenever possible, ask the person to indicate exactly where each pain is. The person who complains of stomach pain may point to the left lower quadrant. A headache may turn out to be cervical neck pain when the site is demonstrated. In addition, even pain in an expected location can also indicate a newly developing problem. When a person with a fracture comments regarding increased pain in the cast area, the nurse may discover, by careful questioning regarding the exact location of pain, that a developing infection under the cast is a concern.

The nurse assesses the quality of the pain by asking the patient to describe the pain in words. Words commonly used include sharp, dull, stabbing, cramping, aching, gnawing, burning, throbbing, tender, heavy, "feels like a boil," and "feels like a lot of pressure." The nurse suggests words only if the patient is having difficulty describing the pain and always gives a choice of terms: "Would you describe it as a sharp pain or a dull pain?" Be alert to references or comparisons to past episodes of illness or pain: "It's a lot like the last time I came to the emergency room," or, "Once I had distress like this after a big Italian meal," or, "Of course, I've had stomach problems all my life, but this time it's pretty bad." These kinds of comments can be followed through to obtain a thorough assessment and can help establish whether the individual's pain experience is acute or chronic in nature.

Intensity of pain is also described from the patient's perspective. The nurse lets the patient describe how strong the pain experience is, for example, mild, moderate, or severe. In addition, the nurse can use a numeric scale of 0 to 10, with 0 meaning no pain and 10 being the worst possible pain. The advantage for using a scale is that it is generally understood by the person and provides an individualized measure of pain that the nurse can use to judge pain relief or the worsening of pain for that person. Further, once the scale has been explained, it takes less energy for the patient in pain to respond to the question of where on the scale to make the current rating of pain. For example, the patient who has multiple fractures of one arm may report pain at 7 on the scale. Following administration of an analgesic, when the nurse returns to assess the effectiveness of the intervention in relieving pain, the patient responds to the question by changing the rating to 2 on the scale. Faces on pain scales can be used with children. Such scales consist of a series of different facial expressions. The nurse explains to the child that each face is for a person who feels happy because there is no pain, or hurt, or sad because there is some or a lot of pain. The child is asked to choose the face that best describes the pain experienced. A similar approach can be used with some adults for whom communication is difficult.

It is also important to assess the onset and duration of pain. This is especially important during initial assessments to determine the acuteness or chronicity of the pain but can also elicit helpful information whenever a complaint of discomfort is voiced. The simple question, "When did you start noticing the pain?" may prompt the person to relate a certain position in bed or the ingestion of a particular food or medication to the discomfort he or she is feeling. An aspect that is related to onset and duration is the constancy of the pain, and the individual is certainly the best judge of this. A person being treated for severe diarrhea and fluid and electrolyte imbalance complained of pain around the site of an intravenous infusion. There was no problem apparent to the nurse, but when the question of whether it hurt all the time was asked, the puzzle was solved. It was related that the discomfort started when the most recent intravenous feeding bottle was hung, but was not present when the arm was held in a slightly bent position. The nurse realized that the higher dose of potassium in the most recent bottle was causing the pain, and it was relieved when the person bent his arm and so slowed down the rate of infusion. Rather than subjecting the person to an unnecessary intravenous restart, communication showed that a slower infusion rate, which the physician approved, kept the person comfortable.

Assessment of Stimuli

Aggravating Factors. In assessing pain, the next step following a thorough description of the pain is to identify the aggravating and alleviating factors. Aggravating factors are those that make the pain worse, while alleviating factors are those that reduce pain. The person may be able to identify certain activities, positions, temperatures, or times of day that tend to make the pain more intense. In identifying factors that reduce pain, the nurse will ask what specific pain relief methods the person has used and what has worked for him or her in the past.

Signs of Other Physiologic Changes. Next the nurse examines the site that the person indicates is painful. Examination is done to look for other signs such as heat, redness, swelling, tenderness, abnormal position, or factors that may be causing local irritation. For example, a postoperative patient who complains of pain in the calf of the leg may show additional signs on examination. If a red, firm, tender area is noted, this is reported to the physician for diagnosis of a possible thrombophlebitis.

Signs of Behavioral Changes. In the next step of assessing the pain experience, the nurse describes the behavioral response to pain. In acute pain, the person may be restless, thrashing, rubbing the body part, pacing, tensing muscles, grimacing, wincing on movement, and making other facial expressions of discomfort. Physiologic responses to acute pain include increased heart rate and respirations, as well as increased blood pressure. With a person in chronic pain, the behavioral response is more likely to include a tired-looking, masked facial expression; quiet; increased sleep and rest; and diverted attention. A person in chronic pain will not likely have changes in vital signs. People who have long endured chronic pain, even when it is severe, may have accommodated themselves to the feeling of pain and therefore demonstrate little outward response. Depression often accompanies chronic pain, and this can serve to drain energy. Consequently, the person tends to avoid both displays of pain and speaking of it due to feelings of helplessness, taking on an "Oh, what's the use" attitude. Sometimes there may not be any identifiable affected body part. For example, the pain connected with some disorders of the pancreas is of such a chronic nature that a person may be observed watching television or talking casually on the phone even while experiencing severe pain.

Persons in acute or chronic pain are likely experiencing anxiety. However, manifestations of anxiety, as well as the other behavioral responses to pain, will be individualized by the person. Another point in assessing pain is that some people with acute or chronic pain may not volunteer information about pain, as they assume that the nursing staff knows their situation and need. It may, in fact, be puzzling to patients that some nurses will question them about pain and others never mention it. One person, admitted for a kidney stone, thought that he was expected to have pain only in the late afternoon and evening hours, as the evening shift nurses were the only ones who frequently checked his level of comfort. Others will not rely on the solicitude of the nursing staff and will readily share their response when they are hurting. The nurse incorporates into the assessment an understanding of the individualized experience of pain, and also the very individualized methods of expressing it. The nurse's own behavioral response also affects the patient's expression of pain.

Validation of Focal Stimulus. The final step of assessment of the pain experience is to compare the nursing judgment with the person's impression to see if both people have the same idea as to what is causing the pain. This has been discussed earlier in this text as validating the focal stimulus. An example of this process might be as follows. The nurse says to the patient: "It seems to me that you're a little more uncomfortable today. Is it because you didn't rest well last night?" The patient responds: "Well, that is partly it, but I was out of the back traction most of yesterday having x-rays and I can sure tell the difference today." This is also the time to check what the person thinks will give relief. Recalling that pain is a subjective experience and recognizing that the person is the only authority about his or her pain, the nurse also knows that the patient is the only one to tell whether or not techniques intended to bring comfort have been effective.

When people are hurting, many aspects of normal physiology and human activity and interaction such as eating, moving, walking, sleeping, communicating, and sexual function can become less effective. Thus, pain reflects a compromised adaptation level affecting the other physiologic mode components and adaptive modes. Behavior observed can involve any of the modes. The nursing diagnosis, however, will focus on the pain. Goals and nursing management for addressing all modes affected will be aimed at the relief of the pain.

Hyperactivity

Hyperactivity is the general term given to a group of behaviors also referred to by terms such as attention deficit disorder, hyperkinesis, or minimal brain dysfunction. The last term is used for children with normal or near normal intelligence who show certain behavior patterns or specific learning disabilities. Behaviors most often noted are hyperactivity, short attention span, distractability, and poor impulse control (Rowland, 1984).

Differences in activity levels for infants and children are common. Texts in pediatric nursing (such as Servonsky & Opas, 1987) caution about the need to determine medically whether the child is truly hyperactive or is just a very active child. Marked differences in activity levels of infants range from placid, easygoing infants to those who have periods of calm and periods of greater activity to those who are in constant motion. These differences can be as great as the most active infant having 300 times the motility of the placid baby. Hyperactivity can be evident in an infant's behavior or may not be manifested until the child is a toddler or school-age. In children affected by an abnormal behavior pattern, in its entirety or in part, boys outnumber girls by about four to one.

An infant who is hyperactive may squirm and fidget, be difficult to hold, resist being confined to a crib or playpen, rest infrequently, sleep poorly, and not be able to sit quietly. For the child, behaviors are impulsive and seem uncontrolled. The child's attention span is short and there is difficulty sitting still and responding to discipline. Fidgeting or excessive running may be noted. Sleep difficulties and difficulty learning are a part of the behavioral pattern. The effects of the behavioral pattern often are noted in parents and siblings who may have difficulty coping with the busy, intense activity of the child's boundless energy.

It is likely that a developmental neurologic dysfunction underlies minimal brain dysfunction and attention deficit disorder and the associated hyperactive behavior. Study of these behaviors is complicated because activity levels and attention spans are influenced by the experiences of the child as well as by brain structures. Further, more recent developments in neuroimaging, including PET (positron emission tomography), cannot be used in children because of exposure to radioactive isotopes. Through EEG and PET studies of adults and animals, it has been noted that getting ready to process a visual stimulus quiets the activity of neurons in the visual areas of the brain. When a stimulus appears, for example, an arrow on a screen, the brain's electrical activity in the visual area is increased in amplitude. These observations suggest that, in normal persons, the act of preparing for a target quiets the sensory system. Accordingly, it is hypothesized that attention deficits result in part from a problem in the child's preparatory mechanisms for attention. If this is the case, the child would be less successful in amplifying relevant stimuli so that these stimuli stand out over distracting stimuli. The greater distractibility of the child with the disorder arises because the quieting mechanisms have failed and the important signals are not amplified. The child is distracted from important sensory cues more readily (Posner & Raichle, 1994). Given the effect of the disorder on a child's development, particularly academic and social, families are often in need of support and specific help in handling the child's behavior.

► PLANNING NURSING CARE

Any loss of sensory function can affect the person greatly, that is, a change in this physiologic mode component affects all the adaptive modes. However, as the Roy Adaptation Model clearly emphasizes, people have great capacities to adapt to both internal and external changes. The nurse strives to understand the processes by which the senses play an important role in perceiving and interacting with the world and the related compensatory and compromised processes. Based on this understanding, the nurse can more competently assess and plan care to promote sensory adaptation. It is possible, then, to assist persons with temporary or permanent sensory losses to achieve and maintain the highest level of adaptation of which they are capable.

In addition to the effect a sensory loss may have on the person, loss of a functioning sense can change the way others, including health professionals, view a person. For example, legally blind persons often report that store clerks, waiters and waitresses, and others rarely address them directly when they are accompanied by a sighted person. In the hospital, a hard-of-hearing person may be labeled as confused or disoriented when he or she does not give what are considered appropriate responses to the queries of hospital staff. The confusion suddenly clears when the nursing staff recognize the person's sense limitation and makes efforts to compensate for the loss.

The application of the nursing process is the formalized way that the nurse makes these assessments and plans appropriate care to promote adaptation and mastery related to the senses. In dealing with the complex processes of the senses, the nurse promotes the person's adaptation, as in other adaptive mode components, by careful assessment and diagnosis, as well as mutual planning to set goals and select interventions. Evaluation then is based on comparing the reassessment of behaviors with the established goals.

Nursing Diagnosis

Diagnosis in the physiologic mode component of the senses proceeds in the same way as discussed throughout this text. The data from the nursing assessment of behaviors and stimuli are interpreted in the statement of a nursing diagnosis. One method for stating a nursing diagnosis according to the Roy model is for the nurse to identify a cluster of observed behaviors and the most relevant stimuli. An example of a nursing diagnosis for a 5-year old boy who has just started kindergarten is: "child will not stay seated in the classroom, runs constantly at recess, does not follow directions, and sometimes falls asleep related to probable medical diagnosis of attention deficit disorder and inconsistency in child care while single mother works."

Another way of stating a nursing diagnosis is to identify a summary label from an established classification list. Using the diagnostic label, the nurse communicates the judgment regarding the clinical situation in a way that most clearly represents the essence of the problem.

In Chapter 3, two classification lists based on the Roy Adaptation model were described, indicators of positive adaptation and commonly occurring adaptation problems. In Table 10–2, the diagnostic categories based on the Roy model for the senses are related to the diagnostic labels approved by the North American Nursing Diagnosis Association (Rantz & LeMone, 1997). The most common diagnosis related to the senses from the NANDA list is sensory–perceptual alteration (specify as to visual, auditory, kinesthetic, tactile, or olfactory). In a given clinical situation, each summary label can be described better by adding a statement of the relevant stimuli. For example, a school-aged child may have a diagnosis of "altered visual sensation due to recent, sudden, and permanent loss of sight in one eye by being struck with a baseball that caused retinal damage." In time, a positive adaptation diagnosis for a hyperactive child may be "increasing effectiveness of integrating sensory input related to consistent plan for quieting techniques used by mother, teacher, and grandmother."

Sometimes an experienced nurse makes a nursing diagnosis based on the Roy Adaptation Model by using a commonly accepted term that summarizes a behavioral pattern when more than one mode is affected by the same stimuli. An example is: "sensory disturbance of overload related to same-day surgery."

TABLE 10–2 NURSING DIAGNOSTIC CATEGORIES FOR THE SENSES

Positive Indicators of Adaptation	Common Adaptation Problems	NANDA Diagnostic Labels
• Effective processes of sensation	• Impairment of a primary sense • Potential for injury • Loss of self-care abilities • Stigma	• Sensory–perceptual alterations (visual, auditory, kinesthetic, gustatory, tactile, olfactory)

• Effective integration of sensory input into information	• Sensory overload and deprivation
	• Sensory monotony or distortion
	• Potential for distorted communication
	• Pain
	   Acute
	   Chronic
		• Pain
		• Pain, chronic

• Stable patterns of perception, ie: interpretation and appreciation of input	• Perceptual impairment	• Sensory–perceptual alterations (as above)
• Effective coping strategies for altered sensation	• Ineffective coping strategies for sensory impairment	• Defensive coping • Impaired verbal communication • Impaired adjustment • Ineffective individual coping

Sensory input, that is, all the stimuli received by the senses, varies in both amount and predictability. Continuous input of meaningful sense cues is necessary for adaptive human behavior. Sensory disturbance occurs when a person is receiving cues at either end of the continuum of absolute reduction in sensory stimulation (sensory deprivation) or increased stimulation to the point of too much (sensory overload). Qualitatively, input ranges from stimuli that have no order or predictability (distortion) to stimuli that are never-changing, repeated, and continuous (monotony). The amount of deprivation, overload, distortion, or monotony that affects a given person depends on the person and the other factors of the situation. In Roy model terms, this means the effect of sensory input depends on the person's integrity of adaptive modes, adaptation level, and other stimuli.

Specific examples of variation of sensory input (focal stimuli changes) that nurses may encounter are deprivation (blindness, eye patches, deafness, isolation, and traction), distortion (one eye patched, scarred cornea, partial deafness, tinnitis, and strange hospital noises), overload (same-day surgery and special care units), monotony (same position and respirator). Behavioral responses to sensory deprivation extend from mild to extreme. Mild reactions to reduced or increased sensory input included boredom, restlessness, irritability, fatigue, drowsiness, mental confusion, and occasional anxiety. In more extreme cases—for example, when researchers have placed subjects in a black, soundproof box—drastic cognitive responses include delusions, primary process thinking, and inability to think. Emotionally, the participants became labile, or unstable. Perceptual hallucinations were frequent. One important contextual factor influencing the behavioral response to variation in sensory input was the amount of concurrent social contact. In the black box experiments, the participants had less drastic effects if they were in contact with the experimenter.

If input through one modality is reduced, for example, if the eyes are patched, then input in other modalities are contextual stimuli. One researcher found that eye-patched patients with hearing impairments had greater reactions to the deprivation than eye-patched patients with normal hearing. Others have noted that immobility at the time of deprivation increases its effect. Some studies have shown that certain drugs have been precipitating factors in responses to deprivation.

Some investigators have validated the expectation that length of time of deprivation is significant. For patients whose eyes were patched for less than 24 hours, only 35 percent had one or more mental symptoms. However, when the time was increased, as in the case of long-term healing of a serious eye injury, 100 percent had one or more symptoms of deprivation. One study found that knowledge of the anticipated length of time of deprivation also lessens the symptoms. Residual factors which may possibly affect behavioral responses to variations in sensory input are: age (older persons seem more susceptible), gender (women seem to tolerate disturbance longer than men), and personality factors (for example, the compulsive person has a greater need to structure the environment).

Goal Setting

In setting goals using the Roy Adaptation Model, the nurse makes a clear statement of outcomes expected for the person as a result of nursing care. This statement is mutually developed when possible and stems from the nursing diagnosis. A clear goal statement is one that contains the behavior of focus, the change or stability expected, and the time frame for achieving the goal.

In dealing with altered sensation, the nurse considers both short- and long-term goals. Often a long-term goal is made up of several successive short-term goals. Given an example of a child with blindness in one eye, the clinic nurse may establish with the child and his mother the goal that he will travel to and from school safely by himself one day in a given week. The long-term goal is that he will be independent in participating safely and effectively in classroom and school activities. Each goal will have appropriate stategies planned to meet the goal.

The outcome criteria established by the American Association of Neuroscience Nurses (AANN) (Mitchell, Hodges, Muwaswes & Walleck, 1988) for persons with uncompensated sensory deficits, particularly of vision, hearing, and tactile sensation, are as follows.

- The individual communicates a sense of comfort and security within the environment.
- The individual uses assistive devices and compensatory techniques correctly.
- The individual sustains no burns, falls, wounds, or pressure injuries.

The nurse then proceeds to develop and implement appropriate strategies to address each goal.

Intervention

Whereas the goal of the nursing care plan focuses on the behaviors noted in the nursing assessment, interventions are based on the related stimuli that have been assessed. Although management of the focal stimulus is a preferred method of promoting adaptation, the loss may be focal and many sensory losses cannot be altered. Nursing interventions thus deal with the person's total experience, comprised of focal, contextual, and residual stimuli. These are the stimuli that affect the person's experience of altered sensation. In understanding the person's total experience, the nurse can better design appropriate interventions.

One example of nursing intervention relates to the stimuli involved in the diagnosis for the 10-year-old boy with recent loss of vision in one eye and the goal to facilitate safety and independence in traveling to and from school. Nursing approaches could include providing the child and his parents with a booklet on safety for the partially sighted, determining the distance and terrain to be covered on the way to school, 10 minutes a day practice walking in an area with obstacles, and having his brother accompany him on the first few walks.

For persons with one or more sensory impairments, the AANN lists the following general nursing measures.

- Orient the individual to the environment, utilizing the intact senses.
- Modify the environment and daily routines to include such things as permanent placement of furniture and articles and adaptation of the telephone, door bells, and warning devices.
- Provide detailed information and instruction related to the disability and appropriate compensatory devices.
- Institute appropriate safety precautions such as providing assistance and supervision and eliminating or reducing environmental hazards.

In considering interventions for adaptation problems evolving from sensory deprivation and overload, an especially tangible and immediate change in or management of stimuli is used. When a person is deprived of adequate sensory input (as could happen when a blind or deaf person is placed in an isolation room, is confined in traction, or is on a respirator), the nurse may make direct use of personal contact on a scheduled basis. Television, radio, auidotapes, and judicious choice of roommates and room location are some interventions designed to increase stimulation.

If the adaptation problem evolves from an overdose of stimulation, as can occur with same-day surgery, prolonged outpatient testing procedures, a noisy location on the unit, or intensive-care unit situations, the nurse will again intervene. This time the plan may provide for uninterrupted rest periods, a move to a quieter location, providing a quiet place for patients to rest between tests, and similar measures designed to reduce the amount of new experiences with which the person is confronted in a given time period. This can be especially important for an older person or a person who is confused (see Chap. 12).

To this point, the presentation of nursing interventions has focused on sensory disturbance. Further discussion of nursing interventions focuses on the compromised adaptive processes discussed previously, pain and hyperactivity.

Pain

Pain can be a frightening and, at times, overwhelming experience, not only for the suffering person, but also for others involved in the situation. As difficult as it may be to witness suffering, people in pain cannot be helped when caregivers avoid them. Feeling confident regarding what is effective nursing care for people experiencing pain helps alleviate the nurse's own apprehensions.

It was noted earlier that the gate control theory of pain links the physiologic and psychological events of pain. The resulting explanation for the holistic human experience provides several approaches to intervention in managing pain. At the site of the pain receptors, other receptors can be stimulated to override the nociceptive, or painful, messages. Pain impulses can also be altered in what has been termed the physiologic "gate" in the dorsal horn of the spinal cord. The interconnections of spinal nerve fiber tracts, thalamus, reticular formation, and cortex are the mechanisms for messages to open or close the "gate."

There are a number of options available when relief from pain and discomfort is the goal. Based on the cause of the pain, the nurse selects one or more interventions. Common pain-relieving activities are listed in Table 10–3. These are particular ways of managing the focal and contextual factors contributing to the pain experience. It should be emphasized that the importance of more than one intervention is often overlooked. The person with incision site pain from a bowel resection may require an intramuscular analgesic, but a short ambulation to relieve gas accumulation also may be warranted. A refreshing bath, a lotion back rub, and some local heat or cold application may be the best combination for a person experiencing a flareup of spinal osteoarthritis.

The context in which the pain management strategies are presented is important to their effectiveness. People want relief and the nurse always suggests interventions to the patient in a positive manner, conveying the idea that pain relief is the specific goal. Even when individuals have to be denied what they see as a relief measure, a positive approach can help, as in the following example. A person was seen in the emergency room at 2:00 AM with

TABLE 10–3 COMMON PAIN-RELIEVING ACTIVITIES

1. General comfort measures
   - Repositioning person in bed or wheelchair
   - Tightening sheets, realignment of pillows, covers
   - Changing dressings
   - Warm or cool baths or showers
   - Back rubs
   - Decreasing movement or ambulation
2. Local application of heat or ice
3. Relaxation exercises
4. Imagery
5. Biofeedback
6. Distraction
7. Use of self-proximity, touch, and reassurance
8. Pharmacologic management with opioids
   - Oral
   - Rectal
   - Intravenous
   - Subcutaneous
   - Intramuscular
   - Transdermal
   - Epidural
   - Intrathecal and intraventricular
9. Adjuvant analgesics
   - Nonsteroidal anti-inflammatory drugs
   - Corticosteroids
   - Tricyclic antidepressants
   - Anticonvulsants
   - Oral and parenteral local anesthetics
   - Psychotropics
10. Anesthetic blocks

the medical diagnosis statement, "rule out appendicitis." The emergency room physician wrote orders for close observation, intravenous fluids, and "no pain medication until seen at 6 AM by surgeon." The patient asked the nurse for a shot for pain. Instead of responding flatly that she could not give the medication, the nurse carefully explains that potent medications would mask symptoms and make the process of medical diagnosis more difficult. Other measures that the nurse could use include staying with the patient for several minutes and incorporating such comments as the following in their conversation: "You'll be able to rest better now that the initial diagnostic work is finished. I'll check on you frequently throughout the night, but I feel that you'll be able to sleep now. You were dehydrated and the intravenous fluid will take care of that problem."

Drug therapy is often used in control of pain. Nurses have the responsibility for making judgments about drug administration, giving the medication, and teaching patients about their drugs, as well as about the use of other pain-relieving measures. Analgesics are common drugs of choice when pain relief is the goal, even though they treat only the symptom of pain and not the cause. Analgesics are classified in several ways: narcotic or nonnarcotic, addictive or nonaddictive, prescription or over-the-counter, strong or weak, and peripheral or central acting. An ideal analgesic would have the strength matched to the intensity of the pain, be nonaddicting, and have few side effects. Peripheral-action drugs interfere with the transmission of painful stimuli from body sites, whereas central-acting drugs alter perception of, and consequently responses to, pain on a cortical level. Narcotics, such as morphine, are the more potent of the oral and intramuscular agents. They interact with the opiate receptors in the body. The nonnarcotic agents, such as aspirin, acetaminophen (Tylenol, Datril, Tempra), and aspirin-like nonsteroidal anti-inflammatory drugs such as ibuprofen (Motrin, Advil, Nuprin), are considered less strong and do not have opiate receptor affinity. However, specific properties of these drugs such as anti-inflammatory action make them very effective for certain painful conditions, arthritis, for example.

More detailed information about the properties of analgesics and about other drug therapies for pain can be found in pharmacology resources. Although morphine is an addictive narcotic for some people, fears about addiction, by the patient in pain or health care workers planning pain relief interventions, are generally misplaced. This issue has intensified with high social concern for drug abuse and its consequences for the individual, family, and community. Melzack (1990) notes that concern over addiction has led many nations in Europe and elsewhere to outlaw virtually any uses of morphine and related substances. Many caregivers in countries where morphine is legal for medical therapy, including the United States and Great Britain, are afraid of turning patients into addicts and therefore deliver amounts that are too small or spaced too widely to adequately control pain. Melzack notes that undertreatment leads to the tragedy of needless pain and suffering. Based on numerous studies that validate the distinction, Melzack urges health care workers to distinguish between the addict who craves morphine for its mood-altering properties and the psychologically healthy patient who takes the drug only to relieve pain.

Based on this concern, the U.S. Agency for Health Care Policy and Research (AHCPR) issued a set of guidelines related to the management of acute pain. These recommendations are summarized in Table 10–4.

Nursing judgment of a high order is used when medications are part of planned interventions for pain relief. This is especially true when several options are prescribed. There may be oral and intramuscular (IM) preparations ordered, several different drugs, or various doses for the same drug. Consider the case of a 34-year-old man admitted to an orthopedic unit after sustaining several fractures and various lacerations during a motorcycle accident. After surgery to insert a pin and cast application, his pain relief medication orders were as follows: Demerol 75 to 100 mg IM every 3 to 4 hours for severe pain,

TABLE 10–4 AHCPR SUMMARY RECOMMENDATIONS FOR ACUTE PAIN

1. *Promise patients attentive analgesic care.* Patients should be informed before surgery, verbally and in printed format, that effective pain relief is an essential part of their treatment.

2. *Chart and display assessment of pain and relief.* A simple assessment of pain intensity and pain relief should be recorded on the bedside vital sign chart or a similar record that encourages easy, regular review by members of the health care team and is incorporated in the patient's permanent record.

3. *Define pain relief levels to trigger a review.* Each institution should identify pain intensity and pain relief levels that will elicit a review of the current pain therapy, documentation of the proposed modifications in treatment, and subsequent review of its efficacy.

4. *Survey patient satisfaction.* At regular intervals defined by the clinical unit and quality assurance committee, each clinical unit should assess a randomly selected sample of patients who have had surgery within 72 hours. Patients should be asked their current pain intensity, the worst pain intensity in the past 24 hours, the degree of relief obtained from pain management interventions, and satisfaction with relief and the staff's responsiveness.

5. *Analgesic drug treatment should comply with several basic principles.*
   a. Nonopioid "peripherally acting" analgesics: Unless contraindicated, every patient should receive an around-the-clock postoperative regimen of an NSAID.
   b. Opioid analgesics: Analgesic orders should allow for the great variation in individual opioid requirements, including a regularly scheduled dose and "rescue" doses for instances in which the usual regimen is insufficient.

6. *Specialized analgesic technologies,* including systemic or intraspinal, continuous or intermittent opioid administration or patient controlled dosing, should be governed by policies and standard procedures that define acceptable levels of patient monitoring and appropriate roles and limits of practice.

7. *Nonpharmacologic interventions.* Cognitive and behaviorally based interventions include a number of methods to help patients understand more about their pain and to take an active part in its assessment and control. These interventions are intended to supplement, not replace, pharmacologic interventions. Staff should give patients information about these interventions and support patients in using them.

8. *Monitor the efficacy of pain treatment.* Periodically review pain treatment procedures, using the institution's quality assurance procedures.

Source: Acute Pain Management Guideline Panel, 1992.

Demerol 50 to 75 mg IM every 3 to 4 hours for moderate pain, Visteril 50 mg IM may be added to Demerol doses as needed, Tylenol 10 grains orally every 4 hours as needed, and Mylanta 30 cc orally every 4 hours as needed.

Judgments involve differentiating between moderate and severe pain, deciding if Vistaril will be of help to this person, administering Tylenol and Mylanta when the need is assessed, and determining the appropriate interval between each injection of Demerol in the context of the pain experience at that time. In addition to assessing the kinds of discomfort the person is experiencing at a given time, other factors are relevant to nursing judgments. They are the exact hour and amount of the last pain medication and how it affected him, how he perceives the pain, and his size. The typical as-needed drug order essentially means that the drug is given only after the pain returns. Enough evidence has now been collected to demonstrate that this approach, based on the fear of addiction, is not valid (Melzack, 1990). Rather, there is another, more humane way to treat pain, which was pioneered in the treatment of cancer patients and is slowly gaining broader acceptance. In this approach, the pain is controlled continuously by doses that are given regularly, according to a schedule that has been determined to prevent recurrence of the individual's pain. With this preventive administration of medication before pain becomes extreme, patients seem to require fewer doses and are better able to resume regular activities earlier (Curtis, 1986).

Other interventions for pain include acupuncture, transcutaneous electrical nerve stimulation, distraction, relaxation and biofeedback, imagery and hypnosis, and enrollment in a pain control center. The latter has provided innovative help to people troubled by chronic, incapacitating pain. These centers emphasize the proper use of nutrition, medication, exercise, relaxation techniques, and insight therapy. A multidisciplinary team helps the person make changes in attitude and lifestyle. The goal is to divert the main focus of the person's life away from the pain. The end result can be a lifestyle and self-concept that is more satisfying for the person, and yet realistic about the physical pain, which cannot be totally eliminated.

Hyperactivity

Managing the environment of a hyperactive child involves interventions that are both preventive and reactive. Preventive interventions are environmental modifications used to reduce stimuli that can contribute to the problem behavior. Some contextual stimuli that can be managed for the hyperactive child include amount of noise, movement, or other persons who may be particularly stimulating. The nurse can help families provide a home atmosphere that has decreased stimuli, for example, busy wallpapers, curtains, and fabrics are best avoided. Sparse, smooth-lined furnishings can be helpful. Reactive interventions teach the child more appropriate ways to deal with his or her own behavior. Strategies include learning self-regulation, listening, and problem-solving skills. For example, for children of school age, it is particularly important that nurses, parents, physicians, and teachers work together in assessing the child's needs and planning a consistent approach to care. Teamwork is facilitated by common understandings of the nature of the problem and the plan for care. The nurse can provide encouragement and support during diagnosis and the time it takes to develop, modify, and maintain an effective plan for care.

Manuals of interventions are available for both teachers and parents which list specific interventions for given behaviors. An example of the goals and objectives set up for the specific behavior "Does not listen to what other students are saying" is as follows.

- Goals: (1) The student will improve listening skills in nonacademic settings. (2) The student will attend to what other students say.
- Objectives to meet the goals include: (1) The student will maintain eye contact when other students are speaking on two out of three occasions. (2) The student will listen quietly when other students are speaking on one out of two occasions. (3) The student will repeat

what other students have said with 25 percent accuracy. (4) The student will respond appropriately to what other students say on one out of four occasions.

For this behavior, one manual (McCarney, 1994) lists 21 interventions, with the first being to make certain that the student's hearing has been recently checked. It is then recommended that the student be reinforced for listening when spoken to by other students (for example, making eye contact, putting aside materials, answering students). The student may be given a tangible reward such as classroom privileges, line leading, passing out materials, or 5 minutes free time. The student may also be given an intangible reward such as praise, a handshake, or a smile for listening to what other students are saying. A third intervention is to reinforce the students in the classroom who listen to what other students are saying. The fourth intervention directs the teacher or parent to speak to the student to explain what the student is doing wrong (for example, failing to listen to what other students are saying) and what the student should be doing (for example, listening to other students when they speak to him or her and listening to other students when they speak to a group).

Given the complexity and constancy of intervention plans, the parents need constant support and encouragement. The nurse can suggest safe, age-related play and social activities. Reassurance that the child's behavior is not willful and that the hyperactivity may decrease or cease in adolescence can be comforting to parents. Parents sometimes need release time provided by a reliable substitute caregiver. Three or four hours, a couple of times a week, may decrease the frustrations of parents who are constantly implementing a plan for given behaviors of hyperactivity. Referral to national and local support groups may be helpful as parents can offer much support and firsthand suggestions for these families.

Evaluation

The effectiveness of nursing interventions is evaluated by determining whether or not the goals of the plan for care have been accomplished. The preset goals identified the behavior of focus, the change or stability desired, and the time frame. Consider the goal described earlier for the child with a recent loss of sight in one eye: "The child will travel to and from school safely by himself one day this week." The behavior of interest is the child's trips to and from school. If he has, in fact, made at least one trip by himself this week without injury, the goal has been accomplished. If this goal was not accomplished, the nurse will assess the situation further to see if all relevant factors in designing the intervention have been considered. For example, in spite of his stated eagerness to try this task, the child may be more afraid than he will admit, particularly if he thinks older boys will take advantage of his vision limitation. Another possibility is that the interventions have not been used long enough.

The child may need more practice navigating on his own street with someone nearby to give feedback and warn him if he is about to make a mistake.

In evaluating interventions for pain, the main criterion is pain relief. As indicated earlier, the patient is the authority on the pain experience and the report of relief is the most important behavioral indicator. The person is also observed for decrease in nonverbal cues of discomfort, for example, clenched teeth, tightly shut lips, furrowed brow, biting the lower lip, grimacing, and rhythmic or protective body movements. Relief may be partial and the intervention may need to be modified in some way. For example, the person may require a larger dose of analgesic, increased ambulation, more frequent position changes, reinforcement of relaxation techniques, or a combination of interventions to obtain more complete relief. In addition, the nurse will evaluate whether or not the person is experiencing any negative side effects from the intervention, such as decreased respirations from an analgesic or pressure on a body part from special positioning.

► SUMMARY

This chapter has focused on the senses as a component of the physiologic mode and channels for receiving information and thus interacting with the environment by way of complex neurologic networks. The theoretical basis for understanding the basic life processes of the senses, particularly vision, hearing, and feeling, were presented briefly and assessment factors were identified. Compensatory processes of sensation were identified and two examples of compromised processes, pain and hyperactivity, were discussed. Then the nursing process based on the Roy Adaptation Model was applied using nursing diagnoses related to the senses, goal setting, interventions, and evaluation.

► EXERCISES FOR APPLICATION

1. For 2 hours, restrict the use of one of your senses by patching one eye. Go about your usual activities and after the 2 hours, write down any difficulties you had. Include any particular emotional reactions related to these difficulties or the experience in general.

2. Spend a few minutes reflecting on the greatest intensity or degree of physical pain you have ever felt. Describe this experience to a friend.

3. Devise a way to assess pain in a school-aged child.

► ASSESSMENT OF UNDERSTANDING

Questions

1. The three primary senses described in this chapter were vision (V), hearing (H) and feeling (F). Label each of the following statements according to the primary sense to which they apply.
   (a) _____ somatosensory pathways
   (b) _____ occipital lobe of the cerebral cortex
   (c) _____ pain
   (d) _____ kinesthesia
   (e) _____ primary auditory cortex
   (f) _____ rods and cones
   (g) _____ touch and pressure

2. Name two first-level assessment parameters (behaviors) for each of the three primary sense processes.
   (a) Vision: _____ and _____ (b) Hearing: _____ and _____ (c) Feeling: _____ and _____

3. In this chapter, six questions for general assessment of stimuli related to sensory processing were presented. What were those questions? List all six.
   (a) _____
   (b) _____
   (c) _____
   (d) _____
   (e) _____
   (f) _____

4. Identify one compensatory process related to each of the primary senses.
   (a) Vision:_____
   (b) Hearing:_____
   (c) Feeling:_____

5. Identify three commonly recurring adaptation problems that apply to all three primary senses.
   (a) _____
   (b) _____
   (c) _____

Situation:

A patient has just had surgery to remove a tumor between the inner ear and the brain stem (acoustic neuroma). He has lost hearing on the affected side. He complains of distorted sound, being unable to tell the direction of sound, being fearful of adequately monitoring his environment, and difficulty in relating to his grandchildren because he cannot understand what they are saying.

6. State a nursing diagnosis for this patient.

7. Derive a goal statement that contains the behavior of focus, the change expected, and the time frame involved.

8. Give at least five basic considerations for nursing judgment when administering medication for pain relief.

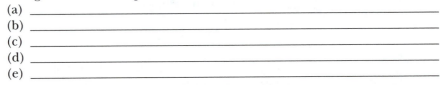

(a) _____

(b) _____

(c) _____

(d) _____

(e) _____

9. Which is the most important criterion for evaluating whether or not nursing interventions have achieved the goal of pain relief?
   (a) the person's statement of comfort
   (b) the time and amount of medication given

Feedback

1. (a) F, (b) V, (c) F, (d) F, (e) H, (f) V, (g) F

2. (a) Vision: Two of: visual tests, functional examination, internal examination.
   (b) Hearing: Two of: auditory screening tests to measure sensitivity and discrimination, evidence of other difficulties (faulty speech, inattentiveness, unresponsiveness, withdrawal in social situations).
   (c) Feeling: Two of: sensation behaviors (response to light touch, joint movement identification, pin prick and dull object to test pain sensation, test of temperature detection, test for symmetry of sensation).

3. (a) Is the impairment temporary, permanent, or is this unanswerable at the current time?
   (b) Is the impairment recent or long standing?
   (c) Is more than one impairment present?
   (d) How does the person view the loss of function?
   (e) How is the person affected in the current environment of home, work, school, clinic, or hospital and moving from one place to another?
   (f) What is the person's level of knowledge, the knowledge needed, and readiness for teaching?

4. (a) prescribing of glasses, use of large-print books
   (b) lip reading or sign language
   (c) using oven mitts when removing hot objects from the oven, wearing rubber gloves in hot dishwater, good skin care processes for people with reduced feeling in hands and feet

5. Any three of: impairment of a primary sense, potential for injury or loss of self-care abilities, potential for distorted communication, stigma, sensory monotony or distortion, sensory overload or deprivation, acute pain, chronic pain, perceptual impairment, ineffective coping strategies for sensory impairment.

6. Examples of nursing diagnoses: Uncompensated auditory deficit, or, Stated difficulty dealing with environment and important relationships due to sudden, recent, and permanent loss of hearing in one ear.

7. Example of a goal: Within the next week, the patient will report enjoying a visit with his grandchildren when he gave them the opportunity to be at the level of his hearing ear and to see his new device for transmitting sound from the deaf side to the hearing ear.

8. Any of the following: the location of the pain, the source, onset and duration, constancy, intensity and type as reported by the person, person's experience of this pain and previous experiences, whether a combination of approaches can bring relief, size of the person, exact time and amount of last pain medication administration, as well as evaluation of relief obtained, and the type of medication available.

9. a

▶ **REFERENCES**

Bates, B. (1991). *A guide to physical examination* (3rd ed.). Philadelphia: Lippincott.

Bullock, B. L., & Rosendahl, P. P. (1992). *Pathophysiology: Adaptations and alterations in function* (3rd ed.). Philadelphia: Lippincott.

Burrell, L. O., Gerlach, M. J. M., & Pless, B. S. (1997). *Adult nursing: Acute and community care* (2nd ed.). Stamford, CT: Appleton & Lange.

Cassell, E. J. (1989). The relationship between pain and suffering. In Hill, C. S., Fields, W. S. (Eds.), *Drug treatment of cancer pain in a drug-oriented society: Advances in pain research and therapy* (Vol. 11, p. 61). New York: Raven Press.

Guyton, A. (1992). *Human physiology and mechanisms of disease* (4th ed.). Philadelphia: Saunders.

Hill, C. (1987). Sensory functions and alterations. In Servonsky, J., & Opas, S. (Eds.), *Nursing management of children* (pp. 1221–1261). Boston: Jones and Bartlett.

Kolb, B., & Whishaw, I. (1985). *Fundamentals of human neuropsychology* (2nd ed.). New York: Freeman.

Marks, R. M., & Sachar, E. J. (1973). Undertreatment of medical inpatients with narcotic analgesics. *Annals of Internal Medicine, 78,* 173.

McCaffery, M. (1979). *Nursing management of the patient with pain* (2nd ed.). Philadelphia: Lippincott.

McCaffery, M. (1997). Pain management handbook. *Nursing 27(4),* 42–45.

McCaffery, M., & Beebe, A. (1989). *Pain: A clinical manual for nursing practice.* St. Louis: Mosby.

McCarney, S. B. (1994). *The attention deficit disorders intervention manual.* Columbia, MO: Hawthorne Educational Services.

Meiss, R., & Tanner, G. (1982). Sensory receptors. In Selkurt, E. (Ed.), *Basic physiology for the health sciences* (pp. 115–159). Boston: Little Brown.

Melzack, R. (1990, February). The tragedy of needless pain. *Scientific American,* pp. 27–33.

Melzack, R., & Wall, P. (1965). Pain mechanisms: A new theory. *Science, 150,* 971.

Melzack, R., & Wall, P. (1970). Psychophysiology of pain. *International Anesthesia Clinics, 81(1),* 3.

Melzack, R., & Wall, P. (1989). *The challenge of pain* (rev. ed.). New York: Penguin.

Mitchell, P. H., Hodges, L. C., Muwaswes, M., & Walleck, C. A. (Eds.). (1988). *American Association of Neuroscience Nurses' Neuroscience nursing: Phenomena and practice* (pp. 501–515). Norwalk, CT: Appleton & Lange.

Posner, M. I., & Raichle, M. E. (1994). *Images of mind.* New York: Scientific American Library.

Rantz, M. J., & LeMone, P. (Eds.). (1997). *Classification of nursing diagnoses. Proceedings of the 12th conference NANDA.* Glendale, CA: CINAHL Information Systems.

Rowland, L. P. (1984). *Merritt's textbook of neurology* (7th ed.). Philadelphia: Lea & Febiger.

Roy, Sr. C. (in press). Alterations in cognitive processing. In Stewart-Amidei, C., Kunkel, J., & Bronstein, K. (Eds.), *American Association of Neuroscience Nurses' Neuroscience nursing: Human responses to neurologic dysfunction* (2nd ed.). Philadelphia: Saunders.

Servonsky, J., & Opas, S. (Eds.). (1987). *Nursing management of children.* Boston: Jones and Bartlett.

Thorpe, D. M. (1990). Comprehensive pain care: The relief of pain and suffering. *Dimensions of Oncology Nursing, 4(1):* 27–29.

11

FLUID, ELECTROLYTE, AND ACID–BASE BALANCE

The maintenance of fluid, electrolyte, and acid–base balance is identified in the Roy Adaptation Model as one of four complex processes associated with the physiologic mode. Maintenance of these substances in correct proportion is vital for the integrity of the individual.

In this chapter, the basic life processes associated with fluid, electrolyte, and acid–base balance are addressed. Although many body systems play roles in these processes, the major role of the kidney in the maintenance of this balance, through the processes of filtration, reabsorption, and secretion, is addressed. In particular, the complex processes associated with the maintenance of fluid balance, electrolyte balance, and acid–base balance are the topics of focus. With each of these complex processes, the parameters for assessment of behaviors and stimuli affecting them are explored. Illustrations of compensatory and compromised processes are also discussed. Finally, guidelines for planning nursing care by formulating nursing diagnoses, establishing goals, selecting interventions, and evaluating nursing care are described.

► OBJECTIVES

After studying this chapter, the reader will be able to do the following:

1. Describe the basic life processes associated with the need for fluid, electrolyte, and acid–base balance as presented in this chapter.

2. Identify important first-level assessment parameters (behaviors) of the basic life processes associated with fluid, electrolyte, and acid–base balance.

3. List second-level assessment parameters (common stimuli) that affect fluid, electrolyte, and acid–base balance.

4. Describe one compensatory process associated with fluid, electrolyte, and acid–base balance.

5. Name and describe two situations of compromised processes of fluid, electrolyte, and acid–base balance.

6. Develop a nursing diagnosis, given a situation related to fluid, electrolyte, and acid–base balance.

7. Derive goals for an individual with ineffective fluid, electrolyte, or acid–base balance in a given situation.

8. Describe nursing interventions commonly implemented in situations of ineffective fluid, electrolyte, and acid–base balance.

9. Propose approaches to determine the effectiveness of nursing interventions.

▶ KEY CONCEPTS DEFINED

Acidosis: A decrease in arterial blood pH (excess of hydrogen ion concentration) related to accumulation of acid or loss of base.

Alkalosis: An increase in arterial blood pH (deficit of hydrogen ion concentration) related to accumulation of base or deficiency of acid.

Calcemia: Pertaining to calcium in the blood.

Electrolytes: Substances that break down into ions when in solution.

Fluids: Internal body fluids located within (intracellular) and outside (extracellular) body cells in various parts of the body not available for general body use, for example, joint fluid or pericardial fluid (third space fluids).

Filtration: A passive process occurring in the glomerulus of the kidney wherein blood plasma is filtered and proteins and blood cells, too large to pass through the membrane, remain behind.

Homeostasis: The maintenance of stable internal environment of the body.

Hyper: A prefix meaning excess or above normal value.

Hypo: A prefix meaning deficit or below normal value.

Kalemia: Pertaining to potassium in the blood.

Natremia: Pertaining to the sodium in the blood.

Osmolarity: Concentration of solutes in a solvent as expressed per unit of weight (kg) of the solvent.

Reabsorption: The reclamation of useful substances (for example, water, glucose, amino acids, ions) from the filtrate back into the blood during the process of blood purification in the kidney.

Secretion: The movement of substances (hydrogen and potassium ions, creatinine, ammonia) from the blood into the filtrate (reabsorption in reverse).

pH: A measure of hydrogen ion concentration and, thus, of acidity or alkalinity.

▶ COMPLEX PROCESS OF FLUID, ELECTROLYTE, AND ACID–BASE BALANCE

Adaptation relative to fluid, electrolyte, and acid–base balance is referred to as the process of homeostasis. Marieb (1994) defined *homeostasis* as the maintenance of a stable internal environment of the body. A wide variety of body systems including the respiratory, circulatory, gastrointestinal, renal, nervous, and endocrine systems play a regulatory role in the maintenance of fluid, electrolyte, and acid–base balance. However, the major responsibility rests with the kidneys. The reader is referred to texts on anatomy and physiology for basic information about the physiologic structures addressed in this chapter.

The kidneys function to maintain the purity and constancy of internal fluids. They process gallons of fluid each day, filtering out wastes and excess ions and returning needed substances to the blood. They regulate the volume and chemical makeup of the blood by achieving proper fluid, electrolyte, and acid–base balance.

Three processes are involved in the filtering of blood and the formation of urine. They are filtration, reabsorption, and secretion. Kidneys filter over 150 L of blood plasma in 24 hours through glomeruli into the tubules which, in turn, process the filtrate by taking substances out of it (reabsorption) and adding substances to it (secretion).

Filtration is a nonselective, passive process which occurs in the glomerulus. The filtration membrane filters blood plasma; proteins and blood cells are too large to pass through and remain behind. Normal blood pressure is required to force plasma out of the blood and into the tubules (filtrate formation).

Reabsorption pertains to the reclamation of useful substances (for example, water, glucose, amino acids, ions) from the filtrate back into the blood. Reabsorption begins and is mostly accomplished in cells of the proximal convoluted tubule, although some reabsorption occurs by osmosis. Most reabsorption depends on an active transport process, which uses very selective membrane carriers. There are many carriers for substances needing to be retained (such as glucose and amino acids) and few for waste products (such as urea, creatinine, and uric acid). The ions retained or excreted depend on the body's needs at the time with respect to pH and electrolyte composition of the blood.

Secretion pertains to the movement of substances (hydrogen and potassium ions, creatinine, ammonia) from the blood into the filtrate (reabsorption in reverse). This process is important for ridding the body of substances (certain drugs, for example) that have not been filtered already.

The kidneys play four major roles associated with fluid and electrolyte balance.

- The excretion of nitrogen-containing wastes (urea, uric acid, creatinine)
- Maintaining water balance
- Maintaining electrolyte balance
- Maintaining acid–base balance of the blood

Excretion was reviewed in Chapter 7. In this chapter, the remaining three processes are reviewed.

► FLUID BALANCE

Fluids within the body can be intracellular, extracellular, or third space fluids. Within the body, water serves as the universal solvent in which electrolytes and nonelectrolytes are dissolved. The concentration of these solutes in water influences fluid balance between intracellular and extracellular compartments. As Marieb (1994, p. 461) describes:

> To maintain blood composition, the kidneys must . . . maintain water and electrolyte balance by absorbing more or less water and ions in response to hormones [hormonal stimulation]. ADH [Antidiuretic hormone] increases water reabsorption and conserves body water. Aldosterone increases tubular reabsorption of sodium and water and decreases tubular reabsorption of potassium.

The concentration of solutes in water influences fluid balance between intracellular and extracellular compartments. Water is taken into the body in the form of beverages and moist food and is a product of metabolism. Water is lost from the body through excretion of urine and feces, perspiration, and respiration. The thirst mechanism regulates intake. Plasma *osmolarity*, the concentration of solutes as expressed per unit of weight (kg) of solvent, triggers the thirst mechanism and the release of ADH from the hypothalamus. Output of water is regulated by the kidneys. As Burrell (1992, p. 101) points out,

"Regardless of large variations in intake, individuals with normal kidney function are able to maintain normal [fluid] balance by secreting either dilute or concentrated urine."

▶ ELECTROLYTE BALANCE

Electrolytes are substances (salts) that break down into ions when in solution. Thus, electrolyte balance addresses concentrations of salts within the body. The major elements forming salts within body fluids are sodium, potassium, and calcium.

Sodium plays a central role in fluid and electrolyte balance by controlling extracellular fluid volume and water distribution in the body. Changes in plasma sodium levels affect plasma volume and blood pressure as well as the volumes in the intra- and extracellular fluid compartments.

Sodium regulation involves a variety of neural and hormonal mechanisms. Aldosterone from the adrenal cortex constitutes a complex hormonal influence in the process of sodium balance by enhancing sodium reabsorption by the kidneys (water follows the movement of sodium by osmosis). Antidiuretic hormone (ADH), produced in the posterior pituitary and stimulated by the hypothalamus, increases the permeability of the collecting tubules of the kidney and enhances water reabsorption. In addition, pressoreceptors in the heart respond to changes in blood volume and stimulate the hypothalamus and posterior pituitary in the production of ADH.

Potassium is required for normal neuromuscular functioning and metabolic activity. The role of potassium in the synthesis of protein is particularly important. Even a slight alteration in potassium levels affects neurons and muscle fibers. In turn, there can be profound effects on other body functions such as cardiac muscle function and cognitive function.

Regulation of potassium is accomplished primarily by renal mechanisms. When concentrations of potassium fall below normal levels, the kidneys conserve potassium by reducing its secretion. There is, however, limited ability of the kidneys to retain potassium. Thus, ingestion of appropriate levels of potassium is important. Three major factors determine the rate and extent of potassium secretion: tubule cell potassium content, aldosterone levels, and the pH of the extracellular fluid.

Most body calcium is found in the bones but a small percentage is required in the extracellular fluid for normal clotting of blood, cell membrane permeability, and secretory functions. Muscular excitability also is affected by calcium.

Calcium is regulated by parathyroid hormone and its antagonist, calcitonin (produced by the thyroid gland). Parathyroid hormone affects calcium release from bone, absorption of calcium by the small intestine, and kidney reabsorption of calcium.

Other minor elements such as magnesium and chloride have important functions within the body. Their actions are complex and often poorly understood. Further information about these elements and those previously described is contained in physiology resources.

▶ ACID–BASE BALANCE

The acid–base status of body fluids is related to the concentration of hydrogen ions and is described in terms of *pH,* normal values of which range from 7.35 to 7.45. Concentration of hydrogen ions is regulated by chemical buffers in the blood, the respiratory center in the brainstem, and renal mechanisms. Buffer systems are important in resisting a change in pH in one or more fluid compartments, while respiratory and renal mechanisms rid the body of excess acid or retain hydrogen ions.

According to Marieb (1994, p. 461), the kidneys must:

> maintain acid–base balance by failing to reabsorb excess bases, by actively secreting excess H⁺, and by retaining bicarbonate ions. Chemical buffers do their part by temporarily tying up excess H⁺ or bases and the respiratory centers modify blood pH by retaining CO_2 (which decreases the pH) or by eliminating more CO_2 from the blood (which increases blood pH). Only renal mechanisms can remove metabolic acids and excess bases from the body.

Full discussion of the complex processes related to fluid, electrolyte, and acid–base balance is not within the parameters of this text. A basic physiology source, for example, Marieb (1994), reviews the intricacies of these processes.

Assessment of Behavior

The nurse caring for a person must have an understanding of behavioral norms indicating fluid, electrolyte, and acid–base balance and must be a skilled observer. The nurse is in an excellent position, due to frequent contact with the person, to assess both subtle and overt behaviors and changes in these behaviors indicating ineffective body responses. It is easier to prevent imbalances if the nurse has knowledge of stimuli that influence these intricate processes. The nurse then uses this knowledge to predict and monitor the person for potential imbalances.

After reviewing the person's history, the nurse proceeds with a systematic assessment of fluid, electrolyte, and acid–base balance. In this case, the basic needs and complex processes associated with the physiologic mode of the Roy Adaptation Model serve as a guideline for the assessment.

Oxygenation

Related to the need for oxygenation are behaviors indicative of respiratory and circulatory function within the body. The particular behavioral manifestation will depend on the stimuli. For example, cardiac arrhythmia can be a manifestation of potassium excess in the blood. Problems with blood volume are manifest in the characteristics of the pulse and blood pressure. Therefore, assessment of fluid, electrolyte, and acid–base balance as related to the need for oxygenation would involve assessment of the pulse, blood pressure, respirations, and change in skin color.

Nutrition

Associated with nutrition need and related to fluid, electrolyte, and acid–base balance are appetite, thirst, symptoms of nausea and vomiting, and the condition of the tongue. Increased thirst can be indicative of excessive amounts of sodium or potassium in the body. A dry, furrowed tongue signals a deficit in fluid volume in the body.

Elimination

The amount and characteristics of urinary output, intestinal output, and bowel activity are important behaviors related to fluid, electrolyte, and acid–base balance. Urinary output is an important indicator of fluid volume while diarrhea can influence both fluid volume and electrolyte balance. Levels of intake and output in situations of fluid, electrolyte, and acid–base imbalance constitute important behavioral indicators. A decrease in bowel sounds evident on abdominal auscultation can indicate problems with potassium levels in the body.

Activity and Rest

Imbalances in fluid, electrolyte, and acid–base balance will also affect the person's need for activity and rest, and their report of how they are feeling. Complaints of fatigue, malaise, drowsiness, restlessness, agitation, and irritability may be behavioral indicators of ineffective adaptation related to electrolytes, particularly where calcium levels are concerned. Disruptions in bone integrity also can indicate calcium problems.

Protection

Related to the processes of physiologic protection is the condition of the skin, and the skin, in turn, reflects fluid, electrolyte, and acid–base balance. The nurse would expect to find abnormalities in skin temperature, turgor, and color in situations of fluid volume alterations. Peripheral and peri-oral sensation can be affected by calcium deficits, with patients reporting "tingling" of fingers or lips. Expected findings with decreases in fluid volume are diminished reflexes and decreased tearing and salivation.

Neurologic Function

Fluid, electrolyte, and acid–base imbalance can result in neurologic manifestations including belligerence, apathy, confusion, disorientation and headache, and progressive alteration in the functioning of the central nervous system.

Laboratory Examination

An important behavioral validation in the assessment of fluid, electrolyte, and acid–base balance is the results of laboratory tests, in particular, those related to concentrations of elements and ions in the blood and urine. Urine is normally clear, yellow, and usually slightly acidic, but its pH value varies widely. Substances normally found in urine are nitrogenous wastes, water, and various ions (always sodium and potassium). Substances not normally found in urine include glucose, albumin (or other blood proteins), blood, pus, white blood cells, and bile. Hemoglobin and hematocrit levels are important indicators of blood volume and specific gravity of urine is an important indicator of body sodium level.

Once the nurse has completed the behavioral assessment of fluid, electrolyte, and acid–base balance, a tentative judgment as to whether the behaviors are adaptive or ineffective is made. As identified in Chapter 3, normal values are available to guide this judgment, as are general expectations relative to the identified behaviors. In other situations, pronounced regulator activity with cognator ineffectiveness may provide the key to the identification of ineffective adaptation. By obtaining an indication of whether the person is maintaining an appropriate balance of fluids, electrolytes, and acids and bases, priorities can be established with respect to the next level of nursing assessment, namely, the assessment of stimuli.

Assessment of Stimuli

With the assessment of stimuli, the nurse gathers data about the factors influencing the behaviors identified in the assessment phases of the adaptation nursing process. This includes the important factor of the body's adaptive ability to maintain the regulatory processes of fluid, electrolyte, and acid–base balance as well as the coping strategies the person uses to maintain or change behaviors.

Integrity of the Physiologic Mode

Of the common stimuli affecting fluid, electrolyte, and acid–base balance, lack of integrity of some aspect of the physiologic mode is the most common source of disruption. In particular, disease pathology associated with acute or chronic illness or injury is frequently the focal stimulus causing ineffective processes of fluid, electrolyte, and acid–base balance.

Consider the example of disruption of skin integrity from a burn. The subsequent loss of extracellular fluid and release of cellular potassium has pervasive effects on body homeostasis. Excessive calcium in the body can result from the breakdown of bone calcium in pathologic conditions such as metastatic cancer of the bone, multiple myeloma, or leukemia. With renal disease, the kidney has limited or no ability to excrete hydrogen ions, potassium, or water. Diabetes is another chronic condition that can adversely affect hydrogen ion concentration within the body. Deficient aldosterone production by the adrenal glands is an acute condition that results in loss of sodium and conservation of potassium. Each of these situations has a profound effect on fluid, electrolyte, and acid–base balance and adaptation.

Stimuli that produce significant changes in blood pressure and volume include, for example, prolonged vomiting or diarrhea, excess perspiration, blood loss, severe burns, wound drainage, and pathologic vasodilation associated with bacterial shock. These stimuli serve to increase blood osmolarity. Through increased concentration of urine and increased water reabsorption, the body attempts to adapt by increasing blood volume.

Medical Interventions

Fluid, electrolyte, and acid–base imbalance may be instigated by the administration of medications or other medical regimens. For example, excessive administration of intravenous solutions can overload the body with fluids. Use of potent or inappropriate diuretic medications without fluid replacement results in loss of fluid, potassium, and sodium. To assist with this problem, some diuretics have been developed with the feature of enabling potassium conservation within the body. Overuse of antacids and laxatives and gastrointestinal suctioning also serve to disrupt electrolyte balance, the former inhibiting the absorption of vital elements and the latter contributing to excessive loss.

Cognator Effectiveness

Cognator effectiveness, as associated with the person's knowledge level, may constitute a stimulus contributing to the fluid, electrolyte, and acid–base imbalance in situations where there is inappropriate use of the medical interventions. For example, a person may be precipitating excessive intestinal absorption of calcium with the overuse of vitamin D. Or the person's dietary intake may be deficient in one or more of the vital elements, either because of lack of knowledge about a balanced diet or disorders such as anorexia.

Developmental Stage

In the very young and the elderly, fluid, electrolyte, and acid–base balance are particularly influenced by body size and makeup, as well as developmental changes. In children, as compared with adults, water accounts for a greater proportion of total body mass, which makes it easier for them to lose fluid. In the neonate, 75 percent of body weight is body water, and the proportion of extracellular to intracellular fluid is greater. Further, on a weight basis, the turnover of water in children is five times greater than that of adults. In addition, the surface area to volume ratio is proportionally greater in children; thus fluid loss through evaporation is potentially greater. Older adults may lack essential electrolytes because of poor nutrition related to a variety of factors such as inadequate dental care, decreased salivation, limited budget for food, and social isolation. In addition, water intake can also be a problem because the thirst mechanism becomes less effective with age. Older people may also limit fluid intake in the late afternoon and evening in an attempt to avoid having to get up to go to the bathroom at night.

Environmental Factors

Environmental factors such as intense heat or inaccessibility of water also affect the body's ability to maintain fluids, electrolytes, and acids and bases in appropriate proportion.

Once the stimuli influencing fluid, electrolyte, and acid–base balance have been identified, the nurse proceeds to suggest whether they are focal, contextual, or residual in their effect on the person's physiologic integrity. The focal stimulus is the one most immediately confronting the person. The stimuli identified represent possible focal stimuli for the complex processes influencing fluid, electrolyte, and acid–base balance. Contextual stimuli are all other internal or external stimuli evident in the situation and contributing to the behavior caused by the focal stimulus. Residual stimuli represent those stimuli whose effect on the individual has not been or cannot be validated.

Within the processes of influencing fluid, electrolyte, and acid–base balance, certain behaviors can be stimuli for other behaviors in some situations. For example, vomiting can be classified as a behavior since it constitutes an action under specified circumstances. However, vomiting can also be considered a stimulus where fluid, electrolyte, and acid–base balance is concerned since persistent vomiting can lead to excessive fluid loss and imbalance in vital elements needed by the body. At times, it may not be clear as to whether a particular activity is a behavior or a stimulus and, in many cases, it may indeed be both. Since the remainder of the nursing process is contingent on factors identified in both parts of the assessment, it may be of value to document the factor as both a behavior and a stimulus to ensure that the concept is not lost as the nursing process proceeds. Experience will clarify the most appropriate method of documenting when such dilemmas are encountered in the assessment of the patient.

▶ COMPENSATORY ADAPTIVE PROCESSES

Roy's concept of the regulator subsystem can be described in the phrase "the wisdom of the body," which means the automatic self-regulation of physiologic processes. Further, the thinking and feeling person, by way of cognator activity, can do much to affect any component of the physiologic mode, and this includes the complex processes associated with fluid and electrolyte balance. Regulator and cognator abilities, then, are important internal stimuli for the person. These subsystems activate compensatory adaptive processes that extend the effectiveness of behavior in reaching the goals of adaptation.

One particular illustration of a regulator activity relates to the functioning of the kidney. If large amounts of water are lost through the lungs, in perspiration, or in the stool, the kidneys compensate that loss by excreting less, more highly concentrated, urine. When intake is excessive, kidneys excrete generous amounts of diluted urine. When blood volume drops, due to hemorrhage, excessive sweating, or diarrhea, for example, arterial blood pressure drops and this ultimately results in a decreased amount of filtrate formed by the kidneys. The change in blood composition stimulates osmoreceptors in the hypothalamus which, in turn, signal the posterior pituitary to release antidiuretic hormone, the effect of which is to prevent excessive water loss in the urine. As more water is returned to the blood stream, blood volume and blood pressure increase to normal levels and only small amounts of very concentrated urine are formed.

An illustration of a compensatory cognator response associated with the complex processes of fluid, electrolyte, and acid–base balance is that of artificial renal dialysis. In some situations, the kidneys are unable to carry out their normal functions due to damaging kidney infections, physical trauma, chemical poisoning, or inadequate blood delivery to the kidneys (arteriosclerosis). The body quickly becomes contaminated with poisonous wastes. In these cases, dialysis with the use of an artificial kidney can be used to prevent death. Some people become totally dependent on dialysis and, as a result, are very knowledgeable about the process, when it is indicated, and how their lifestyle must be adapted to accommodate this compensatory adaptive process.

► COMPROMISED PROCESSES RELATED TO FLUID, ELECTROLYTE, AND ACID–BASE BALANCE

Fluid Imbalance

Disturbances of fluid balance in the body can be described in terms of excessive water loss (dehydration), excessive intercellular water retention, and accumulation of fluid in the interstitial compartments (edema). Water volume is closely tied to sodium levels since sodium functions as a magnet for water, controlling extracellular fluid volume and water distribution in the body.

Electrolyte Imbalance

Disturbances in electrolytes are described with combinations of prefixes and root words: *hyper* meaning excess (above normal) and *hypo* meaing deficit (below normal); kalemia (pertaining to potassium), natremia (pertaining to sodium), and calcemia (pertaining to calcium). A decrease in sodium ion concentration in the blood (hyponatremia) inhibits the release of antidiuretic hormone and allows more water to be excreted in the urine. An increase in sodium levels (hypernatremia), such as caused by decreased blood volume, stimulates the release of antidiuretic hormone and results in less water in the urine.

Potassium excess in the extracellular fluid (hyperkalemia) increases neuron and muscle fiber excitability and causes depolarization. Deficits (hypokalemia) cause hyperpolarization and nonresponsiveness. Both situations can lead to abnormal cardiac rhythm and cardiac arrest. Confusion is the manifestation in the brain of these situations of potassium imbalance.

Low levels of calcium (hypocalcemia) result in increased excitability and muscle tetany. High levels (hypercalcemia) inhibit neuron and muscle cell activity.

Acid–Base Imbalances

Abnormalities in acid–base balance can be respiratory (associated with the respiratory system control of pH) or metabolic (control that is nonrespiratory in nature) and result in acidosis or alkalosis. Marieb (1994) described acidosis as "a drop in arterial pH below 7.35" (p. 451). This represents a higher than optimal H^+ concentration for the functioning of most body cells. Alkalosis occurs whenever the pH of arterial blood rises above 7.45, representing an abnormally low hydrogen ion concentration in the extracellular fluid. Respiratory acidosis occurs when gas exchange in the lungs is hampered by disease or inadequate inspiration. The result is the accumulation of carbon dioxide in the blood. Alkalosis occurs when carbon dioxide is released in excessive amounts, for example, through hyperventilation. Acidosis results in central nervous system depression and can result in coma and death. Alkalosis results in overexcitement of the nervous system and can lead to muscle tetany, extreme nervousness, convulsions, and respiratory arrest leading to death.

► PLANNING NURSING CARE

Fluid, electrolyte, and acid–base balance are priority requirements for an individual's physiologic adaptation. In applying the nursing process, the nurse makes a careful assessment of behaviors and stimuli related to these complex processes. In assessing factors influencing fluid, electrolyte, and acid–base balance, regulator and cognator effectiveness in initiating compensatory processes is also considered. Based on this thorough first- and second-level assessment, the nurse makes a nursing diagnosis, sets goals, selects interventions, and evaluates care.

Nursing Diagnosis

Assessment data of behaviors and related stimuli are interpreted and used in establishing a nursing diagnosis. By using the Roy Adaptation Model, the nurse can state diagnoses as specific behaviors with the stimuli that are most relevant or may employ summary labels to convey complex concepts in abbreviated terms.

Roy has developed a typology of indicators of positive adaptation related to fluid, electrolyte, and acid–base balance (see Table 3–2). Included in the typology are stable processes of water balance, stability of electrolytes in body fluids, balance of acid–base status, and effective chemical buffer regulation. It is important to recognize situations of effective adaptation so that these can be maintained or enhanced. In fluid, electrolyte, and acid–base balance, a nursing diagnosis illustrating adaptation could be, "stable processes of fluid, electrolyte, and acid–base balance due to adequate hydration, good nutritional status, and integrity of other physiologic components."

Commonly recurring adaptation problems defined within the Roy Adaptation Model include dehydration; edema; intracellular fluid retention; shock; hyper- or hypo- calcemia, kalemia, or natremia; acid–base imbalance; and ineffective buffer regulation for changing pH.

In situations of fluid, electrolyte, and acid–base disruption, it is important that the essence of the disruption be conveyed in the nursing diagnosis, which then provides direction for subsequent steps of the nursing process. This is facilitated by identification of the specific behaviors that are of concern and the relevant stimuli that are influencing them. An example of this type of nursing diagnosis could be, "urinary output of 5 mL in 8 hours due to no oral fluid intake, traumatic injury to leg with excessive loss of body plasma, and lack of fluid replacement."

A disruption in fluid, electrolyte, and acid–base balance would likely yield many nursing diagnoses relating to each of the ineffective behaviors. A detailed approach, as described, may facilitate thorough interpretation of the data.

The use of a summary label to develop a nursing diagnosis is often an effective way of communicating a cluster of behaviors to experienced nurses. The concept of "shock" might be such a diagnosis, for example. The diagnosis statement could be, "shock due to hemorrhage from gastric ulcer." Much information is contained using the terms "shock" and "hemorrhage" that would provide meaningful direction for the experienced nurse, but may be less meaningful and provide less direction for the person with less clinical and theoretical background.

In Table 11–1, the Roy model nursing diagnostic categories for the complex processes of fluid, electrolyte, and acid–base balance are shown in rela-

TABLE 11–1   NURSING DIAGNOSTIC CATEGORIES FOR FLUID, ELECTROLYTE, AND ACID–BASE BALANCE

Positive Indicators of Adaptation	Common Adaptation Problems	NANDA Diagnostic Labels
• Stable processes of water balance	• Dehydration • Edema • Intracellular water retention • Shock	• Fluid volume excess • Fluid volume deficit • Risk for fluid volume deficit
• Stability of electrolytes in body fluids	• Hyper- or hypo- calcemia, kalemia, or natremia	• Altered (specify type) tissue perfusion (renal, cerebral, cardiopulmonary, gastrointestinal, peripheral)
• Balance of acid–base status	• Acid–base imbalance	
• Effective chemical buffer regulation	• Ineffective buffer regulation for changing pH	

tion to nursing diagnosis labels approved by the North American Nursing Diagnosis Association (Rantz & LeMone, 1997).

In situations of fluid, electrolyte, and acid–base imbalance, it is tempting for the nurse to focus on the pathophysiology involved rather than the behaviors and stimuli that are related to what is happening physiologically in the person's body. Knowledge of pathophysiology is important to assist the nurse in the identification of behaviors and stimuli related to fluid, electrolyte, and acid–base balance but, with the framework that the Roy Adaptation Model provides, behaviors and stimuli pertain to the person's behavioral manifestation of the problem and the factors that appear to be causing it. In turn, the nursing diagnosis also focuses on behaviors and stimuli rather than on the pathophysiologic condition(s). Once the nursing diagnosis is formulated, the nurse proceeds to the fourth step of the nursing process, goal setting.

Goal Setting

Based on thorough assessment and understanding of adaptation problems related to fluid, electrolyte, and acid–base balance, the nurse sets goals in terms of outcomes for the person. A complete goal statement includes the behavior of focus, the change expected, and the time frame in which the goal is to be achieved. Relative to the situation involved, goals may be long-term or short-term.

In the example provided, a patient was observed to have only 5 mL of urinary output in an 8-hour period. This is considered to be ineffective behavior when compared to the normal and expected urinary output of a healthy person. A goal for this person could be, "The patient's urinary output will increase within the next hour." This would constitute a short-term goal, the behavior of which is "urinary output," the change expected is "increase," and the time frame is "the next hour."

Consider a situation where a person has been diagnosed with "diarrhea due to excessive use of laxatives." A long-term goal in this situation may be, "The person will have regular bowel functioning without the use of laxatives within a 2-week period." Here the behavior is "bowel functioning," the expected change is designated by "regular" and "without the use of laxatives," and the time frame is "within a 2-week period."

Generally, the goal of the nurse relative to fluid, electrolyte, and acid–base balance is to reestablish an adaptive state of balance. This goal is operationalized by the identification of the specific goals that address each of the ineffective and potentially ineffective behaviors identified.

Another goal during the acute phase of fluid, electrolyte, and acid–base imbalance is to protect the individual from any potential injury or untoward occurrence. In this respect, the importance of anticipating potential problems associated with the person's condition is evident.

The necessity of involving the person, where possible, in the establishment of the goals is a principle that must be remembered if the goals are to be realistic and the person is to be committed to their attainment. The nurse then proceeds to identify and implement nursing interventions to assist the person in achieving the behavioral goals.

Intervention

The intervention step of the nursing process according to the Roy Adaptation Model depends on the identified stimuli as the nurse either promotes or reinforces the stimuli, or takes action to change or delete them. Just as the focus of goal setting is the person's behavior, the focus of intervention is the stimulus influencing the behavior. Thus, according to the Roy Adaptation Model, intervention is the management of stimuli and involves either altering, increasing, decreasing, removing, or maintaining them.

In the previous situation involving the patient with limited urinary output in 8 hours, interventions could focus on the oral fluid intake, the injury to the leg, and the lack of fluid replacement. All of these are stimuli identified in the nursing diagnosis. By identifying and analyzing possible approaches, the nurse selects the approach with the highest probability of achieving the goal. Administering oral fluids may resolve the problem but if surgery is imminent, oral intake may jeopardize the scheduling of the procedure.

It so happens that the injury to the leg is scheduled for surgical repair. To assist with the management of this stimulus, the nurse would be involved in preparing the person for the operating room. Intravenous replacement may be something that could be started immediately. The nurse may be involved in initiating the infusion and in monitoring its administration and subsequent effect on the patient.

In many situations of fluid, electrolyte, and acid–base imbalance, the nurse will be involved in the administration of intravenous fluids. The type of fluid, its rate of administration, and the additives will depend on the patient's situation, condition, size, and cause of the problem. For example, Ringer's lactate is frequently administered in situations of hypovolemic shock. Types of fluid include electrolyte and glucose solutions, blood and blood products, and plasma substitutes. The intravenous site must be carefully prepared and then monitored to ensure that the apparatus is intact and that direct access to the circulatory system is maintained. In addition, the site of access must be given meticulous care since it is a direct point of entry for bacteria into the blood stream.

In compromised fluid, electrolyte, and acid–base balance, ongoing monitoring of the individual in all aspects of the physiologic mode is of utmost importance. As medications are administered, alertness for reactions and drug interactions must be maintained. These actions point to the importance of initial assessment for allergies or chronic conditions for which medications are taken. Intake and output of fluids must be carefully monitored and recorded and symptoms associated with the underlying physiologic disorder must be assessed. This situation illustrates once again that the nursing process is ongoing and simultaneous, with interventions being carried out as first and second levels of assessment are in progress.

Throughout the care process, emotional support must be provided for the individual and family. Because of the urgency of situations of fluid, electrolyte, and acid–base imbalance, and the involvement of other health team members in the assessment and treatment of the physiologic disruption causing the problem, it is important for the nurse to keep in mind and respond to the individual's needs and to function as an coordinator and integrator of the activities taking place.

In an artificially linear nursing process, following the implementation of the nursing interventions, their effects on the individual's behavior are evaluated. This is accomplished in the sixth and last step of the nursing process, evaluation.

Evaluation

Evaluation involves judging the effectiveness of the nursing interventions in relation to the person's adaptive behavior, that is, whether the person has attained the behavior stated in the goals. The nursing interventions would be identified as effective if the person's behavior is in accordance with the stated goal. If the goal has not been achieved, the nurse identifies alternative interventions or approaches by reassessing the behavior and stimuli and continuing with the other steps of the nursing process.

In considering the previously identified goal, "The patient's urinary output will increase within the next hour," the nurse, in evaluating the effectiveness of the intervention, would measure the urinary output within the hour. Had there been no urinary output, the absence of urine would be an indication that the patient was not progressing toward the goal and that the behavior continued to be ineffective. This would necessitate immediate action on the part of the nurse with prompt and continued reassessment and further intervention.

In this situation, the patient was scheduled for surgical intervention. It would be important that the concern about urinary output be communicated to the care team in the operating room, so that the observation initiated on the unit would continue during the surgical procedure. This points to the importance of effective communication, verbal and written, so that continuity of care is maintained even though the involved health care team members change.

► SUMMARY

This chapter has focused on the application of the Roy Adaptation Model to the complex physiologic processes associated with fluid, electrolyte, and acid–base balance. An overview of these basic life processes was provided along with the identification of parameters for assessment of behaviors and stimuli. Illustrations of innate and learned adaptive compensatory responses related to fluid, electrolyte, and acid–base balance were described and examples of compromised processes were provided. Finally, guidelines for planning nursing care through the formulation of nursing diagnoses, goals, and interventions were explored, and evaluation of nursing care was described.

► EXERCISES FOR APPLICATION

1. Develop a tool to assist you with the assessment of fluid, electrolyte, and acid–base balance. In the tool, address important behavioral indicators and stimuli that commonly affect fluid, electrolyte, and acid–base balance.

2. Using the tool developed in exercise 1, assess your own status relative to fluid, electrolyte, and acid–base balance. Reread the relevant sections of this chapter to identify the adequacy of your tool.

► ASSESSMENT OF UNDERSTANDING

Questions

1. The kidneys play a major role in the maintenance of fluid, electrolyte, and acid–base balance within the body. Which of the following constitute functions of the kidney?
   (a) the excretion of nitrogen-containing wastes
   (b) maintaining water balance
   (c) maintaining electrolyte balance
   (d) maintaining acid–base balance

2. In assessment of behavior related to the complex physiologic processes of fluid, electrolyte, and acid–base balance, which mode(s) is/are of particular concern?

3. List five common stimuli that lead to fluid, electrolyte, or acid–base imbalance.
   (a) _____
   (b) _____
   (c) _____
   (d) _____
   (e) _____

4. Label the following compensatory processes as indicative of regulator (R) or cognator (C) activity.
   (a) _____ the commitment to drink 8 glasses of water each day
   (b) _____ adherence to a sodium-restricted diet
   (c) _____ decrease in filtrate formation in kidney

(d) _____continuous ambulatory peritoneal dialysis (CAPD)

(e) _____thirst

5. In list A are compromised processes of fluid, electrolyte, acid–base balance. Match them to the descriptors in list B.

List A	**List B**
(a) _____ acidosis	1. excess level of potassium in the blood
(b) _____ hypocalcemia	2. sodium values of blood above normal
(c) _____ dehydration	3. calcium level in blood is below normal range
(d) _____ alkalosis	4. accumulation of fluid in interstitial compartments
(e) _____ hypernatremia	5. excessive water loss
(f) _____ edema	6. a decrease in arterial blood pH
(g) _____ hyperkalemia	7. accumulation of base in arterial blood

Situation:

Joe is a 20-year-old diabetic patient admitted to the hospital after having a "24-hour flu" with nausea, vomiting, and headache. On assessment, the nurse identifies that he has not eaten or had anything to drink in 2 days. He reports scant urinary output twice in the last 24 hours.

6. Construct a nursing diagnosis consisting of a statement of behavior within one mode with its most relevant influencing stimulus.

7. Derive a goal related to the nursing diagnosis you developed in item 6.

8. Management of which stimulus(i) might assist in achievement of the goal set in the previous item?
   (a) The management of the nausea and vomiting by securing an order for antiemetic medication.
   (b) The management of the diabetic condition by investigating blood sugar level.
   (c) The management of intake with intravenous infusion.

9. If the goal developed in item 7 was "The patient will have a urinary output of 50 mL within 4 hours," what would be the key to evaluating the effectiveness of the intervention?

Feedback

1. a, b, c, and d

2. the physiologic mode

3. (a) integrity of the physiologic mode
    (b) medical interventions
    (c) cognator effectiveness
    (d) developmental stage
    (e) environmental factors

4. (a) C, (b) C, (c) R, (d) C, (e) R

5. (a) 6, (b) 3, (c) 5, (d) 7, (e) 2, (f) 4, (g) 1

6. Example of nursing diagnosis: "Decreased urinary output due to inadequate intake of fluids," or "Inadequate intake due to nausea and vomiting."
7. Example of goal: "The patient will have increased urinary output within 8 hours."
8. Any or all responses may apply.
9. The measurement of urinary output in 4 hours.

▶ REFERENCES

Burrell, L. O. (1992). *Adult nursing in hospital and community settings.* Norwalk, CT: Appleton & Lange.

Marieb, E. N. (1994). *Essentials of human anatomy and physiology* (4th ed.). Redwood City, CA: Benjamin/Cummings.

Rantz, M. J., & LeMone, P. (Eds.). (1997). *Classification of nursing diagnoses. Proceedings of the 12th conference NANDA.* Glendale, CA: CINAHL Information Systems.

▶ ADDITIONAL REFERENCES

Gordon, M. (1995). *Manual of nursing diagnosis 1995–1996.* St. Louis: Mosby.

Servonsky, J., & Opas, S. (Eds.). (1987). *Nursing management of children.* Boston: Jones and Bartlett.

Sims, L., D'Amico, D., Stiesmeyer, J., & Webster, J. (1995). *Health assessment in nursing.* Redwood City, CA: Addison-Wesley.

12

NEUROLOGIC FUNCTION

Neurologic function plays a key role in a person's adaptation. Both the regulator and the cognator subsystems are based on the processes of neurologic function. Intact neural channels affect regulator processing. Similarly, perceptual and information processing, learning, judgment, and emotion are cognator processes with a neurologic basis. Understanding of the complexities of neurologic processes is rapidly growing in the multidisciplinary neurosciences. This chapter focuses specifically on how this knowledge can help the nurse understand the thinking, feeling, moving, and interacting person who is adapting within the changing world. This physiologic mode component contributes to the holistic functioning of the person. Two basic life processes that are key to neurologic function are cognition and consciousness. Assessment of behaviors and stimuli related to cognition and consciousness are outlined in this chapter. Compensatory strategies that act to maintain neurologic function are identified. Examples of compromised processes are discussed with a focus on memory deficits and decreased level of consciousness. Planning nursing care with nursing diagnoses, goals, interventions, and evaluation is described for this physiologic mode component. Emphasis is placed on promoting integrated thinking and feeling processes to promote health.

▶ OBJECTIVES

After studying this chapter, the reader will be able to do the following:

1. Describe the basic life processes associated with the neurologic function as presented in this chapter.

2. Identify important first-level assessment parameters (behaviors) of the basic life processes associated with neurologic function.

3. List second-level assessment parameters (common stimuli) that affect neurologic function.

4. Describe one compensatory process associated with neurologic function.

5. Name and describe two situations of compromised processes of neurologic function.

6. Develop a nursing diagnosis, given a situation related to neurologic function.

7. Derive goals for an individual with ineffective neurologic function in a given situation.

8. Describe nursing interventions commonly implemented in situations of ineffective neurologic function.

9. Propose approaches to determine the effectiveness of nursing interventions.

▶ KEY CONCEPTS DEFINED

Action potential: Rapid changes in the cell membrane potential of the neurons associated with potassium within the cell and sodium outside the cell.

Cognition: A broad term encompassing the human abilities to think, feel, and act.

Coma: The state of unconsciousness from which a person cannot be aroused to make purposeful responses.

Consciousness: Level of arousal and awareness, including orientation to the environment and self-awareness.

Integrated neural functioning: Integrated brain activity that is a result of the fact that centers for many functions are widely distributed and interconnected throughout the brain.

Memory deficit: Decrease in ability to process one's experience by storing and retrieving information.

Neural plasticity: The adaptive capacities of the central nervous system; the ability to modify its own structural organization and functioning.

Neuron: Structural and functional unit of the nervous system that carries information in the form of impulses.

Synapse: The junction point of one neuron to the next; site of neurotransmitter activity.

► COMPLEX PROCESSES OF NEUROLOGIC FUNCTION

All neurologic functioning, and the basic life processes of cognition and consciousness in particular, depend on the *neuron* as the structural and functional unit of the nervous system. Messages are carried throughout the body in the form of impulses through a succession of neurons. Anatomically, the links between neurons are highly organized in the complex structures of the nervous system. Figure 12–1 illustrates the major components and Table 12–1 lists the structures of the nervous system. They are the central nervous system with the major divisions of the brain and the spinal cord, and the peripheral nervous system that is made up of 12 pairs of cranial nerves and 31 pairs of spinal nerves (see Table 12–2).

The functioning of the peripheral nervous system has afferent and efferent components. The efferent component includes what is called the autonomic nervous system. Activation of the autonomic nervous system (ANS) occurs mainly by centers located in the spinal cord, brainstem, and hypothalamus. The relationship of two divisions of the autonomic nervous system to the cranial and spinal nerve structures is seen in Figure 12–2. The ANS is commonly considered the essential neurogenic regulatory system for maintaining the internal environment of the body at an optimal level, called homeostasis (Selkurt, 1982). The significance of the autonomic activity can be seen in Table 12–3, which describes the effects of sympathetic and parasympathetic action on the body organs. Nerve signals are transmitted throughout these structures by *action potentials,* that is, rapid changes in the cell membrane potential of the neurons. These events, action potentials, can be understood by the physics related to potassium within the cell and sodium outside the cell (explained further in basic physiology texts).

The nerve signals spread in the nervous system by way of the synapses. The *synapse* is the junction point from one neuron to the next. Some of the most recent and significant discoveries in the neurosciences relate to studies of the chemical synapses of the central nervous system. This work involves the identification of neurotransmitters that are secreted by the first neuron at a synapse. In turn, this chemical acts on receptor proteins in the membrane of the next neuron to excite it, inhibit it, or modify its sensitivity in some other way. The synapses, then, can perform selective functions (Guyton, 1992) in carrying the nerve signals through the system. Significant research on identifying neurotransmitters and their selective activity is contributing greatly to understanding neural activity. Neurologic function is carried out by way of a complex network of neuronal circuits for the transmitting of the nerve sig-

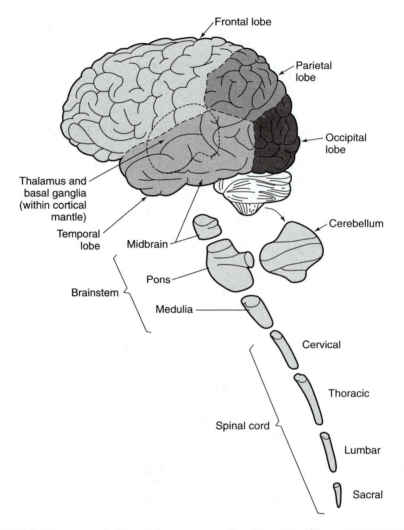

FIGURE 12–1. Major components of the central nervous system. *(From Cohen, D. H., & Sherman, S. M. (1988). The nervous system. In Berne, R. M., & Levy, M. N. (Eds.),* Physiology *(p. 74). St. Louis: Mosby. Redrawn from Kandel, E. R., & Schwartz, J. H. (1981).* Principles of neuroscience. *New York: Elsevier Science Publishing Co. Used with permission.)*

nals. One way to examine the general design of this complex network is to look at the major functions it fulfills. These include the sensory division (see Chap. 10), the motor division (see Chap. 8), the division for processing of information, and the division for storage of information (Guyton, 1992). The latter two divisions are discussed in this chapter as the process of cognition. Further, the particular process of human consciousness is described as a related life process.

TABLE 12–1   STRUCTURES OF THE NERVOUS SYSTEM

Central Nervous System	Peripheral Nervous System
Brain	**Basic structures**
Cerebrum	Cranial nerves
Cerebellum	Spinal nerves
Medulla	
Spinal cord	**Functional networks**
Cervical	Afferent
Thoracic	Receptor neurons[a]
Lumbar	Pathways of flexion[a]
Sacral	Swallowing reflexes[a]
	Efferent
	Somatic
	Autonomic

[a] Examples of afferent functioning.

TABLE 12–2   SUMMARY OF CRANIAL AND SPINAL NERVES AND THEIR FUNCTIONS

Cranial Nerves	Function	Spinal Nerves	Function
I. Olfactory	Sense of smell		Sensation, movements and sweat secretions by muscles in regions:
II. Optic	Visual acuity		
III. Oculomotor	Pupils and extraocular eye movement (EOM)	C1-5	Neck
		Phrenic Plexis	Diaphragm
IV. Trochlear	Eye movements	C5-7	Shoulder, arm
V. Trigeminal	Facial sensation and jaw movement	C5-8	Forearm
		C7–8	Hand
	Corneal reflex (used more frequently in assessing the comatose patient)	L1–5 and S1	Pelvis
		L2–5 and S1, 2	Thigh
		L4–5 and S1, 2	Leg
VI. Abducens	Eye movements	S1, 2	Foot
VII. Facial	Facial movement and taste sensation (anterior two thirds of tongue)	S3, 4, 5	Perineum
		S2, 3	Bladder
VIII. Acoustic	Gross hearing		
IX. Glossopharyngeal	Gag reflex and ability to swallow		
X. Vagus	Cardiac regulation Gastric secretion		
XI. Spinal accessory	Head movements		
XII. Hypoglossal	Tongue movements		

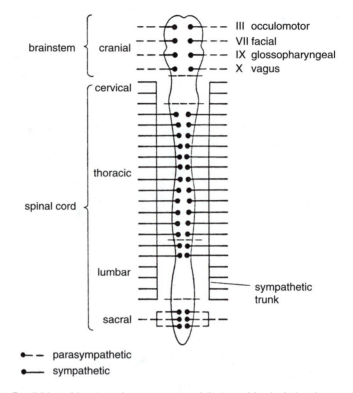

FIGURE 12–2. Two divisions of the autonomic nervous system relative to cranial and spinal cord nerves. *(From Vander, A. J., Sherman, J. H., & Luciano, D. S. (1980).* Human physiology. *New York: McGraw-Hill. Used with permission.)*

► COGNITION: PROCESS AND ASSESSMENT

In today's society, the processing of information is a major resource both for the individual and for any group. The world is rapidly changing and requires purposeful and changing interactions and responses. The human nervous system acts as a control mechanism for such interactions and responses. It literally receives millions of bits of information from different senses, integrates and interprets these, and initiates a response. The incredible speed of the processing is seen at every level of function, from the pupillary reflex of the eye, to the quick evasive action when spotting a hazard on the road, to the sensing of the tone of a group on entering a room. The complexity of processing is seen, for example, when a nurse cares for a dying patient. The nurse is able to take in more than bits of information; rather the nurse experiences with the person the gamut of emotions that lie in the meaning of life and its ultimate purpose for both of them.

The complex transmitting of signals as described earlier is just the beginning of human activities that provide meaning to life experiences. The in-

TABLE 12-3 FUNCTIONS OF THE AUTONOMIC NERVOUS SYSTEM DESCRIBED BY EFFECTS ON BODY ORGANS

Organ	Effect of Sympathetic Stimulation	Effect of Parasympathetic Stimulation
Eye:		
Pupil	Dilated	Constricted
Ciliary muscle	Slight relaxation	Constricted
Glands:		
Nasal	Vasoconstriction and slight secretion	Stimulation of copious (except pancreas)
Lacrimal		secretion (containing many enzymes for
Parotid		enzyme-secreting glands)
Submandibular		
Gastric		
Pancreatic		
Sweat glands	Copious sweating (cholinergic)	None
Aprocrine glands	Thick, odoriferous secretion	None
Heart:		
Muscle	Increased rate	Slowed rate
	Increased force of contraction	Decreased force of contraction (especially of atrium)
Coronary arteries	Dilated (β_2); constricted (α)	Dilated
Lungs:		
Bronchi	Dilated	Constricted
Blood vessels	Mildly constricted	Dilated
Gut:		
Lumen	Decreased peristalsis and tone	Increased peristalsis and tone
Sphincter	Increased tone (most times)	Relaxed (most times)
Liver	Glucose released	Slight glycogen synthesis
Gallbladder and bile ducts	Relaxed	Contracted
Kidney	Decreased output and renin secretion	None
Bladder:		
Detrusor	Relaxed (slight)	Excited
Trigone	Excited	Relaxed
Penis	Ejaculation	Erection
Systemic arterioles:		
Abdominal muscle	Constricted	None
	Constricted (adrenergic α)	None
	Dilated (adrenergic β_2)	
	Dilated (cholinergic)	
Skin	Constricted	None
Blood:		
Coagulation	Increased	None
Glucose	Increased	None
Basal metabolism	Increased up to 100%	None
Adrenal medullary	Increased secretion	None
Mental activity	Increased	None
Piloerector muscles	Excited	None
Skeletal muscle	Increased glycogenolysis	None
	Increased strength	

From Guyton, A. (1987). Human physiology and mechanisms of disease (p. 443). Philadephia: Saunders. Used with permission.

tegrated higher process of cognition that emerges makes it possible for one to connect past experiences with the present and relate both past and present to the future. This process is particularly important since it acts as a regulator of life events. Furthermore, in the Roy Adaptation Model, understanding cognitive and emotional processing by the cognator subsystem is essential to understanding and relating to the adapting person.

Cognition is a broad term encompassing the human abilities to think, feel, and act. It is most frequently described as information processing. Models of information processing have developed from early applications such as telephone switchboards in the 1940s to recent computerized cellular data exchange without wires. Basically, these models describe input, central processing, and output stages. A given model may emphasize one stage more than another depending on the purpose of the model. Das and colleagues (Das, 1984; Das, Kirby, & Jarman, 1975, 1979; Molloy, Das, & Pierce, 1990) developed an information integration model based on studies by Luria (1973, 1980) of head injury patients. In this model, the structure is the brain, the processes are neuropsychological, and the knowledge base is provided by the experience and education of the person.

Roy (1988) proposed a related nursing model for cognition (see Fig. 12–3). This model draws from knowledge in the neurosciences and from observations in neuroscience nursing practice. The inner circle lists basic internal processes of arousal and attention, sensation and perception; coding and concept formation, memory and language; and planning and motor response. These functions are dependent on the brain structure neurologically and neurochemically. The model shows that the basic cognitive processes occur within a field of consciousness. *Consciousness* (discussed in further detail later in the chapter) is characterized by both arousal and awareness, particularly awareness of self. The environment for cognitive processing is based on an understanding of environment as defined in the Roy Adaptation Model. More specifically, the environment for cognitive processing includes focal stimuli as immediate sensory experience, and contextual and residual stimuli, considered primarily in terms of education and experience. The broken lines in the figure indicate the permeability between the stimuli fields.

The circles of the model highlight contemporary views in both nursing and cognitive science that the individual is a participant and partner in the developmental process. Cognitive processing abilities throughout the life span are subject to interactional factors and multiple and mutual influences. Development involves biologic aspects, or maturation, and environmental factors, such as learning opportunities. Rather than age affecting development at a steady pace, this interactive model also implies individual participation, historical, social, biologic, and environmental influences. Children and the elderly have a much greater degree of variability in expression of cognitive abilities, and have less well studied and inherently more difficult to understand cerebral organization for cognitive processes. Children are subject to growth spurts and developmental stages and lags. Changes associated with aging can be either primary and nonpathologic such as alterations in sensory

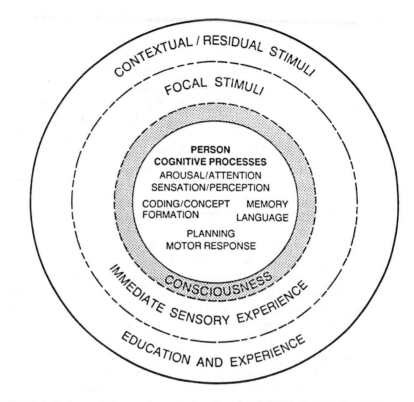

FIGURE 12–3. Nursing model for cognitive processing. *(From Roy, C. (1988). Alterations in cognitive processing. In Mitchell, P. H., Hodges, L. C., Muwaswes, M., & Walleck, C. A. (Eds.), American Association of Neuroscience Nurses' Neuroscience nursing: Phenomena and practice (p. 188). Norwalk: Appleton & Lange. Used with permission.)*

functioning, or secondary and pathologic, such as changes associated with Alzheimer's disease.

A principle basic to Roy's cognitive processing model is *integrated neural functioning*. This principle notes that brain activity is integrated due to centers for many functions being widely distributed and interconnected throughout the brain. Integrated neural functioning is manifested in several ways. Knowledge of exactly how thinking and feeling processes occur at the neurologic level is limited, but increasing. Scientists continue to pursue the question and one major conclusion is that it appears that many brain areas participate and interact in these processes. Cortical and subcortical areas are involved and processes of consciousness, attention, and perception are intimately interrelated.

The principle of integrated neural functioning is operating when the person selects important stimuli from among all possible stimuli present and then channels these stimuli to the relevant brain centers for an appropriate response. Increasingly, data are being presented to show that relevant brain centers for many functions are distributed throughout the brain. Mountcastle (1979, 1997) reviewed a century of work that used various approaches to obtain functional maps of the brain, and then made conclusions based on recent data from newer methods of brain mapping. Mountcastle recognized that each area of the cortex has distinctive layers and columns of cells; however, each also has its own unique set of extrinsic connections. Columns in areas located at some distance from one another, but with some common properties, may be linked by long-range connections within the cortex. Through these widely and reciprocally interconnected systems, integrated activity is the very essence of brain function. Mountcastle's conclusion supports Luria's (1980) insights gained from 40 years of working with head injured patients from World War II. The principle of integrated neural functioning calls into question the notion of localization (functions located in specific structures), lateralization (separate functions for each cerebral hemisphere), and stimulus–response learning (responses from reflexes chained together).

The brain's unique power is due mainly to its ability to store information, that is, to code a representation of experience for future use. An early scientist in the field, Lashley (quoted in Pribram, 1969), reviewed the experimental evidence related to how the brain goes about storage and retrieval. Lashley concluded, somewhat wryly, that on the basis of available evidence, learning and remembering were obviously impossible. Later Willis and Grossman (1981) identified that from what is known about higher processing functions, the storage of information is a function of the brain as a whole. Central higher functions are thought of as producing a structural or electrophysiologic change in the brain. This change is called the memory trace. Various models are used to study the processes that produce the memory trace, the processes for gaining access to the trace, for recalling it to consciousness, and for producing motor activity. The hippocampus may be involved in processes of sorting, assembling, and supplying information, for example, with sensory information that is emotionally significant. Further, metabolic activity, or protein synthesis, may be important in these central processes. The holistic formulation of cerebral function is useful in nursing assessments and interventions related to cognition.

Assessment of Behavior

Assessments of neurologic function, and cognition in particular, are at times subtle and often critical for all the goals of adaptation from survival through mastery and the person and environment transformations of increasing adaptation. The detail and outcome of an initial cognitive assessment varies according to the person's condition. For example, a nurse in the emergency room may assess confusion and unclear speech in an elderly person with other significant neurologic signs and summon a neurologist for diagnosis of a stroke. The nurse in a well-baby clinic may be observing the developing integrated neural activity of a child over time, making detailed assessments of sensory, motor, and cognitive functioning, and using these data in planning care with the family.

In assessing the basic life process of cognition, the major concepts in Roy's nursing model of cognition in Figure 12–3 can be helpful. The previously described model of cognition with input, central processing, and output processes forms the structure for the assessment. Consciousness and sensory and motor evaluation are also important components in the assessment of neurologic function and these are described elsewhere: consciousness in the next section of this chapter, and sensory and motor evaluation in Chapters 8 and 10.

Ways to assess information processing and storing of memories are diverse. Each approach is based on understanding the organization of cognitive functions and of how these processes take place. Major functions of cognition are outlined in Table 12–4, based on the nursing model for cognitive processing. The nurse collects meaningful data during interview and observation, particularly including a careful history of change in cognition over time. Behaviors for each processing function are noted in a global way. Family members' reports and patient observations of functioning provide important clinical data needed for nursing care planning as well as for medical diagnosis.

TABLE 12–4 MAJOR FUNCTIONS OF COGNITIVE PROCESSING WITHIN A NURSING MODEL

Input Processes
Arousal and attention
  Selective attention
  Speed of processing
  Alertness
Sensation and perception
  Primary sense processing
  Pattern recognition
  Naming and associating

Central Processes
Coding
  Registration
  Consolidation
  Synthesis
Concept formation
  Integrated recognition
  Abstraction and flexibility
  Calculation
Memory
  Simultaneous
  Successive
Language

Output Processes
Planning
Motor response
  Motor planning
  Initiating action
  Regulating action

Nursing assessments related to integrated neurologic functioning lead to identifying dysfunctions that have an impact on daily living (Cammermeyer, 1988). Specific deficits and behavioral manifestations of each of the functions listed in Table 12–4 are described in detail by Roy (in press).

Behavioral assessment of input processes focuses on two major areas: arousal and attention, and sensation and perception.

Input Processes

Arousal and Attention. Behaviors associated with arousal and attention tend to be apparent during the history-taking process. The person's orientation is evident in responses to such questions as "What is your name?" and, "Where do you live?" Other behavioral aspects include selective attention, the speed with which the person processes information, and the alertness demonstrated with such behaviors as response to direct commands.

Sensation and Perception. Sensation and perception include behaviors related to primary sense processing, pattern recognition, and naming and association. The assessment of primary senses has been addressed in other chapters, particularly Chapter 10. Pattern recognition can be assessed by asking the person to select specific shapes to fit into receptacles of the same shape, for example. Naming and association can be assessed by asking simple questions to test for recognition of objects or pictures.

Central Processes

The second assessment area associated with the cognition model is that of central processing. The four aspects included in this area are coding, concept formation, memory, and language.

Coding. Coding includes the registration, consolidation, and synthesis of information. Are the events underway being noticed by the person and is the response within the realm of expectations under the circumstances? Is the person able to perform direct commands and is there evidence of spatial orientation?

Concept Formation. Evidence of concept formation is associated with integrated recognition, abstraction and flexibility, and calculation abilities. To what extent can the person comprehend the complexities of that which is occurring in the environment? Abstraction and flexibility can be assessed by asking the person to explain a proverb or to identify similarities or differences between two objects. The ability to perform mathematical calculations is a further indication of the person's cognitive processing of concepts.

Memory. Memory can be viewed in terms of simultaneous and successive memory. Evidence of the person's memory processing will be evident during the history-taking process and the ability to relate past medical problems. A test of memory is the person's ability to repeat four numbers in reverse order. Remembrance of significant dates can also be an indicator of integrity of the person's memory.

Language. The person's language capabilities are an important indicator of cognition. What are the characteristics of speech—flowing, spontaneous, rhythmic, clear enunciation, normal tone? Is the use and understanding of vocabulary at an expected level?

Output Processes

The third assessment area of cognition is output processes. Included in this is the assessment of the person's capabilities associated with planning and with motor responses.

Planning. Planning involves the ability of the person to anticipate future possibilities and to appropriately determine actions required to effectively adapt. Evidence of judgment and insight would be indications of intact planning processes leading to realistic and achievable actions. The person's inability to act in terms of the future would indicate ineffective cognition as it pertains to the ability to plan.

Motor Response. Motor response includes the aspects of motor planning, initiating action, and regulating action. Is the person able to appropriately sequence motor activities to accomplish a task? Do his or her extremities respond to intentions formulated in the mind? For example, a person might will to move the right arm, but does that action happen physically as intended? At times, the debilitated elderly require prompting to help with initiating action. They may appear unable to feed themselves, but when helped to initiate the activity, are able to carry on independently. Regulation of action deals with the ability to appropriately sequence motor activity and to perform the action in consecutive and consistent steps. Many people with degenerative disease of the nervous system, such as Huntington's chorea, are unable to regulate their physical movements, with resulting jerky and random physical actions.

An assessment can be made of each one of these functions by observing the person involved in one ordinary task. For example, the nurse assesses the normal cognitive processing of a toddler when the child reaches out and calls for mother. The mother has been selected out from other stimuli in the room; the child perceives that she is there, recognizes a pattern, and makes an association. Coding, early concept formation, memory, and language have all been involved and the motor response follows.

For more specific screening of level of functioning, a number of tests exist that are appropriate for clinical use. For example, the Mini-Mental State (MMS) (Anthony, LeResche, Niaz, Von Korff, & Folstein, 1982; Folstein, Folstein, & McHugh, 1975) tests orientation, registration, attention, calculations, recall, and language. It takes 5 minutes to administer and has proven reliable in identifying dementia and psychiatric disorders. By noting subtle difficulties that a person is having in information processing, the nurse can identify needs for formal neuropsychologic evaluation. The person's frustration in ordinary situations or making excuses for simple mistakes can be initial cues of difficulties with cognition.

Assessment of Stimuli

The identification of factors that contribute to changes in neurologic status, and cognition in particular, is part of the nursing assessment of this physiologic mode component. As with behavioral assessment, the nurse can contribute significant information about the circumstances surrounding changes in cognitive functioning. On initial presentation, the nurse talks with the patient, family, or witnesses to the onset of ineffective behaviors. In the case of an automobile accident, did the person lose consciousness first and then collide with another car? Was the homeless person found hallucinating on the street complaining of dizziness or deprived of meals with adequate protein? Did a painter simply fall from the ladder or did he clutch at his chest first? The focal and contextual stimuli can be related to the person's medical condition or, in fact, stem from the person in any of the four modes of adaptation. In the examples discussed, we see the kaleidoscopic characteristic of the model, with behaviors becoming stimuli and one stimulus affecting another.

Pathophysiology

Often a given neurologic medical diagnosis is the focal stimulus for the changes in cognitive behavior observed by the nurse. For example, blood collecting in the subdural space from head trauma will affect the person's ability to identify what day it is and where the person is. Trauma, infection, neuromuscular disease, vascular disturbances, and developmental disorders result in varying degrees of cognitive deficits, as well as other neurologic deficits.

A vascular spasm may cause a brief and temporary headache that has little effect on the person's cognition and adaptive potential. On the other hand, conditions such as cerebrovascular accidents (strokes) and multiple sclerosis can result in extensive changes that require great and prolonged efforts to maximize adaptive potential through the use of cognition. Similarly, the nurse recognizes that various treatment modalities, including medication and surgery, affect the cognitive processes. For example, drugs categorized as anticonvulsants, cerebral vasodilators, and narcotic analgesics all affect level of arousal. Dramatic changes related to cognition follow certain forms of treatment. For example, surgical intervention can result in the cessation of formerly intractable seizures, with periods of inability to process information.

Blood Gases and Hemoglobin Levels

Two of the laboratory indicators that have the greatest immediate effect on cognition are arterial blood gases and hemoglobin levels. The partial pressure of carbon dioxide ($Paco_2$) in the arterial blood and oxygen Pao_2 affect cerebral blood flow which, in turn, influences alertness and the ability to process information. Similarly, if hemoglobin is low, the oxygen-combining capacity of the blood is reduced and cerebral hypoxia is exacerbated, with possible confusion. If the hemoglobin is above normal, there is a greater tendency for clot formation, resulting in vascular obstruction and, therefore, ischemia and cognitive changes.

Nutritional Status

Nutritional status can affect cognition and neurologic functioning. For example, the nurse considers that obesity increases the risk of hypertension and having a cerebrovascular accident. Similarly, certain nutritional deficits affect neurologic status. For example, thiamine deficiency results in disturbances in the metabolism of nerve tissue. The tissue is then unable to appropriately utilize carbohydrates, resulting in the neurologic manifestations of weakness, muscle pain, and tenderness. The output part of cognitive processing is affected. Fluid intake can also affect neurologic status. For example, decreased fluid intake results in reduced intracranial pressure; increased intake hastens recovery in certain neurologic infections. These changes can affect cognitive deficits that have resulted from the pathology.

Activity and Rest

In neuromuscular disruptions, activity can either exacerbate or relieve particular behavioral manifestations of the condition. For example, tremors in Parkinson's disease decrease with activity and increase with rest. The distressing behavior of increased muscular fatigability in myasthenia gravis increases with activity and decreases with rest. Although coughing is an important activity after many surgeries, it is inadvisable in many cranial surgeries, because it increases intracranial pressure. Deep breathing and turning instead can promote adaptive ventilation.

The nurse can use knowledge about positioning to enhance cognitive, neurologic, and adaptive functioning. For example, after a thrombotic or embolic cerebrovascular accident, keeping the patient in a side-lying position decreases the risk of aspiration. Keeping the head of the bed low for the first few days may promote cerebral circulation. Keeping the head of the bed slightly elevated and the head in alignment with the body are important for the patient with increased intracranial pressure. If the head is out of alignment with the body (that is, the body is flat and the head turned to the side), venous return from the brain is impaired and intracranial pressure increases further.

Stress

The neuroendocrine and behavioral response to stress is discussed in Chapter 13. Some specific applications of this concept as it affects cognitive and neurologic adaptation are noted here. Stressors can take the form of painful procedures, emotional trauma, or a lowered body resistance from fatigue and malnutrition. Such stress factors serve as a stimulus for aggravating cognitive and neurologic changes. For example, the noxious stimulation such as suctioning or a venipuncture can cause intracranial pressure to increase. As this pressure increases, we see that cognitive behavioral manifestations may worsen, lethargy progressing to stupor, for example. In neuromuscular disruptions such as multiple sclerosis and myasthenia gravis, stress factors of fatigue, malnutrition; cold, damp weather; and even pregnancy can exacerbate the behavioral manifestations of those diseases and neuromuscular weakness.

Knowledge

Stress can result from inappropriately negative expectations of a neurologic medical diagnosis. If so, anxiety, fear, depression, and hopelessness may result. Expectancies are related to knowledge level. For example, a brain tumor erroneously signifies death to many. In fact, death occurs only in some cases. Paralysis may signify sterility, which is not usually the case in the female. It is therefore essential that the nurse have knowledge about the particular disruption being observed and understand the specifics of the individual case and medical prognosis. The effective exchange of information between doctor and nurse can be a key factor in the patient's developing realistic self-expectations.

For all neurologic conditions, the nurse must assess the patient's and family's understanding. Assessing this stimulus is important for the intervention phase of planning care. Information is given according to the level of comprehension. Teaching is initiated when the acute period has subsided and learning readiness is evident; for example, when there is lack of denial of medical facts, lack of excessive anxiety, and pain is under control. Teaching measures include an exploration of what one should expect in terms of physiologic changes as well as modifications in self-concept, role function, and interdependence. To prevent complications or possible recurrence of the neurologic problem, the nurse informs the family and the individual of behaviors to report to the physician. Adjustments to changes in neurologic functioning can be made more successfully, and with less stress, when the person can distinguish between expected bodily changes and indications of complications. The nurse helps clarify these expectations.

Physical Environment

Altered cognition often results from changes in the physical environment. The environment can positively or negatively affect cognition. In the case of a disoriented person, the hospital environment itself can greatly accentuate ineffective behavior. Artificial lighting, the noise of foreign machinery, and altered time schedules all contribute to a person's confusion. Once such persons are medically stable, returning them to the familiar surroundings of their homes can promote cognitive adaptation. Noise is an important stimulus, as it can further increase intracranial pressure. Even the lack of clutter in the environment serves as a stimulus. In the case of a person who has had a cardiovascular accident, uncluttered surroundings in the home or hospital promote the behavior of orientation.

Self-concept Mode

An adaptive self-concept is of utmost importance in dealing with chronic neurologic impairments, particularly those affecting cognition. Once the individual has been able to grieve the loss of function, integration of a new body image is essential. This reintegration is necessary to move forward with the tasks of rehabilitation. An adaptive body image can make the difference between one's relearning to walk, speak, and generally live up to one's potential, or being prone to progressive debilitation.

Role Function Mode

Within the role function mode, developmental level is considered a determinant of one's primary role. In the context of this chapter, specific neurologic conditions, and their effect on cognition, are more common at certain ages than others. For example, multiple sclerosis and head trauma occur most frequently in the young adult, whereas Parkinson's disease and cerebrovascular accident occur more frequently in the older adult. Disorientation is more prevalent in the elderly due, in part, to sensory impairments, vascular degeneration, and selective changes in neurotransmitters.

Interdependence Mode

The interdependence adaptive mode highlights the importance of significant others and support systems in the life of an individual. For the person with difficulties in cognitive functioning, family members hold unusual prominence in the person's ability to cope with these changes. Many of the behaviors associated with changes in cognition are chronic. Situations of altered communication ability, muscular weakness, and disorientation require a great deal of patience. If the family or significant others offer support and understanding, this can act as a stimulus to enhance the person's ability to cope. In some instances, the family may not be able to change a particular behavioral manifestation of neurologic dysfunction (such as progressive muscular weakness in Duchenne's muscular dystrophy), but their support can help prevent complications in all four adaptive modes. With the encouragement of the family, the person may be better motivated to strengthen new muscle groups as other muscles are affected. This action not only affects the physiologic mode in helping to prevent the complications of inactivity, but the person's self-concept is better maintained. Similarly, feelings of independence are encouraged as the person is better able to carry out some of the responsibilities of previous roles by the simple fact of being more physically mobile.

Whenever possible, the nurse assists the cognitive and neurologically impaired persons to maintain their role in the family. For the paralyzed individual, cognitive processes such as contributing to family decision making are promoted. The nurse assists the family in identifying the remaining adaptive behaviors and promoting these. If neurologic impairments are irreversible, the nurse assists the family in preventing complications and, if genetic influences are known, may discuss counseling with the family.

The nurse who is assessing stimuli affecting a person's cognitive and neurologic functioning then carefully considers the family and significant other relationships that are primary factors influencing how the person will be able to deal with changes in function.

► CONSCIOUSNESS: PROCESS AND ASSESSMENT

Consciousness has been defined as an awareness of the internal and external environment. Theoretically consciousness includes two components: arousal, the awakeness of the person; and content, the interpretation of internal and external environment (Crigger & Strickland, 1985). Consciousness also is a significant process associated with the person's ability to adapt or self-regulate. This significance is based on the role of consciousness in the perception of sensory input and the central process of registering information. Human activity is much more than output of a highly complex physical system. It cannot be understood solely in terms of musculature and neurocircuits. Activity stems from what is called intentionality. A person's intentions stem from such things as needs, motives, values, and beliefs that are built into human consciousness.

The neurologic basis for consciousness is a complex interaction involving the cerebral cortex, subcortical structures including the hypothalamus, and brainstem centers. If any of these structures is damaged or disconnected from the other two, an altered state of consciousness results. The alert state requires the neural activity of the ascending reticular activating system of the brainstem communicating with both cerebral hemispheres. Similarly, feedback from the cerebral cortex of both hemispheres into the reticular activating system of the brainstem is necessary for consciousness.

There is much about human consciousness that still is considered a mystery in terms of scientific explanation. Yet what began as a philosophic debate has been studied in many related sciences. The result is encouraging progress in understanding the importance of consciousness—of self, values, and action. Eccles (Eccles & Robinson, 1985) notes that there is strong support for the hypothesis that the supplementary motor area of the brain is the sole recipient area for mental intentions that lead to voluntary movements. Dennett (1991), however, insists that consciousness is a mode of action of the brain as a whole rather than a subsystem. The philosopher Kant (Kemp, 1979), describes a person as a subject who is responsible for one's actions. Self-consciousness is necessary to monitor and regulate behavior. To be self-conscious is to have knowledge of oneself. Self-consciousness involves knowledge, not just of one's physical state, but also of inner reality. Consciousness as an awareness of an inner reality includes the reality of mental states and activities. Persons can recognize that they are angry, happy, or believes or hopes in something. Churchland (1988) points out that this suggests different degrees of self-consciousness, since the ability to discriminate subtly different types of mental states presumably improves with practice and increasing experience. From the perspective of transpersonal psychology, Wilber (1997) presents a model of a spectrum of consciousness that moves from basic levels of matter to body, mind, soul, and then to spirit. As people move from one level to another, they are reborn into new, deeper, and wider spheres of consciousness at each stage.

The expansion of introspective consciousness is generally viewed as a good thing both for the individual and for the society. As noted earlier, nurse-authors such as Newman (1994) view health as expanding consciousness. Scientists such as Churchland and Wilbur suggest how one might improve or enhance introspective access. Eccles describes the two-way flow of consciousness in a discussion of voluntary movement, freedom of will, and moral responsibility. Eccles (Eccles & Robinson, 1985) cites a transcendent importance of recognizing that by using thought, the person can influence the operation of the neural mechanisms of the brain. In this way people can bring changes in the world for good or ill. Eccles uses the simple metaphor that the conscious self is in the driver's seat. Life can be regarded as successive patterns of choice that lead to the feeling of fulfillment, with resulting happiness that comes to a life centered on meaning and purpose. The Roy Adaptation Model's philosophic assumptions clearly recognize the ideal that each person is to have the maximum freedom to realize her or his potential. This ideal stems from the belief that human life has common meaning, purpose, and destiny.

Assessment of Behavior

Unequivocally, the major assessment factor to determine neurologic status is level of consciousness. It has been said, "The brain does not fail unannounced." Rather, a predictable set of behaviors occurs and can be identified. Slight changes in level of consciousness are significant. Increasing forgetfulness or slight lethargy may be the first behavioral indicators of increasing intracranial pressure.

Level of Consciousness

Level of consciousness can be classified in a number of ways. Mitchell (1988) notes that the amount and kind of stimulus required to arouse a person and the nature of the response are basic dimensions used in all classifications. Therefore these are the key factors to assess. One approach that quantifies arousal is the Glasgow Coma Scale, or GCS (Jennett & Teasdale, 1977), which has become the most frequently used approach in the acute care setting.

The behaviors noted at regular intervals are eye opening, verbal response, and motor response. The examiner's voice is the stimulus, but if there is no response, then pressure can be applied to the person's finger tip. The best response in a given time period determines the score because this has been found to be the most reliable score. The maximum cumulative score of 15 indicates a fully conscious, alert person, whereas the minimum score of 3 indicates coma. *Coma* is also described as the state of unconsciousness from which a person cannot be aroused to make purposeful responses.

Figure 12–4 shows how a person's GCS can be noted on a flow sheet and the level of progress determined and evaluated over time. At the same time, the nurse may note a decrease in score, which indicates worsening of neurologic status requiring rapid attention.

Motor Response

The quality of motor response is an important behavioral indicator of neurologic status. Neurologic control of basic motor functioning is tested first by asking the person to squeeze the examiner's two hands simultaneously. Then the person is asked to push both feet against the nurse's hands (if in bed)

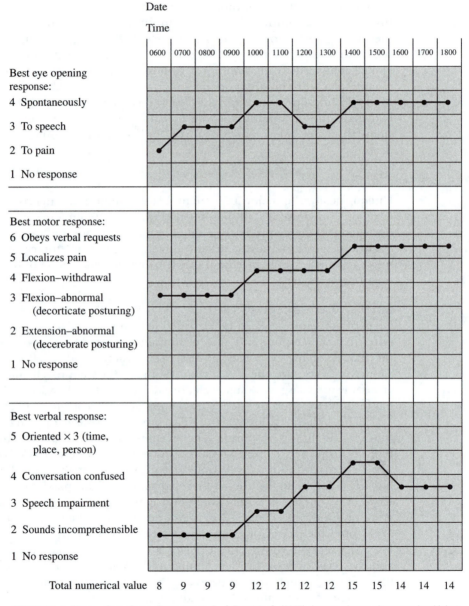

FIGURE 12–4. Glasgow Coma Scale. *(From Jennett, B., & Teasdale, G. (1977). Aspects of coma after severe head injury. Lancet, 1(8017), 878–881. Used with permission.)*

and equality of strength is noted. The general equality of all movements is also noted, as decreased muscle strength is a frequent behavioral indicator of neurologic disruptions.

Response to Pain

If consciousness is impaired, the quality of motor response to pain is particularly important. This can be evaluated during a routine procedure that includes the use of a noxious stimulus, such as endotracheal suctioning. The following possible responses to pain are listed in order of increasingly disrupted neurologic functioning.

1. Purposeful movement. Movement is made away from the pain stimulus.
2. Nonpurposeful movement. A random movement is made in response to pain.
3. Decorticate rigidity. The legs extend and rotate internally with the feet plantar flexed. The arms adduct and are pulled in to the chest with the wrists and fingers flexed. This indicates the interruption of cortical motor fibers but intact pathways through the brainstem.
4. Decerebrate rigidity. As in decorticate posturing, the legs extend, the arms extend, the wrists and fingers are flexed. This indicates the disruption of motor fibers in the midbrain and brainstem.

Decorticate and decerebrate posturing may at first be unilateral and then become bilateral, the former being less serious. At first, the posturing may occur only with noxious stimulation. As the dysfunction increases, the posturing is continual. With severe neurologic dysfunction, there is no response to pain. This is usually a grave sign.

Orientation and Level of Awareness

Consciousness has been referred to as involving both level of arousal and awareness. Awareness includes the level of orientation and level of self-awareness. Oriented persons know time, place, person, and purpose, that is, where they are, their name, and why they are there. The confused person appears dazed and in varying degrees, either continuously or intermittently, is not oriented to time, place, person, or purpose.

Consciousness as self-awareness is reflected in the person as an individual as well as in relationships with others. The nurse observes the person's mood, expressions, grooming, mannerisms, and speech. Behaviors of the self-concept, role function, and interdependence modes are relevant for this assessment.

Vital Signs

Changes in vital signs are manifestations of changes in levels of consciousness, particularly when the situation has become severe. Blood pressure initially demonstrates an increase in systolic pressure with widening of the pulse pressure. This is followed by a sudden decrease in systolic pressure. Pulse rate first slows but then becomes rapid and thready as increased intracranial pressure continues. Changes in respirations indicate deterioration in the patient's condition. Body temperature may vacillate between hyperthermia and hypothermia.

Assessment of Stimuli

The identification of factors that contribute to changes in neurologic status and level of consciousness, in particular, is part of the nursing assessment of this complex adaptive process. As with behavioral assessment, the nurse can contribute significant information about the circumstances surrounding changes in the level of consciousness.

Situational Circumstances

On initial presentation, the nurse talks with the patient, family, or witnesses to the circumstance that prompted the change in level of consciousness. Was there a traumatic event? Did the person express any perceptions, such as a severe headache, prior to the change in consciousness? Or has the change been insidious and gradual? Responses to these questions can lead to further ideas about contributing factors. For example, it may be reported that the person experienced a seizure just prior to the onset of the change in level of consciousness.

Physiologic Status

Disruptions in physiologic integrity can, at times, contribute to altered levels of consciousness. Lesion, trauma, tumor, electrolyte imbalance, or degeneration can cause decreased level of consciousness.

It is important that the patient be examined for signs of injury. Trauma to the brain can result from blunt force, penetrating wounds, contusion opposite a point of impact, or a fracture at the base of the skull. The resulting tissue damage can result in changes in level of consciousness.

Noxious Substances

In some situations, the ingestion of noxious substances can be the cause of altered levels of consciousness. The person's breath is smelled for the odor of alcohol, acetone, or other chemicals such as glue, kerosene, carbon tetrachloride, or gasoline. In some cases, drug use may be suspected. It is important to establish when the last dose was consumed.

Medical Interventions

There is some swelling of the brain after neurosurgery and this can affect levels of consciousness for a limited period of time. Monitoring for signs of decreasing levels of consciousness is important during this period to identify any complications such as intracranial bleeding or infection. The use of some sedatives such as tranquilizers and medications for sleep, particularly in the elderly, can inadvertently affect level of consciousness. Similarly, doses of steroids and anticonvulsants need to be monitored for the effect on the level of alertness and responsiveness. Sometimes coma is purposefully induced on a trial basis using barbiturates in a patient who has increased intracranial pressure that has not responded to conventional therapy. The therapeutic principle is that the immediate decrease in cerebral blood flow and brain metabolism will be beneficial. This treatment has been useful in reducing intracranial pressure for patients with head injury, Reye's syndrome, encephalitis, and cerebral hemorrhage (Hickey, 1992).

Pathophysiology

Conditions such a meningitis, hydrocephalus, and stroke can underlie changes in the level of consciousness. In addition, degenerative diseases including Parkinsonism, Huntington's chorea, and Alzheimer's disease can affect the person's level of consciousness.

▶ COMPENSATORY ADAPTIVE PROCESSES

A major compensatory adaptive process to preserve cognitive and neurologic functioning is *neural plasticity*. Plasticity refers to modification of structures with functional changes. Neural plasticity refers to the adaptive capacities of the central nervous system—its ability to modify its own structural organization and functioning. One can think of plasticity as a second fundamental property of the nervous system. According to the first property, a nerve excitation makes a rapid change that leaves no trace. Plasticity, on the other hand, permits enduring and functional changes to take place. The enduring changes of the developing nervous system have three specific characteristics. These plasticities occur at critical periods, can last over a lifetime, and seem to lack what is usually defined as motivation and reinforcement for their establishment. A well-studied example of molding the structure and function of the nervous system by environmental changes is the development of vision and hearing in animals. Limiting sensory input at a given time can result in lack of later ability to have full use of a given sense. Plasticity is greater in early years, with multiple new patterns of structure and function possible. The reservoir of plasticity decreases across the life span. Still, recent studies are focusing on plasticity of the adult brain, the aging brain, and particularly the person with brain injury.

There is evidence of greater potential for retaining and restoring nervous system functional effectiveness than was previously thought (Bignami, Bloom, Bolis, & Adeloye, 1985; Diamond, Johnson, & Ingham, 1975; and Finger & Stein, 1982). Many mechanisms of neural plasticity have been identified, including sprouting of remaining nerve fibers after injury. Following acute injury to the central nervous system, there are immediate decreases in the function of neurons in other areas of the brain or spinal cord caused by decreased input, shock, and other factors. Functional recovery from these remote effects is possible as a result of synaptic reactivation of neurons and this is facilitated by rehabilitation (Gouvier, Ryan, O'Jile, Parks-Levy, Webster, & Blanton, 1997). Though study in this area is incomplete, the knowledge that neural plasticity exists provides incentive for nursing research and practice in this area of promoting adaptation with neurologically injured patients at all phases of recovery.

► COMPROMISED PROCESSES OF NEUROLOGIC FUNCTION

Adaptation problems can result when any of the processes related to neurologic function are disrupted. Two specific examples of compromised adaptive processes related to neurologic function are discussed here. Memory deficit is a commonly occurring problem associated with cognitive processes. Similarly, decreased levels of consciousness is a significant compromised process of neurologic function.

Memory Deficit

A deficit in the ability to process experience by storing and retrieving information is generally termed *memory deficit*. Memory deficits stem from the complex working systems for reception, coding, and storage of information, as well as retrieval of information. As noted earlier, brain structures such as the hippocampus may be involved in particular stages, for example, sorting, assembling, and supplying information that is emotionally significant. Short-term changes in synaptic function have been identified in work on habituation and conditioning, but how such changes might be converted into long-term memory lasting for years is not known. The role of metabolic activity or protein synthesis in these processes is a broad area of study. It has been noted that an overriding principle of cognitive processing is the integrated functioning of the brain as a whole. This characteristic makes the memory storage and retrieval processes most sensitive to changes that occur throughout the brain.

Focal stimuli for memory deficits include metabolic changes, infection, tumors, seizures, stroke, and toxic reactions. The retrieval process seems most affected by these pathologies. The memory disturbance that generally follows closed head injury has particular characteristics. These patients may have a period of coma followed by a period of confusion. During the length of these two intervals, current events have not been stored. This time frame is commonly called the period of posttraumatic amnesia and its duration is often used as an index of closed head injury severity.

Degenerative brain pathology, as sometimes occurs in alcoholism and other drug use, has long been known to produce defects of memory. Korsakoff's syndrome describes a cluster of six characteristics of this type of pathology (Talland, 1965). They are:

1. Anterograde amnesia, in which patients are unable to form new memories.
2. Retrograde amnesia, that is, the patients have global impairment of remote memory for most of their adult life.

3. Confabulation, where information is made up to cover up memory loss.
4. Meager content in conversation indicated by little spontaneous conversation.
5. Lack of insight that is particularly difficult because patients are virtually unaware of their memory deficit.
6. Apathy manifested by indifference and incapacity to persevere in ongoing activities.

Alzheimer's disease is another degenerative brain disorder that has generated interest for both clinical and scientific reasons. It accounts for about 50 percent of patients diagnosed as demented and it provides a good model for the study of senility in general. Changes in the brain structures, including neuronal loss in the temporal lobe and brainstem, are being studied. Further research relates neurochemical changes, particularly the cholinergic system. This condition leads to marked deficits in memory, language, and perception, as well as symptoms of depression. Losses generally occur in stages of mild, moderate, and severe.

Persons with memory deficits can be deprived of the richness of their own past. They can feel lost in the unfamiliar world of the here and now. They are suspicious of what may happen to them because of the inability to understand and predict events as yet unfolding. Adaptation problems related to memory can occur transiently, as in concussion, or for a prolonged period as with Alzheimer's disease. The deficit can be continual or intermittent. It can have qualitative aspects such as defective spontaneous recall, lack of ability to integrate information into a whole as a basis for a modulated response, or conceptual inflexibility. In general, the nurse can be working with a diagnosis of memory deficit, but always recognizing that observations of behaviors and stimuli, together with updated knowledge in the field, provide the basis for planning care.

Decreased Level of Consciousness

Changing pressures within the cranium affect the level of consciousness because the skull is a nonflexible bony structure. The brain takes up 80 percent of the space inside the skull. Cerebrospinal fluid and the blood in the cerebral arteries and veins occupy the remainder of the space. A change in the volume of any one of these components brings about compensatory changes to maintain intracranial pressure (ICP) at a normal level. However, if pressure within the skull increases, there is little room to accommodate the change. Increased intracranial pressure (IICP) refers to an increase in pressure in the subarachnoid space where cerebrospinal fluid (CSF) circulates around the brain and spinal cord and in the ventricles. One bodily mechanism to attempt adaptation by immediately relieving IICP is brain herniation, that is, the brain protruding into another compartment or area, taking advantage of any spaces where brain structures meet. The brain itself is not rigid and can make shifts with fairly predictable patterns, each associated with characteristic clinical signs. This compensation is usually short lived, however, and quickly becomes life-threatening.

The several compartments of the cranium are separated by sheets of dura. Pressure shifts brain tissue from one area where pressure is high to another where pressure is lower. There are three major patterns of brain shift (Plum & Posner, 1982). Shifts across the intracranial cavity force the brain tissue under the dura that divides the two hemispheres (midline shift). In downward displacement, the hemispheres and the basal nuclei go through the tentorium where the midbrain passes (central herniation). Displacement and compression of blood vessels further contribute to disturbance of ICP and to cerebral hypoxia. Severe brainstem changes result. Finally, there is herniation through the foramen magnum where all the structures are being pulled downward (uncal herniation). The latter is signaled by warnings from structures that lie outside the brain parenchyma. Of particular clinical importance is the fact that the third cranial nerve, which controls pupil response and extraocular eye movements (EOM), may be caught between swollen structures and ligaments. Thus, the lethal effects of compression of the medulla can be prevented by the nurse's observation of a change in the size of the pupil of the eye. In assessing the behavior of decreased level of consciousness, the nurse notes the related neurologic signs that indicate changes in intracranial pressure. Figure 12–5 shows the sequence and progression of behavioral responses to IICP. In this case, accurate observations of behaviors are used to identify the relevant stimuli for patients with decreased intracranial adaptive capacity (Mitchell, 1988). Nursing judgments in these acute situations can be life-saving.

A patient can have the diagnosis of decreased level of consciousness due to increased intracranial pressure. The anatomic basis for consciousness is divided into two regions: the cerebral hemispheres above the tentorium and the reticular formation of the brainstem extending from the midpons through the diencephalon. Understanding this problem requires an understanding of the condition of increased intracranial pressure (IICP). This condition can be seen in many neurologic disruptions, such as central nervous system tumors, brain abscess, hydrocephalus, aneurysms, and traumatic brain injury with contusions or hematoma.

► **PLANNING NURSING CARE**

Neurologic function is an important requirement for an individual's adaptation in all of the four modes. In applying the nursing process, the nurse makes a careful assessment of behaviors and stimuli related to the complex processes of cognition and consciousness. In assessing factors influencing neurologic function, regulator and cognator effectiveness in initiating compensatory processes is considered. Based on this thorough first- and second-level assessment, the nurse makes nursing diagnoses, sets goals, selects interventions, and evaluates care.

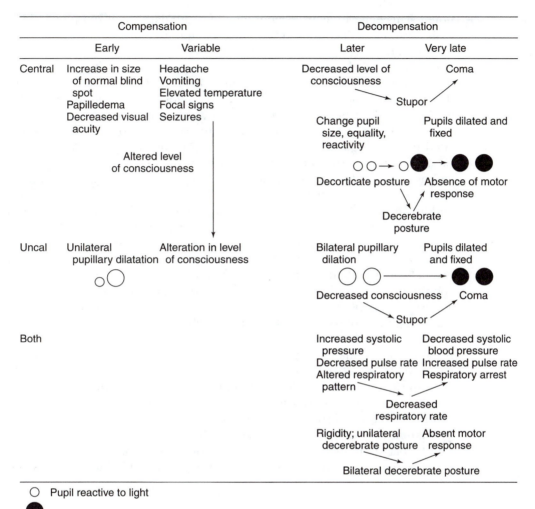

	Compensation		Decompensation	
	Early	Variable	Later	Very late

Central	Increase in size of normal blind spot Papilledema Decreased visual acuity	Headache Vomiting Elevated temperature Focal signs Seizures
		
		 Altered level of consciousness
			Decreased level of consciousness
			     Stupor
			
			 Change pupil size, equality, reactivity
			
			 Decorticate posture
			   Decerebrate posture
				Coma
				
				 Pupils dilated and fixed
				
				 Absence of motor response

Uncal	Unilateral pupillary dilatation	Alteration in level of consciousness	Bilateral pupillary dilation Decreased consciousness Stupor	Pupils dilated and fixed Coma
Both			Increased systolic pressure Decreased pulse rate Altered respiratory pattern Decreased respiratory rate Rigidity; unilateral decerebrate posture Bilateral decerebrate posture	Decreased systolic blood pressure Increased pulse rate Respiratory arrest Absent motor response

○ Pupil reactive to light

● Pupil nonreactive to light

FIGURE 12–5. Behavioral responses of supratentorial IICP; classified by stage of appearance and herniation syndrome. *(From Moidel, H. (1976). Nursing care of the patient with medical surgical disorders (p. 868). New York: McGraw-Hill. Used with permission.)*

Nursing Diagnosis

Assessment data of behaviors and related stimuli are interpreted and used in establishing a nursing diagnosis. The nurse prepared to use the Roy Adaptation Model can state diagnoses as specific behaviors with the stimuli that are most relevant or may employ summary labels to convey complex concepts in abbreviated terms.

During the nursing assessment of neurologic function, the nurse notes the positive functioning of this intricate system of thinking, feeling, moving, and interacting. At the same time, changes in functioning and any deficits are noted. This behavioral assessment together with data about stimuli provides a basis for nursing diagnoses in this mode component.

Because of the subtleties of behavior changes that are important, Roy's first method of diagnosis is often the most appropriate, that is, statement of the behavior with the relevant stimuli. For example, the nurse might note that the 13-year-old in her 6th day of coma following a car accident has flickered her eyelids when the overhead lights were turned on.

Roy has developed a typology of indicators of positive adaptation related to neurologic function (see Table 12–5). Included in the typology are: (a) affective processes of arousal and attention; sensation and perception; coding, concept formation, memory, and language; and planning and motor response; (b) integrated thinking and feeling processes; and (c) plasticity and functional effectiveness of developing, aging, and altered nervous system. It is important to recognize situations of effective adaptation so that these can be maintained or enhanced. Commonly recurring adaptation problems include decreased level of consciousness, defective cognitive processing, memory deficits, instability of behavior and mood, ineffective compensation for cognitive deficit, and potential for secondary brain damage. The NANDA diagnostic labels (Rantz & LeMone, 1977) are listed in the last column and include: high risk of secondary brain injury; altered level of responsiveness, decreased; altered level of responsiveness, heightened; altered level of responsiveness, inappropriate behaviors and moods; and uncompensated cognitive deficit (specify type of deficit).

In situations of neurologic disruption, it is important that the essence of the disruption be conveyed in the nursing diagnosis in such a manner as to provide direction for subsequent steps of the nursing process. This is facilitated by identification of the specific behaviors that are of concern and the relevant stimuli that are influencing them. An example of this type of nursing diagnosis could be "changes in vital signs associated with increased intracranial pressure."

TABLE 12–5 NURSING DIAGNOSTIC CATEGORIES FOR NEUROLOGIC FUNCTION

Positive Indicators of Adaptation	Common Adaptation Problems	NANDA Diagnostic Labels
• Effective processes of arousal and attention; sensation and perception; coding; concept formation, memory, language; planning, and motor response	• Decreased level of consciousness • Defective cognitive processing • Memory deficits • Instability of behavior and mood	• High risk of secondary brain injury • Altered level of responsiveness: decreased • Altered level of responsiveness: heightened
• Integrated thinking and feeling processes	• Ineffective compensation for cognitive deficit	• Altered level of responsiveness: inappropriate behaviors and moods
• Plasticity and functional effectiveness of developing, aging, and altered nervous system	• Potential for secondary brain damage	• Uncompensated cognitive deficit (specify)

This diagnosis pertained to a young adult male in the emergency unit following a motor vehicle accident. Although he arrived unconscious, he regained consciousness but was disoriented. He was conversing and following commands but could not recall anything about the accident. He described severe headache, visual disturbances, dizziness, and a sense of nervousness. As the time progressed, his headache worsened, he developed drowsiness and confusion, difficulty in thinking, and ultimately, he had a seizure. A medical diagnosis of subdural hematoma was made following an MRI scan and surgical intervention was initiated. Other nursing diagnoses applicable in this situation might be "decreased level of conscious due to signs of increased intracranial pressure associated with head trauma."

Goal Setting

In using the Roy Adaptation Model, goal setting involves working with the patient and family to establish clear outcomes for nursing care. A complete goal statement includes the behavior of focus, the change expected, and the time frame in which the goal is to be achieved. Goals can be long term or short term and these time frames are relative to the situation involved. However, when working with patients with disorders of the nervous system, characteristically the goals tend to take the extremes of being very immediate, as in critical care, or very long term, as in rehabilitation and care of the elderly.

For the young man with decreased level of consciousness due to increased intracranial pressure, the general goal of care is to minimize intracranial pressure and prevent secondary brain injury and complications of coma, with eventual progression to a higher level of responsiveness. Prevention of secondary brain injury includes the following process criteria identified by the AANN Standards (Mitchell, 1988):

1. To identify the individual's baseline level of brain function, including responsiveness, size and reaction of pupils, brainstem reflexes, respiratory rate, and behavior.
2. To institute measures to promote cerebral perfusion, including avoiding hypoxia, hypercapnia, hypo- or hypertension.

An example of a specific goal for the young man described previously who has decreased level of consciousness due to increased intracranial pressure can be stated, "Within 30 minutes, the cause of the increased intracranial pressure will be identified and steps will be initiated to alleviate the pressure." The behavioral focus of the goal is the intracranial pressure, the change expected is that it will be alleviated, and the time frame is 30 minutes.

Another goal example pertains to a longer-term situation: a person with memory deficit. The general goals of nursing care are to provide for safety and other basic needs, to establish a sense of trust and confidence, to help the person and family understand the person's abilities and limitations, to improve memory function, and to develop and use methods to compensate for deficits. A specific goal for the family of a person with Alzheimer's disease might be: "Before the nurse's home visit next week, the husband will devise two ways to remind his wife not to go outdoors alone and at that time will report on the effectiveness of their use." The focus of the goal is on the husband's development and use of effective memory devices for his wife's safety. The criteria will be whether two methods were devised that worked. The time frame is 1 week.

Intervention

Interventions are carried out to meet the stated goals. According to the premises of the Roy model, altering the stimuli that make up the adaptation level is a way to promote adaptation. Managing focal stimuli is often the intervention of choice when dealing with neurologic functioning, and these cover a wide range of the person's internal and external environment. Nutritional and fluid intake can be altered according to its effect on neurologic functioning, for example, limiting fluids after cranial surgery. Another example of managing focal stimuli is providing tactile and auditory stimulation for the patient in a coma.

Contextual and residual stimuli can also be the focus of interventions to broaden the range of coping ability. Measures to reduce stress and fatigue are used to minimize the neuromuscular weakness of exacerbation of such conditions as multiple sclerosis and myasthenia gravis, as well as to control episodes of seizure activity in persons with epilepsy. While teaching a mother specific exercises for her child with cerebral palsy, the nurse may also refer her to a support group for parents of children with disabilities to help her manage other contextual and residual factors affecting the situation.

Some of the key interventions related to the nursing diagnoses discussed will be outlined. Basic medical-surgical textbooks and books on the neurosciences for nurses and other clinicians can be consulted for other specific interventions related to neurologic functioning and all its complexities in the many situations of normal development and disruptive changes that the nurse may see.

In a situation of decreased level of consciousness due to increased intracranial pressure such as that described previously, the nurse recognizes the significance of the intracranial pressure and carries out the following interventions:

1. The first priority is to maintain an open airway, adequate ventilation, and circulation.
2. Observe and report slight neurologic changes, especially changes in pupils, motor response, verbalizations, and vital signs.
3. Maintain a quiet environment.
4. Elevate the head of the bed 30 degrees with the head in alignment with the body (turning the head alone can result in constriction of

vessels in the neck and decrease venous blood return from the brain).

5. Prevent sudden increases in pressure, as from vigorous coughing, isometric exercises (contraction and relaxation of a muscle without mechanical work), or straining during defecation, which can bring on the Valsalva maneuver.

6. Minimize emotional and physical trauma (spaced family visits with instructions given to avoid emotional upsets).

Varying degrees of coma require attention to all physical nursing measures. In the acute situation relating to the motor vehicle accident victim, interventions with which the nurse would be involved include organizing and preparing for diagnostic assessment and ultimately emergency surgical intervention. In emergency circumstances such as that described, preoperative teaching involving the patient is not possible. Rather, conscientious neurologic assessment continues and physical preparations for surgery are made. Immediate transport is necessary and preparation of the operative site would be accomplished in the operating room. Much of the attention of the nurses will be directed toward the family members, their understanding of the situation and the required surgery, and the expected outcomes. In any situation where family are unexpectedly called to the emergency room, and particularly when neurosurgery is involved, the nurse is mindful of the stress and emotions involved. Reinforcement of explanations provided by the surgeon will probably be necessary. Postoperatively, nursing interventions will be directed at the prevention and recognition of complications; evaluation of neurologic status; prevention, recognition, and control of increased intracranial pressure; supportive care; and, in the longer term, rehabilitation.

In situations of ongoing unconsciousness, it is the nurse's responsibility to prevent complications of the comatose state, such as decubiti, stomatitis, and atelectasis. The patient is turned and repositioned every 2 hours and given back massage. Turning alternates the pressure on different areas of the skin as well as enhancing ventilation. Various devices such as gel pads, egg crate mattresses, sheepskin, alternating pressure pads, and waterbeds help prevent decubiti. An alternating pressure mattress is particularly effective because pressure in various areas is frequently altered. A rubber doughnut placed around the decubitus actually complicates matters by creating further decubiti. This is caused by the increased pressure on the skin beneath the doughnut. The nurse uses foot supports or a foot board to prevent foot drop, that is, falling of the foot due to flexor paralysis of the ankle.

If the eyes are open and blinking is absent, artificial tears can be used, but patching protects the eyes better. A usual approach is to wet eye patches in a sterile water or saline solution and gently cover the eyes with the lids closed. The nurse removes the patches to do pupil checks and allow for possible sensory input for short periods. In cases of coma, a neurologic assessment is done every 2 to 4 hours. For cranial nerves, checks are done on III (pupils), V (corneal reflex), and IX and X (swallow and gag). Any voluntary movements and responses to pain are noted. A check is made for the plantar reflex. As in all other conditions, an open airway is a priority concern. The patient's trachea is suctioned if breath sounds are congested or the airway obstructed. The nurse assesses for incontinence and abdominal or bladder distention. Mouth care is provided every 2 hours to prevent infection, such as stomatitis, respiratory tract infection, and aspiration. The nurse explains to the patient what is being done, and never discusses a negative prognosis at the patient's bedside. The sense of hearing is often present although no other neurologic faculties appear intact.

The interventions for memory deficits will be tailored to the particular person, to the deficit noted, as well as to the person's remaining abilities. The nurse works with the family to plan care for the person. Both family and nurse will avoid confusing the person with details beyond the immediate. They can provide frequent reassurance when the person shows fear of the unfamiliar. Developing a sense of trust and confidence can be enhanced by simple measures such as putting the name of the primary care nurse readily in view at the patient's bedside or attached to the person if ambulatory. Useful, orienting information is given often, such as the time of day or how long until the next meal or bedtime. Simple routines for care in daily living are developed and used. The steps for dressing can be written out. A daily schedule is posted or put on audio tape for those with vision problems or attached to the armrest of a wheelchair for those up in the chair.

The nurse and other caregivers use a calm, matter-of-fact approach when the patient needs the same information given repeatedly or when there are signs of confabulation or lack of insight. The person also can be guided toward productive and satisfying activity after simple self-care needs are met. For example, the list of daily activities may include watering a plant. The particular plant listed is changed according to which plant needs to be watered and the patient is not burdened with having to remember which plant was done the day before.

For some persons, it may be necessary to provide protection and supportive supervision. Structures such as doors and stairwells will be checked and altered to prevent unsupervised wandering and falling. The psychological comfort of the environment can be enhanced by activities such as reminiscent groups. In the long-term care of people with memory deficits, especially those that are progressive, the nurse may recommend resources to provide relief for caregivers. The nurse can be helpful as a knowledgeable and caring person when a family needs assistance with the issues related to long-term institutional care.

Earlier in this chapter, the principles of integrated neural functioning and neural plasticity were described. Based on evidence that multiple networks in the brain can carry on the same function, and that there are possibilities for modifying central nervous system structural organization and function, in many conditions there is hope for recovering or improving memory function following brain injury, particularly in the younger person (Bach-Y-Rita, 1978). People who suffer brain injury from stroke or head injury present difficult problems of memory deficit and levels of recovery are often uncertain. There can be continued inability to remember conversations or instructions, telephone numbers, written material, television shows, or even faces for several months after the stroke or accident. The person may lose track of speech in mid-sentence. This is especially true if there is any distraction or interruption such as a phone ringing or someone speaking and interrupting the train of thought.

In designing interventions for improving memory, two principles that have already been mentioned are used, that is, they are individualized to the person and to the deficit. The nurse is in a good position to do this especially for the settings where these persons will be (Sisson, 1988). Based on frequent contact with patients and their families, the nurse observes the specific deficits and reactions to them. In this way, meaningful and individualized intervention techniques and strategies can be developed.

In some settings, the nurse also has available formal evaluation of memory deficits by the health care team including members with neuropsychology knowledge. In other cases, the nurse bases care primarily on the nursing assessment of the memory deficit. Interventions are further individualized by the total nursing assessment, which includes the influences of the other adaptive modes. A specific factor might be tolerance to fatigue; for example, immediately after head injury, a 10-minute session of memory exercises at the bedside may be the patient's limit, and when working with young adult male patients (representing nearly 80 percent of the head injury population), one can devise memory exercises using playing cards so that the activity is more acceptable to patient's primary role.

A final major principle in designing interventions for improving memory is that the efforts of the nurse, family, and other health care personnel are based on a specific theoretical approach to understanding cognitive function. The notion of integrated brain functioning and the model of an information processing system can be helpful here. The Das–Luria model has been used by Roy (1989) to further define a proposed cognitive information processing model. In the work of these authors (Das, Kirby, & Jarman, 1975, 1979; Luria, 1973, 1980), the basic information-processing functions of sensory input, perception, memory, concept formation, and output have simultaneous and successive properties. Simultaneous means that the input is received all at once such as seeing the picture of a house and synthesizing the separate parts of it into a whole. Successive processing refers to processing elements in serial order. For example, in hearing human speech, one hears one word after another and makes a sentence from the order of words.

The same simultaneous and successive dimensions are present in planning functions as well. One can think of solving the task of drawing a line through a maze. If the maze formation is very simple, one can see the whole and quickly generate and execute the program for solving the task. If, however, it is a complex maze, then parts of the maze are taken in serial order while the planning functions of searching, comparing, hypothesizing, and verifying are carried out.

Based on this particular understanding of cognitive processing, the memory aids to promote retraining can be planned to activate simultaneous and successive processing. For example, capitalizing on the dimension of simultaneous processing, the person can be taught to recall family members using a photo album. The person is asked to repeat aloud several times the name of a given person in a picture, seeing the entire face, speaking the name, and hearing it at the same time. The name is then used in a meaningful statement. For example, "Aunt Louise is my mother's sister." The name is further associated with a characteristic obvious in the picture, such as "Aunt Louise has red hair."

A simple method of using successive processing to improve memory is to have lists of words that the person repeats after the examiner. The list becomes increasingly long and is varied from words that are similar in some way to those that have no similarities. Another technique can be to have a deck of playing cards in which one card at a time is laid down in front of the person. The next card is taken off the deck and placed on top of it. The person is asked to identify the card before the last card on the stack when the caregiver stops dealing. As the person's memory improves, the instructions can be made more difficult by having the person name the second card back or the third card back.

Simultaneous and successive processing practice (Roy, 1989) can be used with a specific deficit such as recalling place names, as in an example of a person who cannot remember the name of the city of residence. This practice involves a set of simple exercises in which families can be involved. The simultaneous strategies are used with a map as the stimulus to learn the name of the city. Then, an additional strategy is to have the person color the area of the city on the map. Sometimes many rehearsals of the task are required. Pictures of readily familiar landmarks of the city that contain the city's name are obtained, and then the name is placed on a card. The patient learns to match the name card with the landmark and says the name of the landmark including the name of the city each time.

There is a rapidly growing literature on memory retraining. Many different perspectives are represented. The nurse can help families evaluate any particular programs they might be considering, especially when these would add great expense to the already heavy financial burden of illness. Computer programs have not yet proven effective and most professionals in the field caution that they will never replace the human being who sits with the patient and provides support as well as feedback on performance. By increasingly understanding how the brain is operating, how memory functions, and how the person has been affected by brain damage, the nurse can creatively help design simple and useful strategies both for daily care of the person with memory deficits by compensating for these and for improving memory function by stimulating simultaneous and successive processing in memory tasks.

Evaluation

Evaluation involves judging the effectiveness of the nursing interventions in relation to the person's adaptive behavior, that is, whether the person has attained the behavior stated in the goals. The nursing interventions would be identified as effective if the person's behavior is in accordance with the stated goal. If the goal has not been achieved, the nurse identifies alternative interventions or approaches by reassessing the behavior and stimuli and continuing with the other steps of the nursing process. Since the goals include the behavior to be focused on, a change or level of stability expected, and a given time, these are the dimensions for judging effectiveness.

In the goal stated earlier as: "Within 30 minutes, the cause of the increased intracranial pressure will be identified and steps will be initiated to alleviate the pressure," the goal would have been achieved if, half an hour later, a diagnosis had been established and steps were underway to intervene. Following the surgery to alleviate the subdural hematoma, further short- and long-term goals would be developed as postoperative care is undertaken. Initially, these would be very short term in nature. For example, "Within the next hour, intracranial pressure will remain stable and within acceptable levels." The evaluation of this goal would rest with the signs of IICP and perhaps intracranial monitoring of pressure levels. As the situation stabilizes and time passes, longer term goals would be developed and continually evaluated in response to the patient's postoperative condition.

Some goals related to memory deficits are particularly difficult to evaluate. The nurse again will use the notion of short-term and long-term goals. Remembering that some neurologic functions are intact or recovering and that some are functioning at a slower pace can help caregivers to be patient with the long process involved. The nurse recognizes, and helps the family to recognize, that improvement may take place only subtly, over long periods of time, and not in steady progression, but with days of better and worse functioning.

► SUMMARY

This chapter focused on the complexities of neurologic processes and how this knowledge can help one understand the thinking, feeling, moving, and interacting person who is adapting within the changing world. Two basic life processes presented as key to neurologic function were cognition and consciousness. Assessment of behaviors and stimuli related to cognition and consciousness were outlined in this chapter. Compensatory strategies that act to maintain neurologic function were identified. Two examples of compromised processes, memory deficits and decreased level of consciousness, were discussed. Planning nursing care involving nursing diagnoses, goals, interventions, and evaluation were described, with particular emphasis on consciousness and memory.

▶ EXERCISES FOR APPLICATION

1. Devise a brief assessment tool for the cranial nerves. Use this tool to assess normal function of a colleague. While doing the assessment, have a mental image of the neural pathways that are operating.

2. Write down at least five different sources of information that come to you each day and think about what it might feel like to be in this environment without the ability to process it selectively.

3. Describe how a person with severe memory deficits might be affected in each of the adaptive modes: physiologic, self-concept, role function, and interdependence.

▶ ASSESSMENT OF UNDERSTANDING

Questions

1. Name the two basic life processes associated with neurologic function as identified in the Roy Adaptation Model.
   (a) _____
   (b) _____

2. Identify three behaviors associated with the assessment of cognition and consciousness.

   Cognition

   (a) _____
   (b) _____
   (c) _____

   Consciousness

   (a) _____
   (b) _____
   (c) _____

3. Identify ten stimuli that affect neurologic function. These may be related to either cognition or consciousness.
   (a) _____   (f) _____
   (b) _____   (g) _____
   (c) _____   (h) _____
   (d) _____   (i) _____
   (e) _____   (j) _____

4. Neural plasticity was provided as an example of a compensatory process associated with neurologic functioning. Describe neural plasticity.

   _____
   _____
   _____

5. Two compromised processes of neurologic function were discussed in this chapter: memory deficits and decreased level of consciousness. Label the following descriptor as associated with either memory deficits (MD) or level of consciousness (LC).
   (a) _____ deficit in restoring and retrieving information
   (b) _____ brain herniation is an associated compensatory process
   (c) _____ a critical situation that can lead to death
   (d) _____ focal stimulus may be seizure, stroke, or toxic reactions
   (e) _____ may result from increased intracranial pressure
   (f) _____ may involve degenerative brain pathology associated with alcoholism

Situation

Jeffery McClure is the 45-year-old father of two children who lives in a rural area about an hour's drive from a major city. He has been diagnosed with epilepsy since he was in his teens. Although multiple treatment regimens have been attempted (control with medications, surgical intervention), his seizures are not under control and intermittently he will have a seizure at home. The nurse involved with the family is interested in helping Jeffery's wife and children to know what to do when Jeffery is having a seizure.

6. Develop two nursing diagnoses related to the situation described—one focusing on Jeffery and the other focusing on the family members.
   (a) Focused on Jeffery: _____
   (b) Focused on the family: _____

7. State goals related to the situation described with specific focus on the nursing diagnoses formulated.
   (a) _____
   (b) _____

8. List nursing interventions designed to achieve the goals specified in item 6b.
   (a) _____
   (b) _____

9. Describe how evaluation of the nursing interventions would be accomplished and how further steps of the nursing process would proceed.
   (a) _____
   (b) _____

Feedback

1. (a) cognition
   (b) consciousness

2. Cognition: any three of the following: arousal and attention, sensation perception, coding, concept formation, memory, language, planning, motor response.
   Consciousness: any three of the following: level of consciousness, motor response, response to pain, orientation, and level of awareness,

3. Any ten of the following: pathophysiology, blood gases and hemoglobin levels, nutritional status, activity and rest, stress, knowledge level, physical environment, self-concept, role function, interdependence, situational characteristics.

4. Neural plasticity is considered to be a fundamental property of the nervous system. It refers to enduring modification of structures within the nervous system to develop or preserve cognitive and neurologic function. These modifications occur at critical periods, can last a lifetime, and seem to lack motivation and reinforcement for their establishment. Plasticity is greater in early years, with multiple new patterns of structure and function possible. There is also increasing evidence for retaining and restoring nervous system functional effectiveness including sprouting of remaining nerve fibers after injury. The reservoir of plasticity decreases over the life span.

5. (a) MD, (b) LC, (c) LC, (d) MD, (e) LC, (f) MD

6. Sample nursing diagnoses:
   (a) Compromised safety related to uncontrolled epileptic seizures and lack of success of treatment regimens.
   (b) Anxiety and uncertainty regarding appropriate actions during seizures due to lack of knowledge.

7. Suggested goals:
   (a) Within 1 week, Jeffery will consistently employ safety precautions to enhance his personal safety in the event of a seizure.
   (b) At the time of Jeffery's next seizure when family members are present, they will demonstrate actions to support Jeffery's safety during and after the seizure.

8. Possible interventions:
   (a) Assess Jeffery's knowledge level about epilepsy and his recurring seizures; eliminate misconceptions and provide correct information; assist in contacting agencies that can provide information and sup-

port, reassurance, and socialization with others facing the same problem; involve him in the development of a treatment plan aimed at taking medications as prescribed, avoiding situations that precipitate seizures, and adjusting his lifestyle (e.g., no driving) while maintaining self-esteem.

(b) Encourage family to discuss their feeling of fear or shame, and assist them in dealing with the constant stress associated with the seizures; instruct them as to what actions to take while the seizure is in progress; point out important observations to be made both before, during, and following the seizure; explore safety precautions associated with daily lifestyle.

9. Evaluation: Nursing interventions would be judged successful if the goals were achieved. Specifically,

(a) Within 1 week, Jeffery has instituted safety precautions to enhance his personal safety in the event of a seizure. He is no longer driving, he is taking his medications regularly and as prescribed, and he is getting lots of rest and avoiding situations that precipitate seizures. Jeffery identified symptoms that occurred just prior to the seizure. Further nursing care involved exploring further the significance of these and his preferred actions when they were evident.

(b) During the occasion of Jeffery's next seizure, his family members were able to support him by staying with him, easing him to the floor, placing a padded tongue blade between his teeth before they were clenched, loosening his collar and belt, turning him on his side, not restraining him, and reassuring and reorienting him when the seizure ended. They observed carefully actions that occurred during the seizure and were able to report on his behavior, mood, and comments prior to the seizure. The intervention was judged effective and further information was provided in answer to questions that were raised by family members.

► REFERENCES

Anthony, J. C., LeResche, L., Niaz, U., Von Korff, M. R., & Folstein, M. F. (1982). Limits of the mini-mental state, a screening test for dementia and delirium among hospital patients. *Psychological Medicine, 12,* 397.

Bach-Y-Rita, P. (1978). *Recovery of function: Theoretical considerations for brain injury rehabilitation.* Toronto, Lewiston, New York, Bern, Stuttgart: Hans Huber Publishers.

Bignami, A., Bloom, F. E., Bolis, C. L., & Adeloye, A. (1985). *Central nervous system plasticity and repair.* New York: Raven Press.

Cammermeyer, M. (1988). Assessment of cognition. In Mitchell, P. H., Hodges, L. C., Muwaswes, M., & Walleck, C. A. (Eds.), *American Association of Neuroscience Nurses' neurological nursing: Phenomena and practice* (pp. 155–169). Norwalk, CT: Appleton & Lange.

Churchland, P. M. (1988). *Matter and consciousness, a contemporary introduction to the philosophy of mind.* Cambridge, MA: MIT Press.

Crigger, N. J., & Strickland, C. C. (1985). Selecting a nursing diagnosis for changes in consciousness. *Dimensions of Critical Care Nursing, 4(3),* 156.

Das, J. P. (1984). Intelligence and information integration. In Kirby, J. (Ed.), *Cognitive strategies and educational performance* (pp. 13–31). New York: Academic Press.

Das, J. P., Kirby, J. R., & Jarman, R. F. (1975). Simultaneous and successive synthesis: An alternative model for cognitive abilities. *Psychological Bulletin, 82,* 87–103.

Das, J. P., Kirby, J. P., & Jarman, R. F. (1979). *Simultaneous and successive cognitive processes.* New York: Academic Press.

Dennett, D. C. (1991). *Consciousness explained.* Boston: Little, Brown.

Diamond, M. C., Johnson, R. E., & Ingham, C. A. (1975). Morphological changes in the young adult, and aging cerebral cortex, hippocampus, and diencephalon. *Behavioral Biology, 14,* 163–174.

Eccles J., & Robinson, D. N. (1984). *The wonder of being human, our brain and our mind.* New York: Free Press.

Folstein, M. F., Folstein, S. E., & McHugh, P. R. (1975). Mini-mental state, a practical method for grading the cognitive state of patients for the clinician. *Journal of Psychiatric Research, 12,* 189.

Finger, S., & Stein, D. (1982). *Brain damage and recovery: Research and clinical perspectives.* New York: Academic Press.

Gouvier, W. D., Ryan, L. M., O'Jile, J. R., Parks-Levy, J., Webster, J. S., & Blanton, P. D. (1997). Cognitive retraining with brain-damaged patients. In Horton, A. M., Jr., Wedding, D., & Webster, J. (Eds.), *The neuoropsychology handbook* (2nd ed.). New York: Springer.

Guyton, A. (1992). *Human physiology and mechanisms of disease* (4th ed.). Philadelphia: Saunders.

Hickey, J. (1992). *The clinical practice of neurological and neurosurgical nursing* (3rd ed.). Philadelphia: Lippincott.

Jennett, B., & Teasdale, G. (1977). Aspects of coma after severe head injury. *Lancet, 1(8017),* 878–881.

Kemp, J. (1979). *The philosophy of Kant.* Oxford: Oxford University Press.

Luria, A. R. (1973). *The working brain: An introduction to neuropsychology.* New York: Basic Books.

Luria, A. R. (1980). *Higher cortical function in man.* New York: Basic Books.

Mitchell, P. H. (1988). Consciousness: An overview. In Michell, P. H., Hodges, L. C., Muwaswes, M., & Walleck, C. A. (Eds.), *American Association of Neuroscience Nurses' Neuroscience nursing: Phenomena and practice* (pp. 57–66). Norwalk, CT: Appleton & Lange.

Molloy, G., Das, J., & Pierce, A. (1990). Some developmental trends in children's information processing strategies. *Psychological Reports, 66,* 443–448.

Mountcastle, V. B. (1979). An organizing principle for cerebral function: The unit module and the distributed system. In Schmitt, F. O., & Worden, F. G. (Eds.), *The neurosciences.* Cambridge, MA: MIT Press.

Mountcastle, V. B. (1997). The columnar organization of the neocortex. *Brain, 120,* 701–722.

Newman, M. (1994). *Help as expanding consciousness* (2nd ed.). New York: National League for Nursing Press.

Plum, F., & Posner, J. (1982). The diagnosis of stupor and coma. Philadelphia: Davis.

Pribram, K. H. (1969). *Brain and behavior 3: Memory mechanisms* (p. 7). Baltimore: Penguin Books.

Roy, C. (1988). Altered cognition: An information processing approach. In Mitchell, P. H., Hodges, L. C., Muwaswes, M., & Walleck, C. A. (Eds.), *American Association of Neuroscience Nurses' Neuroscience nursing: Phenomena and practice* (pp. 185–211). Norwalk, CT: Appleton & Lange.

Roy, C. (1989). Nursing care in theory and practice: Early interventions in brain injury. In Harris, R., & Rees, R. (Eds.), *Recovery from brain injury: Expectations, needs, and processes* (pp. 95–110). Northfield, South Australia: Institute for the Study of Learning Difficulties, South Australian College of Advanced Education.

Roy, C. (in press). Alterations in cognitive processing. In Stewart-Amidei, C., Kunkel, J., & Bronstein, K. (Eds.), *American Association of Neuroscience Nursing's neuroscience nursing: Human responses to neurologic dysfunction* (2nd ed.). Philadelphia: Saunders.

Selkurt, E. E. (1982). *Basic physiology for the health sciences.* Boston: Little, Brown.

Sisson, R. (1988). Alterations in memory. In Mitchell, P. H., Hodges, L. C. , Muwaswes, M., & Walleck, C. A. (Eds.), *American Association of Neuroscience Nurses' Neuroscience nursing: Phenomena and practice* (pp. 171–183). Norwalk, CT: Appleton & Lange.

Talland, G. A. (1965). *Deranged memory.* New York: Academic Press.

Wilber, K. (1997). *The eye of spirit.* Boston: Shambhala.

Willis, W., Jr., & Grossman, R. (1981). *Medical neurobiology: Neuroanatomical and neurophysiological principles basic to clinical neuroscience.* St. Louis: Mosby.

► ADDITIONAL REFERENCES

Burrell, L. O., Gerlach, M. J. M., & Pless, B. S. (1997). *Adult nursing: Acute and community care* (2nd ed.). Stamford, CT: Appleton & Lange.

Boss, B. J. (1993). The neurophysiological basis of learning: Attention and memory implication for SCI nurses. *SCI Nursing, 10,* 121–129.

Brooks, N. (1984) *Closed head injury: Psychological, social, and family consequences.* Oxford: Oxford University Press.

Brooks, N. (1992). Psychosocial assessment after traumatic brain injury. *Scandinavian Journal of Rehabilitation Medicine, 26(Suppl.),* 126–131.

Pi Lambda Theta, San Jose Area Chapter. (1983). *Helping head injury and stroke patients at home: A handbook for families.* San Jose, CA: Pi Lambda Theta.

Posner, M., DiGirolamo, G., & Fernandez, D. (1997). Brain mechanisms of cognitive skills. *Consciousness and Cognition, 6,* 267–290.

Taylor, J., & Bellenger, S. (1980). *Neurological dysfunctions and nursing intervention.* New York: McGraw-Hill.

13

ENDOCRINE FUNCTION

Endocrine function is the last of the complex processes identified in the Roy Adaptation Model. The endocrine system, in close association with the autonomic nervous system, integrates and maintains all the body's physiologic processes to promote normal growth, development, and maintenance of structure and function. In this dual regulatory system, nervous system actions that are acute and of short-term duration are supplemented by slower and longer hormonal actions, permitting precise control of body functions. Even minute changes are recognized immediately and effective adaptation is accomplished. When all interrelated endocrine processes are running smoothly, adaptive behaviors are observed. However, when one component is disrupted, other parts of the endocrine system, the physiologic mode, and the person as a whole may be affected.

This chapter provides an overview of the endocrine system and includes a description of the component glands and their related functions. Emphasis is placed both on its functions as a single system and its interaction with other body processes, particularly the nervous system, in maintaining physiologic integrity. Knowledge of endocrine structure and functioning serves as a basis for assessing the person's behavior and the significant stimuli influencing that behavior. Illustrations of innate and learned adaptive responses to compensate for ineffective processes related to endocrine function are described. Examples of compromised processes are discussed. Finally, guidelines for planning nursing care by formulating diagnoses, establishing goals, selecting interventions, and evaluating nursing care are described.

► OBJECTIVES

After studying this chapter, the reader will be able to do the following:

1. Describe the complex processes associated with endocrine function.

2. Identify important first-level assessment parameters (behaviors) for the complex processes of endocrine function.

3. List second-level assessment factors (common stimuli) affecting endocrine function.

4. Describe one compensatory process related to the complex processes of endocrine function.

5. Name and describe two situations of compromised processes of endocrine function.

6. Develop a nursing diagnosis, given a situation related to endocrine function.

7. Derive goals for an individual with ineffective endocrine function in a given situation.

8. Describe nursing interventions commonly implemented in situations of ineffective endocrine function.

9. Propose approaches to determine the effectiveness of nursing interventions.

► KEY CONCEPTS DEFINED

Endocrine glands: Small collections of specialized tissue located in widely separated regions of the body that release substances (hormones) into the blood for transport to the site of influence.

Exocrine glands: Specialized tissues that release substances into a duct for transport to the site of influence.

Hormonal stimulation: The initiation of hormone secretion by another hormone.

Hormones: Secretions of endocrine glands that function as chemical messengers with regulatory effects on specific anatomic structures and physiologic processes.

Humoral stimulation: The initiation of hormone secretion by the changing composition of body fluids.

Negative feedback mechanisms: The chief means of regulating blood levels of hormones wherein hormone secretion is triggered by some stimulus; then rising hormone levels inhibit further release.

Neural stimulation: The initiation of hormone secretion by nerve fiber signals.

Stress: The transaction between the environmental demands requiring adaptation and the individual's cognator and regulator coping processes; involves the body's neuroendocrine responses that Selye (1976) termed the general adaptation syndrome (GAS).

Target organ or tissue: The anatomic destination of a hormone wherein physiologic response is produced.

▶ COMPLEX PROCESSES OF ENDOCRINE FUNCTION

The endocrine system is composed of the *endocrine glands,* small and unimpressive collections of specialized tissue located in widely separated regions of the body. Marieb (1994, p. 266) names the endocrine glands as: pituitary, thyroid, parathyroid, adrenal, pineal, thymus, pancreas, the gonads (ovaries or testes), and the hypothalamus (actually part of the nervous system). Although other tissues and organs (for example, the heart, lungs, kidneys, stomach, and small intestines) perform minor endocrine functions, the focus of this chapter will be on the glands listed above.

Initially, distinction is made between exocrine and endocrine glands. *Exocrine glands* produce substances which are released into a duct for transport to the site of action. An example is the exocrine pancreas, which releases digestive enzymes into the duodenum through the pancreatic duct. The exocrine glands are not included in this consideration of endocrine function.

The endocrine glands, on the other hand, secrete one or more *hormones,* chemical messengers with regulatory effects on specific body parts or organs, directly into the bloodstream, where they are transported to, and ultimately influence, other anatomic structures and physiologic processes. The sites of destination for hormones are termed *target organs* or *tissues.*

According to Marieb (1994), the major processes controlled by hormones include "reproduction; growth and development; mobilization of body defenses against stressors; maintenance of electrolyte, water and nutrient balance of the blood; and regulation of cellular metabolism and energy balance" (p. 264). The glands of the endocrine system, with the hormones they release, their principal sites of action, and the processes they influence are outlined in Table 13–1.

Each hormone is unique, yet all hormones have some characteristics in common. In general, endocrine hormones are secreted in small amounts.

TABLE 13–1 ENDOCRINE SYSTEM IN SUMMARY

Endocrine Glands and Hormones	Principal Site of Action	Principal Processes Affected by the Hormone
Anterior Pituitary		
Growth hormone (GH)	General	Growth of body cells, soft tissues, bone, and cartilage
Thyroid-stimulating hormone or thyrotropin (TSH)	Thyroid	Growth and secretory activity of the thyroid gland
Adrenocorticotropin (ACTH)	Adrenal cortex	Growth and secretory activity of the adrenal glands
Follicle-stimulating hormone (FSH)	Ovaries	Development of follicles and secretion of estrogen
	Testes	Development of seminiferous tubules, spermatogenesis
Luteinizing hormone (LH) or interstitial cell stimulating hormone (ICSH)	Ovaries	Ovulation, formation of corpus luteum, secretion of progesterone
	Testes	Growth of male testes, secretion of testosterone
Prolactin (lactogenic hormone) (LTH)	Mammary glands	Secretion of milk, maintenance of corpus luteum and progesterone secretion
Melanocyte (MSH)	Skin	Pigmentation
Posterior Pituitary		Acts as storage area for hypothalamic hormones
Antidiuretic hormone (ADH) (vasopressin)	Kidney arterioles	Reabsorption of water, regulator of osmolarity; blood pressure
Oxytocin (pitocin)	Uterus	Contraction of uterine muscles, facilitates migration of sperm in uterus
Hypothalamus		
Releasing hormones	Anterior pituitary	Controls release of hormones stored in posterior pituitary, released upon nerve impulse from hypothalamus
Thyroid		
Thyroxine (T_4) and triiodothyronine (T_3)	General	Regulates catabolic phase of metabolism, metabolic rate of all cells, and body heat production; influences growth and development; insulin antagonist
Thyrocalcitonin (calcitonin)	Bone	Inhibits bone reabsorption, lowers blood level of calcium and phosphorous
Parathyroids		
Parathyroid hormone (PTH)	Bone	Regulates plasma calcium and phosphorous levels, promotes bone reabsorption, increases absorption of calcium

TABLE 13–1 ENDOCRINE SYSTEM IN SUMMARY (CONT.)

Endocrine Glands and Hormones	Principal Site of Action	Principal Processes Affected by the Hormone
Thymus		
Thymosin	Lymph nodes	Lymphocyte development during childhood
Pineal		
Melatonin	Gonads	Regulation of day and night cycle, sexual maturation
Adrenal Cortex		
Mineralocorticoids (aldosterone)	Kidney	Reabsorption of sodium, elimination of potassium, ammonium, and magnesium; maintenance of volume status
Glucocorticoids	General	Maintains blood glucose level by increasing gluconeogenesis and decreasing rate of glucose utilization by cells
Androgens and estrogens	General	Preadolescent growth spurt of secondary sexual characteristics
Adrenal Medulla		
Epinephrine (adrenalin)	Cardiac muscle, smooth muscle, glands	Stimulator of receptors in physiologic response to stress; emergency functions same as stimulation of sympathetic nervous system: increases blood pressure, cardiac output, blood glucose levels, and myocardial contraction; dilates bronchioles
Norepinephrine	Organs innervated by the ANS	Most potent stimulator of the receptors in the physiologic response to stress, increases peripheral resistance, increases blood pressure
Pancreas		
Islets of Langerhans		
Insulin	General	Lowers blood glucose levels, decreases glycogenolysis, gluconeogenesis, and ketogenesis, increases glycogenesis, decreases protein catabolism
Glucagon	Liver	Mobilizes glycogen stores, raises blood sugar levels, glycogenolysis
Somatostatin	General	Lowers blood sugar by interfering with release of growth hormone and glucagon

TABLE 13–1 ENDOCRINE SYSTEM IN SUMMARY (CONT.)

Endocrine Glands and Hormones	Principal Site of Action	Principal Processes Affected by the Hormone
Ovaries		
Estrogen	Reproductive system	Development of secondary sexual characteristics, repair of the endometrium after menstruation
Progesterone		Development of breast tissue and endometrium, maintains pregnancy, competes with aldosterone at level of renal tubule
Testes		
Testosterone	Reproductive system	Development of male secondary sexual characteristics, normal functioning of male reproductive system

They cause an alteration in cellular activity by either increasing or decreasing the rate of normal metabolic processes. Although the precise change depends on the specific hormone and the cell type, hormones generally have one or more of the following three actions.

1. Plasma membrane permeability (electrical state) is changed.
2. Enzyme function is altered (activation or inactivation).
3. Genetic material is stimulated to produce instructions for making particular enzymes.

The extent of hormonal action varies among hormones. One, such as thyrocalcitonin, may have only regional effects while another, like thyroxine, exerts its effect pervasively over all metabolic processes in the body. *Negative feedback mechanisms* are responsible for the regulation of hormones. Specifically, hormone secretion is initiated by internal or external stimuli. The resulting rise in level of hormone in the body inhibits further hormone release.

Most hormonal action is initiated by one of three categories of stimuli: hormonal, humoral, or neural. *Hormonal stimulation* involves the initiation of hormone release by another hormone. For example, the hypothalamus releases hormones that stimulate the anterior pituitary to release hormones. These, in turn, stimulate other endocrine organs to secrete hormones. *Humoral stimulation* refers to changing levels of certain ions and nutrients in body fluids. Decreasing blood calcium level prompts the release of parathyroid hormone (PTH). As calcium levels increase, the stimulus is diminished. *Neural stimulation* involves nerve fibers in the initiation of hormone release. An example of this is the sympathetic nervous system stimulation of the adrenal medulla to release norepinephrine and epinephrine during periods of stress.

Although each endocrine gland can be viewed as a separate unit with its own independent functions, the various glands also function interdependently. As illustrated previously, the release of hormones from one gland often influences hormonal release from other glands. Similarly, a disturbance in one endocrine gland is likely to incur a disturbance in others. For example, a decrease in the release of thyroid stimulating hormone (TSH) by the anterior pituitary gland causes the thyroid gland to secrete less thyroxin and triiodothyronine.

Earlier mention was made of hormone production in locations other than the major endocrine organs. Several examples of this are provided. Prostaglandins are released from plasma membranes in response to local irritation. Their effects range from vasoconstriction to enhancing blood clotting to increasing the digestive secretions in the stomach. Erythropoietin is produced in the kidney in response to hypoxia. It stimulates the production of red blood cells in the bone marrow. The placenta produces hormones (human chorionic gonadotropin, estrogen, progesterone, human placental lactogen, and relaxin) that maintain pregnancy and prepare for the process of delivery.

A full discussion of the complex structures and functions related to functioning of the major endocrine glands and other endocrine processes and structures is beyond the parameters of this text. The reader is directed to basic anatomy and physiology and specialty nursing science textbooks for a more in-depth presentation.

Assessment of Behavior

As was the case with neurologic function, integrity of endocrine function, or lack thereof, has profound effects on physiologic integrity as a whole and the ultimate functioning of the individual in all of the other modes. In addition, disruptions of the endocrine system are often long term in nature. The role of the nurse in assessment and supportive nursing interventions is to contribute to the promotion of integrity of the whole person over time.

Since endocrine hormones affect the functioning of all the needs and processes inherent in physiologic integrity, the nurse must implement an overall appraisal of the individual's physiologic integrity when carrying out a nursing assessment of adaptive and ineffective behaviors related to endocrine function. The nurse uses the skills of interviewing, observation and inspection, and measurement of internal and external behaviors to gather both subjective and objective data in each of the components of the physiologic mode. The focus is not only on the patient's current status in each area but also on any changes over time noted by the person. Behaviors reflective of endocrine dysfunction in one or more of the physiologic mode components may be evident. The behavior manifested depends on the characteristics of the focal stimuli. The physiologic needs and complex processes identified in the Roy Adaptation

Model provide a framework for assessment of behavior in relation to endocrine functioning.

Oxygenation

In assessing oxygenation as related to endocrine functioning, the nurse considers the person's mental status as well as respiratory and circulatory functioning. Initially, level of consciousness and mental status are noted. The person's predominant mood, memory, degree of alertness, and thought patterns are important indicators of endocrine disruption. Depression, agitation, or psychoses are sometimes evident. Lability of moods and irritability may be associated with excessive ACTH.

Blood pressure and pulses are affected by many hormones and alterations from normal patterns can be indicative of dysfunction. Hypertension can be related to fluid retention associated with excessive ACTH. Increases or decreases in heart rate and rhythm or changes in heart sounds can result from alterations in thyroid hormone. Percussion of the chest can provide evidence of an enlarged heart, sometimes a result of alterations in growth hormone, thyroid hormone, or insulin.

Respirations are assessed for increase or decrease in rate. Tidal volume (affected by insulin) is measured. Changes in voice or speech are important to note. Percussion of the chest can provide evidence of pleural effusion, sometimes evident in alterations in thyroid hormone.

Activity and Rest

Endocrine functioning also affects a person's need for activity and rest. Aspects for assessment include energy level, sleep patterns, coordination and extent of body movements, and the presence of abnormal behaviors. Generalized weakness is commonly reported by people who have alterations in adrenocorticoid, thyroid, insulin, and pituitary hormonal levels.

Nutrition

The person's appetite, amount and type of food intake, and weight changes are all indicators of endocrine functioning associated with nutrition. A decrease in body weight in the absence of voluntary caloric restriction or a marked general increase in exercise suggests the presence of underlying hormonal dysfunction. Truncal obesity can indicate altered levels of cortisol.

Bowel sounds are auscultated; they are affected in disruptions of thyroid hormone or insulin. Palpation of the abdomen can indicate an enlarged liver or ascites, also influenced by the same hormones.

Fluid, Electrolyte, and Acid–Base Balance

Fluid, electrolyte, and acid–base balance is often altered in endocrine dysfunction. Assessment of these complex processes addresses the person's desire for fluid, status of the mucous membranes, and the presence of abnormalities such as diaphoresis and edema. Mineralocorticoids secreted by the adrenal glands play a major role in elimination or retention of body fluid through their influence on the kidney.

Elimination

Elimination, in terms of the amount, characteristics, and patterns of urinary and intestinal output, are assessed relative to endocrine functioning. For example, the volume, timing, and frequency of urinary output is an important indicator of diabetes mellitus. The constituents of urine are important in diagnosing conditions of adrenocorticoid hormonal alteration. The report of tenderness in the kidney area can be indicative of an underlying pathophysiologic problem.

Protection

Relative to the need for protection, assessment data reflecting endocrine functioning relate to both the nonspecific and the specific defense processes—characteristics of the skin, hair, and nails and the body's ability to withstand and recover from infections. Areas of focus include skin characteristics (color, texture, moisture, turgor, and depth), pigmentation distribution, tanning ability, tendency to bruise, presence of acne or straie, and rate of wound healing. The person's hair is assessed for color, amount, texture, distribution over the body, and how easily it can be broken. Nail characteristics, such as growth, texture, and smoothness, reflect endocrine functioning. For example, abnormal behaviors resulting from an elevation of thyroxine are warm, damp, soft-textured skin; silky hair; loosening of the nail from the nail bed; and absence of forehead wrinkling. In situations of excessive glucocorticoid secretion, the skin becomes very friable and capillary fragility increases dramatically. The person bruises easily and purple-red striae can be present on the abdomen, breasts, shoulders, and buttocks.

The inflammatory response is influenced by the glucocorticoids. For example, cortisol is thought to limit both the inflammatory response and the immune response. Any evidence of changes in these aspects is important to note.

The Senses

Endocrine functioning can also be assessed by looking at the status of the person's senses. The alteration of ability in the senses (hearing, touch, vision, and smell) can be indicative of endocrine problems. Hearing loss and decreased night vision can indicate thyroid dysfunction. Exophthalmus and eye lid tremor, retraction, or lag can also be evident in such situations. Retinal problems occur with insulin disruptions.

Other behaviors to note are the presence of abnormal sensations such as pain and intolerance to temperature changes. Diminished sensory responses to stimuli in the lower extremities and neuropathies of the bladder and bowel are associated with decreased insulin production.

Neurologic Function

Assessment of neurologic function is another aspect involved in the first level of assessment related to endocrine function. Level of consciousness and mental function and presence of tremors or seizures are all important indicators. Functioning of the central nervous system is also assessed. For example, tremors of the tongue and extremities may be evident in situations of thyroid disruption. Level of consciousness is affected by thyroid hormone, aldosterone, parathyroid hormone, and insulin. In hyperthyroidism, actions of the central nervous system increase, resulting in nervousness, restlessness, decreased attention span, and fatigue. For people with epilepsy, seizures worsen. In situations of hyperparathyroidism, changes in mental function can range from fatigue and loss of initiative to acute psychoses.

Structural Development

Other assessment areas to consider involve the structural development of the body's skeletal system, soft tissues, and organs. The body's skeletal structure is affected profoundly by levels of growth hormone, thyroxine, and triiodothyronine. Therefore, assessment of endocrine functioning considers the person's skeletal and soft-tissue development in relation to age, predicted growth, and body proportions. For example, decreased linear bone growth is associated with decreased thyroxine levels. An increased rate of linear bone growth, with premature closure of the epiphyseal centers and altered body proportions, can be related to decreased levels of androgen or growth hormone. Other indicators of growth hormone dysfunction are the development of a progressive underbite or space between the lower teeth.

An increase and redistribution of soft tissue is associated with high levels of adrenocorticoid hormones. In cases of an increase in thyroid hormones, the thyroid gland is noted to be larger, tender, and sometimes asymmetrical in shape. Facial appearance is an important factor associated with thyroid or cortisol problems. In fact, many endocrine disorders have associated facial characteristics that are often diagnostic keys to the underlying problem.

Similarly, the growth and development of the person's reproductive structures and their related functioning is dependent on adequate endocrine hormones. Alterations in the size and shape of genitalia, libido, secondary sexual characteristics, onset of menarche and menopause, and penile erectile functioning are indicators of endocrine functioning. For example, reduced output of follicle stimulating hormone (FSH) and luteinizing hormone (LH) can result in breast and uterine atrophy in females and reduced beard and testes size in males.

Other Adaptive Modes

There may be evidence of endocrine dysfunction in one or more of the other adaptive modes. Self-concept is often affected by disruptions in cortisol, testosterone, thyroid hormone, and insulin levels. This situation may, in turn, have an impact on role function and interdependent relationships.

Laboratory Tests

Because of the multiple functions of the endocrine system, various tests are used to determine whether disruption of this regulating system is present and, if so, to help in identifying the factors influencing the person's ineffective behaviors. These tests are of two general types. The first are tests involving direct measurement of the concentration of various hormones or antibodies specific to chemical groups or conformations of hormones in the plasma, blood, or urine. Examples of these are bioassay of thyroid hormone and chemical assay of cortisol and PTH levels. The second are tests in which indirect methods of measuring hormonal concentration are used, such as the urine test for 17 ketogenic steroids and the thyroid stimulation test.

A careful analysis of the person's behavior in each of these areas is essential as the basis of a realistic, individualized nursing care plan. The nurse must determine if a particular behavior is adaptive, requires supportive interventions, or is ineffective, necessitating management of stimuli. This judgment is made by considering each behavior in light of the indicators of effective adaptation. Just as the foundation of a house serves as a basis for the rest of the structure, the data gathered and decisions made at this stage of assessment determine the merit and success of the subsequent nursing care plan.

Assessment of Stimuli

The second component of the assessment of the complex process associated with endocrine function is the identification of the focal, contextual, and residual stimuli influencing the behaviors observed in the first level of assessment. As evident in the previous discussion, the focal stimulus for the observed behaviors was primarily compromised processes of endocrine function. Other factors that exert an influence, both in situations of compromised processes and in adaptive situations, include developmental stage, family history, ethnicity, environmental conditions, medical interventions, the person's knowledge level, and the integrity of other modes. As with the other needs and complex processes, compensatory processes are also important considerations.

Developmental Stage

The person's developmental stage is an important factor for consideration when assessing stimuli related to endocrine function. Certainly, there are normal developmental changes that occur in each of the developmental phases. At puberty, there is marked development of the secondary sexual characteristics, for example. In addition, many endocrine disruptions tend to become evident at certain ages. Although type II diabetes mellitus may occur at any age, its onset is usually after age 30.

As Hancock (1997, p. 1083) pointed out, most endocrine glands show altered function with advancing age. In fact, endocrine disorders are most common in persons 40 to 50 years of age. Anatomically, atrophy of glands occurs (for example, the pituitary), but the significance of this is not clear. In other situations, such as that of the ovary, the target tissue fails to respond to the stimulating hormone. Most clinical findings are nonspecific, however, and as Hancock (1997, p. 1084) observed, almost all early clinical findings can be attributed to aging, if the inclination exists.

Family History

Because of the hereditary nature of some disruptions in endocrine function (type II diabetes mellitus, for example), it is important to inquire about the health patterns of other family members. In situations where endocrine disruptions have been present for other family members, it is important to explore the person's understanding of what these situations entailed.

Ethnicity

The person's ethnicity is an important consideration in the second level of assessment of endocrine function. For example, type I diabetes mellitus is more common among whites than African Americans. Type II is more common in women than men and in African Americans, Hispanics, and Native Americans than whites (Moriarty, 1997, p. 1147).

Environmental Conditions

Contextual stimuli, such as external environmental conditions, frequently augment the effects of the focal stimuli. For example, the internal temperature changes noted in dysfunction of the thyroid gland may be increased by changes in environmental temperature and humidity. Similarly, the lassitude evident in hypothyroidism may be accentuated by a socially impoverished milieu.

Health Care Interventions

Medical and nursing interventions designed to assist the person in adapting to a disease process contribute additional contextual stimuli. For example, medications are one group of stimuli that tend to compound difficulties in adapting. It is not unusual for a person to be receiving an antibiotic, a corticosteroid, and an analgesic all at the same time for an endocrine-related condition. Each of these drugs has a desired effect on the focal stimulus (glandular dysfunction); however, they may have associated adverse effects which affect other endocrine glands and neuroendocrine integrating mechanisms.

Other interventions related to the treatment of ineffective behaviors in another mode can have a negative impact upon endocrine function. These include diet, exercise, availability of fluids, and activity level.

Surgical intervention is often an approach selected to deal with disruption of endocrine function. Certainly, this creates a significant stimulus for the person that requires adaptation. The surgical process, if utilized, is an important consideration for all steps of the nursing process and may, for a time, be the focus of a significant amount of nursing activity.

Knowledge Level

In situations of endocrine disruption, the person's knowledge level about the condition is an important stimulus. This is particularly evident in the case of diabetes mellitus. Does the person understand the interrelationship of diet, exercise, and insulin and know the symptoms of imbalance and the actions to take if such occurs? Is the importance of consistent and conscientious monitoring of blood glucose levels understood?

The individual's level of understanding about the situation is important in any disruption of the endocrine system. Frequently, medications will be used to treat the condition. It is important that the person have a thorough understanding of the actions, interactions, and side effects of the substances that are being consumed.

Integrity of Other Modes

Previously mentioned were the potential behaviors that may be observed in situations of endocrine disruption, particularly in relation to the person's self-concept. It is easy to understand how disruptions in endocrine functioning could contribute to problems in role function and interdependence, as well.

What is not so clear, although there is increasing evidence to indicate a linkage, is the influence that psychosocial disruptions have on physiologic functioning and on the endocrine system, in particular. For this reason, it is important to identify situations of a psychosocial nature that could be having an effect on the person physiologically.

► COMPENSATORY ADAPTIVE RESPONSES

Viewed as an adaptive system (see Chap. 2), the person has innate and acquired ways of responding to the changing environment. Further, Roy conceptualizes these complex adaptive dynamics as the coping processes of the regulator and cognator subsystems. One particular illustration of regulator compensatory abilities associated with endocrine function relates to the neuroendocrine stress response.

Although both the cognator and regulator subsystems determine the body's total response to environmental stimuli, that part of the adaptation response associated with endocrine function is located within the regulator coping processes. The major parts of the regulator subsystem are the neural, chemical, and endocrine components. All three are activated in response to a major stimulus. The perception–psychomotor part is considered neural in nature and this overlaps with the cognator coping processes. It serves to connect the two processes, thereby allowing physiologic response to influence cognitive responses and vice versa. The remaining two components of the regulator coping processes, chemical and endocrine responses, act together to regulate the body's physiologic response to stress.

Stress was defined by Roy and McLeod (1981) as the transaction between the environmental demands requiring adaptation and the individual's cognator and regulator coping processes. The stress response is the process that results from any physical or psychological stimulus disturbing the adaptive state (Andrews & Roy, 1986). The term *stressor* is viewed as synonymous with Roy's notion of the focal stimulus.

Selye (1976) proposed that the body's physiologic response can take two forms. The first response form, the local adaptation syndrome (LAS), occurs when the body is confronted by a local stimulus and only one organ or part of the body reacts. One example is the inflammatory response or immune response. The neuroendocrine mechanisms are not activated during this process. The second response pattern, the general adaptation syndrome (GAS), occurs whenever a collective of body systems is threatened or the person undergoes prolonged periods of stress. The GAS is a neuroendocrine response involving primarily the sympathetic branch of the autonomic nervous system and the pituitary, adrenal, and thyroid glands. The body's neuroendocrine responses to stress (GAS) in which the hypothalamus and medulla oblongata are activated in response to a sensory stimulus, such as severe pain, are outlined in Figure 13–1.

Selye (1976) suggested that both the GAS and the LAS develop in three distinct stages. First is the alarm reaction stage, when the whole body's neuroendocrine defenses against the stimulus, regardless of whether it is bacteria or verbal abuse, are alerted and mobilized to protect the body. The second stage of resistance is when the body attempts to cope by limiting the stimulus' effects to the smallest possible area. The last stage is the stage of exhaustion, in which the body's adaptive ability to resist the stressor becomes exhausted.

The phases vary in duration and intensity in relation to the strength of the stimulus that initiated the stress response. For example, a brief, sudden, unexpected noise may elicit only very brief unmeasurable responses reflective of the alarm phase. The stress response does not continue into the resistance or exhaustion phases. On the other hand, a major surgical operation may produce more measurable, prolonged responses of the second and third phases.

In addition to regulator compensatory responses, the cognator subsystem plays an important role in adaptation relative to endocrine function. A person with diabetes mellitus provides an example of how a person with a compromised process of metabolism can learn to adapt and compensate. Through education and practice, individuals learn about the important balance among diet, exercise, and insulin. They learn how to regulate each and can become very effective in maintaining an appropriate balance. They also learn about complications that occur with imbalance, and what to do to intervene at an early stage to avoid more serious complications. Through cognator compensatory processes, many people with diabetes are able to adapt effectively and maintain physiologic and psychosocial integrity.

► COMPROMISED PROCESSES OF ENDOCRINE FUNCTION

Ineffective endocrine behaviors are most commonly caused by compromised processes of endocrine function, frequently associated with the interruption or dysfunction of the negative feedback mechanisms. Hancock (1997, p. 1075) identified four sources of such disruption.

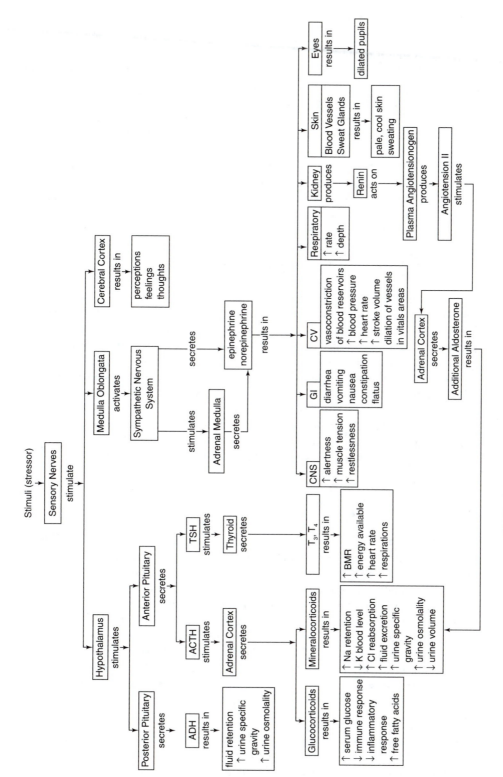

FIGURE 13–1. Neuroendocrine mechanisms response to stressful stimuli.

1. A gland develops the ability for function autonomously; the negative feedback mechanisms are no longer influential. Hyperfunction develops. An example of this situation is hyperthyroidism.
2. A gland is absent or defective for congenital, acquired, or surgical reasons; thus, it no longer adequately responds to stimulation. Hormonal deficits occur. Surgical intervention for a glandular tumor can cause such complications.
3. Cells of target tissues or organs increase or decrease in their sensitivity to hormonal stimulation. Hypo- or hyperfunction develops. For example, diabetes mellitus is considered to be related to a loss of cell sensitivity to insulin.
4. Prolonged suppression of glandular function by administration of its hormone product (such as steroids from the adrenal cortex) can result in acute deficit upon its withdrawal.

As with other cells of the body, those of the endocrine glands are susceptible to trauma, vascular interference, autoimmune disorders, infection, and neoplasm. The functional and structural changes in endocrine glands precipitated by these stimuli take similar forms regardless of the specific gland affected.

Hormonal disturbances are characterized by either hyposecretion or hypersecretion of a hormone, or an imbalance between or among hormones. Each of these situations is characterized by particular physiologic symptoms and behaviors. Exploration of the specific ramifications associated with each endocrine disorder is beyond the scope of this text. The reader is encouraged to consult a pathophysiology resource for specific descriptions of the physiologic disruptions associated with endocrine function.

▶ PLANNING NURSING CARE

In applying the nursing process to the complex processes of endocrine function, the nurse makes a careful assessment of behaviors and stimuli. In assessing factors influencing endocrine function, regulator and cognator effectiveness in initiating compensatory processes is considered. Based on this thorough first- and second-level assessment, the nurse formulates a nursing diagnosis, sets goals, selects interventions, and evaluates care.

Whereas stress was previously identified as a compensatory process, when it remains unresolved, stress becomes a compromised process. This compromised process affects the person as a whole. Nursing and related literature contributes to understanding the process of stress and its effects.

Nursing Diagnosis

Development of nursing diagnoses associated with endocrine regulation is accomplished in the same way as in the other areas of the physiologic mode. One method involves a statement of the person's behaviors together with the influencing stimuli. Another method makes use of summary labels. Nursing diagnoses may reflect either adaptive or ineffective behaviors. In the former case, a sample nursing diagnosis states, "Normal development of secondary sexual characteristics due to effective endocrine functioning."

In the case of ineffective behaviors, a multitude of nursing diagnoses may result. The endocrine system is closely interrelated with other body systems; therefore, a disturbance in one endocrine regulating mechanism is likely to precipitate disturbances in others. Problems commonly occur in one or several of the following areas: cardiac output, comfort, safety, nutrition, self-concept, protection, activity and rest, elimination, coping abilities, compliance, fluid volume balance, knowledge level, cognitive processes, and stress tolerance. A nursing diagnosis illustrating ineffective behaviors is "Intolerance to heat, increased appetite with weight loss, frequent diarrhea, fine hand tremors, weakness, clumsiness, fatigability, and nervousness associated with thyroid hyperactivity."

It is also possible to construct a nursing diagnosis using a summary label that captures clusters of behaviors. This method is used by experienced nurses to communicate significant amounts of information in one phrase. As identified in Chapter 3, there are five indicators of positive adaptation identified in the Roy Adaptation Model.

1. Effective hormonal regulation of metabolic and body processes.
2. Effective hormonal regulation of reproductive development.
3. Stable patterns of closed-loop negative-feedback hormone system.
4. Stable patterns of cyclical hormone rhythms.
5. Effective coping strategies for stress.

Likewise, five commonly recurring adaptation problems are identified.

1. Ineffective hormone regulation
2. Ineffective reproductive development
3. Instability of hormone system loops
4. Instability of internal cyclical rhythms
5. Stress

A nursing diagnosis stated with the use of a summary label reads, "Instability of menstrual cycle related to dietary restriction and excessive exercise." (This situation is frequently evident in young women engaged in competitive sports.) Both the behavior and the stimuli stated in this example of a nursing diagnosis communicate a wealth of information to an individual experienced in adaptation problems associated with endocrine function. However, for the inexperienced person, the more detailed expression of behaviors and stimuli is more meaningful.

The use of a summary label when more than one mode is affected by the same stimulus is often an effective way of communicating a cluster of behaviors. For example, the concept of "stress" might be such a diagnosis—one word captures a multitude of behaviors and stimuli. The diagnosis statement could be "stress associated with too many demanding commitments and too little time."

In Table 13–2, the Roy model nursing diagnostic categories for the complex processes of endocrine functioning are shown with the one related nursing diagnosis label approved by the North American Nursing Diagnosis Association (Rantz & LeMone, 1997).

In situations of endocrine dysfunction, it is tempting for the nurse to focus on the pathophysiology involved rather than the behaviors and stimuli that are related to what is happening physiologically in the person's body. Knowledge of pathophysiology is important to assist the nurse in the identification of behaviors and stimuli related to endocrine dysfunction, but with the framework that the Roy Adaptation Model provides, behaviors and stimuli pertain to the person's behavioral manifestation of the problem and the factors that appear to be causing it. In turn, the nursing diagnosis also focuses on behaviors and stimuli rather than on the pathophysiologic conditions(s). A well-written nursing diagnosis aids in setting priorities and establishing direction for the next step of the nursing process, goal setting.

Goal Setting

Each step of the nursing process focuses on the individual's behavior, the stimuli influencing that behavior, or both. With the nursing diagnosis, the statement developed included both the behavior and the stimulus. With the goal setting step, the focus is on the person's behavior. Each goal identifies a behavior that is to be addressed.

Many endocrine dysfunctions have a chronic as well as an acute phase. Thus, the goal setting process includes both long- and short-term goals, each of which states the behavior of focus, the change expected, and the time frame in which the goal is to be achieved.

The following statements provide examples of possible goals for a person with activity intolerance related to a decrease in metabolic rate secondary to hypothyroidism. "Throughout the next several days, the person will develop a list of factors that increase fatigue." "Within 1 week, the person will

TABLE 13–2   NURSING DIAGNOSTIC CATEGORIES FOR ENDOCRINE FUNCTION

Positive Indicators of Adaptation	Common Adaptation Problems	NANDA Diagnostic Labels
• Effective hormonal regulation of metabolic and body processes	• Ineffective hormone regulation	• Altered growth and development
• Effective hormonal regulation of reproductive development	• Ineffective reproductive development	
• Stable patterns of closed-loop negative-feedback hormone system	• Instability of hormone system loops	
• Stable patterns of cyclical hormone rhythms	• Instability of internal cyclical rhythms	
• Effective coping strategies for stress	• Stress	

demonstrate an increase in activity tolerance, decreased signs of fatigue and dyspnea on exertion, and will independently perform activities of daily living." Each of these goals indicates the behavior of focus, the change desired, and the associated time frame.

Consider a situation where an 11-year-old boy demonstrates the behaviors of excessive urination, excessive hunger and thirst, rapid weight loss, and weakness and is diagnosed with type I diabetes mellitus. He requires a daily injection of insulin, balanced carefully with diet and exercise, to control metabolic processes. Goals related to the situation could be "Within 1 week, the boy will select foods according to the guidelines recommended by the American Diabetes Association"; or "Within 2 weeks, the child will demonstrate the ability to do his own blood glucose testing"; or "Within 1 month, he will be able to calculate, prepare, and administer his own insulin."

In order to be effective in guiding the progress of the individual, goals must be established in collaboration with the person involved. As with each step of the nursing process, the individual must be an active participant, where possible, to insure that accurate and relevant information is obtained, that it is interpreted appropriately into nursing diagnoses, and that achievable and relevant goals are established. This is the only way that interventions that will assist in achieving effective adaptation can be determined.

The identification of nursing interventions is the next step of the nursing process as described in the Roy Adaptation Model.

Intervention

The intervention step of the nursing process according to the Roy Adaptation Model focuses on the stimuli affecting the behavior identified in the goal setting step. The intervention step is thus the management of stimuli and this involves either altering, increasing, decreasing, removing, or maintaining them.

In the previous situation involving the boy recently diagnosed with type I diabetes mellitus, the stimuli affecting the observed behaviors involves the balance between diet, exercise, and the action of insulin within the body. Thus, interventions would be directed to these areas of influence.

Dietary modifications for the diabetic person address optimum nutrition, maintenance of ideal body weight, control of the plasma glucose level, prevention of complications of the disease, and individualizing the meal pattern to accommodate the person's lifestyle. Exercise is an important consideration that can help keep the manifestations of diabetes under control. The intricacies of insulin administration (concentration; modifications; onset, peak, and duration of action; complications; administration; and monitoring and control by glucose testing) involve the development of knowledge, skills, and attitudes, an educational challenge for both the individual and the nurse.

All of the above interventions focus on stimuli (diet, exercise, levels of insulin) that are causing the ineffective behaviors for the person. As with many other endocrine function disturbances, the problems tend to be long-term challenges for the individual. Many interventions relate to the person's knowledge level and understanding about the problem to equip them to make the necessary adaptations on an ongoing basis. Knowledge about crisis situations associated with acute episodes is also very important. The young man with diabetes requires knowledge about many serious acute complications such as hyperosmolar nonketotic coma, diabetic ketoacidosis, hypoglycemia, and infection. The same holds true for many other situations of endocrine disruption. It is not within the parameters of this text to explore endocrine disorders in more depth. The reader is referred to pathophysiology resources and nursing practice textbooks for further information.

Evaluation

Evaluation involves judging the effectiveness of the nursing interventions in relation to the person's adaptive behavior, that is, whether the person has attained the behavior stated in the goals. The nursing interventions would be identified as effective if the person's behavior is in accordance with the stated goal. If the goal has not been achieved, the nurse identifies alternative interventions or approaches by reassessing the behavior and stimuli and continuing with the other steps of the nursing process.

In considering the previously identified goal, "Within 2 weeks, the child will demonstrate the ability to do his own blood glucose and urine testing," the nurse, in evaluating the effectiveness of the interventions would, within 2 weeks, have the boy demonstrate his ability to do glucose and urine testing. Successful demonstration of the processes would indicate that the intervention (probably an educational process) was effective. Similar evaluation could be conducted with respect to the ability to administer insulin to himself.

It is important to recognize that the nursing process and the six steps are ongoing, simultaneous, and overlapping. Although they have been separated and dealt with in an artificially linear manner for discussion purposes, often intervention can be occurring at the same time as first- and second-level assessment is proceeding. Likewise, evaluation occurs on an ongoing basis, being held in mind even when nursing diagnoses are being established and as goals are being formulated.

► SUMMARY

This chapter has focused on the application of the Roy Adaptation Model to the complex physiologic processes associated with endocrine function. An overview of these basic life processes was provided along with the identification of parameters of assessment behaviors and stimuli. Illustration of innate and learned adaptive compensatory responses related to endocrine function were described and examples of compromised processes were provided. Finally, guidelines for planning nursing care through the formulation of nursing diagnoses, goals, and interventions were explored and evaluation of nursing care was described.

The following chapter turns to the self-concept–group identity modes. This mode and the remaining two modes are directly influenced by adaptation in the physiologic mode and, in turn, disruptions in the other modes have physiologic ramifications.

► EXERCISES FOR APPLICATION

1. Recall a recent stressful situation in your life, perhaps an examination or a car accident. Using the behavioral assessment categories in this chapter, list the behaviors you exhibited which reflected activation of your neuroendocrine mechanisms.

2. Create a table with three columns: major endocrine glands, behaviors associated with hyperactivity, and behaviors associated with hypoactivity. Use a pathophysiology or nursing textbook to complete the columns.

Example:

Endocrine Gland	Hypersecretion	Hyposecretion
Anterior pituitary—growth hormone	Giantism—proportional accelerated linear growth Acromegaly—bony and soft tissue growth of extremities	Midgets—very short with adult proportions Dwarfism—normal trunk size with short extremities

► ASSESSMENT OF UNDERSTANDING

Questions

1. In Column B, name the hormone(s) that stimulate(s) the process identified in Column A. In Column C, identify the endocrine gland that secretes it.

Column A Process	Column B Hormone	Column C Secreting Gland
(a) growth of body cells, soft tissue and cartilage	_____	_____
(b) reabsorption of water, regulator of osmolarity, blood pressure	_____	_____
(c) regulates the catabolic phase of metabolism, metabolic rate of all cells, and body heat production	_____	_____

(d) regulates plasma
calcium and phos-
phorous levels _____ _____

(e) reabsorption of
sodium; elimination
of potassium, ammo-
nium, and magnesium _____ _____

(f) emergency response to
stressful situations similar
to sympathetic nervous
system _____ _____

2. Which of the following physiologic components are important areas for assessment of behaviors related to endocrine function? Check the ones that apply.

(a) _____ oxygenation
(b) _____ activity and rest
(c) _____ nutrition
(d) _____ fluid, electrolyte, acid–base balance
(e) _____ elimination
(f) _____ protection
(g) _____ senses
(h) _____ neurologic function

3. Although the focal stimulus in situations of endocrine dysfunction is frequently a pathophysiologic problem, give an example of a situation where disruption in normal processes is caused by another factor.

4. An important regulator compensatory process is termed "the stress response." The body's physiologic response takes two forms: LAS and GAS. Label the following statements according to the form (LAS or GAS) they describe.

(a) _____ stimulus is localized
(b) _____ neuroendocrine response
(c) _____ collective body systems are threatened
(d) _____ only one organ reacts
(e) _____ periods of stress are prolonged

5. No matter what the source of endocrine disruption, the resulting structural and functional changes take similar forms. The observed behaviors are a ramification of either _____ or _____ of the particular hormone.

Situation

Mr. J. is a 66-year-old male who has been recently diagnosed with type II diabetes mellitus. Assessment revealed that he is experiencing excessive urination and is very thirsty. He is very weak and feels light-headed. He states that he is hungry all the time. Since his diagnosis of diabetes, Mr. J. has been following a "special diet"; however, he recently has had several social engagements where he overindulged. Because he has been feeling tired and weak, he has forgone his regular morning and evening walks. When asked about his blood glucose level, he commented that he has not tested it lately since he ran out of supplies. Mr. J. has never attended an educational program for diabetics.

6. Formulate two nursing diagnoses for this situation focusing on specific behaviors and using a summary label.

7. Develop a short-term and a long-term goal statement for Mr. J.

8. Identify two interventions that will address the goals that you developed in item 7.

9. What would be the behavior that would indicate that Mr. J. had achieved the goals developed in item 7?

Feedback

1.

Column B	Column C
Hormone	**Secreting Gland**
(a) growth hormone	anterior pituitary
(b) antidiuretic hormone	posterior pituitary
(c) thyroxine and triiodothyronine	thyroid
(d) parathyroid hormone	parathyroids
(e) mineralocorticoids	adrenal cortex
(f) epinephrine	adrenal medulla

2. all of them

3. Examples:
    Failure to ovulate caused by the administration of birth control pills.
    Menstrual irregularity attributed to strenuous exercise and rigid weight control.
    Unnatural strength and physical development related to the ingestion of steroids.

4. (a) LAS
    (b) GAS
    (c) GAS
    (d) LAS
    (e) GAS

5. hyposecretion, hypersecretion

6. Example of nursing diagnosis: Excessive urination, thirst, weakness, and lightheadedness related to imbalance in diet, exercise, and insulin levels. Hyperglycemia related to inadequate understanding of insulin regulation in relation to diet and exercise.

7. Example of short-term goal: Within 1 hour, Mr. J. will have a blood glucose level within the acceptable range.
Example of long-term goal: Within 1 week, Mr. J. will be regularly monitoring his blood glucose levels and recording them on a chart together with an account of his dietary intake and exercise.

8. The short-term intervention would involve obtaining a blood glucose level and responding appropriately to the situation. If hyperglycemic, he may require fluid replacement and the restoration of control using diet, exercise, and medication. The long-term intervention would involve his attendance at a diabetic instruction class to enhance his knowledge, skill, and commitment to regulating his diet and exercise.

9. Evaluation for the short-term goal would involve retesting of blood glucose levels to determine whether they have responded appropriately and are now within normal limits. Evaluation for the long-term goal would be a chart indicating that Mr. J. was indeed carefully monitoring his diet, exercise, and blood glucose level.

▶ REFERENCES

Andrews, H. A., & Roy, C. (1986). *Essentials of the Roy Adaptation Model.* E. Norwalk, CT: Appleton-Century-Crofts.

Hancock, M. R. (1997). Nursing assessment and common endocrine interventions. In Burrell, L. O., Gerlach, M. J. M., & Pless, B. S. (Eds.), *Adult nursing: Acute and community care* (2nd ed., pp. 1074–1084). Stamford, CT: Appleton & Lange.

Marieb, E. N. (1994). *Essentials of human anatomy and physiology* (4th ed.). Redwood City, CA: Benjamin/Cummings.

Moriarty, D. M. (1997). Disorders of the endocrine pancreas: Diabetes mellitus. In Burrell, L. O., Gerlach, M. J. M., & Pless, B. S. (Eds.), *Adult nursing: Acute and community care* (2nd ed., pp. 1143–1196). Stamford, CT: Appleton & Lange.

Rantz, M. J., & LeMone, P. (Eds.). (1997). *Classification of nursing diagnoses. Proceedings of the 12th conference NANDA.* Glendale, CA: CINAHL Information Systems.

Roy, Sr. C., & McLeod, D. (1981). Theory of the person as an adaptive system. In Roy, Sr. C., & Roberts, S. L. (Eds.), *Theory construction in nursing: An adaptation model* (pp. 49–60). Englewood Cliffs, NJ: Prentice Hall.

Seyle, H. (1976). The stress of life (2nd ed.). New York: McGraw-Hill.

14

SELF-CONCEPT–GROUP IDENTITY MODE

The adaptive mode pertaining to the personal aspect of human systems is termed the self-concept mode for the individual and the group identity mode for collective human systems. These major concepts have been developed in further detail to guide assessment of the effectiveness of adaptation from both individual and group perspectives.

The self-concept mode for the individual focuses specifically on the psychological and spiritual aspects of the human system. The basic need underlying the self-concept mode has been identified as *psychic and spiritual integrity*—the need to know who one is so that one can be or exist with a sense of unity and meaning. Psychic integrity, and the related dimension of spiritual integrity, are basic to health. Adaptation problems in this area may interfere with the person's ability to heal or to do what is necessary to maintain other aspects of health. It is important for the nurse to have knowledge about the self-concept mode in order to assess behaviors and stimuli influencing the person's self-concept.

Self-concept is defined as the composite of beliefs and feelings that a person holds about himself or herself at a given time. Formed from internal perceptions and perceptions of others, self-concept directs behavior. The self-concept mode is viewed in the Roy Adaptation Model as having two components: the *physical self*, including body sensation and body image; and the *personal self*, comprised of self-consistency, self-ideal, and moral-ethical-spiritual self. Some examples of these components include the statement, "I look like I haven't slept in a week!"—a behavioral statement related to body image. The statement, "I know I can figure out how to fix this lamp," illustrates self-ideal behavior.

The group identity mode as related to groups is analogous to the self-concept mode for the individual. It reflects how people in groups perceive themselves based on environmental feedback. The group identity mode is comprised of interpersonal relationships, group self-image, social milieu, and culture. The basic need underlying the group identity mode is termed *identity integrity*—the ability of group members to relate to each other in a manner that indicates awareness of group identity, effectively and efficiently maintains and enhances the identity of the group, and moves it toward goal achievement.

This chapter provides an overview of the self-concept–group identity mode, and the integrated processes of developing self and focusing self associated with psychic and spiritual integrity. For collective human systems, the integrated process associated with identity integrity is shared identity. Compensatory adaptive processes related to self-concept–group identity are discussed and examples of associated compromised processes are explored for both individuals and groups. Finally, the chapter provides guidelines for planning nursing care by formulating diagnoses, establishing goals, selecting interventions, and evaluating nursing care.

► OBJECTIVES

After studying this chapter, the reader will be able to do the following:

1. Describe the self-concept–group identity mode according to the Roy Adaptation Model.

2. Identify important first-level assessment parameters (behaviors) for the self-concept–group identity mode.

3. Identify second-level assessment factors (stimuli) that influence the self-concept–group identity mode.

4. Describe one compensatory process related to self-concept and group identity.

5. Name and describe two situations of compromised processes of self-concept and group identity.

6. Develop a nursing diagnosis, given a situation related to self-concept–group identity.

7. Derive goals for a given situation illustrating ineffective self-concept and group identity.

8. Describe nursing interventions commonly implemented in situations of ineffective self-concept and group identity.

9. Propose approaches to determine the effectiveness of nursing interventions.

► KEY CONCEPTS DEFINED

Anxiety: A painful uneasiness of mind due to a vague, nonspecific threat; threatens a person's sense of self-consistency.

Body image: How one views oneself physically and one's view of personal appearance.

Body sensation: How one feels and experiences the self as a physical being.

Community: A group of persons with some common bond, whether living near one another or not, such as, having the same religious beliefs; or coming from the same country of origin.

Coping strategies: The person's habitual responses used to maintain adaptation; the ways the person functions to maintain integrity in everyday life and in times of stress.

Developing self: Growing self-perceptions based on physical, psychological, and cognitive development, and perceptions of others' reactions to self. These experiences are cognitively organized into self-schemas.

Focusing self: The process of being in touch with the physical and personal self in a way that surfaces hope, energy, continuity, meaning, purpose, and pride to be an individual self within the whole human community; awareness of self, consciousness, and meaning are transformed in person and environment integration, which the person focuses on by way of thinking and feeling.

Group culture: The group's agreed upon expectations, including values, goals, and norms for relating.

Group identity: Shared relations, goals, and values, which create a social milieu and culture, a group self-image, and coresponsibiity for goal achievement.

Identity integrity: In collective human systems, the basic need of the group identity mode; implies the honesty, soundness, and completeness of the group members' identification with the group; involves process of sharing identity and goals.

Life closure: The process through which a person resolves the issue of the meaning of one's life and accepts the reality of eventual death.

Low morale: The state in a group that results from the challenges to the usual tendency toward cohesiveness and failure of the processes for shared identity and evident in low energy for activities related to group goals or relationships.

Moral-ethical-spiritual self: That aspect of the personal self which includes a belief system and an evaluation of who one is in relation to the universe.

Personal self: The individual's appraisal of one's own characteristics, expectations, values, and worth, including self-consistency, self-ideal, and the moral-ethical-spiritual self.

Physical self: The person's appraisal of one's own physical being, including physical attributes, functioning, sexuality, health and illness states, and appearance; includes the components of body sensation and body image.

Psychic and spiritual integrity: On the individual level, the basic need of the self-concept mode; the need to know who one is so that one can be or exist with a sense of unity, meaning, and purposefulness in the universe.

Schema: The structures for encoding and representing information.

Self-concept: The composite of beliefs and feelings that one holds about oneself at a given time; formed from internal perceptions and perceptions of others' reactions.

Self-consistency: The part of the personal self component which strives to maintain a consistent self-organization and to avoid disequilibrium; an organized system of ideas about self.

Self-esteem: The individual's perception of self-worth that is a pervasive aspect of the personal self.

Self-ideal: That aspect of the personal self-component which relates to what the person would like to be or is capable of doing.

Self-schema: Cognitive generalizations about the self derived from past experience that organize and guide the processing of the self-related information contained in an individual's interactions with others.

Sexual dysfunction: Ineffective sexual behavior related to physical or psychological factors; demonstrated by decreased sense of sexual self or aggressive sexual behavior.

Shared identity: The process whereby the members of the group come to common perceptions of the environment, common cognitive and feeling orientations, and shared goals and values.

► SELF-CONCEPT–GROUP IDENTITY PROCESSES

For the individual, self-concept is defined as the composite of beliefs and feelings that a person holds about self at a given time (Driever, 1976). Formed from internal perceptions and perceptions of others' reactions, self-concept is influential in directing behavior. The question, "Who am I?" is so central that the sense of self plays a major part in everything a person does. The self is considered the image that the individual has of oneself as a physical, social, and spiritual or moral being (Gecas, 1982).

In the Roy Adaptation Model, the individual aspect of the self-concept mode is viewed as having two subareas, the physical self and the personal self. The *physical self* includes two components, body sensation and body image. It includes the person's appraisal of physical being, including physical being, including physical attributes, functioning, sexuality, health and illness states, and appearence. *Body sensation* applies to the ability to feel and to experience oneself as a physical being. Statements such as, "I feel sick," "I feel exhausted," or "I feel great!" are examples of body sensation behaviors. *Body image* applies to how one views oneself physically and one's appearance. "I need to lose some weight," "I feel I'm rather attractive," or "I'm not very physically fit," are all behavioral statements related to body image. Figure 14–1 is a diagrammatic representation of the self-concept with two subareas and their components. Body sensation and body image are depicted as the two component parts of the physical self.

The personal self is viewed as having three components: self-consistency, self-ideal, and moral-ethical-spiritual self. *Self-consistency* refers to an organized system of ideas about self. The mind works to make all the ideas in the self system seem to be consistent with, or fit together with, one another. Lecky (1961) identified that through the need for self-consistency, the person strives to maintain a coherent self-organization and avoid disequilibrium. Behavior related to self-consistency can be observed in a person's response to a situation and in verbal statements. Examples are, "I'm a person who is always

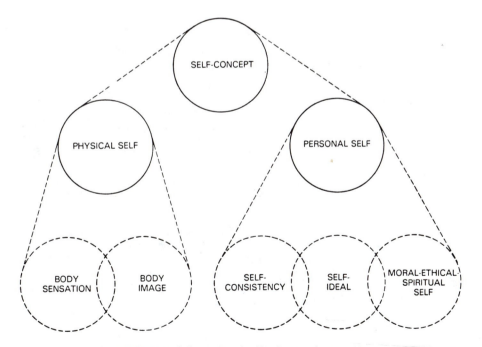

FIGURE 14–1. Self-concept mode with subareas and components.

on time," or "I'm really anxious about my surgery." *Self-ideal* relates to what one would like to be or is capable of doing. "I want to be a nurse," or "I would like to be able to do better in French class," are statements manifesting a person's self-ideal. The *moral-ethical-spiritual self* includes the belief system and an evaluation of who one is in relation to the universe. It is evidenced by such statements as, "I believe that any taking of human life is wrong," or "I believe that my suffering has some part to play in this world." These components will be explored further in developing an understanding of the processes and assessment related to self-concept.

Group identity refers to shared relations, goals, and values that create a social milieu and culture, a group self-image, and co-responsibility for goal achievement. Each concept of the definition can be viewed as the group identity mode subareas and components (see Figure 14–2). These components will be discussed further in considering processes and assessment of group identity.

Focusing specifically on the psychological and spiritual aspects of the person, the basic need of the self-concept mode is *psychic and spiritual integrity*. The need to know who one is so that one can exist with a sense of unity and purposefulness in the universe is the basis of psychic and spiritual integrity. As the underlying need of the self-concept mode, it is the goal of adaptation re-

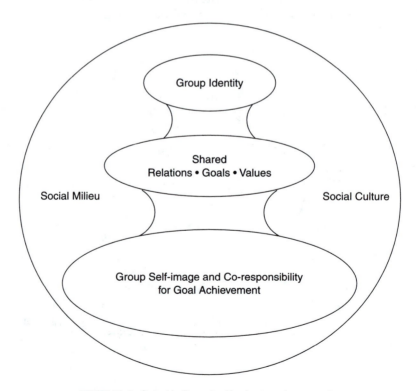

FIGURE 14–2. Group identity mode with subareas and components.

lated to the individual's self-concept. Processes used in creating psychic and spiritual integrity include developing self and focusing self. The basic need underlying the group identity mode is termed identity integrity. *Identity integrity* implies the honesty, soundness, and completeness of the group members' identification with the group. A key process in meeting the need for identity integrity in a group is the broader process of sharing identity and goals.

▶ DEVELOPING SELF: PROCESS AND ASSESSMENT

Both the physical and personal self develop throughout one's life. For the child, the developing self is influenced by increasing physical and thinking capacities and by interactions with others. Piaget (1954), Erikson (1963), and Neugarten (1969, 1979) are developmental theorists who provide understanding of the process of the developing self.

According to Piaget, infants and young toddlers are in the sensorimotor stage, using all their senses and motor skills to define and interpret objects and events. The major cognitive task is to experience triumph over objects. The child's thinking proceeds from directly acting as a whole on the environment to more goal-directed action with an object to make something happen. Between 6 and 12 months, self is seen as separated from objects. In Piaget's preoperational stage, toddlers and preschoolers complete the task of understanding symbols, such as classifying by color, shape, or size. Perceptually, at ages 2 to 5 years, self is the focus and purpose of the world. The child will reject another's viewpoint and be unaware that the other person can have a different viewpoint. Between ages 5 and 8, the child is less egocentric, but will have difficulty comprehending a conflicting viewpoint. The school-age child is in the concrete operational stage of cognitive development and can master classes, quantities, and relations such as time and space. Thinking is limited by relying on experience, and by the limited number and quality of past experiences. Adolescents have formal operations thought processes that include abstract and symbolic relationships. Their view of the world goes beyond the present and the concrete to include future possibilities, abstractions, and contrary-to-fact propositions. Such thinking is used in creating self-consistency, self-ideal, and a moral-ethical-spiritual self.

Parallel to the child's physical and cognitive maturation, the child also explores the world by building relationships. Initial relationships may be with the primary caregiver, for example the mother or father. Gradually, the child interacts and adjusts as a member of a family and a school or play group. The eight maturational crises described by Erikson (1963) are listed in Chapter 4 and are useful in understanding the influence of interaction on psychological development and the developing self-process. The reader is referred to the original author. However, it is not difficult to recognize the influences of reactions of others in such maturational crises as trust versus mistrust, autonomy versus shame and doubt, initiative versus guilt, and industry versus inferiority. In Erikson's maturational theory, particular emphasis is placed on identity emerging between 12 and 18 years of age.

The developmental approach of Neugarten (1979) focuses on the second half of life. In this theory, time, age, and life cycle are key to making a meaningful life story from a life history. The approach has been used to understand development of self in the elderly.

Another theory that provides understanding of the developing self process is work on self-schema and processing information about the self (Markus, 1977). In discussing the information processing of the cognator, the Roy Adaptation Model notes that the amount of stimulation available at any time is greater than a person can process or even attend to. Tendencies to select what to notice, learn, or remember are not random. Rather Markus (1977; Markus & Wurf, 1987) proposes that they depend on some internal cognitive structures that allow the individual to process the incoming information with some degree of efficiency. *Schema* is a term used for the structures for encoding and representing information. *Self-schema* are cognitive generalizations about the self derived from past experience that organize and guide the processing of the self-related information contained in an individual's interactions with others. Self-schemas have been documented in a variety of domains, for example, body weight (Markus, Hamill, & Sentis, 1987), exercise (Kendzierski, 1988), and sexual identity (Markus, Crane, Bernstein, & Siladi, 1982), related to physical self; and academic performance (Garcia & Pintrich, 1994), related to self-ideal.

In the broader self-perception theory of Coombs and Snygg (1959), self is seen as a constellation of self-perceptions. A number of symbolic interaction theorists (Cooley, 1964; Goffman, 1959, 1967; Mead, 1934; Sullivan, 1953) describe that the person bases self-perception on the way in which responses of others are perceived. Mead proposed that the concept of self refers to an individual's awareness of being a distinct entity in society. Although the sense of self is not present at birth, it arises in the process of social experience as the infant, child, and adult relate to other individuals and the wider society. Cooley expanded on this idea by maintaining that a sense of self is the result of social interactions in which one sees one's self reflected in the meanings and evaluations of others. Cooley maintained that the person sees in imagination the other person's judgment of one's self (appearance, for example); and as a result, the person experiences self-feelings, such as pride, satisfaction, or humiliation. However, Mead noted that for the self to develop in its fullest sense, it is necessary not only to take on the attitudes of others directed toward the self, but also to acquire the attitudes of the group and society in which the person holds membership. The individual must therefore be able to comprehend the situation from the standpoint of the generalized other. For example, the teenage girl puts herself in the place of her classmates, "stands in their shoes," and perceives that in their eyes she is fashionable when she wears clothes and makeup like they wear.

Using several theoretical approaches, the *developing self* process can be summarized as growing self-perceptions based on physical and cognitive development, and perceptions of others' reactions to self. These experiences are cognitively organized into self-schemas.

Assessment of Behavior

The five components of the self-concept mode form the basis for behavioral assessment of psychic and spiritual integrity. As the nurse gradually gets to know the patient, there is evidence of behaviors that indicate the developing self processes for both the physical and personal self. Behavior is manifest through the person's appearance relative to such factors as grooming, posture, and facial expression, and through statements the person makes about self. For example, a person may appear pale and drawn and make the comment, "I'm not feeling very well." Both appearance and statement are behaviors related to the component of the physical self, body sensation. Similarly, a person who has brought a rosary into the hospital is telling something about the moral-ethical-spiritual self.

At times, the nurse makes a purposeful assessment by questioning a person relative to self-concept. To do this effectively, the nurse must provide a comfortable and trusting environment for the person since in the nursing assessment of self-concept the person is asked to share some intimate feelings about self. The nurse uses sensitive awareness and observation, interviewing, interaction, and physical assessment skills to assess behaviors in each component of the self-concept mode. In considering assessment of the developing self process, assessment of the physical self is considered most relevant and will be described. Assessment of the personal self is considered in the section on focusing self process.

Assessment of the person's physical self is of primary importance in the promotion of adaptation. Adaptation problems in the area of the self-concept mode, and specifically the physical self component, may interfere with the person's ability to heal and to do what is necessary to maintain and promote health. The two components of the physical self, body image and body sensation, represent categories of behaviors that suggest to the nurse the effectiveness with which the patient will be able to adapt in the situation at hand. In addressing the self-concept component of physical self with the patient, it is important that the nurse understand and be comfortable with a personal physical self and related body image, body sensation, and sexuality. Not only is an adaptive physical self required by the patient in dealing with other adaptation problems, it is a personal requirement for the nurse attempting to assist the patient toward effective adaptation in the self-concept mode. The nurse also provides for privacy and meets the person's immediate needs. Confidentiality is discussed. The nurse tells the person who else, if anyone, will have access to the information. The patient may wish to keep certain aspects of the interview strictly between the nurse and self. The nurse tells the patient whether that is possible in advance and honors the agreement. The nurse does not impose judgments or stereotypes on the person receiving care. Good communication skills including open-ended questions, use of silence, and reflection are used. Questions are related to the individual's need for promoting health and are placed in the realm of common concern. For example, the nurse could say, "Many people are concerned about their sexual activity following colostomy surgery." Campsey (1985) viewed sexuality as a human experience that needs to be explored, experienced, and shared. The person receiving care, however, is often hesitant to bring up the subject. The nurse has the responsibility to show a willingness to deal with issues of sexuality.

Body Sensations

The nurse assesses the infant or nonverbal person's body sensation component by observing or obtaining a report from the nurturing person of facial expressions, body posture, physical tensions, level of relaxation, ease of feeding and eliminating, and depth of sleep. All human beings share sexual feelings as part of body sensations (Calderone & Ramey, 1982). The person experiences pleasurable sexual sensations from the time of birth, or possibly before. Human sexuality involves far more than the sex act and reproduction. Sexuality involves who and what we are as male and female, how we get that way, how we feel about it, and how we deal with each other about it. Dreams, fantasies, ideals, pleasure, and laughter are involved.

Once the young person has become fairly verbal, the nurse can add questions related to the assessment of body sensations. The nurse assesses the person's knowledge, needs, preferences, losses, and any effects of a medical condition or treatment in the area of sexuality. Examples of such questions are listed in Table 14–1. The nurse adapts the questions into his or her own words. The person's developmental level and personal communication style are also taken into consideration. The nurse uses accurate terminology and checks with the person receiving care for mutual understanding of terms being used. The body sensation behaviors are the observations listed, as are the individual's responses to the questions. For example, the person may state, "I feel_____(strong, weak, sexually responsive, faint, pained)." The nurse validates any hunches drawn from observation. For instance the nurse might say, "I see your brow is furrowed and your jaw is clenched. What are you feeling now?"

The importance of helping people identify their body sensations is noted in an example of research-based nursing intervention. One program of research has shown that if the nurse prepares a patient for a procedure, such as introduction of a nasogastric tube, by describing the physical sensations that will be felt, the person is better able to cope with the procedure and cooperate with what needs to be done (Johnson & Leventhal, 1974).

Body Image

Body image behaviors, how the body looks to oneself and how one feels about how the body looks and functions, is assessed next. Part of body image is identifying the self as male or female. The Adaptation Model deals with gender identification in the role function mode, primary role. Sex role identification is discussed here as related to the body image component of physical self-concept. The nurse makes direct observations of the person's posture, carriage, and level of personal hygiene and grooming. A complete physical assessment including pelvic, Pap, and breast examinations for women and

TABLE 14–1 ASSESSMENT OF BEHAVIOR OF THE PHYSICAL SELF COMPONENT

Characteristics	How to Elicit Behavior	How Behavior Is Manifested
Body sensation: how the body feels to the self.	How do you feel physically?	I feel (strong, weak, tired, rested, etc)
Sensations allow one to experience the body.	What physical sensations are you experiencing?	I feel (cold, warm, pained, sexy, etc) Facial expression Muscular tension
Sensations allow one to experience the self as a sexual being.	How often do you have sexual feelings?[a]	I have sexual feelings (daily, weekly, never, etc)
	How do you usually deal with your sexual feelings?	I usually (ignore them, masturbate, make love, etc)
	How satisfied are you with your methods of dealing with your sexual feelings?	I am (fairly satisfied, not satisfied at all, etc)
Body image: how one feels about the body; how one's body looks to the self.	Describe how you see yourself physically.	I am (slim, fat, well-built, tall, pretty, ugly, etc)
Level of satisfaction with appearance.	What aspects of your physical appearance do you like?	I like (my height, my hair, my smile, etc)
	What, if anything, would you like to change about your appearance?	I would like to change (my weight, my teeth, etc)
	How do you feel about your appearance?	I feel (pretty good, upset since this surgery, etc)

[a] When the person does not bring up the subject of sexuality, the nurse decides if specific questions are indicated. Questions are asked in the context of the person's health situation.

Content of Table 14–1 is based in part on Cho, J. M. (1998). Nursing process manual: Assessment tools for the Roy Adaptation Model. Glendale, CA: Polaris Press.

genitourinary examination for men is included, when relevant and appropriate. The nurse may perform this examination or obtain the information from the written record. Detailed information on how to do a physical assessment can be found in textbooks on physical assessment. During the physical exam, the nurse has the opportunity to talk with the person about any concerns and questions and to teach about self-awareness and self-care. Based on these observations and the list of questions in Table 14–1, the nurse asks open-ended questions to identify body image behaviors. Taking into consideration the person's health care situation and cues from the person, the nurse decides whether or not to carry out a detailed assessment of sexuality. The person's responses as well as the nurse's observations are noted as body image behaviors. The identified behaviors can be judged to be adaptive or ineffective. Adaptive behaviors contribute to the person's psychic and spiritual integrity. Ineffective behaviors detract from or prevent formation and maintenance of the person's integrity. On completion of the assessment of physical self behaviors, the nurse is ready to assess the factors influencing those behaviors.

Assessment of Stimuli

The following discussion of stimuli will be divided into seven categories of common influencing factors based on theories related to the developing self process. The summary that follows briefly describes each of the categories and suggests ways to elicit the information.

Physical Development

Age and degree of physical development affect self-concept as abilities change and control of bodily functions change. All the normal changes of growth and development are stimuli for the physical self behaviors. The human body is continually changing, and these changes require alterations in the sense of physical self. As the nervous system matures, the infant learns to roll over, sit, crawl, stand, and walk. Further growth leads to the physical changes of puberty. Continuing development brings on the initially subtle and then more evident changes of aging. All of these events affect the person's concept of self. The nurse is aware of normal growth and development theory and applies it when identifying physical self stimuli.

In addition, physiologic behaviors are reviewed. These provide important stimuli for the physical self component of the self-concept mode. The applicable physiologic mode behaviors are considered stimuli for the physical self component. For example, the person's height, weight, color and distribution of hair, muscular strength, skin condition, ability to control bodily functions, and neurologic function all influence how the person perceives and feels about the body. The nurse using the Adaptation Model completes the physiologic mode assessment using direct observation, physical assessment skills, and review of the written record. The information gained in assessment is useful in understanding the stimuli, or factors, affecting the physical self component.

Stages of Cognitive Development

Newer models of life-span development place emphasis upon the role of the individual as a participant and partner in the developmental process throughout life (Horton, 1990). Cognitive development involves many interacting factors, for example, biologic aspects that include genetic makeup and maturation. In addition, environmental factors, including social interaction, learning, and culture are involved. All of these factors interact and can affect cognitive development throughout the life span. Although Piaget's (1954) model was developed in studying children, it can be useful in describing stages of cognitive development that are relevant to understanding the developing physical self. Sensorimotor, preoperational, concrete, and abstract stages of thinking can be assessed by the nurse in both adults and children. A simple task to differentiate between concrete versus abstract reasoning is to draw a bottle that is tilted toward one side and half filled with water. To be classified as using abstract reasoning, the person must be able to explain that the water is drawn level with the floor because of gravity's pull on the water. The level of thinking greatly affects how one perceives the self physically in the physical world.

Interaction With Primary Caregivers

The formation and maintenance of a sense of physical self is influenced profoundly by the reactions of primary caregivers. The infant gains information about self through body sensations (Montagu, 1986). Perception of touch from the nurturing person(s) as gentle, warm, and physically supportive leads to a sense of security in the infant. Consistent responses by the caregivers to the child's sensations of hunger and discomfort of position, need for touch, fatigue, and wet or dirty diapers also leads to a sense of security within the body. The nurse observes interactions between the young person and the primary caregiver when possible to gain information in this category. Questions are used to gather this earlier information from persons who are adults. For example, the nurse might ask, "What do you know about how your parents reacted to you when you were a baby?" An overweight, unemployed female adult stated, "My father never held me during my first year of life. Mother told me he was so disappointed that I wasn't a boy that he could hardly look at me. He still calls me Sam, never Samantha."

The young child's sense of physical self is influenced by the caregivers providing names and values to the parts, sensations, and functions of the body. Mothers play the age-old game of pointing and naming body parts with the growing infant. Comments such as, "Is your nasty gut hurting you again?" or "Are you feeling pressure in your gut? Maybe you will go to the bathroom soon," help shape how the person feels about body sensations and functions. Studies have shown that physiologic arousal is the same for fear, joy, anger, and emotional attraction. It has been suggested that the interpretation of these sensations as distinct feelings of fear, joy, anger, or emotional attraction is due to input provided by others (Kleinke, 1978). The values and feelings the primary caregivers have about their own body sensations and images are communicated to the child. Some people simply never talk about physical sensations and functions. Other people talk about them indirectly using euphemisms. Some people are able to talk openly and frankly about their bodily functions. The child's developing sense of physical self is influenced by the verbal and nonverbal—what is said as well as what is not said—messages of caregivers. The nurse gathers data in this category by direct observation when possible. Questions also are used to gather these data from the person and significant others.

Reactions of Others

The person's experiences of other people's reactions, including the influence of culture related to having certain physical characteristics, abilities, and sensations, strongly influence the formation of physical self behaviors. From the moment of birth and even before, parents apply societal standards to the individual. The pregnant woman might say, "I'm glad I know it's a boy, but he kicks so hard, I know he's going to be aggressive." Comments at the delivery of a newborn might include statements such as, "Too bad you had another girl," or "He's so tiny he'll never make a football player." Each society and culture values certain physical attributes. The values are communicated by others' reactions, but also by way of myths, legends, fairy tales, books, television, movies, magazines, and advertising. The individual who inherits desirable physical characteristics is rewarded while the person who does not lacks rewards and often receives negative input. The North American culture values the young, slim, firm, well-proportioned female body and the tall, muscular, male body. The ideal is infrequently the reality.

Further, a primary view of the human body in Western societies for a long time has been that of an object, a machine which should perform to the "owner's" wishes. A level of mistrust, annoyance, and ignorance about bodily functions has pervaded the culture. Advertising promises that taking certain over-the-counter drugs will let the individual complete a full day's activities despite a cold or flu. Professional athletes take drugs to kill the pain of injury and continue playing. The message is, "Don't feel sick and you won't be sick," in fact, "Don't feel." A study by Amann-Gainotti (1986) demonstrated the lack of knowledge about body structure and function. This study found that many adolescent girls do not know the source of menstrual blood. Western culture has long taught individuals to be cut off from true awareness and understanding of their own body sensations and functions (Johnson, 1983). Recently, there has been a movement in health promotion to unite body, mind, and spirit and to be aware of the physical self. In light of this mixed cultural situation, the nurse may need to be very sensitive and patient when interviewing the person concerning physical self behaviors and stimuli. The person may have limited ability to discuss physical self data due to lack of information. The interview may be a beginning experience of someone truly wanting to know how the body feels and is integrated into who one is as a person.

Also from a cultural perspective, reflected by reactions of others, religious groups teach certain attitudes about body image, function, and sexuality. For example, masturbation, abortion, and homosexuality are not accepted in the religious teachings of the Orthodox Jews, Roman Catholics, and traditional Protestants. In some traditions, including Middle Eastern, intercourse is reserved only for marriage. Some liberal branches of Protestant religions may sanction any activity or behavior that is considered healthy and does not harm another person. The nurse is aware of the keen impact of reactions of others and of cultural norms, including religion, on the developing self and uses open-ended questions to obtain information from the individual about how such experiences have influenced that person's sense of physical self.

Maturational Crisis

Erikson (1963) described eight psychosocial stages of development human beings go through from birth to death in old age (see Chap. 4). Likewise, Neugarten (1979) focuses on the maturational tasks of the second half of life. Each stage challenges the individual to resolve a maturational crisis. A person moves through the stages at an individual rate. No crisis is ever completely resolved. As life events unfold, the person has the opportunity for the reworking of each crisis. The nurse uses knowledge from theories, such as Erikson's and Neugarten's, and direct questions to assess this category of stimuli affecting the developing self process.

Perception and Self-schema

Over time, a perception of self results from the individual's interpretation of all the various interactions with others and the environment. According to Coombs and Snygg (1959), a core or inner cell of self-concept is formed of perceptions about self which are the most vital, fundamental aspects of the individual. The interactions with primary caregivers, and rewards, sanctions, and responses of others within the culture are internalized. Attempts to organize, summarize, or explain one's own behavior in a particular domain result in development of cognitive structures about the self that are called self-schema. *Self-schema* are cognitive generalizations about the self that organize and guide the processing of the self-related information contained in the individual's social environment. They represent the way the self has been differentiated, and as individuals have repeated experiences of a certain type, their schema become increasingly resistant to inconsistent or contradictory information. This issue is discussed later in this chapter as the tendency to self-consistency. If a person has a developed self-schema, the person can make judgments about self with relative ease (for example, "I know I can handle the diet changes needed for my health."), can report behavioral evidence about a given domain (for example, identify body image characteristics), and anticipate future behavior in the domain (for example, "I am the kind of person who bounces back fairly quickly; this surgery won't keep me down."). The nurse asks questions to elicit the person's perception of physical self and observes whether or not the data reflect a self-schema.

Coping Strategies

Coping strategies are defined as the person's habitual responses used to maintain adaptation. When assessing the physical self component, the nurse seeks information from the individual regarding usual practices for maintaining a positive sense of physical self. For example, many people do regular physical workouts. Some people have grooming routines such as hair dresser appointments that help maintain a positive sense of self. Eating a specific diet and taking certain nutritional supplements and vitamins may give the person a sense of well-being. Disruption of any of these and other routines might threaten the person's sense of physical self.

The seven categories of influencing factors are not all-inclusive. The nurse uses other applicable theories and information for determining stimuli affecting physical self behaviors. Behaviors in the other three adaptive modes can serve as stimuli for physical self behaviors. Stimuli may contribute or not contribute to an adaptive developing self process. The nurse may wish to label the identified stimuli as to the effect upon the self-concept. During the intervention phase, stimuli that are making a positive contribution will be maintained and enhanced, and those that are not will be altered or eliminated when possible.

► **FOCUSING SELF: PROCESS AND ASSESSMENT**

The self-concept involves both stability of the self over time and consistency, unity, and organization of self. A number of theorists discuss stability of self from varying perspectives. The term selected for the theoretical commonalities is the *focusing self* process. Focusing implies being in touch with the physical and personal self in a way that surfaces hope, energy, continuity, meaning, purpose, and pride to be an individual self within the whole human community in its struggle for peace, unity, and balance (McMahon, 1993). Focusing involves a process of awareness of who one is and of one's place as an individual among other people in society. It moves beyond individualism to perceiving self as part of the common patterns and integral relations of persons and the earth, as noted in the assumptions of the Roy Adaptation Model for the 21st century (see Chap. 2).

In psychology in the mid-20th century, there was a focus on behaviorism. Some theorists began to see the need to focus study on the uniqueness of the person. Lecky (1945, 1961) proposed the theory of self-consistency from an attempt to conceive of a person as a unique and dynamic whole whose most significant characteristic is individuality. Self-consistency, as discussed by other theorists as well, refers to the organization of ideas and attitudes about self which is acquired through the transaction between the person and environment (Elliott, 1986; Rogers, 1961). Lecky asserts that through the demands of self-consistency, the person strives to maintain a consistent self-organization and avoid disequilibrium. In discussing Lecky's work, Zhan (1994) notes that the most constant factor in one's experience is the self and the interpretation of one's own meaning—the kind of person one is and the place one occupies in the world.

Another theory related to self-consistency is Festinger's theory of cognitive dissonance. This theory has been elaborated by others and reflects the individual's efforts to minimize perceived discrepancies between the self-concept and other aspects of experience (Festinger, 1962; Markus & Zajonc, 1985; Rosenberg, 1968). This theory is discussed further as a compensatory adaptive process. Andrews (1990) adds the proposition that people reconfirm their self-concept through current social interaction. Self-consistency has been identified as the result of striving for unity or integrity during the transaction between person and environment (Beck, 1976; Lecky, 1961; Rogers, 1961). Inconsistency in self-organization results in discomfort and disturbance. The individual uses cognitive processes to reduce tension and to maintain a consistent self. Antonovsky (1986) describes the result of these processes as a sense of coherence. Coherence is described as a sense of global orientation of the extent to which one has a dynamic feeling of confidence.

Both self-esteem and self-preservation are motives discussed by Rosenberg (1965, 1979). *Self-esteem* is a pervasive aspect of the self-concept and relates to the worth or value the person holds of self. In describing areas of self-concept, Rosenberg describes dimensions, which include self-attitudes of continuity, consistency, clarity, and accuracy; and structure, referring to the values or criteria used to assess different self-attributions. Erikson (1968) described identity as "a subjective sense of an invigorating sameness and continuity" (p. 19).

In discussing the creative self, Zohar (1990) notes the human capacity to support unity of consciousness and the construction of relational wholes. The person is capable of creative self-reflection in dialogue with the environment. Zohar adds that the concept of morality is created in response to the person's need for an integrated picture of appropriate social behavior. Whereas the middle of the 20th century advocated the view of the person as a unique individual, entering the 21st century, the unity of patterns of person and environment is noted. People share a destiny with the universe and are responsible for mutual transformations. Quoting Zohar (1990), and other authors who look at persons in relation to a purposeful universe, Roy has made the foci of assumptions for the 21st century mutual complex person and environment self-organization and a meaningful destiny of convergence of the universe, persons, and environment in what can be considered a supreme being or God (see Chap. 2).

Focusing is the process whereby the person is in touch with the physical and personal self. One is comfortable with body sensations and body image as part of the total self. Self-consistency is maintained and self-ideal and the moral-ethical-spiritual self are transformed in human consciousness. Awareness of self, consciousness, and meaning are elements of person and environment integration, which the person focuses on by way of thinking and feeling.

Assessment of Behavior

In assessing the focusing self process, the nurse considers the components of the personal self aspect of self-concept. Personal self behaviors are expressed in verbalization of thoughts and feelings as well as in actions. An individual's view of self cannot be inferred from observing only a few behaviors. A thorough assessment is done before a nursing diagnosis can be made. To obtain the assessment data, as in assessing the physical self, the nurse creates an atmosphere in which the person feels safe to express thoughts and feelings. The attitude of the nurse does much to set the tone of safety or lack thereof. Since feelings are the subjective response of the individual, there are no good, bad, right, or wrong feelings. Laughing, crying, raging, shaking, and talking are expressions of feelings. The tension of unexpressed feelings is contained within the person. It is possible to feel very angry, for example, without raging or even talking about it. Such suppression of feelings, however, ties up psychic energy and interferes with the ability to do other things, such as think clearly and heal. In terms of the Roy model, this is cognator ineffectiveness. The nurse who conveys an accepting, nonjudgmental attitude can facilitate the expression of feelings and enhance cognator effectiveness. The nurse needs to be in touch with personal feelings and have an appropriate outlet for feelings. When this is the case, the nurse will be able to listen to the expression of feelings by the other person without imposing personal reactions.

Another aspect in creating a safe environment for the person is the ability to state clearly and directly the purpose of an interaction. For example, the nurse might say, "I am going to spend some time talking with you about your thoughts and feelings about yourself. Since each person is different and responds differently to (giving birth, surgery, or cancer, for example), it is important for me to understand how you are feeling now. That way I can plan with you care based on your needs and wishes." The actual wording will vary for the individual situation. The time and place of an interview and other nurse–patient interactions will be planned appropriately. The person who is in pain, for example, cannot attend to questions relating to the personal self. If the person is in a room with other people present, it may not be possible to attend to a nursing interview. The immediate physiologic needs and the need for privacy must be met prior to beginning a personal self assessment. Table 14–2 lists the subcomponents of personal self, how to elicit behaviors, and how the behaviors may be manifested. The nurse will find the words that are appropriate to the actual setting and communication style of those involved. Nonverbal behaviors of posture, facial expression, tone of voice, eye contact are noted. The personal self is also reflected in planning, developing moral values, and making decisions consistent with the self. Once the personal self behaviors are identified, the nurse makes an initial judgment as to whether

TABLE 14–2   ASSESSMENT OF BEHAVIOR OF THE PERSONAL SELF COMPONENT

Characteristics	How to Elicit Behavior	How Behavior Is Manifested
Self-consistency: personality traits; how one views self in relation to actual performance or response to situation.	How would you describe yourself as a person? What are your personal characteristics?	I am (a smart person, a person of strong will, like a child, not worthwhile, etc)
Self-ideal: what one would like to be or do related to what one is capable of being or doing.	What are your aspirations for yourself as a person? What would you change about yourself if you could?	I would like to be (someone who makes a difference, famous, a strong person, etc) I would change (how I lose my temper, my inability to do math, my sense of not belonging anywhere, etc)
Moral-ethical-spiritual self: one's sense of self in relation to one's sacred, ethical beliefs; how self is viewed in relation to one's value system, beliefs about "rightness" or "wrongness"; evaluator of "who I am."	How would you describe your spiritual beliefs? How do your spiritual beliefs affect your view of self? How do you measure up to your own standards of right living? How do you evaluate yourself? from doing as I believe, etc)	I believe in (God, a higher being, natural order, etc) I go to (church, AA meetings, the mountains, etc) I like to (read certain books, meditate, practice yoga, etc) I am (pretty consistent, a long way I tend to be (hard on myself, patient with myself, pretty happy with myself, etc)

Source: Based on Cho, J. M. (1998). Nursing process manual: Assessment tools for the Roy Adaptation Model. Glendale, CA: Polaris Press.

each behavior is effective or ineffective. Adaptive behaviors promote survival, growth, reproduction, mastery, and person and environment transformations, including transcendence. Another criterion for judging behaviors as adaptive or ineffective is the extent to which the behaviors lead to the realization of the individual's goals relative to the ideal self. Assessment of stimuli is the next step in understanding the focusing self process.

Assessment of Stimuli

Identifying the influencing factors, or stimuli, related to the focusing self process helps in understanding the personal self. The theories related to personal self-concept, as discussed, provide the categories to be covered in the second level of assessment. Six general categories of influencing factors are described and examples are provided of how to collect data. The order in which the categories are assessed and the type of data collected will vary according to the individual situation. For a young child, observations of interactions with the environment and consistency of behavior may be used more frequently than interview questions on values of self-attributes, for example.

Transaction Between Person and Environment

Interactions of the person with the environment is a key concept of nursing, and of the Roy Adaptation Model in particular. Looking to the future, Roy has redefined adaptation as the process and outcome whereby the thinking and feeling person uses conscious awareness and choice to create human and environmental integration. The particular function of person and environment interaction as a stimulus to the focusing self process raises it to a new concept, that of transaction. Interaction means to act upon each other. Transaction adds the notion that both are changed in the process and integration and mutual transformation are possible. People are, in their essential makeup, composed of the same "stuff" and held together by the same dynamics as those which account for everything else in the universe. Swimme and Berry (1992) note that, "To be is to be related, for relationship is the essence of existence. . . . Nothing is itself without everything else" (p. 77).

An example of how nurses include the environment in assessment is given by Carnevalli and Thomas' (1993) definition of nursing diagnoses. The authors expand the focus from human responses to include the situation, the context surrounding the person, and the responses. In using the Roy model to assess the effect of transaction between person and environment, the nurse observes how the person and environment change each other and whether the pattern leads toward integration. On the other hand, the nurse notes whether or not the person finds the environment toxic to self and, in turn, is toxic to the environment. Data suggest that environmental stability plays an important role in self-concept stability (Demo, 1992). Newman (1994) notes that it is the pattern of our lives (transactions of person and environment) that identifies us, not the substance that goes into making up that pattern. Identifying patterns of the whole and helping people to deal with them is important developing knowledge in nursing. Both nurse-scholars, including Roy and Newman, and nurses in practice will contribute to this knowledge by insightful observations of patients in their life experiences.

Striving for Unity or Integrity

Theorists who discuss the importance of self-consistency postulate a striving for unity or integrity (Elliott, 1986; Lecky, 1961). The striving for unity or integrity may well be an innate human quality that affects adaptation in the self-concept mode as well as in the other adaptive modes. Through a consistent striving for self-organization, the person avoids imbalance and discomfort. Identifying the need for balance of the inner self as related to health is reflected in many traditions of both Eastern and Western healing.

Confirmation Through Social Interaction

The focusing self process is influenced by confirmation through social interaction, and particularly by observing the reactions of others. The work of the interactionist theorists, Cooley, Mead, and Sullivan, as identified in the discussion of the physical self, forms the basis of this stimulus. In essence, these theories state that individuals start to think of self in the ways in which they perceive that others view them. For example, the person who is repeatedly told, "You are thoughtless of others," may incorporate a sense of being a selfish person. In the same way, if the person holds this view, new situations will be interpreted in a way that confirms this concept of self. If the nurse comments that the patient in the next bed is very ill, a person with this background of social interactions may immediately believe that he or she has been disturbing the patient. Once a person reaches adulthood, the messages significant others have given regarding a person's personal value have been incorporated into the self-concept.

Interviewing the individual can provide data on factors influencing the focusing self process. Again, family members have a significant impact on the formation and confirmation of self-concept. The nurse assesses the family's influence on the person's self-concept in this category. Sample questions are: Who are the family members? What is the family's value of the individual? Who does the person receiving care feel particularly close to in the family? Does the person get the same message from all family members? Does the person believe that confirmations of self are realistic or sometimes could be misinterpretations? Is the person able to accept new data of positive interpretations of self? Not all of these data will be available or relevant for every patient. When possible, the nurse will also interview any significant others who are available and will observe the patient's social interactions.

Consciousness of Person and Environment Meanings

Awareness of self, consciousness, and meaning are elements of person and environment integration which the person focuses on by way of thinking and feeling. Which personal characteristics are valued is determined in part by cultural and social norms. Race, sex, class, religion, and other societal discriminations affect the individual's concept of self. The nurse assesses the person's awareness of what significant people in his or her life expect, what the individual values as expected of her or him, and how these compare with social values and the current situation. The nurse may discover factors influencing changes in the person's current sense of self as different from the original ideal self. The situation of illness itself will be a stimulus for changes in the personal self, especially self-consistency and self-ideal. Helping the person find new meaning in an altered physical or personal self may be a focus for nursing care.

Value of Self Attributes

Rosenberg (1979) discussed self-esteem as a motive and noted that within the self-concept there are values or criteria used to assess different self-attributions. *Self-esteem* has been defined as that pervasive aspect of the personal self component that relates to the worth or value the person holds about the self (Driever, 1976). How one establishes the worth of personal attributes influences the focusing self process. Elliott (1986) reports an empirical link between self-esteem and self-consistency among young people ages 8 to 19 years. Other data suggest that self-evaluation is represented by a "moving base-line" from which situational fluctuations emerge (Demo, 1992). Further, self-evaluation generally becomes more favorable through the life span.

In earlier work on the Roy Adaptation Model, Driever (1976) defined low self-esteem as a negative feeling of self-worth that handicaps a person's ability to adapt to the environment. The nurse may recognize many manifestations of low self-esteem including the following: withdrawal from others; decrease in spontaneous behavior; appearance of sadness, anxiety, or discouragement; feelings of isolation; inability to express or defend oneself; avoidance of situations of self-disclosure or notice; sensitivity to criticism; self-deprecation; denial of successes or accomplishments; rumination about problems; and seeing the self as a burden to others. Teaching the building of self-esteem in children is an important part of pediatric nursing (Servonsky & Opas, 1987). Being aware of levels of self-esteem and their effect on the person is significant in all of clinical nursing practice.

Coping Strategies

Another category of stimuli the nurse will consider is the person's coping strategies. *Coping strategies* are the ways the person functions to maintain integrity in everyday life and in times of stress. Some of these are habitual and learned over time and others may be developed in a new situation, based on general tendencies of the cognator and regulator. It is important to find out if the person has previously faced an experience similar to the current one and how that experience was dealt with. Data in this category are obtained by interviewing the person and significant others. A research instrument to measure coping strategies derived within the Roy model currently is being tested by Roy and colleagues. Research using the Roy Adaptation Model, discussed in Chapter 18, identifies some of the patterns of coping used by given patient populations.

There are other factors that influence an individual's process of focusing self. As the nurse interviews and interacts with the person receiving care, data may arise that do not fit in the specified six categories but which do influence the person's processes related to the personal self. These additional data are included in the assessment as well and used to plan nursing interventions. When obtaining stimuli assessment data, the nurse refers back to the information obtained in the behavioral assessment as much as possible. For example, the nurse might say, "You mentioned earlier that you feel you are a strong and capable person (self-consistency behavior). How have people that you interact with regularly helped you feel that way about yourself?" Such a question will probably elicit stimuli assessment data under the category confirmation through social interaction. The nurse phrases the questions specifically to help keep the person focused on the current situation. In that manner, the nurse obtains the data needed to plan nursing interventions. Influencing factors contribute to effective adaptation or may exert an influence toward ineffective adaptation. It may be helpful to identify the effect that each stimulus has on the person. The benefit of doing so is evident in the step of planning interventions.

▶ SHARED IDENTITY: PROCESS AND ASSESSMENT

In the group identity mode, a major process of adaptation is shared identity. Studying shared identity involves studying more than individual self-concepts and people relating to one another as members of groups. Some authors, following Lewin (1948), who was an early theorist on small-group interaction, note that goal-directed behavior of individuals, groups, organizations, nation-states, or any other large-scale social system is a function of the perceived external environment and of the shared cognitive, emotional, motivational, and normative orientations of members of these social systems (Rabbie & Lodewijkx, 1996). *Shared identity,* then, is the process whereby the members of the group come to common perceptions of the environment, common cognitive and feeling orientations, and shared goals and values. Topics related to shared identity, such as interpersonal relations, the importance of communication, family interaction, and the infrastructure for collectives, are found in Chapter 16 in discussion of the interdependence adaptive mode. The consideration here is on the shared identity of voluntary personal and professional groups.

The term *group culture* is used to describe the group's agreed-upon expectations that include values, goals, and norms for relating (Kimberly, 1997). The expectations are shared and result in patterned behavior relevant to the group's relation to its environment and to interaction of its members among themselves and with outsiders.

Communal sharing is another term related to the process of shared identity. Communal sharing is a relationship of equality in which people are merged for the purposes of the group, so that individual selves are not distinct (Fiske, 1991). People attend to being a member of the group and have a common sense of identity in which individuality is not marked. Emphasis is placed on the common characteristics that brought the group together. What is important to individuals is membership in the group and the boundaries that contrast the group members with outsiders. The group members have a sense of solidarity, unity, and belonging. Fiske notes that they identify with the collectivity and think of themselves as being all the same in some significant respect, not as individuals but as "we."

Relevant theory and practice in nursing moves beyond the concept of communal sharing by describing a particular kind of group culture based on women's experiences. The culture described by Chinn (1995) emphasizes that the realization of the individuality of each group member enables the shared identity of the group, rather than that the individual identity becomes secondary to group identity. The author uses the acronym, PEACE, to discuss effective ways of relating in all kinds of groups and communities. PEACE is both intent and process and is rooted in women's ancient wisdom. Chinn notes that the close link between values and action can be referred to as "doing what we know, and knowing what we do." The process Chinn outlines is an effort to describe the values of women's ways of making peace in groups, and the skills, actions, and abilities that go with those values. The author draws from the experiences of women's groups dedicated to transformation to present a process represented by five words. Use of the process requires conscious awareness of the group interaction and commitment to particular values, and the congruent actions, of the ways in which individuals can choose to relate to one another.

The PEACE intent and process described by Chinn (1995) articulates the values reflected in the assumptions of the Roy Adaptation Model and can be viewed as a process for shared identity. The words chosen to describe the process are praxis, empowerment, awareness, consensus, and evolvement. Praxis refers to thoughtful reflection and action that occur in synchrony, in the direction of transforming the world. In praxis, values are made visible through deliberate action. Empowerment includes growth of personal strength, power, and ability to enact one's own will and love for self in the context of love and respect for others. It requires listening to the senses as well as listening intently and actively to others, consciously taking in and contributing to the strength of the group. Chinn describes awareness as an active, growing knowledge of self and others, and the world in which one lives. It means a heightened awareness of the present moment, and also a transcendent awareness that sees beyond the moment to the past and the future. This awareness makes one conscious of the contradictions in the world. One example might be that what is defined as "peace" is often "war," such as being silent at a meeting only to rant and rave afterwards. Consensus is an active commitment to group solidarity and group integrity; it focuses on cooperation and collectivity. This commitment requires an internal attitude that welcomes differences of opinion and an openness to self-reflection. In the process described by Chinn, evolvement means a commitment to growth in which change and transformation are conscious and deliberate. Growth and transformations of the group happen in cycles and are valued and celebrated by the group.

Knowledge about how groups share identity, and what groups are important to a person, is useful in planning individual nursing care. In addition, the knowledge of shared identity can help nurses contribute to the effectiveness of groups in which they participate, from hierarchical institutions to committees and self-help groups. Insights from the theories related to the shared identity process are useful in assessing behavior and stimuli related to this integrated life process in groups.

Assessment of Behavior

First-level assessment of the group identity mode includes assessing behaviors of shared identity in groups. Assessment can be made by direct observation and by reports from persons in the group. The nurse assesses the patterns of behavior relative to the group's common perceptions of the environment, common cognitive and feeling orientations, and shared goals and values. Since patterns are being assessed, the assessment is done over time, not as a single observation or report. Each group has its own particular structure and purpose that gives rise to the group culture. However, some generalizations can be made about assessing behavior patterns and particular applications will be made to assessing the shared identity in groups built on the group culture described by Chinn (1995).

Perceptions of Environment

An important consideration in assessing patterns of shared identity is to understand how the group defines the boundaries between members of the group and nonmembers. In a school, does the work group include faculty and staff of a department? Are the tenured-track faculty and clinical faculty considered the same group? On the hospital administrative team, are vice presidents for all services included in a group, or is the vice president for nursing included in a separate group with other nurse administrations in the institution? Behaviors of shared identity include the group's common understanding of who are internal and who are external. Other ways of describing environment are discussed further when stimuli for shared group identity are considered.

Chinn (1995) identifies that the ideal may be that all groups based on PEACE processes seek to be open to all who wish to join them. There can be a dilemma, however, in balancing the desire to remain open to new thoughts and integrating diversity within the group, and yet remaining effective in accomplishing the work of the group. Chinn suggests that the group consider openness as relative and changing rather than as a choice between open or closed. For example, as the tasks of the group change, a natural flow of movement occurs with people both leaving and joining the group, possibly on a temporary basis. A group responsible for a given task, for example, operating a volunteer respite service, can set up times when membership is open and new volunteers can be oriented and introduced as members of the group.

Cognitive and Feeling Orientations

Whether the group members share common cognitive and feeling orientations is important behavioral evidence of shared identity. The group identifies which orientations are important to the group. For example, a group working on repealing death penalty laws may welcome people who have differing reasons for their support of the group, some humanitarian and others, religious. Still, belief in the need to repeal the laws and the emotional energy to work toward this goal are the relevant common orientations.

Chinn (1995) provides a list of questions about the congruence of intent and actions that are the most relevant cognitive and emotional orientations in the culture of groups based on PEACE processes. These can be used, and modified, for assessing groups, and oneself, when a group is built on similar principles. They include the following questions.

- Do I know what I do, and do I do what I know? (praxis)
- Am I expressing my own will in the context of love and respect for others? (enpowerment)
- Am I fully aware of myself and others? (awareness)
- Do I face conflicts openly and integrate differences in forming solutions? (consensus)
- Do I value growth and change for myself, others, and the group? (evolvement)

Goals and Values

Shared identity process can also be assessed by observing, directly or indirectly, the patterns of behavior related to goals and values. Group goals are simply defined as goals upon which the members agree. Kimberly (1997) relates goals to values by noting that individuals accept a goal for the group when they can relate it to one or more of their values. A group goal can express an individual goal at a more concrete level. The group defines the goals and values that are relevant to its shared identity, and these are based on what defines the group as a group and on the shared cognitive and emotional orientations. Goals and values prescribe behavior related to goal attainment. For example, a group working on repeal of death penalty laws may decide that group members will be involved in activities related to collecting studies of the effects of the death penalty, lobbying efforts, media contacts, and public education. Shared identity is strong when group actions focus mainly on commitment to common values and attainment of group goals.

In an analysis of group action, Chinn (1995) introduces the concept of power, noting that power is the energy from which action arises. Chinn notes clearly, however, that the power within PEACE groups is different from power as it is usually understood. In patriarchal terms, power refers to the capacity to impose one's will on others and often involves manipulating or controlling others. Chinn clarifies that the kind of power required to create and live within PEACE reflects an ideal where the focus shifts to underlying values associated with the exercise of power. What is valued in groups established on PEACE principles is the capacity to be in harmony with others and with the earth, and to join others in directing collective energies toward a future that the group seeks together. Strategies for use of this kind of power are familiar to nurses. However, often they are not recognized as power because they contrast sharply with patriarchal power and they are not yet common modes of action in many groups. One example Chinn provides of the contrast in the two types of power is of the power of hierarchy compared to the power of unity. The power of hierarchy depends on a linear chain of command where layer upon layer of responsibilities are subdivided into separate and discreet areas of responsibility. The power of unity values thoughtful deliberation of the group and emphasizes integrating the variety within the group. The group shares the responsibility for decision making and for acting on those decisions in a network of equals. Understanding these distinctions, nurses can assess behaviors related to shared identity processes in groups based on PEACE principles by evaluating group actions indicating values related to the use of power. These insights can be helpful in assessing behavior of any group.

Assessment of Stimuli

Based on a behavioral interaction model for studying groups (Rabbie & Lodewijkx, 1996), particular stimuli that affect shared identity of groups are selected for discussion. These include demands and distance, external social environment, and leadership and responsibility.

Demands and Distance

Demands and distance refer to the problems posed for a group to solve and whether or not the group has face-to-face interaction. Often a situation stimulates a group to form based on common interests in the situation. The intrusion of the profit motive in health care systems in the United States has led to creation of ad hoc groups of physicians and nurses concerned about the quality of care. The civil rights movement, and the many groups working on this issue, in the United States in the 1960s was a reaction to the reality of segregation, and the less apparent effects of pervasive racial prejudice and intolerance.

Group action is often dependent on face-to-face interaction. For example, the PEACE groups described by Chinn (1995) are based on members being physically present with each other, at least some of the time. However, some authors have shown that individuals in the same social category can coordinate their actions with one another in responding to external demands (Rabbie & Lodewijkx, 1996). The North American Jewish community acted as a group to support, financially and morally, the new country of Israel more than 50 years ago. Today, video and Internet conferencing are changing the definitions of group interactions. The distance between members of a group and how the group bridges that distance are important stimuli for shared identity.

External Social Environment

The external social environment refers to the group's perception of changes in the behavior of other people or groups with whom the group interacts. If a given department in the health care agency perceives that it is being targeted for budget cuts by the administration, this becomes a powerful external stimulus for the members of the department to strengthen their shared identity. The staff of the department will develop strategies to attain common perceptions of the situation and will share beliefs and feelings. Based on this interaction, they will develop shared goals and values.

In relation to the external social environment, Chinn (1995) addresses the challenges faced when introducing PEACE processes into existing groups influenced by hierarchical structure. Overcoming institutional expectations for established roles and behaviors is not easy. Chinn suggests that a beginning can be made by the group introducing the change making a conscious commitment to a value that they freely choose. The group then chooses one PEACE process to focus on as a starting point. For example, the power of unity, referred to earlier, can be a constant focus whereby the group actively seeks to understand differing perspectives that each person brings. Allowing time for each person to speak often is in conflict with tightly scheduled agendas of meetings. However, gradually, members of the group can ask to hear what others think. Chinn notes that change may be slow and invisible and suggests that forming a group outside of the institution may be helpful in sustaining the efforts to create institutional change. Nurses are accustomed to working with opposing value structures, but sometimes are not as skilled at how to make changes. Chinn's work offers some alternatives.

Leadership and Responsibility

In the literature on group processes and structures, there is much discussion about how authority structures develop in groups and the effect they have on group behaviors. In assessing factors influencing shared identity then, the issue of authority in the group is an important consideration. As noted, the goals and values determine the actions of the group. Attaining the goals requires creating some division of labor. Even in the simple group action of holding a meeting, someone may secure the place to meet, another may send out notices, and someone else may volunteer to take minutes of the meeting. Some theorists of group processes note that, based on what people do in the group, positions emerge. Some positions relate directly to goal attainment. Other positions relate to coordinating the goal-directed activities of the others and thus become authority positions (Kimberly, 1997). The group sets limits on how much discretion the authority person has with respect to such activities as redefining the group goal, establishing norms, changing positions of people in the group, or allocating new members to positions. Authority operates differently based on the goals and values of the group, but the pattern of leadership and responsibility that emerges in a group clearly has an effect on the shared group identity.

In working with PEACE groups, Chinn (1995) recommends rotating leadership and responsibility. The process of rotating leadership means more than having a different leader for each meeting. Chinn notes that the rotation process turns over to each member of the group the rights and responsibilities for leadership, tasks, and decisions. A convener may begin a meeting, but after that, whoever is speaking is the leader. The person who is speaking passes leadership simply by calling the name of the next person who indicates readiness to speak. During the discussion, each person makes notes of personal thoughts and ideas about what others are saying. The group listens carefully and allows people to complete their thoughts before indicating a desire to speak. The notes taken by each person facilitate the process of rotating leadership and are a personal tool to remain in touch with one's own thoughts while others are speaking. They can be a personal journal of experiences in the group. Based on the goals of the group, it may also be necessary to have at least one person record minutes of the meeting. A PEACE group at times rotates responsibilities to a task group. The group determines the responsibilities of the task group and provides direction that helps the task group accomplish its work in concert with the goals and values of the total group. The task group is then accountable to bring its work back to the larger group.

Assessing behavior and stimuli in groups is a skill that will increase as the nurse's knowledge and experience in group process grows. There is significant literature in nursing and in related fields, particularly social psychology and organizational behavior, to facilitate this growth.

▶ COMPENSATORY ADAPTIVE PROCESSES

The self-concept–group identity mode has many compensatory processes, based on the richness and flexibility of personal strengths within each individual and the sharing of these capabilities within groups. As defined earlier in this book, compensatory processes represent the adaptation level at which the cognator and regulator, or stabilizer and innovator, have been activated by a challenge to the integrated life processes. Three compensatory processes selected for discussion are grieving, cognitive dissonance, and community cohesion.

Grieving

Grief recovery has been called a neglected growth process. When a loss occurs, or a person considers to face death, the cognator and regulator are activated with the possibility of reaching higher levels of adaptation and person and environment transcendence. From this perspective, grieving losses and life closure are considered compensatory processes of adaptation. Loss as it applied to the physical self-component is any situation, either actual or potential, in which part of the body or a body function is altered in such a way that it no longer has the qualities that render it valuable. The series of emotional responses that occur following the perception or anticipation of a loss is grief. In the broadest sense, grieving can be applied to any situation in which loss is involved. Common losses in the four adaptive modes include loss of physical function; loss of sense of self, including facing death; loss of role function; and loss of interpersonal relationships. When the compensatory process of dealing with loss is not successful, problems of compromised adaptation, such as body image disturbance, powerlessness, or unresolved loss, may result.

Life is filled with losses and grieving is a natural response. Grieving is not a pathologic process, but rather can bring healing and a higher level of personal integrity and transformation. In the literature, the process of grieving is viewed as consisting of four stages.

1. Shock and disbelief
2. Apprehending the loss
3. Attempting to deal with the loss
4. Final restitution and resolution

The nurse's role in helping the person effectively use this compensatory process is a significant part of nursing care. Table 14–3 outlines the stages of grieving a loss and lists samples of expected behaviors, common stimuli, and common nursing approaches at each stage. The nurse can be helpful to the grieving person through sensitivity to the meaning of the situation for the individual, purposeful interviewing, and validating hunches from observation and theory.

As discussed in relation to the developing self process, the work of mastering one stage of development prepares the ground for the work of the next stage. The tasks of a stage are never achieved completely. Until the end, life affords opportunities to resolve developmental issues at yet higher levels. Related to the process of grieving is the process that Dobratz (1984) has defined as *life closure*. The process of life closure is the ultimate opportunity to rework previous issues in the full development of the personal self.

Life closure, the process through which a person resolves the issue of the meaning of one's life and accepts the reality of eventual death, is a normal part of the life cycle. Erikson (1963) identified the crisis of this last stage as ego integrity versus despair. Ego integrity involves accepting one's life as it has been. Despair includes fear of death and the feeling that time is too short and that one's life should have been lived differently.

Beginning the process of life closure is often a response to the aging and death of parents. Interacting with parents in the last months of their lives forces the person to confront personal feelings about aging and death. Parents are a strong link to the individual's past. Death of the parents marks the end of a segment of life and leaves the individual next in line for death (Silverstone & Hyman, 1976). Death of siblings, spouse, or peers may also stimulate facing one's own death. The physical changes of aging also serve as stimuli for the process of life closure. The relatively constant adult physical self-image is challenged by changes in appearance, function, and stamina

TABLE 14–3 STAGES OF GRIEVING A LOSS

Expected Behaviors	Common Stimuli	Common Nursing Approaches

Stage 1: Shock and Disbelief (lasts minutes to days)
Statements indicating fact of the loss has not been apprehended: "Oh, I can't believe it's true"
Verbal report of stunned numb feeling
Blank facial expression
Sitting motionless and dazed
Little or no attention to the surroundings
Automatic carrying out of routine
Verbal expression of intellectual acceptance and making plans for dealing with the loss
Inability to look at part of the body affected by the loss
	Focal
	  Need to protect self from being overwhelmed by painful feelings
	Contextual
	  Suddenness of the news of the loss
	Residual
	Other circumstances surrounding the loss—eg, physical illness, need to support others affected by the loss
		Be present—use touch to communicate caring and presence
		Tell the person you are there to help
		Refrain from making judgments
		Provide for privacy
		Allow denial—don't agree or refute it
		Ask the person to talk about current feelings
		Provide for contact with significant others
		Provide for physiologic needs

Stage 2: Apprehending the Loss
Sighing
Verbal report of slight sense of unreality
Verbal report of intense subjective distress
Expression of anger at the circumstances and desire not to be bothered
Crying
Behaviors of fear and anxiety:
  Report of loss of strength
  Report of emptiness in chest or epigastrium
  Report of tightness in throat
  Appetite changes
  Weight loss
  Report of inability to sleep
  Inability to engage in organized activity
Report of a sense of emotional distance from others
Feeling of emptiness
Searching for lost object
Feelings of guilt and shame
Beginning ability to talk about the reality of the loss: "I guess it's really happening"
Beginning ability to look at and touch the part of the body affected by loss
	Focal
	  Mention or thought of the lost object
	Contextual
	  Presence of other people
	  Importance of the lost object
	  Degree of ambivalence toward the lost object
	  Ability to tolerate and express painful feelings
	  Response of significant others
	Residual
	  Cultural norms of how to grieve
		Be present and listen
		Gently remind person of reality
		Provide for privacy
		Tell the person the responses of this stage are normal and expected
		Reflect, paraphrase, use silence to encourage expression of feelings
		Use all the above approaches with significant others
		Notify clergy of person's choice

TABLE 14–3 STAGES OF GRIEVING A LOSS (CONT.)

Expected Behaviors	Common Stimuli	Common Nursing Approaches
Stage 3: Attempting to Deal With the Loss (the main work occurs intrapsychically and takes months to years) Report of preoccupation with lost object or function Waves of sadness and crying Feelings of despair Talk about the lost object and experiences with it prior to the loss Expression of feelings of loss of intactness and wholeness of self Report of altered body sensations— eg, itching feeling in a leg that has been amputated Development of physical illness Carrying out of self-care routine— looking at and touching the affected part of the body	Focal Contemplation of future without the lost object Contextual Importance of the lost object Degree of ambivalence toward the lost object Spiritual beliefs Number of and degree of resolution of past losses Degree of preparation for the loss Physical and psychological health of the person Ability to tolerate and express painful feelings Amount of guilt felt Age of the person Residual Cultural prescription of how to grieve Contemplation of the unexpected experience of grief itself	Be present and listen Tell person it is normal to feel sorrow, guilt, anger, helplessness Use open-ended questions to elicit expression of feelings Refrain from making judgments Ask the person to talk about the meaning of the lost object Ask person to talk about past losses—how it felt, what helped, how it was resolved Remind person it takes time to go through grieving process Use touch to communicate presence and caring Ask person about spiritual beliefs Involve clergy person as requested by person Apply above approaches to significant others
Stage 4: Final Restitution and Resolution Expression of interest in alternatives for the lost object or function Ability to talk about the loss experience without bitterness and guilt	Focal Level of success or completion of previous stages of grief Contextual All stimuli listed above Residual All stimuli listed above	Active listening techniques Help person problem-solve how to form new patterns of functioning and relating Refrain from judging Point out person's strengths and gains

Source: Data drawn in part from three books on nursing diagnosis: Carpenito, L. (1985). *Handbook of nursing diagnosis*. Philadelphia: J.B. Lippincott; Gordon, M. (1985). *Manual of nursing diagnosis*. New York: McGraw-Hill; Kelly, M. A. (1985). *Nursing diagnosis source book*. E. Norwalk, CT: Appleton-Century-Crofts; and from Chapter 18 "Loss" by Marjorie H. Buck In *Introduction to nursing: An adaptation model* (2nd ed.) by Sister Callista Roy. Englewood Cliffs, N.J.: Prentice-Hall, Inc., 1984, pp. 337–352.

brought on by aging. Similarly, illness raises questions of a changing self and of personal mortality. Pain, disability, and chronic health issues in late middle age and the older years cause the person to stop and rethink his or her view of life, self, and the universe. Cultural views and the person's perception of aging and death also influence dealing with life closure.

In Western society, there still is reticence to talk about death. Kübler-Ross (1969) and many succeeding researchers have found that dying people are overwhelmingly grateful to have someone listen to their thoughts and feelings. With an understanding of the assumptions of the Roy Adaptation Model, the nurse is prepared to assist people to reminisce about their lives and previous experiences and to recognize the meaningfulness of the pattern of their lives. The nurse confirms the person in assurance that life has pattern and meaning, that one is united with other people in the context of a meaningful universe, and that, in a spiritual sense, all persons and creation share a common destiny. Purposeful communication using reflecting, paraphrasing, open-ended questions, and active silence will promote an effective life review.

The nurse will need to be comfortable with the subject of loss, death, and dying to help others achieve greater personal integrity in the processes of grief and life closure. Reading literature, attending classes and workshops, and sharing personal feelings with family and friends helps the nurse to be prepared to assist the person with grief and life closure and with finding meaning in loss and death. The nurse respects each individual and the unique process of grieving and life closure. The nurse takes cues from the person as to when it is time to enter into, and at times to continue, the process of grieving or of life closure. The nurse continually conveys a willingness to listen and provides help and support by making eye contact, sitting down, and reflecting comments from past conversations.

Cognitive Dissonance

Cognitive balance is a concept that has been used in many theories of self-concept and group identity, as has been noted. Cognitive dissonance (Festinger, 1962) is the term frequently used to indicate a particular process of cognitive balancing that occurs after a difficult decision is made by an individual or group. Decisions, by their nature, involve alternatives, doubt, ambivalence, and conflict. Perhaps more than one alternative is attractive to the individual or different alternatives are attractive to different members of the group. Dissonance is created by considering the choices. A class of nursing students may be discussing a change in uniforms for acute care settings, or in the dress code for home visits and outpatient settings. The longer and stronger the discussion, the more ambivalence will be created, leading to a state of cognitive dissonance. When the alternatives are under consideration, the individual members of the group feel a mixture of negative and positive emotions related to different choices. The dissonance is a continuous source of tension, and the individual or group attempts to reduce it in a number of ways. For example, once the decision is made, there is a tendency to begin valuing the selected choice even more than before. This process is a way the individual or group copes with the doubts and skepticism generated during the discussion. The students may focus on the comfort and ease of care of the new uniforms selected, rather than that there was a difference of opinion about color. Living with a decision is made easier by emphasizing the positive aspects of the choice.

Community Cohesion

As noted, people form groups for a variety of reasons, both personal and professional. A *community* is a group of persons with some common bond, whether living near one another; having the same religious beliefs; or perhaps coming from the same country of origin, but not necessarily living in close proximity in the country of immigration. Some authors note that when people form a community, there is a natural tendency toward cohesion. This is a predictable outcome of the group identity and, if not taken to excess, can lead to positive effects for the individual and the group. Cohesiveness has been defined as the extent to which the features of the group bind the members to it. The bases of cohesiveness include: the liking or attraction among members, similar norms and values, the effective pursuit of goals, and maintaining good working relations (Kimberly, 1997).

Individual members of a community enjoy the link that exists between them and the group. The support, trust, and affection among the community contributes to personal growth, even if there is an occasional expression of hostility, dissatisfaction, or frustration. Cohesion has been called the "glue" that causes the members to remain in the community even when there are pressures or influences to leave it. For the community, the benefit is that cohesive groups usually enjoy low turnover and high participation because members desire continuation of the group and its commitment to common goals. Cohesion enhances group norms, and norms contribute to cohesion. The Boy Scouts of America and, particularly, the local scout troop, is a voluntary community. It is reported (Powers, 1998) that the fastest growing group of Boy Scouts, which now number nearly 5 million, are blacks and Latinos from poor urban neighborhoods. They are drawn to what scouting offers—structure, identity, attention, camaraderie, recognition, and positive role models. In return, the eager recruits have revitalized the Boy Scout movement in the cities.

► COMPROMISED PROCESSES OF SELF-CONCEPT–GROUP IDENTITY

When there is inadequate integration of life processes and ineffective compensatory life processes related to self-concept–group identity, compromised processes occur and the third adaptation level results in adaptation problems. Difficulties can occur in any or all of the processes of self-concept–group identity. Three examples of compromised processes are discussed here: sexual dysfunction and anxiety (related to the individual) and low morale (related to groups, either personal or professional).

Sexual Dysfunction

Sexual dysfunction, an adaptation problem of the physical self, is defined as ineffective sexual behavior related to physical or psychological factors. The term sexual dysfunction is used when the person identifies a problem with sexuality or when antisocial sexual behavior results in harm to others (Kelly, 1985). Thus the person may demonstrate sexual dysfunction in one of two ways—verbalization of decreased sense of sexual self or aggressive sexual behavior.

Decreased sense of sexual self is revealed by the person's comments. Several factors inherent in the experience of illness contribute to this compromised adaptation process. The pathophysiology of disease, medications, and particularly chemotherapy may contribute directly to the physiologic sexual response. Factors during hospitalization that affect the sense of sexual self include asexual hospital gowns, hospital routines, procedures that invade and assault the person's body, lack of privacy, and the interruption of the regular routine of work, hobbies, recreation, and social interactions.

Asking for personal information about the nurse, such as address, telephone number, and social and sexual life is considered aggressive sexual behavior. Attempts to touch the nurse's body, seductive comments and jokes, or unnecessary exposing of the genitals are other aggressive sexual behaviors. Such behaviors by the patient may be precipitated by discomfort with lack of privacy, uncertainty about the effects of illness or surgery on sexual functioning, and feelings of helplessness to control life in the face of illness. Lack of information and clarity about sexuality may also affect sexual dysfunction, both decreased sense of sexual self and the use of aggressive sexual behaviors.

Anxiety

One of the most common compromised processes related to the personal self is anxiety. *Anxiety* is the result of anything that threatens a person's sense of self-consistency and is defined as a painful uneasiness of mind due to a vague, nonspecific threat. A mild or brief moderate anxiety response can activate the person to confront and cope with a threatening event in an adaptive way. At this level, anxiety is considered a compensatory process. A recurrent, prolonged, or severe anxiety response, on the other hand, may hinder the individual's attempt to adapt to the environment. Anxiety as a compromised process uses needless energy and is ineffective in integrating one's experiences into the personal self-concept. A thorough assessment of behaviors and stimuli is made before the nursing judgment of anxiety as an adaptation problem can be reached.

The behaviors indicative of anxiety are complex, individual, and diverse. They often mimic behaviors of other adaptation problems. Some of the behavioral reactions that can be associated with anxiety are identified within each of the adaptive modes. In the physiologic mode the person may manifest any of the following: constant activity, sleep disturbances, cold clammy skin, alopecia, dry mouth, dilated pupils, voice tremors and pitch changes, trembling, difficulty concentrating, amenorrhea, difficulty breathing, tachycardia, palpitations, loss of appetite or overeating, nausea and vomiting, flatus, constipation or diarrhea, polyuria, and increased perspiration.

Changes specific to self-concept mode components that may occur in anxiety include: changes in sex drive and performance; disgust with one's body; decreased self-care and hygiene; sadness and crying; pseudo-cheerfulness; denying of feelings; inner preoccupation; negative self-talk; rumination about problems; angry outbursts; and talking of fear, apprehension, and worry. Effects of anxiety on the role function mode include inability to make decisions, difficulty doing simple tasks, difficulty meeting responsibilities, and decreased interest in usual roles. In the interdependence mode, the anxious person often expresses feeling alone and isolated.

The focal stimulus for anxious behaviors is the perceived threat. Common stimuli include experiences of loss, actual or anticipated; sudden changes in lifestyle, positive or negative; assault; invasive procedures; disease; unknown or fatal prognosis in illness; rapid or extreme changes in role function; disruptive family life; history of past anxiety states; unconscious conflict; unmet needs; and transmission of another person's anxiety to the individual.

When anxiety is at a compromised level, the nurse works with the person toward three general goals.

1. The person will verbalize feeling anxiety and that this is ineffective in meeting other goals and needs.
2. The person will verbalize insight into the nature and source of the anxiety.
3. The person will demonstrate the ability to cope effectively with the anxiety.

How to develop specific goals for adaptation problems is discussed later as part of the nursing process.

Low Morale

Morale is defined simply as the state of mind of a person or group as exhibited by confidence, cheerfulness, and productivity. *Low morale* in a group is a state resulting from challenges to the usual tendency toward cohesiveness and failure of the processes for shared identity. Manifestations of low morale are evident in low energy of the group for activities related to the goals of the group or to maintaining group relationships. Complaints about small issues multiply and individuals retreat to self-interests. The members of the group are no longer interested in putting energy into sharing cognitive and emotional orientations. Commitment to values and goals of the group become less active and intense.

There are many factors that can precipitate low morale in a group, or lead to its insidious development. Changes in any of the three stimuli considered relevant to shared identity may be responsible for changes in morale. If demands on a group increase without the resources to meet the demands, frustrations can evolve quickly into low morale. If ways to communicate over distance are altered, there may be a gradual erosion of morale in the group. When a group that has met annually about common research interests loses funding to travel, they may find that alternate ways of sharing do not create the same joy and productivity.

In the discussion of the group's perception of changes in behavior of other people or groups, it was noted that this can lead to efforts to strengthen shared identity. The example was given of a department perceiving that they are being targeted for budget cuts by the administration. In this situation, if the perceptions turn out to be validated by layoff notices to one third of the staff, and if all efforts to deal as a group with the issue are ineffective, then low morale is a likely consequence. The cycle of low morale continues downward as changes are implemented and the demands of greater workloads are placed on fewer staff.

Leadership and how responsibility and accountability are distributed are key factors in enhancing or lowering morale. One of the most devastating blows to group morale is a leader's inequitable distribution of responsibility and accountability for group goals. If even one nurse on a given unit consistently receives lighter patient loads and never attends unit meetings, resentment and the powerlessness to explain or change the situation leads to low morale in the whole group. Perhaps equally distressing for the group is the situation in which goals are altered by the leader without consulting the group. Many nurses have experienced the low morale resulting when a health care agency is purchased by a larger corporation and new leadership changes the philosophy and mission of the institution by announcement in a newsletter. The problems resulting from low morale provide a real threat to any group, and certainly affect the type of patient care nurses can provide when it occurs in a health care setting. Nurses may also meet many patients whose health issues are exacerbated by low morale resulting from the many changes occurring in contempory work settings.

▶ PLANNING NURSING CARE

In applying the nursing process to the self-concept–group identity mode processes, the nurse makes a careful assessment of behaviors and stimuli. In assessing factors influencing self-concept, regulator and cognator effectiveness in initiating compensatory processes is considered. With respect to collective human systems and group identity, stabilizer and innovator effectiveness is an important consideration. The presence of compromised processes of adaptation becomes a nursing priority. Based on thorough first- and second-level assessment, the nurse formulates nursing diagnoses, sets goals, selects interventions, and evaluates care.

Throughout this section on planning nursing care, the situation of Wanda K. is used for illustrative purposes. Wanda is a professional nurse educated at the graduate level. For 2 years, she has occupied an administrative position in a long-term care hospital and is responsible for resident care within the facility.

For the past year, her job has been filled with challenges and conflict. The leadership in the organization has been in the process of making significant changes in the way in which they administer the hospital. In addition, a funding crisis has necessitated frequent and disruptive changes in operating plans.

Wanda expressed to a trusted colleague that she has lost interest and pleasure in her job. For 2 months, she has not been sleeping well and has felt a general lack of energy. She is also beginning to doubt her capabilities as a nurse and administrator. She states, "Every day looks gray and gloomy," "I don't enjoy anything in life anymore," and "I know I am not doing well at my job."

When she first assumed her position, Wanda was part of a newly constructed administrative team. The administrative leadership at the hospital voiced commitment to a process of organizational change characterized by an environment of empowerment, decentralized decision making, innovation, mutual respect, and effective stewardship of resources. Wanda was fully committed to the established direction and wholly supportive of the administrative vision.

Within a short time, however, it became apparent that, although her boss talked about these values and principles, his actions were precisely opposed to the direction and vision. He was disrespectful of members of his administrative team, did not support them in their roles, continued to make autocratic decisions, and could not be relied on to follow through on commitments, thus compromising the performance of the others. As a result, the management team split into two factions: one group who continued to support and persevere with the described vision and another segment who took their lead from the chief executive.

Wanda was highly committed to the values and goals identified in the vision and worked with her staff team in a manner which reflected them. This, however, led to problematic situations when the resident care staff had recommendations regarding a particular action, yet the chief executive insisted on controlling the direction of the decision. It seemed that Wanda could do nothing right. At times, she would be in tears at meetings and at other times appeared very reluctant to contribute. Her question of her trusted colleague was, "What should I do?"

Nursing Diagnosis

Development of nursing diagnoses associated with self-concept–group identity is accomplished in the same way as in the other adaptive modes. One method involves the statement of the behaviors together with the influencing stimuli; another method makes use of summary labels.

Nursing diagnoses may reflect either adaptive or ineffective behaviors. In the situation of Wanda K., a sample adaptive nursing diagnosis states, "Help-seeking behaviors (a coping strategy to deal with threats to self) arising from a positive relationship with a trusted colleague." The request for help (behavior) is influenced by a previous and ongoing supportive relationship (stimulus).

In the case of ineffective behaviors, a multitude of nursing diagnoses may result. As the self-concept–group identity mode is closely interrelated with the other modes, a disturbance in one is likely to precipitate disturbances in others. For example, for Wanda, a diagnosis might be "Feelings of insecurity and worthlessness due to lack of support and respect from boss and powerlessness related to the dissonance in practiced values." The relationship between the individual and the environment is evident in this diagnosis.

It is also possible to construct a nursing diagnosis using a summary label that captures a cluster of behaviors. This method is used by experienced nurses to communicate significant amounts of information in one phrase. As identified in Chapter 3, there are a number of indicators of positive self-concept adaptation identified as summary labels in the Roy Adaptation Model. Indicators for the physical self include positive body image, effective sexual function, psychic integrity with physical growth, adequate compensation for bodily changes, effective coping strategies for loss, and effective process of life closure. For the personal self, the indicators are stable pattern of self-consistency, effective integration of self-ideal, effective processes of moral-ethical-spiritual growth, functional self-esteem, and effective coping strategies for threats to self.

Likewise, commonly recurring adaptation problems are identified: for the physical self—body image disturbance, sexual dysfunction, rape trauma syndrome, and unresolved loss; and for the personal self—anxiety, powerlessness, guilt, and low self-esteem.

Similarly, indicators of positive adaptation have been identified for group identity. They are effective interpersonal relationships, supportive culture, positive morale, principle-based relationships, and value-driven relationships. Commonly recurring adaptation problems for group identity include ineffective interpersonal relationships, oppressive culture, low morale, abusive relationships, and valueless relationships.

Considering the collective system involving the administrative team in Wanda's situation, a nursing diagnosis using a summary label might be, "Oppressive culture due to dissonance between stated values and those practiced by the chief executive." Both the behavior and the stimulus stated in this example communicate a wealth of information to nurses experienced in adaptation problems associated with self-concept or group identity. However, for the inexperienced person, the more detailed expression of behaviors and stimuli is more meaningful.

Use of a summary label when more than one mode is affected by the same stimulus is often an effective way of communicating a cluster of behaviors. For example, depression might be such a diagnosis. One word captures a multitude of behaviors and stimuli. The diagnosis statement could be, "depression due to work-related problems."

In Table 14–4, the Roy model nursing diagnostic categories for integrated processes of self-concept–group identity are shown in relation to nursing diagnosis labels approved by the North American Nursing Diagnosis Association (Rantz & LeMone, 1997).

Goal Setting

Each step of the nursing process focuses on the individual or collective system's behavior, the stimuli influencing that behavior, or both. With the nursing diagnosis, the statement developed included the behaviors and stimuli. With the goal-setting step, the focus is on behavior. Each goal identifies a behavior that is to be addressed.

TABLE 14–4 NURSING DIAGNOSTIC CATEGORIES FOR SELF-CONCEPT–GROUP IDENTITY

Indicators of Adaptation	Common Adaptation Problems	NANDA Diagnostic Labels
• Positive body image	• Body image disturbance	• Body image disturbance
• Effective sexual function	• Sexual dysfunction	• Sexual dysfunction
• Psychic integrity with physical growth	• Rape trauma syndrome	• Ineffective denial
• Adequate compensation for bodily changes	• Unresolved loss	• Anticipatory grieving
		• Dysfunctional grieving
• Effective coping strategies for loss		• Posttrauma response
		• Rape trauma syndrome: compound reaction, silent reaction
• Effective process of life closure		
• Stable pattern of self-consistency	• Anxiety	• Rape trauma syndrome
• Effective integration of self-ideal	• Powerlessness	• Altered sexuality patterns
• Effective processes of moral-ethical-spiritual growth	• Guilt	• Personal identity disturbance
	• Low self-esteem	• Chronic low self-esteem
• Functional self-esteem		• Situational low self-esteem
• Effective coping strategies for threats to self		• Self-esteem disturbance
		• Spiritual distress (distress of the human spirit)
• Effective interpersonal relationships	• Ineffective interpersonal relations	
• Supportive culture	• Oppressive culture	• Potential for enhanced spiritual well-being
• Positive morale	• Low morale	
• Group acceptance	• Stigma	• Hopelessness
• Principle-based relationships	• Abusive relationships	• Powerlessness
• Value-driven relationships	• Valueless relationships	• Anxiety
		• Fear

Many self-concept–group identity problems have a chronic as well as an acute phase. Thus, the goal-setting process includes both long- and short-term goals, each of which states the behavior of focus, the change expected, and the time frame in which the goal is to be achieved.

The following statement provides an example of a possible goal for the situation concerning Wanda: "Within 1 week, Wanda will voice enhanced confidence in her capabilities and self-worth." From the perspective of the group, a goal might be, "Within 6 months, all members of the administrative team will consistently demonstrate the hospital's articulated values and goals."

In order to be effective in guiding progress, goals must be established in collaboration with the person involved. As with each step of the nursing process, the individuals, where possible, must be active participants to ensure that accurate and relevant information is obtained, that it is interpreted appropriately into the diagnoses, and that achievable and relevant goals are established. This is the only way that interventions can be determined that will assist in achieving psychic and spiritual integrity for the individual, or identity integrity where groups are concerned.

After formulating goals, the nurse proceeds to the identification of nursing interventions, the next step of the nursing process as described in the Roy Adaptation Model.

Intervention

The intervention step of the nursing process according to the Roy Adaptation Model focuses on the stimuli affecting the behavior identified in the goal setting step. The intervention step is thus the management of stimuli and this involves either altering, increasing, decreasing, removing, or maintaining them. At the same time, the nurse may help the person or group to use effective coping strategies to strengthen compensatory processes. A review of the stimuli affecting adaptive life processes and the discussion of compensatory processes earlier in the chapter provides insight into specific interventions aimed at psychic and spiritual integrity for individuals and identity integrity for groups.

In Wanda's situation, the focal stimulus appears to be the behavior of her boss. However, given his place in the organizational structure, his removal from the situation is unlikely. In general, such situations in organizations can rarely be handled that straightforwardly. Certainly, the situation in which Wanda finds herself is problematic and the interventions must be directed at changing the situation. It may be possible to alter the behavior of her boss. Perhaps a conversation with him expressing the assessed dissonance of his behavior with the stated values and goals would result in a change. As it happens, such conversations have been attempted with no resolution. Because of her own deep values, changing her own beliefs and behavior is not an option for Wanda as a way to remove the dissonance. At some point, if the situation remains unresolved, Wanda may have to look at removing herself from the situation by finding another place of employment. Each of these approaches is an attempt to alter the stimulus causing the observed behaviors.

Evaluation

Evaluation involves judging the effectiveness of the nursing interventions in relation to the person's or collective's adaptive behavior, that is, whether the behaviors stated in the goals have been achieved. The nursing interventions are effective if the behavior is in accordance with the stated goal. If the goal has not been achieved, the nurse identifies alternative interventions or approaches by reassessing the behavior and stimuli and continuing with the other steps of the nursing process.

The previously identified goal was stated as, "Within 1 week, Wanda will voice enhanced confidence in her capabilities and self-worth." Indications of progress toward this goal would be Wanda talking with her friend about her increased confidence in her abilities and her self-esteem. She may state, "I know that I am working constructively with my staff and that my actions reflect the stated values for the hospital." Or she may say, "The problems exist because my boss is not 'walking the talk.' Unless that dissonance is resolved, the problems will continue and this goes way beyond me and my capabilities."

From the perspective of the collective human system, in this case the administrative team, consider the previously stated goal, "Within 6 months, all members of the administrative team will consistently demonstrate the hospital's articulated values and goals." Evaluation of achieving this goal may involve an interview with all members of the administrative team. Questions related to unity of approach and commitment to goals and values would be addressed. Perhaps in that interval, some members of the team would have changed. Evidence of goal achievement would be affirmation that, indeed, all members of the team are assessed to be reflecting the articulated values and goals in their interactions. Or there may have been agreement that the vision as stated was not achievable and alterations would have been made in how people agree to work together.

It is important to recognize that the nursing process and the six steps are ongoing, simultaneous, and overlapping. Although they have been separated and dealt with in an artificially linear manner for discussion purposes, intervention is often occurring at the same time as first- and second-level assessment is proceeding. Likewise, evaluation occurs on an ongoing basis, being held in mind even when nursing diagnoses are being established and as goals are being formulated. Another consideration of overlap in the nursing process is that both individual and collective may be considered at the same time in planning nursing care. Competency in using the adaptation model at individual and group levels comes with increasing knowledge and experience.

► SUMMARY

This chapter has focused on the application of the Roy Adaptation Model to the self-concept–group identity mode. An overview of two processes—developing self and focusing self—associated with psychic and spiritual integrity for the individual, and shared identity associated with identity integrity for collective human systems, was provided along with identification of parameters for assessment of behaviors and stimuli. Illustration of compensatory processes related to self-concept–group identity were described and examples of three compromised processes, sexual dysfunction, anxiety, and low morale, were provided. Finally, guidelines for planning nursing care through the formulation of nursing diagnoses, goals, and interventions were explored and evaluation of nursing care was described.

► EXERCISES FOR APPLICATION

1. Draw an illustration to portray each of the various aspects of the self-concept–group identity mode. Try to include all the components and the associated integrated processes.

2. Select one aspect of the physical or personal self component of self-concept and create questions that would be appropriate for assessment of stimuli related to that particular aspect.

▶ ASSESSMENT OF UNDERSTANDING

Questions

1. The basic need underlying the self-concept–group identity mode is _____ for the individual and _____ for the collective human system. The two subareas of the self-concept mode are:
   (a) _____ which includes two components, (1) _____, and (2) _____.
   (b) _____ which includes (1) _____, (2) _____, and (3) _____.

2. Fill in the following table with respect to the assessment of behavior in the self-concept–group integrity mode.

Integrated Process	Assessment Parameter	Examples of Behavior to Be Noted
a. Developing self		1.1
		1.2
		1.3
	1.	2.1
	2.	2.2
		2.3
b. Focusing self		1.1
		1.2
		1.3
	1.	2.1
	2.	2.2
	3.	3.1
		3.2
		3.3
		3.4
c. Shared identity		1.1
		1.2
		1.3
	1.	2.1
	2.	2.2
	3.	2.3
		3.1
		3.2
		3.3

3. Identify the following stimuli as being associated with the integrated processes of developing self (DS), focusing self (FS), or shared identity (SI). Note all that apply.
   (a) _____ physical development

(b) _____ demands and distance
(c) _____ perception and self-schema
(d) _____ transaction between person and environment
(e) _____ coping strategies
(f) _____ striving for unity or integrity

4. Which of the following could be considered compensatory processes related to self-concept–group identity?
   (a) the tendency of people to select mates who have the similar physical characteristics
   (b) integrating a loss into one's physical self-concept
   (c) prolonged ambivalence about a decision
   (d) liking or attraction among members of a group
   (e) considering mortality when a parent dies

5. Identify one compromised process of self-concept–group integrity related to each of the following components.
   (a) physical self _____
   (b) personal self _____
   (c) shared goals and values _____

Situation:

Stella Marinez is a 20-year-old Mexican-American woman who is a junior nursing student at a university in the Midwest. She has been a good student and is delighted to be in her first clinical placement. However, during her second week, she was caring for a person with a gangrenous arm. She fainted and had to be taken to the student infirmary. Stella began to confide in a trusted colleague, a graduate nursing student whose clinical placement overlaps her own. Stella indicated to her colleague that she was concerned about not feeling well and how this was affecting her work.

Physically, Stella is tiny. She is 5 feet and 1 inch tall and wears size 6 clothing. When school started in the fall, she was proud to have diminished to a size 2. She admits that she has given up her meal pass since she doesn't eat that much. Stella prefers to do heavy exercise during the meal breaks.

During her younger years, Stella's closely knit family were migrant workers who moved from Texas to California to Oregon with the crops. She has an older and a younger brother who were always very protective of her when they worked in the fields. At one point, the family received an unexpected inheritance from a grandmother in Mexico. This enabled the family to purchase a small adobe house in the Imperial Valley in California and to become involved in the dried fruit industry. Stella was able to stay in one location during high school and, during this time, she did very well in her studies. Stella realized that she wanted to be a nurse when she was helping her mother care for a dying relative. A high school counselor was helpful in her successful admission to a university nursing program.

During the past summer, Stella went home from the university to spend time with her family. There, she began to date the older brother of a friend, a man 10 years her senior. Her family was not in favor of this relationship and told her that he was too old for her and that he would only break her heart. The man's sister warned Stella not to trust her brother. After about 6 weeks of an intense relationship, the man suddenly broke off any association with Stella. Within the week, he announced his engagement to another woman, a tall, slim Anglo-American of his own age. She was a person that he had been involved with while Stella was away at school, but who had been out of town in the early summer.

In her hurt and disappointment, Stella returned to the Midwest early stating, "It's a small town back there and I don't want everyone looking at me." She joined the university gym and began vigorous exercise morning and evening as well as running at noon when she could.

6. Formulate a nursing diagnosis for the above situation using two methods.
   (a) _____
   (b) _____

7. Construct a goal for Stella.

   _____

8. Since interventions are focused on stimuli, what interventions could be used to alleviate the situation described, considering the following stimuli.
   (a) loss of significant other (male friend)
   (b) perceptions and self-schema
   (c) coping strategies

9. How would you evaluate achievement of the goal you established in item 7?

   _____

Feedback

1. psychic and spiritual integrity, identity integrity
   (a) physical self, (1) body image, (2) body sensation
   (b) personal self, (1) self-consistency, (2) self-ideal, (3) moral-ethical-spiritual self

2. a.1. Body sensations: 1.1 facial expressions, 1.2 body posture, 1.3 physical tensions, 1.4 ease of feeding and eliminating [as examples]
   a.2. Body image: 1.1 gender, 1.2 posture, 1.3 carriage, 1.4 level of personal hygiene, 1.5 grooming [as examples]
   b.1. Self-consistency: 1.1 how a person describes self, 1.2 how the person behaves over time, 1.3 what about self the person most wants to protect [as examples]

b.2. Self-ideal: 2.1 expressing satifaction at meeting own goals, 2.2 expressions of ongoing goals for self [as examples]

b.3. Moral-ethical-spiritual self: 3.1 description of spiritual beliefs, 3.2 religious or spiritual practices, 3.3 consistency of beliefs and behavior, 3.4 contentment with self [as examples]

c.1. Perceptions of environment: 1.1 definition of group boundaries, 1.2 who are considered outside the group, 1.3 how the group incorporates new members [as examples]

c.2. Cognitive and feeling orientations: 2.1 common beliefs, 2.2 common feelings, 2.3 congruence of intent and actions [as examples]

c.3. Goals and values: 3.1 goals agreed on by the group, 3.2 values agreed on by the group, 3.3 use of power in the group [as examples]

3. (a) DS, (b) SI, (c) DS, (d) FS, (e) DS, (f) FS

4. b, d, e

5. (a) sexual dysfunction
   (b) anxiety
   (c) low morale

6. Examples of nursing diagnoses:
   (a) Deterioration in health and stamina due to minimal intake and severe exercise
   (b) Disconnection from support systems related to perception that significant others (family and friends) were critical of her choices

7. Example of a goal: Within 1 week, Stella will voice acknowledgment that her coping strategies of minimal intake and severe exercise are compromising her health and her career goals (self-ideal).

8. Possible interventions:
   (a) Encourage expression of feelings, thoughts, and questions about the experience.
   (b) Explore events surrounding her short-term relationship that are having a negative effect on Stella's self-concept. As details are recalled, Stella may come to realize that current thoughts and feelings about self are based on distorted self-ideal or misinterpretations of others' reactions.
   (c) Talk therapy may help Stella to understand the potential complications associated with the coping strategies she is using.

9. Stella will acknowledge that her lack of intake and severe exercise are causing her health to deteriorate and may interfere with her ability to finish her nursing education and achieve her career goals. She will initiate steps to get further help.

► **REFERENCES**

Amman-Gainotti, M. (1986). Sexual socialization during early adolescence: The menarche. *Adolescence, 21,* 703–710.

Andrews, J. D. W. (1990). Interpersonal self-confirmation and challenge in psychotherapy. *Psychotherapy, 27(4),* 485–504.

Antonovsky, A. (1986). The development of a sense of coherence and its impact to stress situations. *The Journal of Social Psychology, 26(2),* 213–225.

Beck, T. (1976). *Cognitive therapy and the emotional disorder.* New York: International Psychiatry.

Calderone, M., & Ramey, J. (1982). *Talking with your child about sex.* New York: Ballantine Books.

Campsey, J. (1985). The sexual dimension of patient care. *Nursing Forum, 22(2),* 69–71.

Carnevalli, D. L., & Thomas, M. D. (1993). *Diagnostic reasoning and treatment decision making in nursing.* Philadelphia: Lippincott.

Chinn, P. L. (1995). *Peace and power: Building communities for the future* (4th ed.). New York: National League for Nursing Press.

Cooley, C. H. (1964). *Human nature and the social order.* New York: Schocken.

Coombs, A. W., & Snygg, D. (1959). *Individual behavior: A perceptual approach to behavior.* New York: Harper & Brothers.

Demo, D. H. (1992). The self-concept over time: Research issues and directions. *Annual Review of Sociology, 18,* 303–326.

Dobratz, M. (1984). Life closure. In Roy, Sr. C. (Ed.), *Introduction to nursing: An adaptation model* (2nd ed., pp. 497–518). Englewood Cliffs, NJ: Prentice-Hall.

Driever, M. (1976). Problems of low self-esteem. In Roy, Sr. C. (Ed.), *Introduction to nursing: An adaptation model* (pp. 232–242). Englewood Cliffs, NJ: Prentice-Hall.

Elliott, G. (1986). Self-esteem and self-consistency: A theoretical and empirical link between two primary motivations. *Social Psychology Quarterly, 49(3),* 207–218.

Erikson, E. H. (1968). *Identity: Youth and crisis.* New York: Norton.

Erikson, E. H. (1963). *Childhood and society* (2nd ed.). New York: Norton.

Festinger, L. (1962). *A theory of cognitive dissonance.* Palo Alto, CA: Stanford University Press.

Fiske, A. P. (1991). *The structures of social life.* New York: Free Press.

Garcia, T., & Pintrich, P. (1994). Regulating motivation and cognition in the classroom: The role of self-schemas and self-regulatory strategies. In Schunk, D., & Zimmerman, B. (Eds.), *Self-regulation of learning and performance: Issues and educational applications* (pp. 129–178). Hillsdale, NJ: Erlbaum.

Gecas, V. (1982). The self concept. *Annual Review of Sociology, 8,* 1–33.

Goffman, E. (1959). *The presentation of self in everyday life.* New York: Anchor.

Goffman, E. (1967). *Interactional ritual.* New York: Anchor.

Horton, A. M., Jr. (Ed.). (1990). *Neuropsychology across the life-span: Assessment and treatment.* New York: Springer Publishing.

Johnson, D. (1983). *Body.* Boston: Beacon Press.

Johnson, J. E., & Leventhal, H. (1974). Effects of accurate expectations and behavioral instructions on reactions during a noxious medical examination. *Journal of Personality and Social Psychology, 2,* 55–64.

Kelly, M. A. (1985). *Nursing diagnosis source book: Guidelines for clinical application.* E. Norwalk, CT: Appleton-Century-Crofts.

Kendzierski, D. (1988). Self-schemata and exercise. *Basic and Applied Social Psychology, 9,* 45–59.

Kimberly, J. C. (1997). *Group processes and structures: A theoretical integration.* Lanham, MD: University Press of America.

Kleinke, C. (1978). *Self-perception: The psychology of personal awareness.* San Francisco: Freeman.

Kübler-Ross, E. (1969). *On death and dying.* New York: Macmillan.

Lecky, P. (1945). *Self-consistency: A theory of personality.* New York: Island Press.

Lecky, P. (1961). In Thorne, C. F. (Ed.), *Self-consistency: A theory of personality.* Hamden, CT: The Shoe String Press.

Lewin, K. (1948). *Resolving social conflicts.* New York: Harper & Row.

Markus, H. (1977). Self-schemata and processing information about the self. *Journal of Personality and Social Psychology, 35(2),* 63–78.

Markus, H., Crane, M., Bernstein, S., & Siladi, M. (1982). Self-schemas and gender. *Journal of Personality and Social Psychology, 42(1),* 38–50.

Markus, H., Hamill, R., & Sentis, K. (1987). Thinking fat: Self-schemas for body weight and the processing of weight relevant information. *Journal of Applied Social Psychology, 17(1),* 50–71.

Markus, H., & Wurf, E. (1987). The dynamic self-concept: A social psychological perspective. *Annual Review of Psychology, 38,* 299–337.

Markus, H., & Zajonc, R. (1985). The cognitive perspectives in sociopsychology. In Lindzey, G., & Aronson, E. A. (Eds.), *Handbook of social psychology* (Vol. 1., 3rd ed.). New York: Erlbaum.

McMahon, E. M. (1993). *Beyond the myth of dominance: An alternative to a violent society.* Kansas City, MO: Sheed & Ward.

Mead, G. (1934). *Mind, self and society.* Chicago: University of Chicago Press.

Montagu, A. (1986). *Touching: The human significance of the skin* (3rd ed.). New York: Harper & Row.

Neugarten, B. (1969). Continuities and discontinuities of psychological issues in adult life. *Human Development, 12,* 121–130.

Neugarten, B. L. (1979). Time, age, and the life cycle. *The American Journal of Psychiatry, 136(7),* 887–894.

Newman, M. (1994). *Help as expanding consciousness* (2nd ed.). New York: National League for Nursing Press.

Piaget, J. (1954). *The construction of reality in the child* (M. Cook, trans.). New York: Basic Books.

Powers, J. (1998). The proud colors of Troop 63: Eager to belong, black and Latino youngsters at Cathedral thrive under Boy Scouts' urban renewal. *Boston Globe,* May 7, D1, D6.

Rabbie, J. M., & Lodewijkx, H. F. M. (1996). A behavioral interaction model: Toward an integrative theoretical framework for studying intra- and intergroup dynamics. In Witte, E., & Davis, J. H. (Eds.), *Understanding group behavior: Small group processes and interpersonal relations* (Vol. 2 , pp. 255–294). Mahwah, NJ: Erlbaum.

Rantz, M. J., & LeMone, P. (1997). *Classifications of nursing diagnoses. Proceedings of the 12th conference NANDA.* Glendale, CA: CINAHL Information Systems.

Rogers, C. (1961). *On becoming a person.* Boston: Houghton Mifflin.

Rosenberg, M. (1965). *Society and adolescent self-image.* Princeton, NJ: Princeton University Press.

Rosenberg, M. (1968). Discussion: The concept of self. In Ahelson, R., Aronson, E., McGuire, W., Newcomb, T., Rosenberg, M., & Tannebaum, P. (Eds.), *Theories of cognitive consistency: A sourcebook* (pp. 384–389). Chicago: Rand McNally.

Rosenberg, M. (1979). *Conceiving the self.* New York: Basic Books.

Servonsky, J., & Opas, S. (Eds.). (1987). *Nursing management of children: A textbook.* Boston: Jones and Bartlett.

Silverstone, B., & Hyman, H. (1976). *You and your aging parent.* New York: Pantheon.

Sullivan, H. S. (1953). *The interpersonal theory of psychiatry.* New York: Norton.

Swimme, B., & Berry, T. (1992). *The universe story.* San Francisco: Harper.

Zhan, L. (1994). Cognitive adaptation processing and self-consistency in the hearing impaired elderly (Doctoral Dissertation, Boston College, 1993). *Dissertation Abstracts International, 54,* 4086B.

Zohar, D. (1990). *The quantum self: Human nature and consciousness defined by the new physics.* New York: Quill/Morrow.

► **ADDITIONAL REFERENCES**

Breakwell, G. (1986). *Coping with threatened identities.* London: Methuen.

Cathcart, R. S., Samovar, L. A., & Henman, L. D. (Eds.). (1996). *Small group communication: Theory and practice* (7th ed.). Madison, WI: Brown & Benchmark.

Hall, B. A. (1997). Spirituality in terminal illness: An alternative view of theory. *Journal of Holistic Nursing, 15(1)*, 82–96.

Napier, R. W., & Gershenfeld, M. K. (1993). *Groups: Theory and experience* (5th ed.). Boston: Houghton Mifflin.

Ryan-Wenger, N. M. (1992). A taxonomy of children's coping strategies: A step toward theory development. *American Journal of Orthopsychiatry, 62(2)*, 256–263.

15

THE ROLE FUNCTION MODE

The role function mode focuses specifically on the roles people occupy in society. The basic need underlying the role function mode has been identified as social integrity for the individual and role clarity for the human group or collective. For the individual, *social integrity* involves the need to know who one is in relation to others so that one can act. For groups, *role clarity* includes the need to understand and commit to fulfillment of one's specified role within the group.

As emphasized previously in this book, inherent in the view of a person as an adaptive and holistic system is the understanding that human life processes are interrelated and capabilities or issues in one area of the person's functioning will affect adaptation in another. If a person is experiencing problems concerning an occupied role, the effects may be manifest in the ability to heal and to maintain and promote health. Health and illness experiences, in turn, affect role performance. Similarly, the effectiveness of role function in groups makes a contribution to the health of society. The role function mode provides the opportunity to focus specifically on how individuals and groups interact within societies. The philosophic assumptions of the Roy model speak to the social nature of people by emphasizing common purpose and meaning for human existence within the convergence of the universe (Roy 1988, 1997a). The reciprocal relationship between society and the person is integral to both the philosophic and scientific assumptions of nursing and the Roy model in particular. Therefore, social adaptation is as much of a concern to the nurse as physiologic and psychological-spiritual adaptation.

This chapter provides an overview of the role function mode of the Roy Adaptation Model for individuals and groups, including description and theoretical bases of the mode. From the theoretical background, integrated life processes are explored along with assessment of behaviors and stimuli for each process. Compensatory and compromised adaptive processes related to the role function mode are identified and discussed. Planning nursing care illustrates application of understanding of the role function mode to nursing diagnoses, goal setting, interventions, and evaluating nursing care.

► OBJECTIVES

After studying this chapter, the reader will be able to do the following:

1. Describe the role function mode according to the Roy Adaptation Model.

2. Identify important first-level assessment parameters (behaviors) for the role function mode.

3. Identify second-level assessment factors (stimuli) that influence the role function mode.

4. Describe one compensatory process related to the role function mode.

5. Name and describe two situations of compromised processes of role function.

6. Develop a nursing diagnosis, given a situation related to role function.

7. Derive goals for a given situation illustrating ineffective role function.

8. Describe nursing interventions commonly implemented in situations of ineffective role function.

9. Propose approaches to determine the effectiveness of nursing interventions in the role function mode.

► KEY CONCEPTS DEFINED

Aggregate role set: The complement of associated positions in a given group; includes all roles available within the group.

Developing roles: The process of adding new roles as one matures through life; involves learning the expectations of the roles.

Expressive behavior: The feelings and attitudes held by the person about role performance.

Instrumental behavior: Goal-oriented behavior; role activities the person performs.

Integrating roles: The process of managing different roles and their expectations.

Outgroup stereotyping: Situation in which people fail to relate to individuals with their own abilities and talents as the best candidates for given roles.

Primary role: An ascribed role based on age, sex, and developmental stage; it determines the majority of behaviors engaged in by a person during a particular growth period of life.

Role: The functioning unit of society; each role exists in relation to another.

Role acquisition: The assumption of a new social position with the performance of behaviors expected of one occupying that social role.

Role clarity: For groups, the basic need of the role function mode; the need to understand and commit to fulfill expected tasks, so that the group can achieve common goals.

Role conflict: Inconsistent expectations held by a person, or by other persons, for a given role in one's role set (intrarole conflict) or by inconsistent expectations among the roles of the person's role set (interrole conflict).

Role distance: Certain behaviors associated with the role are not compatible with self-concept; instrumental and expressive behaviors differ in kind and number.

Role expectations: Beliefs held by society in general, by an individual, or by those in complementary roles, about what is appropriate behavior associated with a role.

Role failure: A situation in which a person occupying a role has an absence of expressive or instrumental behaviors or those behaviors are ineffective.

Role mastery: Indicates that a person demonstrates both expressive and instrumental behaviors that meet social expectations associated with role set.

Role-taking: A process of looking at or anticipating another person's behavior by viewing it within a role attributed to the other; basing one's interaction on the judgment about the other's role; focuses on the meaning that the acts have to both persons in a role interaction.

Role transition: Growth in a new role with increasing effectiveness of expressive and instrumental role behaviors.

Role set: The particular complex of roles which an individual holds simultaneously; the total number of roles one has developed at a given time.

Secondary role: A role that a person assumes to complete the tasks associated with a developmental stage and primary role.

Social integrity: For individuals, the basic need of the role function mode; the need to know who one is in relation to others so that one can act.

Tertiary role: A role that is freely chosen by a person, temporary in nature, and often associated with the accomplishment of a minor task in a person's current development.

▶ ROLE FUNCTION PROCESSES

A *role* has been defined as the functioning unit of society. Each role exists in relationship to another. For example, the parent role relates to a child; the employer role, an employee; and the nurse role, a patient. Associated with each role are expectations about how a person behaves toward a person occupying the complementary position. Theories about roles, then, seek to explain behavior as actions taken in accordance with agreed-upon expectations for persons occupying given positions. Individuals play roles in relation to each other and as members of groups, as well. The basic needs of the role function mode are *social integrity,* accomplished for the individual by knowing who one is in relation to others, namely, the roles occupied and the associated societal expectations, so that one can act appropriately; and *role clarity,* accomplished for the members of a group by understanding and commitment to fulfill expected tasks, so that the group can achieve common goals. Social integrity and role clarity represent the underlying needs of the role function mode.

There are many approaches to role theories, but basically these are divided into two types, structural and interactional. Structural role theories are based on structural–functional approaches to persons in society such as those developed by Parsons and Shils (1951). Similarly, Linton (1945) saw roles as emphasizing structural components of societies and, because they were associated with social status in social systems, they were of a relatively fixed nature. Interactional approaches to role theory draw upon symbolic interactionism based on Mead (1934) and those who followed him. This theory emphasizes socialization through taking the role of the other. Today, there is an effort by scholars to bridge the gap between these theoretical approaches and to see them as complementary. Structural approaches look at the broad perspective of people within positions in society, and interactional approaches look at ways that people negotiate meanings while interacting in given role situations. The theoretical bases of the role function mode is illustrated in Figure 15–1.

An illustration of the two approaches and how they work together can be seen in the example of a nurse beginning in a new position at an outpatient clinic of a health care center. During an orientation session, the new

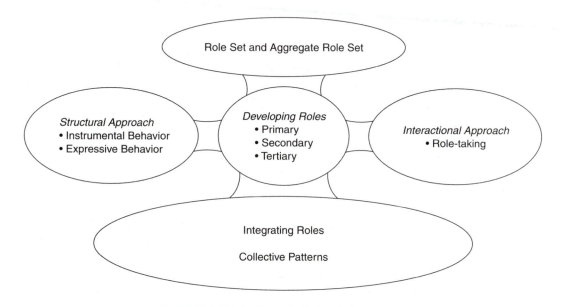

FIGURE 15–1. Role function mode with theoretical components.

employee is introduced to policy and procedure manuals that describe role expectations for behavior as related to the interdisciplinary team and to patients. The nurse is beginning to build a picture of structural role expectations in the different positions she holds in the organization. Later that day, while she is taking a break in the cafeteria, her unit director approaches and sits beside her. The new employee immediately identifies certain aspects of their mutual roles. She is aware that she will be expected to refer to this person as a resource in solving difficulties in her nursing practice. The nurse is also aware that the unit director will conduct her first performance evaluation. The interaction that follows between the two nurses in reciprocal roles is how the meaning of the roles is worked out. When the unit manager begins the conversation by commenting on the school of nursing from which the new employee graduated, the nurse interprets this as a friendly way of getting acquainted, beyond their roles in the structure. She responds from this perception of the other's behavior and the two begin comparing their educational and professional work backgrounds.

Both structural and interactional approaches are useful in understanding adaptation in the role function mode. The role function mode deals specifically with the person's place in society and how the person interacts in reciprocal roles and roles in groups. The goals of the mode are social integrity and role clarity. Processes used to create social integrity and role clarity are developing roles, role-taking, and integrating roles.

▶ **DEVELOPING ROLES: PROCESS AND ASSESSMENT**

Developing roles refers to the process of adding new roles as one matures through life. The process involves learning the expectations of the roles. In addition, within a given stage in life, additional new roles are acquired. *Role acquisition* is the assumption of a new social position with the performance of behaviors expected of one occupying that social role. *Role expectations* consist of beliefs held by society in general, the individual, and those in complementary roles about what is appropriate to do or not to do. Each time a new role is added, the person experiences the process of developing a role. The total number of roles one has developed at a given time is defined within the role function mode as the person's *role set*.

A classification of role sets as involving primary, secondary, and tertiary roles has been adopted for use in the Roy Adaptation Model (Banton, 1965; Randell, 1976). A person will have one primary role but will have many secondary and tertiary roles. The *primary role* determines the majority of behaviors that the person engages in during a particular period of life. It is determined by age, sex, and developmental stage (Erickson, 1963). (See Table 15–1.) Examples of primary roles are 5-year-old preschool male, 16-year-old adolescent female, and 70-year-old mature adult male. The association of age, sex, and developmental stage in labeling the primary role enables the identification of specific role expectations in relationship to the developmental stage and to social processes.

Secondary roles are those that a person assumes to complete the tasks associated with a developmental stage and primary role. For example, a 25-year-old young adult male or female may be faced with the task of being able to nurture, support, and provide for spouse and children. Secondary roles that are assumed related to this task could be husband or wife, father or mother,

TABLE 15–1 DEVELOPMENTAL STAGES AND SOCIAL PROCESSES RELATED TO DEVELOPING ROLES

Age (years)	Developmental Stage	Social Process
Birth–1½	Infant: trust vs. mistrust	Society contributes to the individual
1½–3½	Toddler: autonomy vs. shame	Society contributes to the individual
3½–6	Preschool: initiative vs. guilt	Society contributes to the individual
6–12	School-age: industry vs. inferiority	Individual begins to contribute to society
12–18	Adolescence: identify vs. role confusion	Individual relates to society through peer groups
18–35	Young adult: intimacy vs. isolation	Individual becomes independent member of society and begins to contribute toward the continuance of society by starting a new family
35–60	Generative adult: generativity vs. stagnation	Individual becomes involved with the survival of society through creative works and the guidance of the next generation
60 and on	Mature adult: ego integrity vs. despair	Individual becomes able to incorporate becoming a follower or a leader; sometimes in the sense of being a consultant

and teacher. The last column of Table 15–1 identifies some general social processes expected of secondary roles for the developmental stages. In the example given, the social process involves becoming an independent member of society and contributing to society by having a family. Secondary roles are normally achieved positions as opposed to primary qualities and require specific role performance. Job positions are secondary roles that assume particular importance in most societies because they are highly relevant to the individual's use of time and access to resources. Secondary roles are typically stable and not readily relinquished since they are developed and mastered over a period of time (Nuwayhid, 1984). Problems of role function usually occur in secondary roles and relate to the presence or absence of factors influencing developing roles. This is discussed further in assessment of stimuli relating to developing roles.

Tertiary roles are related primarily to secondary roles and represent ways in which individuals meet their role-associated obligations (Malaznik, 1976). Associated with the role of father might be that of junior football team coach or Boy Scout leader. Tertiary roles are normally temporary in nature and freely chosen by the individual, and may include activities such as clubs or hobbies. Figure 15–2 illustrates the role set for an individual using the classifi-

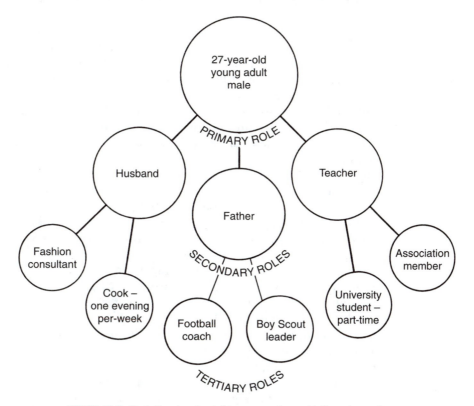

FIGURE 15–2. Illustration of a role set. Primary, secondary, and tertiary roles are shown.

cation of roles discussed. Understanding developing roles involves first identifying the primary, secondary, and tertiary roles in the person's role set.

Further understanding of how role sets develop contributes to understanding developing roles. According to role theorists, role sets are derived from patterns of the division of labor within society (Biddle & Thomas, 1979). Tasks in society, or in a group, are divided according to the specializations needed for the expected behaviors. For example, it is commonly noted that society needs people in the role of doctors to fulfill expectations for the treatment of disease. Society needs nurses to fulfill expectations for understanding the person's experience of health and illness, caring for them, and helping them cope with such life experiences. From the perspective of one individual, listing role sets adds up to listing the responsibilities the person holds based on specialty functions within society. *Role set*, then, means the particular complex of roles that an individual holds simultaneously. These roles will be a combination of primary, secondary, and tertiary roles.

Role sets may also be examined within a group. Secondary and tertiary roles for the individual are enacted within groups. Groups have sets of roles that interact, for example, in the family, husband and wife interact; parents and children interact; children interact with each other; and each of these roles interacts with other family members such as aunts, uncles, cousins, and grandparents. There is a rich literature on role theory within families that can be consulted for further understanding of developing roles in the context of the family.

In a given group, the complement of associated positions is called the *aggregate role set* (based on Biddle & Thomas, 1979, p. 41). For example, family members not only have titles related to the family structure, but also may be involved in any of a variety of roles within a family. These roles include decision making, leisure activities, emotional and physical nurturing, and communication among and between extended family members. The aggregate role set, then, includes all the roles available within the group. The concepts of individual role set and aggregate role set are related since the role set for any individual is drawn from the total aggregate role sets of the groups of which the person is a member.

If a group to which a person belongs changes the division of labor, and consequently the aggregate role sets within the organization, then the role set for a particular person may change. This is the case when health care agencies merge and positions are combined. For example, there may be only one nursing director position for the same-day surgery program in a reorganized health care setting, whereas two persons may have held two like positions in separate settings before the merger. No longer holding this role from the aggregate role set, an individual may have the opportunity to develop a new role, such as consultant. Role sets become the agenda for developing roles, and often successful development of one role provides a challenge for the process of developing other roles.

For an individual, there are multiple possible conflicting expectations within and among the aggregate role sets. For example, a teacher may need to meet with an administrator after school to fulfill an expectation of his developing role as teacher. At the same time, he is expected to arrive on time at a practice field in his role as football coach. This issue is discussed further as the process of integrating roles.

Within the Roy Adaptation Model, a structural approach to roles has been useful in identifying behavioral components to assist in the assessment of developing roles. These components are defined as instrumental and expressive behaviors, and apply to each role the person occupies (Nuwayhid, 1984; Parsons & Shils, 1951).

Instrumental behaviors, or goal oriented behaviors, are those activities persons perform as part of their roles. The person uses strategic behaviors with the goal of *role mastery,* namely, the demonstration of both instrumental and expressive role behaviors that meet societal expectations. Instrumental behaviors are normally physical actions that have a long-term orientation. For example, maintaining a job over time meets social expectations related to supporting a family.

Expressive behaviors, or affective behaviors, involve the feelings and attitudes held by the person about role performance. The goal of expressive behavior is direct or immediate feedback. Expressive behaviors are emotional in nature and result from interactions which enable the person to express these role-related feelings in an appropriate manner. The mother or father brings a surprise home from work to experience the appreciation and delight of the child.

Similar concepts are discussed in recent work by Patterson (1996). He suggests that the structural–functional models tend to distinguish between relatively spontaneous affect or emotion-driven behavior and more managed or deliberate behavior. Spontaneous patterns might be rooted in emotion, but managed patterns are goal oriented or strategic, and consequently, behavior patterns might be independent of affect. Instrumental (goal oriented) and expressive (affective) behavior are thus learned in relation to developing roles of one's role set. These concepts from structural role theory are useful for nursing assessment as related to the integrated life process of developing roles.

Assessment of Behavior

The nurse begins assessment in the role function mode when first meeting the person and is attuned to behaviors that the person might reveal spontaneously. After creating a comfortable milieu, the nurse proceeds with an in-depth first-level assessment related to developing roles.

Identification of Roles

The primary, secondary, and tertiary roles the person occupies, and the associated instrumental and expressive behaviors, form the basis for behavioral assessment of social integrity relative to the developing roles process. In assessing behavior, the nurse begins by identifying the person's age and related primary role. From this information, secondary roles can be projected and, by purposeful questioning, secondary and tertiary roles can be determined together with their relative importance for the person.

Instrumental and Expressive Behaviors

Behavioral assessment would also include the determination of instrumental and expressive behaviors associated with each role. Direct observation of the performance of specific roles can provide further information as to the adaptive process of developing roles.

Consider as an example a 19-year-old young adult female who has just entered college. In addition to the secondary role of student, one can project such roles as daughter, sister, girlfriend, and participant in sports activities. Associated with the role of student are the instrumental behaviors of studying, attending classes, taking exams, writing papers, and participating in laboratory sessions. Expressive behaviors include "sounding off" with peers, complaining to parents about a heavy workload, and rejoicing about exam results with the teacher.

Following identification of the person's set of roles and related instrumental and expressive behaviors, tentative judgments can be made relative to how adaptive the developing role processes are. Adaptive role development behaviors are those that meet role expectations; ineffective behaviors do not meet role expectations. *Role mastery* is the term used to indicate that a person demonstrates both expressive and instrumental behaviors that meet social expectations associated with one's role set. Basically, the nurse assesses whether or not instrumental behaviors are achieving expected goals, and whether expressive behaviors provide satisfaction for the person.

Assessment of Stimuli

The structural approach to roles also provides a basis for second-level assessment, or identifying stimuli that affect the developing role process. In addition to the instrumental and expressive behavioral components, four role performance requirements have been described by Nuwayhid (1984), based on Parsons and Shils (1951). These requirements are viewed as necessary within the social structure to allow a person to develop role behavior, be it instrumental (namely, goal directed) or expressive (feeling based). Other important stimuli include physical makeup and chronologic age, self-concept and emotional state, knowledge of expected behaviors, other roles, role models, and social norms.

Requirements

The four role performance requirements constitute major stimuli for role development; their presence facilitates the person's role development by identifying expected behaviors for each role within the role set. The requirements for role behavior are consumer, reward, access to facilities and circumstances, and cooperation and collaboration. The following example pertains to the sick role (originally described by Parsons, 1964) and to later applications by nurses to the wellness role. Illustrations are provided of the requirements to both instrumental and expressive behaviors.

Associated with the sick role of patient is the instrumental behavior of taking medications prescribed by another and associated with the wellness role is the person's self-initiated health promotion behaviors. The requirements for the behaviors are as follows.

1. *Consumer.* Who or what benefits from the person's performance of role behaviors? For example, the patient in the sick role benefits by taking prescribed pain medication; the well person benefits by doing daily exercise.

2. *Reward.* What rewards does the individual receive for performance of role behaviors? Pain is alleviated and physical mobilization can be increased. In the wellness role, the person who exercises feels an increased sense of well-being.

3. *Access to facilities and set of circumstances.* Are materials or tools available to perform role behaviors? In the sick role, medication is available, as is appropriate equipment for its administration. In the wellness role, the person is able to schedule a time and place to exercise.

4. *Cooperation and collaboration.* To what degree is the individual allowed time and circumstances to perform role behaviors? Medication is brought to the patient in the sick role and time is allowed to elapse before its effect is felt. The person in the wellness role has someone to stay with her child so that she can go to the workout room to exercise.

Expressive behaviors also are associated with development of sick or well roles, as can be noted in further application of the same four requirements.

1. *Consumer.* The need for immediate feedback from an appropriate and receptive person. In some situations, this person is the nurse who is available to care for the patient and assess response to medication. In the wellness role, a friend who is a nurse joins the person for her exercise session.

2. *Reward.* An established network that will provide feedback on role performance. In both illness and wellness cases, the person receives consistent encouragement and feedback from the nurse.

3. *Access to facilities and set of circumstances.* The need to feel that one has what is needed to accomplish the task. The nurse provides time to discuss the person's concern about taking medication or doing exercise.

4. *Collaboration and cooperation.* The positive emotional tone and belief that the setting in which the role is performed provides the climate needed to fulfill the role. Both individuals feel that they are actively involved in decisions related to care and health promotion.

The four requirements of both instrumental and expressive behaviors are important to consider when assessing stimuli influencing role development behaviors. Their presence or absence may serve as focal, contextual, or residual stimuli to the observed behaviors.

Physical Attributes and Chronologic Age

Physical attributes and chronologic age influence which roles a person is suited to occupy. For example, at 19 years of age, a person's learning capabilities permit college study. Certain jobs require given physical capabilities, such as a horse trainer, yet persons with physical disabilities may perform many roles for which their abilities qualify them. For example, it is not unusual to see an office manager or attorney who is confined to a wheelchair because of a neurologic condition that affects the spinal cord but not the brain. In addition, society is redefining age limitations on certain roles. Older persons are allowed to adopt children and second careers are common in later years.

Self-concept and Emotional Well-being

Self-concept, as an adaptive mode, affects developing roles. The role must fit within the person's self-ideal, namely, be something that the person expects of himself or herself. In addition, the person must feel capable of occupying the role and carrying out behaviors expected in the role. An example is a young woman who always planned to go to college and feels capable of undertaking and succeeding in her selected course of study. This self-motivation and confidence affect the individual's capacity or ability to develop the role successfully. The person must also have the emotional well-being to fulfill the role. Taking on one or more new roles can be stressful and a certain amount of emotional resilience facilitates the developing role process. The young woman in the example has no emotional concerns that would hinder her performance as a student. Further, she was active in sports in high school, thus has experience in handling both winning and losing, and has developed the perspective and emotional flexibility associated with such "ups" and "downs."

Knowledge of Expected Behaviors

Because knowing what is expected in a given role is essential to developing the role, the person uses cognator processes to gain knowledge of expected behaviors. In particular, perception, information processing, and learning are important in role development. The young woman beginning college is alert to formal notices such as the school catalogue and communications from the registrar's office. She watches and listens to both faculty members and other students in the early days of classes. She is building both formal and informal knowledge about what behaviors are expected in the performance of her new role. For example, she recognizes that, as a student, she is expected to study, plan ahead on projects, attend and participate in classes, and maintain B average grades to remain in her chosen major.

Other Roles

Expectations of behavior in one role may hinder performance of behaviors in another. It is also relevant that skills learned in one role may facilitate another developing role. Throughout life, there are opportunities for experience in managing a variety of roles. Further, people learn how many and what kinds of roles they can accomplish successfully within the level of stress they are willing to tolerate. Thus, the developing of a new role may be dependent on the person's assessment of their total role set, namely, all other roles. The student in college may decide that she will not compete for a position on a sports team until she has mastered other college roles and resolved expectations from the student and girlfriend roles. Integrating roles is discussed as another process of the role function mode.

Role Models

The number, quality, and responses of role models influence the process of developing roles. Role modeling occurs when a person observes a significant other to attain understanding and emulation of the complexity of behaviors of the other's role. Imitation and trial and error are used in role modeling, without direct reinforcement for imitation. Imitating attributes of others is considered a prevalent type of social role learning. Meleis (1975) notes, however, that in a face-to-face society, role modeling is intensive and ensures accurate and relatively smooth role transitions. Whereas in highly developed, mobile, technical, and nontraditional societies, role modeling is reduced. Nurses have recognized the value of enhancing role modeling as a way of promoting healthy role behaviors (Erickson, Tomlin, & Swain, 1988). In the example of the college student, she can look to her parents, older siblings, and other students as role models for student behaviors. She might begin professional role development by observing which journals her teacher reads.

Social Norms

General rules of conduct for role behavior established by society are referred to as norms. *Norms* represent standards of socially approved and disapproved behavior. Group norms regulate the performance of role behavior within the group as an organized unit. They are the expected behaviors for the group as a system, as well as for each member within the group. Norms can provide an important mechanism for social control of individuals' behavior in society. The tendency to change perceptions, opinions, or behavior in ways that are consistent with group norms is referred to as conformity. Norms usually include sanctions, namely, reward or punishment, for those who do or do not behave within the social or group norm. Norms vary greatly in different cultures, and so too does the extent to which people are expected to adhere to norms. In the past, it was noted that basically there were two different cultural orientations toward persons and their relationships to groups. Some cultures value individualism and the virtues of independence, autonomy, and self-reliance. Other cultures value collectivism and the virtues of interdependence, cooperation, and social harmony. Given cultures vary at different times in the balance expected between individual goals and the good of the group.

Contemporary writers note that rapid changes at the turn of the millennium are creating a global society among the people of the earth. Cultural norms still will vary, but there is increasing emphasis on creating ways that norms and values can be inclusive of the good of the individual, various groups, and future inhabitants of the earth. Zohar and Marshall (1994) note that both individualism and collectivism are mechanistic social models. The authors speak to the social need for commitment to higher common values and note that a community is held together neither by complex calculations of self-interest nor by sets of bureaucratic rules. Rather, it draws on its common culture of collective patterns of thinking, feeling, and acting. The search for meaningful social norms, according to these authors, involves the creative use of both freedom and ambiguity. McMahon (1993) speaks of finding the common ground for a global spirituality and community in the human bodily experience. Roy (1997b) has noted that human participation in transformation is the key to future human development and that nurses are an important part of societal redefining of norms. Chinn's (1995) approach to PEACE groups, described in Chapter 14, is a way of creating social norms based on unity, diversity, commitment, and consensus, rather than culturally established hierarchies. Social norms and the search to redefine norms influence developing roles.

Stimuli other than those discussed above may be relevant in an individual's role situation. These should be considered as additional influencing factors in the second-level assessment. The context and meaning of the individual situation is taken into account using an interactionist perspective. (This perspective is discussed further in the following section.) Once the stimuli influencing the person's developing roles have been identified, the behaviors, in light of the theoretical bases, are evaluated as adaptive or ineffective in maintaining social integrity. Stimuli are identified as focal, contextual, or residual and are labeled as to whether they are exerting a positive or negative influence on the developing role process.

► **ROLE-TAKING: PROCESS AND ASSESSMENT**

Role-taking is a process of looking at or anticipating another person's behavior by viewing it within a role attributed to the other. The person then bases the interaction on a judgment about the other's role. Role-taking is based on symbolic interactionism. In Chapter 14, symbolic interactionism was introduced as a theory related to the developing self-concept. As noted above, the approach also is significant in role theory. Mead (1934) and followers assert that reciprocal social relationships or interactions determine how the mind develops, and that the human individual thinks first of all in social terms. The importance of reactions of others in forming the self-concept has been noted.

In cosmic terms, persons are who they are through participating in the common life of the planet (Zohar & Marshall, 1994). In addition to being a major factor influencing the developing self-concept, interactions with others involve role-taking, a key process of the role function mode. Role-taking focuses on the meaning that the acts have to both persons in a role interaction. A person's role behaviors emerge based on one's own meanings and interpretations of other's meanings.

In early work on the theory of the adaptive modes, Roy (Roy & Roberts, 1981) proposed the significance of the role-taking process in understanding the role function mode. Mead (1934) observed that individuals work out the play of their own role by imaginatively "taking the role of the other." Turner (1979) extended this concept by specifying three standpoints from which the role-taking process takes place. First, the person may simply adopt the standpoint of the person in the other role, such as the person who says, "If I were in her shoes, this is what I would do." In this case, the process is an automatic determinant of behavior. One simply acts from the standpoint of the other. Second, the person may understand the other's standpoint by adopting the standpoint of a third party, such as the person who says, "I know what my mother would do in relating to this person." This process indicates which behavior is expected depending on the inferences made concerning the role of the other. Here, the function of role-taking is to determine how one should act toward the other. Finally, the self may take the standpoint of a purpose or objective rather than a specific directive, such as the person who says, "I want to impress this person and although I'm not sure what would work, I'll try this approach." Here, the person lacks a specific or detailed directive and consequently must shape personal behavior according to what the person judges to be the probable effect of the interaction between the owned role and the inferred role of the other. Turner (1979) described the characteristics of the role-taking process as reciprocal, with every role a way of relating to other roles in a situation; a tentative process (since role-taking occurs in interaction) continuously testing the conception one has of the role of the other; and grouping behaviors into units as a collection of possible actions that are regarded by the self or viewer as belonging together.

In applying an interactionist perspective of role, Meleis (1975) notes that through interaction and role-taking with others, the person's roles are discovered, created, modified, and defined. This is apparent in the earlier example of a nurse in a new position as she develops the meanings of her several roles by interacting with persons in the clinic.

Within groups, interactions lead to roles that may be formal or informal, but all involve a set of expected behaviors (Brehm & Kassin, 1996). Formal roles are generally designated by titles, for example, chairperson, secretary, treasurer. Within the group, this is known as structural identification of roles. Informal roles, or those that develop in an interactional manner, are less obvious but still very influential in the group. Bales (1958), using distinctions similar to those noted before, proposed that regardless of people's titles, enduring groups give rise to two types of roles: an instrumental role to help the group achieve its tasks, and an expressive role to provide emotional support and maintain morale. The same person can fulfill both roles, but often the roles are assumed by different persons in the group. Bales considered that informal roles in groups develop like the pattern of dividing the labor in traditional family roles. Here, the father is responsible for earning a living and the mother acts as the caretaker. Current research notes that men and women who feel equally competent about task performance will adopt roles and the manner in which they behave in groups in ways that are quite similar (Brehm & Kassin, 1996). The research confirms that groups tend to informally develop expressive and instrumental roles. However, it challenges the original assumption that they are gender determined; both men and women adopt either instrumental or expressive roles. An interactionist approach to roles for individuals and groups contributes to nursing assessment of role function.

Assessment of Behavior

First-level assessment of the role function mode, as in other adaptive modes, deals with identifying behaviors. Since the role function mode deals with social integrity and role clarity, behaviors can be viewed from two perspectives: macrocosmic and microcosmic.

In assessing developing roles, emphasis is placed on the more macrocosmic, broader, and long-term process. For example, the identification of a role set takes a broad view of the person's life and social development. The related instrumental and expressive behaviors are viewed as emerging patterns as roles develop. In assessing behaviors of the role-taking process, the perspective is narrowed somewhat to the role-taking experience in a given situation. An individual behavior is described, or a unit of behaviors is grouped. Understanding the person or group within a social context requires significant knowledge and experience for both the broad and narrow views of assessment; the first, because the effort is to summarize much information into a full picture; the other, because it requires insight into the dynamics of meaning between interacting persons. This understanding is developed throughout the nurse's career, but basic principles are provided in this book, so that the nurse can begin to grow in this area of nursing knowledge.

Of particular relevance in assessing role-taking process is for the nurse to understand one's own role-taking behavior in the nurse–patient interaction. A useful exercise for learning about the nurse–patient relationship is called process recording. In process recording, a conversation between the patient and the nurse is written down as closely to verbatim as possible in two columns. A third column is made to the right of the statements for the nurse to write down reflections about the meaning of the interaction. A sample process recording is provided in Table 15–2. Through this type of exercise, the nurse is doing a microcosmic assessment of role-taking behavior. The purpose is to identify the role behavior of one as it affects and is affected by the role behavior of the other.

TABLE 15-2 SAMPLE PROCESS RECORDING TO FOCUS ON ROLE-TAKING BEHAVIOR IN THE NURSE AND PATIENT INTERACTION

Situation: The nurse enters the room where a young mother is with her child who has just been admitted to the pediatric unit of the medical center with fever of unknown origin. The child was born with spina bifida and the mother has been caring for him at home for 5 years.

Nurse	Mother and Child	Reflection on Meaning
Good afternoon, Mrs. Fabien, and Stevie, how are you doing today? I hear you have a fever.	Oh, I am glad you are here, Ms. Moralez. Yes, Stevie's temperature started up on Friday and nothing I do has helped.	The Mom is really feeling frustrated. It seems to help that she recognized me.
Sounds like you have had a hard time. What do you know so far about what is causing the elevated temperature?	Oh, the usual. Anything from urinary tract infection to meningitis.	The long haul is getting to Mrs. Fabien. I see Stevie occasionally when he needs acute care, but for her this is an everyday thing.
Yes, there have been a lot of these problems. But then I see you and Stevie only when something like this happens. For you, Stevie's care is everyday. You do such a good job of meeting his needs.	Yeah. But I don't feel that I do a good job when something like this happens, and we don't know yet how serious it is.	I really can be a support to Mrs. Fabien during this time of diagnosis and treatment. (You know, my sister is expecting a baby in a few weeks; what if her baby has a serious birth defect?) Better respond to what this mother is saying now.
Well, the lab work is started and we should begin to get some answers soon. I am glad you brought Stevie in right away. Your vigilance is his best protection.	Oh, he is just such a good little guy, and a joy for the whole family. I really can't do enough for him. I know we will get through this, too, and I can't tell you how glad I am that you are here. I know you will help get information as soon as possible.	It really helps to have a relationship with the mother from the start. She is counting on me. Maybe I can help not only get through this acute episode, but show her how she can continue to grow in her mothering of little Stevie.

Assessment of Stimuli

Second-level assessment identifies stimuli that affect the role-taking process. Factors that affect the person's perception and behaviors in role-taking include general determinants, social setting, cognator processes, cognitive resources, and social perception.

General Determinants

Just as age, gender, and developmental stage help to determine the role set in a structural approach to developing roles, so too have biology, gender, culture, and personality been noted to be primary influences in the choice of social environments (Patterson, 1996). Choosing a college in a small town or a large city may be based on personal factors, but it will determine some of the dimensions of the social environment. The social environment in turn influences the role-taking interactions that are available. For example, going to college with a twin in a small town may influence the amount and type of one-to-one social interactions with others. Culture also affects who, when, and how often one interacts with others, as is noted in the organizations created by international students.

Social Setting

Social setting is important in promoting or constraining role-taking interaction. In this case, social setting means the conditions under which two persons interact. Consider the example of what characteristics of a setting allow the nurse to enter the process of role-taking as a partner in health care with the patient. The setting, whether hospital room, clinic, or home, will provide privacy for interaction, at least at times. The nurse needs to manage the setting with the patient in such a way as to not feel rushed by other commitments. Further, planning of assignments will include continuity of care by the nurse with the patient over time.

Cognator Processes

Within the social environment of role-taking, the cognator processes of perceptual and information processing and judgment are key. In role-taking, all of one's perceptual awareness and ability to process informational cues is used and, in addition, a judgment must be made about the information to trigger behavior within the interaction. The example of the nurse newly employed at a clinic and meeting her unit supervisor in the cafeteria demonstrates the use of the cognator processes in the role-taking process. The nurse perceives where the nurse administrator sits, her facial expression, body posture, and the words she uses. The nurse processes the perceptions and makes the judgment that the other person is providing an invitation to get acquainted. Thus, she begins sharing educational and professional experiences, rather than asking questions about the procedure manual. Note that the setting, and likely the gender and age, of the other nurse also may be influencing factors for the behavior.

Cognitive Resources

Cognitive resources refer to cognitive capacity available for attending to, processing, and managing concept formation and judgment while in a role-taking situation. Each part of cognator processing requires energy, and regardless of total cognator effectiveness, one must have energy to use this capacity or it is not available for the interaction. Further, when cognitive resources are concentrated on the immediate social situation, they can be distributed among monitoring self, interpreting the role partner, or awareness of the setting or the topic of conversation. A person can be highly motivated to participate in role-taking; however, over time the amount of energy required by the interaction may be draining for either or both persons. Caregiver burden and nurse burnout are two examples described in the nursing literature that illustrate how cognitive resources drained by intense interactions contribute to energy depletion in given roles. Factors that help a person use cognitive resources to promote adaptation in the role-taking process include attentional focus and cognitive effort. Emotions and goals help to increase energy that is needed to focus the attention of cognitive resources on a role-taking interaction. For example, positive attitude, or liking of the other individual, helps to maintain the focus on the other. Similarly, if an important goal is at stake, as in a job interview, then attentional focus is more easily maintained. Similarly, there are many reasons for the person to put more cognitive effort into an interaction. A nurse may be very committed to developing a role as health partner with a particular patient, both because of strong professional commitments as a nurse, and also because of acute awareness of the health consequences for the patient depending on this interaction.

Social Perception

Social perception is a general term for the processes by which people come to understand one another. It is clear that some persons are better at understanding others and this is a major influence on role-taking. Again, skill at social perception is a complex nursing ability and the reader is referred to additional sources for further understanding. In a basic sense, social perception is described as a three-step process (Brehm & Kassin, 1996). Observation of persons, situations, and behavior is the first step. These are the raw data of social perception. Second, there is a process whereby people explain and analyze behavior. To interact effectively with others, it is useful to know how they are feeling and to identify dispositions, namely, more stable characteristics. Attributing certain personality traits, attitudes, and abilities helps a person to predict another's behavior. Basically, we want to infer that a person is friendly and can be trusted. Since people cannot observe these attributes, they must infer them from what a person says and does. The last step of social perception is for the person to integrate observations into a coherent impression of the other person. There are many overt and subtle ways in which impressions create a distorted picture of reality. On early observations, a person may make immediate judgments based on initial cues and this is referred to as "snap judgments." The inferring of attributes about a person may be correct or incorrect. A study of integrated impressions about people was done by showing different groups brief videotapes of 10 women telling the truth or lying about their feelings (Ekman & O'Sullivan, 1991). Among the following observer groups of college students, police investigators, trial judges, and psychiatrists, all scored only slightly better than chance, namely, making the correct judgment between 53 and 58 percent of the time. Only the U.S. Secret Service agents scored better than chance, making correct judgments 64 percent of the time.

Despite the fact that social perception is imperfect, there are ways in which people are more competent as social perceivers. The more experience people have with each other, the more accurate they are; for example, they are more accurate in judgments about friends and acquaintances. Although people are not good at making global judgments, such as knowing what people are like across a range of settings, they can make predictions in given situations. For example, one can predict a co-worker's action on the job, which is more important than being mistaken about the other's personality. Social perception skills can be enhanced in people who learn the rules of probability and logic; for example, taking a statistics course can improve ability to reason about social events. Finally, people can form more accurate impressions of others when motivated by a concern for accuracy and open-mindedness. Nurses can benefit from knowing that understanding of people can be enhanced and the problems of bias can be minimized to the extent that we observe others with whom we interact, make judgments that are reasonably specific, have some knowledge of rules of logic, and are sufficiently motivated to form an accurate impression. Social perception is a potent factor influencing effective role-taking.

► INTEGRATING ROLES: PROCESS AND ASSESSMENT

Each individual has many roles within a role set, and each role has given expectations coming from self, others, and society. The person is often confronted with the need to articulate roles and expectations. Further, within groups, role differentiation requires that members of the group clarify and articulate their role expectations and behaviors. *Integrating roles* is the process of managing different roles and their expectations. Integrating roles provides the function of regulation within individuals, between persons in complementary roles, and among groups members.

Roy (Roy & Roberts, 1981) noted the early work by Merton (1957) in describing six social processes for integrating role sets. First, the person evaluates the relative importance of various statuses. For example, family and job obligations have priority over voluntary associations. Second, the differences of power of those in the role set gives the person a larger measure of autonomy. For instance, if two members of the role set have competing power to impose their will, the individual may choose to whom to respond. Third, Merton describes the situation of the insulation of role activities from observability by members of the role set. If one's activities in another role are not known to a member of one's role set, then the person is less subject to competing pressures. Fourth, observability of conflicting demands by members of the role set may serve to integrate the roles. When contradictions are plain, it becomes the task of members of the role set to resolve the contradictions. Compromise is usually the result. Merton's next consideration is that there is mutual social support among status occupants. Persons in certain statuses form supportive associations, for example, parents of teenagers who are in drug rehabilitation programs. Finally, Merton says that one may delete roles from one's role set. This is discussed later when role failure is considered. However, the person may not be in role failure, but may choose to break off a given role relation to leave greater consensus among role expectations of the remaining role set. For example, after working in a teaching assistant position for a semester, a graduate student may feel that one can better meet student role expectations if not also trying to meet expectations in the teaching assistant role. Thus choosing to leave the position for a semester is a good decision.

Viewing integrating roles somewhat differently, Goode (1960) notes that strain within the functioning role system is associated with activating ways for reducing strain. Two basic techniques are used. First, the person or group manages the role set by compartmentalization, delegation, elimination of role relationships, extension, and barriers against intrusion. Second, the person or group responds by setting or carrying out the terms of the role relationships. Setting the terms leads to role clarity and increases accountability for role performance within the group.

In addition to these regulatory processes, in a system of integrated role sets there is feedback for control of output, or integrated behavior. When a person perceives personal behavior and the behavior of the other in an interaction, this perception acts as feedback to control further role behavior, as noted in the discussion of the role-taking process. Turner (1962) refers to internal validation of the interaction itself. This internal validation lies in the successful anticipation of the behavior of relevant others within the range necessary for the enactment of one's role. External validation derives from the generalized other. It is based on the person's perception of whether the behavior is judged to constitute a role by others whose judgments are considered correct or legitimate. If role behavior is not validated, internally or externally, there will be corrections in the output of role performance. This is another part of the process of integrating roles.

Handel (1979) sees a convergence of structural and interactionist views in providing answers to problems of integrating roles. From the structuralist view, social stability and patterned conduct are explained by structures that lessen the intensity of adverse consequences of conflicting expectations. However, the author notes that there has not been much structural middle-range theory developed to explain how the person copes with conflicting expectations. Interactionists have addressed the negotiation of meaning in interaction as the person's practical solution to the problems generated through conflicting expectations in role sets. Negotiated meanings do not replace conflicting expectations, but coexist with them as a working consensus among the interacting persons or groups concerning how conflicts are to be resolved in given situations. The combined structural and interactional approaches are useful to understanding nursing assessment of integrated roles.

Assessment of Behavior

The behavioral assessment of integrating roles involves identifying an effective pattern of role performance for an individual or group. Major methods of assessment are observations of role behaviors and listening to persons' perceptions of how well they handle integrating role sets. The nurse further identifies whether or not the strategies the person or group uses for role integration seem to be working to their satisfaction. Given the person's role set, does the person integrate expectations for primary, secondary, and tertiary roles? Does the person or group feel comfortable adjusting role expectations frequently? Does the person or group use flexibility in meeting expectations of multiple others and of multiple groups? Does the individual or group identify role strains when they occur? Can they problem-solve for strategies to decrease role strain? When negotiations of meanings of roles or clarification of expectations are needed, are all those involved included in the negotiation? Do the negotiated meanings lead to better role integration and role performance? Are new roles incorporated without undue stress on existing roles? Is the person or group able to feel comfortable with terminating roles? The nurse is aware that it is not conformity to role expectations that is the focus of assessment of integrating roles. Rather the nurse assesses behaviors related to success and satisfaction with integrating roles. Successful integration of roles is observed in effective patterns of role performance. Satisfaction with integration of roles is shown in a joy of achieving expectations and minimizing the strain of competing expectations.

Assessment of Stimuli

Many of the factors that influence the other role processes, developing roles and role-taking, are also stimuli affecting integrating roles. Yet some specific influencing factors can be identified and described briefly. These include size and complexity of role set, cognator processes, and developmental stage of the group.

Size and Complexity of Role Set

If managing many roles and their expectations is the core of integrating roles, then the sheer number of roles is a major influencing factor. The simple illustration in Figure 15–2 gives an example of 10 roles that might be within an individual's role set. The actual number is likely many more. It can be noticed that for many of these roles, there are multiple other persons in the reciprocal roles; for example, a father may relate to several sons and daughters, and to step-children as well. A teacher has many students, and also many groups associated with the teacher role, including administrators, other faculty members and staff responsible for the goals of the school, and parent–teacher groups, who often have a broad range of concerns. These examples of the extensiveness of role interactions relate to only two secondary roles. The number of roles occupied and the expectations of self, multiple others, and society for each role need to be looked at in assessing the factors influencing integrating roles.

In addition to the number of roles, a role set has another characteristic referred to as complexity. Merton (1968) uses the notion of patterns of role sets to illustrate the fact that even a seemingly simple social structure is extremely complex. Complexity in regard to role sets stems from the fact that any individual occupying a particular role set interacts with complementary roles that are differently located in the social structure. Values and moral expectations of those in other statuses may in some measure differ from those of the person in the role. Merton notes, for example, that members of a school board are often in social and economic strata quite different from the public school teacher. A salesperson for an international firm has a highly complex role set, considering the different views of client statuses in different cultures. Complex modern society multiplies the number and complexity of role sets.

Cognator Processes

When integrating roles is a challenge to the person, the cognator process of judgment, particularly using problem-solving and decision-making skills, is most significant. The use of judgment depends on the effectiveness of other cognator processes. Accuracy of perceptual and information processing, relevant learning, and emotional soundness affect judgment processes. However, when assessing factors influencing the person or group's integrating of roles, the nurse will look to the problem-solving and decision-making skills that are being used. These cognator strategies are essential to using any of the social processes identified for integrating role sets and for being able to develop new strategies based on cognitive and emotional strengths of the person and shared within a group. As people interact in groups, the effectiveness of integrating the roles of the group depends heavily on group problem-solving and decision-making skills. For example, a new task may be identified by a group involved in lobbying for better health care when they receive notice of a special legislative hearing on the issue. To respond to the challenge, roles will be adjusted and integrated to accommodate the new task while maintaining focus on their ongoing goal-oriented projects. How the group works together to define and solve the problem of adjusting tasks and role expectations, and how they work together quickly and effectively to make group decisions, has a significant impact on their role integration at this time. In addition, the use of cognator processes will affect the future integration of group roles.

Developmental Stage of the Group

In assessing integrating roles for both individuals and groups, an influencing factor to consider is the developmental stage of a group, or groups, to which the person belongs. Worchel (1996) developed a model of group development from observations of ongoing groups, which he regarded an important consideration in any group-based analysis. This model's stage I was named the stage of discontent, because this period often creates the foundation for group formation. Although groups may be created by other factors, such as a work team, group formation issues need to be examined. Group members may feel alienated at first, and helpless to influence the group; hence, participation may be low and dominated by a few. Stage II may be initiated by a precipitating event. The incident may be relatively minor and unplanned, such as the rumor of pay inequities among the work group, or an emotional outburst by a single group member. The event often surfaces common dissatisfactions and initiates meaningful contact between members. Stage III of group development occurs when the members focus on defining the group and determining its membership. Members become concerned with demonstrating that they are the "in-group." The period of identification incorporates features of group activities referred to as forming, storming, and norming activities (Tuckman, 1965). Stage IV involves group productivity in which identity issues are less apparent and the group sets goals and initiates planning for how to achieve those goals. Processing information revolves around productivity issues. Differentiating members by skills, motivation, and leadership are issues. This leads to stage V, the individual stage. The members begin to demand recognition for their contributions and request resources on the basis of equity rather than equality. The group takes a more cooperative stand toward out-groups because members may be exploring opportunities for themselves in the out-groups. The author describes stage VI as that of decay. As increasing attention is paid to personal needs, the group becomes less important to each person. Subgroups may form and compete for power. The group drifts into a new period of discontent, stage I. These generalizations about stages of group development, or similar considerations, are important for how they affect integrating roles for both individuals and groups.

► COMPENSATORY ADAPTIVE PROCESSES

The role function mode has compensatory processes, just as do the other adaptive modes. As defined earlier in this book, compensatory processes represent the adaptation level at which the cognator and regulator, or stabilizer and innovator, have been activated by a challenge to the integrated life processes. In general, to compensate means to provide a means of counteracting variation to act as an equalizing, counterbalancing force. When a given role function process is challenged in such a way that there is a threat of compromised adaptation, compensatory adaptive processes are activated. As compensatory processes act, the adaptation level is somewhere between the level of integrated processes and compromised processes. Effective compensatory processes increase adaptation level. Two compensatory processes selected for discussion are role transition and role distance.

Role Transition

During role development or role change, the person goes through a process called role transition. *Role transition* is defined as growth in a new role with increasing effectiveness of expressive and instrumental role behaviors. In the case of the maternal role, for example, the new role is one of a series of secondary roles that an individual assumes to meet the developmental tasks of her primary role. It is a continuous and ongoing process. As an individual ages chronologically, the primary role changes; new developmental tasks confront the individual, and new secondary and tertiary roles are assumed in order to meet these developmental tasks. It should be noted that the transition from one secondary role to another secondary role is a much more arduous and time-consuming process than moving from one tertiary role to another.

Tertiary roles, by their nature, are usually temporary and require less emotional and physical involvement than secondary roles.

The individual does not always have a conscious choice about assuming a new role. Many secondary roles can be thrust on the individual by circumstances and the environment. For example, a man who has worked all his life as a taxi driver may have an accident that leaves him unable to drive a taxi, but he may still be able to hold another kind of job. This man, then, has to seek a new job, and perhaps retraining. He did not choose to seek a new secondary role, but his ability to adapt to his new job and make an effective transition to a new secondary role is a challenge to his social integrity. Such challenges are a concern for nurses with respect to promoting integrated adaptive role function.

In assessing the role function mode adaptation of various persons with whom nurses come in contact, they will identify many secondary and tertiary roles that are in transition. After a woman has had a heart attack, she may be able to return to work, but she may have to give up some of her tertiary roles, like being an officer in her district nursing association. Meleis (1975) noted that role transitions require the person to incorporate new knowledge, alter behavior, and change the definition of self in the social context. Specifically, Meleis urged that nurses be aware of developmental, situational, and health–illness role transitions. When people find their accustomed role set in transition, this can be a challenging time that requires nursing intervention to promote adaptation in the role function mode.

As nurses have used the Roy Adaptation Model, they have developed guidelines for evaluating progress in role transition. The person is moving toward effective role transition when adaptive expressive behaviors are exhibited, with a few adaptive instrumental behaviors that partially meet with the social expectations associated with the assigned role. However, the number or quality of the behaviors is not sufficient to indicate an integrated adaptation level relative to role transition. The adaptive behaviors, however, reflect positive movement toward the goal of role mastery. In the initial phase of effective role transition, the behaviors will primarily be expressive behaviors. However, this occurs for a short period of time. Almost immediately, some instrumental behaviors are observable. If the transition is effective, the number and quality of instrumental behaviors will increase over time.

As noted in the literature on role theory, for role transition to occur, certain factors must be present in the environment. These factors are the requirements described previously as stimuli influencing the developing role process. Also, the expressive and instrumental behaviors during role transition are affected by the other major stimuli described. When role transition is less successful, the individual exhibits adaptive expressive behavior but exhibits ineffective instrumental behaviors for a particular role. Unlike the other difficulties in role function, which usually arise from some sort of conflict, difficulty with role transition is usually the result of a lack of knowledge, education, practice, or role models. For example, a new mother experiencing difficulty with transition to the maternal role has the self-concept of mother, wants to be a mother, and may even know what a mother is expected to do, but she does not know how to accomplish the tasks.

Two approaches based on role theory that nurses use to promote role transitions are introduction of role cues (Roy, 1967) and role supplementation (Clarke & Strauss, 1992; Meleis, 1975). In work with mothers who were in role transition in adjusting their mothering roles to interacting with a child in the hospital for the first time, Roy used interactional role theory to develop and test a set of role cues that the nurse used with the mother. The pediatric staff nurse purposefully used three categories of action in interacting with the mother.

1. Congruent orientation, the focus of attention in common with the mother's focus of attention
2. Involvement, by communicating with the mother concerning the child's condition, treatment, or activities
3. Role reference, by which the nurse used words and actions to define for the mother what she might do for her child

The simple approach of role cues has been effective in pediatric nursing. For Meleis (1975), the approach of role supplementation involves any deliberative process whereby role difficulties are identified and the conditions and strategies for role clarification and role-taking are used to promote role transitions. Role supplementation can be used both as prevention, as in working with expectant mothers, or therapeutically, as when the person fails to make progress in role transitions such as reluctance to accept rehabilitation after a major illness or injury. According to Meleis, role supplementation is operationalized for practice and research to include role clarification, role-taking, and role modeling; role rehearsal, reference group, and communication; and interactions. To become an expert practitioner in using these approaches, the reader is referred to the original references.

Role Distance

A second compensatory process in the role function mode is known as role distance. In *role distance,* certain behaviors associated with the role are not compatible with self-concept. The individual experiencing role distance at first appears to be experiencing difficulty with role transition. However, a detailed assessment reveals that the individual's instrumental behaviors in role distance vary greatly in degree and in type of response from the individual in role transition. For example, the individual has the knowledge and experience to perform the instrumental behaviors associated with a role, but does so only when absolutely necessary or when there is no one else around to perform the tasks. The individual functions at a point just above role failure by performing the minimal number of prescribed instrumental behaviors for the role. In role distance, the individual exhibits both instrumental and expressive behaviors appropriate to a particular role, but these behaviors differ significantly from prescribed behaviors for the role (Nuwayhid, 1991; Schofield, 1976).

Perhaps the most significant difference between role distance and the other role function processes is that the role is incompatible with the individual's self-concept. The individual feels uncomfortable because the role is undesirable, either in part or as a whole. This is important to consider because the individual may not reject an entire role, but rather certain behaviors associated with the role that the individual perceives as undesirable. The individual seeks to alleviate this discomfort by exhibiting expressive behaviors that make the role seem unimportant or unworthy. Individuals occupying complementary roles are made to feel uncomfortable in their positions. The individual makes derogatory remarks about the role and jokes, belittles, and constantly speaks out about the role in negative terms. It should be kept in mind that this occurs in degrees. The more undesirable the role, the more numerous, severe, and pronounced are the exhibited expressive behaviors.

When role distance is being used as a compensatory process, the nurse focuses on decreasing the threat or discomfort to the person's self-concept. A simple example is the patient who is joking about the hospital gown while changing for same-day surgery. The nurse can comment casually that although this is not how the person generally appears to the world, in this setting everyone looks like this. The nurse may add that the situation is temporary and the patient will be dressing in the usual attire as soon as possible. In more involved situations of role change, the nurse recognizes that the person basically has two choices to reach a new level of adaptation by reintegrating their role function. The nurse's approach may be to help the person identify these choices, select the one that is best, and act on that choice. If the person is uncomfortable with certain role behaviors because they do not match the self-ideal, then one choice is to delete the role from the role set and focus on other roles more compatible with the self. Another choice is to reexamine the self-ideal in a way that may incorporate the role from which the self is distancing. The basis for a choice generally rests with the value and importance of the role for the person. If this is a highly valued role such as that of new father, or one that is important because it is inevitable, such as living with a chronic illness, then the person may need help identifying and dealing with the discrepancies felt between role behaviors and self-concept. Helping people recognize the choices they can make related to their well-being is a significant part of what nurses can do to promote adaptation. This approach is particularly relevant in actualizing the values and beliefs of the Roy model. The nurse will work to improve effectiveness in working with patients regarding choices for health since such choices are opportunities for personal growth in situations of role distance and many other patient situations.

▶ COMPROMISED PROCESSES OF ROLE FUNCTION

Whenever an individual fails to perform the prescribed behaviors for a role, for whatever reasons, a compromised adaptation level exists. The focal stimulus or immediate cause for the behavior varies according to the processes involved. In some cases, it may be the absence of knowledge, lack of education, or scarcity of role models that lead to compromise. In other cases, the setting, cognator processes, or self-concept may not be adequate to achieve role mastery. A compromised adaptation level may occur in the individual person or aggregate group. It may relate to the macrocosmic view of developing structural roles or to the microcosmic view of role-taking in a given situation.

Role Conflict

Role conflict refers to inconsistent expectations held by a person, or by other persons, for a given role in the role set or by inconsistent expectations among the roles of the person's role set. Role conflict, therefore, can be specified as intrarole conflict and interrole conflict.

In intrarole conflict, the individual fails to demonstrate either instrumental or expressive behaviors, or both, appropriate for a role, as a result of incompatible expectations from self or one or more persons in the environment concerning the individual's expected behavior (Schofield, 1976). For example, Martha S. comes from a traditional Italian Catholic family. She maintains a very close relationship with her mother and is in mastery of her daughter role. Martha is now the mother of a 6-week-old baby girl. She has read, taken classes, and searched the Internet about baby care, and is up to date on the current trends. Martha's mother, however, is old-fashioned, and still believes in keeping the baby's head and feet covered in warm clothing in the middle of summer. Martha's mother's praise and approval are very important to Martha. In performing her role as mother, Martha finds herself performing behaviors that try to meet her own perceptions of the maternal role, and then trying to meet her mother's expectations. As she vacillates back and forth, Martha applies all of her energy trying to accommodate two opposing views of the maternal role. Given this conflict, Martha will not achieve role mastery.

Interrole conflict occurs when an individual fails to demonstrate the appropriate instrumental or expressive behaviors as a result of the role set having one or more roles with expected behaviors that are incompatible. In this situation, the individual is occupying roles that are in competition. An example of interrole conflict would be the case of Louise B. Louise is an electrical engineer who was just promoted at work. She works 10 to 12 hours each day and is in role mastery. Louise delivered a baby boy 8 weeks ago, and she now considers her life total chaos. She wants to be at work to maintain her position and control. At the same time, she wants to be with her baby and be involved with as much of his care as possible. As a result, she is torn between the two roles and is not experiencing mastery in either one.

Role Failure

Role failure differs from role conflict in that the individual fails to exhibit adaptive expressive behaviors. To be successful at role function, the individual must want to assume the role. In *role failure,* the individual does not want to assume the role, and any expressive behaviors that are observed are usually ineffective because they are aimed at pleasing those in complementary roles. The individual has an absence of expressive behaviors or exhibits ineffective expressive behaviors, or has an absence of instrumental behaviors or exhibits ineffective instrumental behaviors for a particular role. The key element in role failure is the individual's desire. If the individual exhibits any adaptive expressive behaviors concerning a role, the individual generally is not in role failure. This is important to remember because when expressive and instrumental behaviors are ineffective, nurses too often label the patient as being in role failure when, really, the behavior is indicative of role transition or role conflict. Role failure does occur, but is likely to be encountered by nurses in advanced clinical practice, such as in complex situations of difficulties with family roles. Role failure is a complex diagnosis in the role function mode and usually involves one or more of the other modes of the Roy Adaptation Model. In role failure, the outcome for an individual or group may be to choose not to fulfill the role. When a volunteer group no longer works toward common goals and the members do not have positive feelings for being together, the group usually disbands. For formal groups with given social responsibilities, as in a family group, the consequences of role failure are more profound. Efforts to resolve role failure are warranted. As in any adaptation problem, thorough first- and second-level assessment can be helpful, and in the role function mode, understanding the effects of the self and interdependence modes are particularly relevant.

Outgroup Stereotyping

A particular adaptation problem in the role function mode that interferes with role clarity has been termed stereotyping. Stereotypes are beliefs that associate certain groups of people with certain types of characteristics and these beliefs then influence judgments of individuals. Stereotyping represents ineffectiveness in all role processes, developing roles, role-taking, and integrating roles. Common illustrations of stereotyping in society, and resulting discrimination and prejudice, are related to gender and race.

The formation of stereotypes begins with the tendency for people to group themselves and others into social categories. Cognitively, it is easier to sort single objects into groups, rather than to think of each as unique. Biologists classify species; nurses classify nursing diagnoses. In some ways, categorizations are useful and adaptive. However, when people are categorized, there is a tendency to misinterpret likenesses and differences (Stanger & Lange, 1994). Groups that the individual identifies with—country, ethnic region, working unit—are called ingroups whereas groups other than one's own are called outgroups. Added to the tendency to social categorization is a common bias called outgroup homogeneity. Put simply, this means that people in the ingroup feel that "we" have interesting and subtle differences between "us," but "they" are all alike. Beliefs about groups that are built on these categorizations tend to be overgeneralized. While stereotypes can offer convenient summaries of social groups, their harmful effects are that they cause people to overlook diversity within categories and lead to inaccurate judgments about particular individuals. Furthermore, stereotypes provide the basis for discrimination and prejudice. Discrimination refers to any behavior directed against persons, often unfairly, based on outgroup membership. Prejudice refers to negative feelings toward others based on group membership. There are mutual links among the three concepts. Stereotypes may cause people to become prejudiced; discriminatory practices may stem from and support stereotypes and prejudice; and prejudiced people may use stereotypes to justify their feelings (Brehm & Kassin, 1996). Role functioning is extremely difficult in a situation of *outgroup stereotyping*. In this situation, people fail to relate to individuals with their own abilities and talents as the best candidates for given roles.

In one theory of gender stereotypes (Eagly, 1987), stereotypes of men as dominant and women as subordinate persist because men occupy higher status positions in society. This division of labor, a product of many factors (biologic, social, economic, and political), leads men and women to behave in ways that fit their social roles. But rather than attribute the differences to these roles, people attribute the differences to the group, that is, gender. Data from the U.S. Census Bureau (1994) report striking sex differences in occupational choices. Further, men and women are judged more favorably when they apply for jobs consistent with gender stereotypes.

Similarly, there are many classic studies of ethnic and racial stereotypes, particularly of African Americans in the United States. Surveys given over the years from the 1950s to the 1980s note that negative images of blacks have decreased (Dovidio & Gaertner, 1986). However, contemporary authors describe modern racism as a form of prejudice that surfaces in subtle ways when it is safe, socially acceptable, and easy to rationalize. According to these theories, many people are racially ambivalent. Generally, people want to see themselves as fair, but they still have deep feelings of anxiety and discomfort in the presence of other racial groups (Hass, Katz, Rizzo, Bailey, & Moore, 1992). Evidence of this ambivalence lies in the fact that many white Americans may speak about principles of racial equality, but in practice they oppose mixed marriages, black political candidates, and racially symbolic policies.

Desegregation of schools was anticipated to be a significant force against outgroup stereotyping. This hope was based on the contact hypothesis, which proposes that direct contact between hostile groups will reduce prejudice under certain conditions. Desegregation has not cured problems of racism because it was also the case that the key conditions of intergroup contact—equal status, personal interactions, the need to achieve a common goal, and social norms that favor intergroup contact—have not been present (Brehm & Kassin, 1996).

Since outgroup stereotyping is socially pervasive and distorts perceptions of individuals, for nurses to interact with people as individuals, they will find ways to deal with stereotyping. Second, nurses can make a difference in promoting role function effectiveness in others by making efforts to decrease stereotyping. Some authors describe stereotypes as being implicit and automatic, or stereotypes as being explicit and controlled. Brehm and Kassin (1996) note that the individual does not need to be trapped into evaluating specific persons in terms of social categories, that is, to use implicit and automatic stereotypes. They quote research that identifies three factors to enable a person to overcome stereotypes and judge others on a more individualized basis (Fiske & Neuberg, 1990). The first factor relates to the amount of personal information one person has about the other. The nurse is in a position to listen to the person's own story and to help others to do the same. Second, the person must have the cognitive resources to focus on the individual member of a stereotyped group. People are more likely to form an impression based on existing stereotypes when they are busy or pressed for time and unable to think clearly about the unique attributes of a single person. Although nurses are often busy, they can strive to maintain their value of the need to focus on the individual within every interaction. The researchers identify motivation as the third factor to alleviate stereotyping. When the person is highly motivated to form an accurate impression of someone, he or she often manages to set aside preexisting beliefs. Common examples are when the person is in an interdependent relationship or needs to compete against the other person. However, by the choice of nursing as a profession, the nurse has the highest motivation possible to overcome stereotyping.

► PLANNING NURSING CARE

In applying the nursing process to the integrated processes of role function, the nurse makes a careful assessment of behaviors and stimuli. In assessing factors influencing role function, regulator and cognator effectiveness in initiating compensatory processes is considered. The presence or absence of compromised processes is also an important matter. Based on this thorough first- and second-level assessment, the nurse formulates nursing diagnoses, sets goals, selects interventions, and evaluates care.

Throughout this section on planning nursing care, two situations are used to illustrate role function: one pertaining to an individual and the other to groups. The first situation involves a 25-year-old young woman, Lin, who recently immigrated to the United States from Korea with her husband. Although she was qualified as a pharmacist in her homeland, her qualifications are not recognized in the United States and she cannot work in her profession. She is currently working in a linen warehouse as a laborer. Although she has made some acquaintances in the Korean community, she does not yet feel as though she has developed close friends. Lin is 6 months pregnant. She is hoping that her mother can come for an extended period to help with her new baby, but those arrangements have not been completed.

The second situation involves two nurses who started their own independent practice business. They identified in their community a health need and market for a service where families could contract with them to "keep an eye" on aging parents by visiting on a regular, agreed-upon basis to ensure that all was well or to assist in accessing required services as necessary. The demand for this service increased so rapidly that more staff were required within a few months. The business continues to grow.

Although many perspectives could be taken in these situations, the focus of the following illustrations will be on role function. First, the nurse identifies the primary, secondary, and tertiary roles occupied by the individual or group with particular attention to the three integrated processes of developing roles, role-taking, and integrating roles. Information about instrumental and expressive behaviors is sought. As stimuli are assessed in second-level assessment, analysis of role performance requirements points to focal, contextual, or residual stimuli that are of importance in planning nursing care. Other important stimuli to be considered were identified earlier in this chapter. The nurse is also continually aware of evidence of compensatory or compromised processes with respect to role function. Based on this thorough first- and second-level assessment, the nurse proceeds to planning nurse care by initially formulating nursing diagnoses.

It is important to note, once again, that the person or group of focus must be involved, where possible, as an active participant in each step of the nursing process. It is only through meaningful involvement that the plans that are established will be realistic and supported by the person for whom they are designed, and ultimately effective in accomplishing the desired outcomes.

Nursing Diagnosis

Development of nursing diagnoses associated with role function is accomplished in the same way as in the other modes. One method involves the statement of the behaviors together with the influencing stimuli; another method makes use of summary labels.

Nursing diagnoses may reflect either adaptive or ineffective behaviors. Consider the situation of the young immigrant woman. In preparation for the baby's arrival, she and her husband have begun to assemble equipment and supplies for the baby. At the linen warehouse where she is employed, there are remnants of fabric that are available at a substantially reduced price. Lin has purchased some of this fabric and is making diapers for the baby. She has also been able to obtain enough fabric for bedding. She and her husband have discovered that baby furniture can be purchased at garage sales at a very reasonable price and they have been spending recent Saturdays searching for needed items. Lin is demonstrating behaviors appropriate to her developing role of mother. A nursing diagnosis capturing these adaptive behaviors could be "Effective instrumental behaviors in anticipation of baby's arrival related to preparatory activities and anticipation of baby's needs."

Each day at work, Lin enthusiastically reports to her co-workers regarding recent accomplishments or acquisitions. This constitutes expressive behavior and can be captured in a nursing diagnosis stating "Appropriate expressive behaviors related to the presence of the four role performance requirements: consumer—co-workers; reward—their interest and enthusiasm; facilities and circumstances—opportunity to socialize at work; and collaboration and cooperation—supportive work environment."

One factor that is causing Lin some concern is the physical distance from her mother. She would really like to be able to speak with her mother for advice and support, yet the distance between them prohibits long telephone conversations. A diagnosis statement that captures this concern is "Absence of mother's advice and support during pregnancy due to mother living in Korea and Lin living in the United States."

Turning to the second situation of the nurses starting an independent practice, a diagnosis statement that captures the circumstances described could be "Thriving business (role/instrumental behavior) due to abundance of consumers wanting to access the services provided." Another way of looking at the situation could involve instrumental behaviors associated with the developing business: "Continually adding staff related to the presence of all four role performance requirements: consumers, rewards, access to facilities and circumstances, and cooperation and collaboration."

The preceding diagnosis illustrations consisted of a statement of behavior together with the influencing stimuli. It is also possible to construct a nursing diagnosis using a summary label that captures clusters of behaviors. This method is used by experienced nurses to communicate significant amounts of information in one phrase. There are eight indicators of positive role function adaptation identified as summary labels in the Roy Adaptation Model.

1. Role clarity
2. Effective processes of role transition
3. Integration of instrumental and expressive role behaviors
4. Integration of primary, secondary, and tertiary roles
5. Effective pattern of role performance
6. Effective processes for coping with role changes
7. Role performance accountability
8. Effective role integration

These summary labels apply to both individual situations and collective human systems or groups. For example, in the first illustrative situation, a diagnosis using a summary label could be "Effective processes for coping with role change related to evidence of instrumental and expressive role performance requirements."

Likewise, six commonly recurring adaptation problems are identified. They are ineffective role transition, prolonged role distance, role conflict, role failure, role ambiguity, and outgroup stereotyping. Consider some further information about the second nursing situation. In one instance, there was a problem when an employee went into a home to check on an elderly couple. The new employee, who was not a nurse, began to give dietary advice when she noticed that the couple was not eating appropriately. She did not understand that she was to alert the nurse to this situation so that a complete assessment could be accomplished. A diagnosis relating to this situation could read "Role ambiguity due to incomplete understanding of role expectations and instances and processes for referral."

The use of a summary label when more than one mode is affected by the same stimulus is often an effective way of communicating a cluster of behaviors. For example, "role failure" is a complex diagnosis that usually involves more than one mode. For the experienced nurse, this label would convey the absence of expressive behaviors related to the role and the understanding that the individual's desire to assume the role is lacking. It would point to the need to look further into the situation for ineffective role transition or role conflict.

In Table 15–3, the Roy model nursing diagnostic categories for the integrated processes of role function are shown in relation to nursing diagnosis labels approved by the North American Nursing Diagnosis Association (Rantz & LeMone, 1997). Once the nursing diagnoses have been established, the nurse proceeds to the next step in the process of planning care, goal setting.

TABLE 15–3   NURSING DIAGNOSTIC CATEGORIES FOR ROLE FUNCTION

Positive Indicators of Adaptation	Common Adaptation Problems	NANDA Diagnostic Labels
• Role clarity	• Ineffective role transition	• Altered role performance
• Effective processes of role transition	• Prolonged role distance	• Caregiver role strain
• Integration of instrumental and expressive role behaviors	• Role conflict—intrarole and inter-role	• Risk for caregiver role strain
• Integration of primary, secondary, and tertiary roles	• Role failure	• Altered parenting
• Effective pattern of role performance	• Role ambiguity	• Risk for altered parenting
• Effective processes for coping with role changes	• Outgroup stereotyping	• Parental role conflict
• Role performance accountability		• Altered family process: alcoholism
• Effective role integration		• Risk for altered parent/infant/child attachment
• Stable pattern of role mastery		• Ineffective management of therapeutic regimen: Individual
		• Noncompliance (specify)
		• Ineffective management of therapeutic regimen: Families
		• Ineffective management of therapeutic regimen: Community

Goal Setting

Each step of the nursing process focuses on the individual's or group's behavior, the stimuli influencing that behavior, or both. With the nursing diagnosis, the statement developed included both behaviors and stimuli. With goal setting, the focus is on behavior. Each goal identifies a behavior that is to be addressed, the change expected, and the time frame in which the goal is to be achieved.

In the situation of the young immigrant woman, Lin, a goal might focus on her continued transition into the role of mother. An example is, "Before the due date for the baby's arrival, Lin will have acquired all the necessary supplies and equipment to care for her new baby." The behavior in this goal relates to the readiness for the baby's arrival in terms of supplies and equipment; the change is that "all" is obtained; and the time frame is "before the due date for the baby's arrival."

Another goal for Lin might pertain to a support system in case her mother is unable to arrange her visit by the time the baby arrives. It may be stated as follows: "Within 1 month, Lin will be developing relationships with other expectant and new mothers in her community." Here the behavior relates to supportive relationships, the change relates to developing these, and the time frame is "within 1 month."

In the second situation of the independent practice agency, a goal related to the nursing diagnosis "Role ambiguity due to incomplete understanding of role expectations and instances and processes for referral" might be, "Within 2 weeks, employees will express confidence in their understanding of role expectations." The behavior in this case relates to employees knowing the expectations for their jobs and fulfilling them, the change is "confidence" versus "uncertainty," and the time frame is 2 weeks.

After formulating goals, the nurse proceeds to the identification of nursing interventions, the next step of the nursing process as described in the Roy Adaptation Model.

Intervention

The intervention step of the nursing process according to the Roy Adaptation Model focuses on the stimuli affecting the behavior identified in the goal-setting step. The intervention step is thus the management of stimuli and this involves either altering, increasing, decreasing, removing, or maintaining them.

In the previous situation involving Lin, the young woman from Korea, one of the goals pertained to her developing a support system with other expectant and new mothers in her community. The stimulus involved in this situation applies to the presence of role performance requirements, a common stimulus associated with effective role development. For example, it is important that this new mother have an established network that will provide support and feedback on her transition into the role of mother. In Lin's situation, it may be possible to involve her in prenatal classes where she will not only obtain additional knowledge regarding childbirth and child rearing, but get to know other women who are expecting babies around the same time. As it happened, there was a Korean nurse involved in presenting the prenatal instruction to the class of expectant parents. This person was able to put Lin in touch with several other Korean immigrants who had just delivered new babies.

In the group illustration, the stimulus of concern was the employee's knowledge of expected behaviors. Since much of her work occurred in isolation from other people with the same role, she did not have the opportunity to observe or question others. Also, the business had not yet developed written guidelines for role performance. These two stimuli were the focus for intervention in this case. A buddy system was developed for the orientation phase of a new employees' experience, and role descriptions, including perimeters of responsibilities, were developed in writing.

The above interventions focused on stimuli (role performance requirements and knowledge of expected behaviors) that were contributing to the illustrated potential or actual role function problem of role ambiguity. The next step of the nursing process returns to focus on the behaviors evident in the situations once the interventions have been applied.

Evaluation

Evaluation involves judging the effectiveness of the nursing interventions in relation to the person's or group's adaptive behaviors, that is, whether the behaviors stated in the goals have been achieved. The nursing interventions are effective if the behavior is in accordance with the stated goal. If the goal has not been achieved, the nurse identifies alternative interventions or approaches by reassessing the behavior and stimuli and continuing with the other steps of the nursing process.

In considering the previously identified goal for Lin, "Within 1 month, Lin will be developing relationships with other expectant and new mothers in her community," if the interventions were effective, Lin would report friendships with other new mothers who are in close proximity to her home. If at the time of evaluation Lin had made no new friends, other approaches would have to be considered to develop a support system for Lin as she develops her new role as a mother.

For the situation with the employee who did not adequately understand her role, the goal was stated, "Within 2 weeks, employees will express confidence in their understanding of role expectations." This goal recognized a problem that pertained to employees in general, even though the specific problem occurred with one individual. The first instance of evaluation could focus on the one employee. Does she now feel comfortable about when she should refer and when she can handle the situation on her own? Do the other employees express confidence in their understanding of role expectations? Perhaps it has been possible to involve them in the development of the guidelines for role performance. The nurse entrepreneurs also will evaluate the effectiveness of the "buddy" experience during orientation in helping new employees understand their role.

It is important to recognize that the nursing process and the six steps are ongoing, simultaneous, and overlapping. Although they have been separated and dealt with in an artificially linear manner for discussion purposes, often intervention is occurring at the same time as first- and second-level assessment is proceeding. Likewise, evaluation occurs on an ongoing basis, being held in mind even when nursing diagnoses are being established and as goals are being formulated.

▶ SUMMARY

This chapter has focused on the application of the Roy Adaptation Model to the role function mode. An overview of the three integrated processes—developing roles, role-taking, and integrating roles—associated with social integrity and role clarity was provided along with the identification of parameters for assessment of behaviors and stimuli. Illustration of innate and learned compensatory responses related to role function were described and examples of three compromised processes (role conflict, role failure, and outgroup stereotyping) were provided. Finally, guidelines for planning nursing care through the formulation of nursing diagnoses, goals, and interventions were explored and evaluation of nursing care was described.

▶ EXERCISES FOR APPLICATION

1. Identify the primary, secondary, and tertiary roles in which you are currently involved.

2. Select one of your secondary roles and list the associated instrumental and expressive behaviors. Assess the requirements for role function of one instrumental and one expressive behavior.

3. Imagine a 45-year-old generative adult male. Project secondary roles for him and formulate appropriate questions or comments that would elicit information about these roles. Speculate about specific behavior related to the role requirements.

▶ ASSESSMENT OF UNDERSTANDING

Questions

1. The three integrated processes associated with the role function mode and as defined by the Roy Adaptation Model are developing roles (DR), role-taking (RT), and integrating roles (IR). Label each of the following statements according to the process to which they pertain.

(a) _____ based on symbolic interactionism
(b) _____ the need to articulate roles and expectations
(c) _____ role set
(d) _____ imaginatively, taking another's role
(e) _____ identifying an effective pattern of role performance
(f) _____ anticipating another person's behavior
(g) _____ adding new roles as one matures

2. Which of the following behaviors would a person exhibit with a nursing diagnosis of ineffective role transition?
   (a) ineffective expressive behaviors
   (b) effective instrumental behaviors
   (c) ineffective instrumental behaviors
   (d) none of the above

3. Column A represents the requirements of instrumental and expressive behavior. Column B represents factors that illustrate the requirements as related to the role of teacher. Label each factor with the requirement it represents.

   Column A

   1. consumer
   2. reward
   3. access to facilities and set of circumstances
   4. cooperation and collaboration

   Column B

   (a) _____ paycheck
   (b) _____ class time
   (c) _____ classroom and supplies
   (d) _____ "prep" time
   (e) _____ students
   (f) _____ curricular materials
   (g) _____ evaluation of performance
   (h) _____ all students pass exams

4. The Roy Adaptation Model describes two compensatory processes associated with the role function mode: role transition (RT) and role distance (RD). Label the following descriptive phrases according to the compensatory process to which they pertain.
   (a) _____ performance of the minimal number of prescribed instrumental behaviors for a role
   (b) _____ closely related to self-concept
   (c) _____ planned or unplanned alterations in accustomed role set
   (d) _____ instrumental behaviors increase over time
   (e) _____ initially, primarily expressive behaviors
   (f) _____ role is viewed as undesirable, in part or in whole
   (g) _____ continuous and ongoing compensatory process
   (h) _____ related to developmental tasks
   (i) _____ role is spoken of in derogatory terms

5. Name the six compromised processes associated with the role function mode as identified in the Roy Adaptation Model.

   (a) _____

   (b) _____

   (c) _____

   (d) _____

   (e) _____

   (f) _____

Situation

Consider an example of a 19-year-old young adult female who has just entered college. In addition to the secondary role of student, one can project such roles as daughter, sister, girlfriend, and participant in sports activities. Associated with the role of student are the instrumental behaviors of studying, attending classes, writing exams and papers, and participating in laboratory sessions. Expressive behaviors include "sounding off" with peers, complaining to parents about the heavy workload, and rejoicing about exam results with the teacher.

Analysis of the role performance requirements (second-level assessment) is as follows:

Instrumental behavior—studying
  1. Consumer: self, significant others, teacher
  2. Reward: gets good grades, passes courses, receives scholarship
  3. Access to facilities and set of circumstances: library is available, evenings are reserved for study time
  4. Cooperation and collaboration: teachers identify important material, boyfriend calls after 9 PM, classmates study at the same time

Expressive behavior—"sounding off" with peers
  1. Consumer: peers
  2. Reward: understanding of peers
  3. Access to facilities and set of circumstances: peers have opportunity to get together after class and in residence situation
  4. Cooperation and collaboration: peers are supportive of each other, all are in the same circumstances

6. Develop a nursing diagnosis that identifies effective adaptation related to the data provided.

7. During her second semester at school, the student experiences a fractured femur as a result of an accident during her sports activities. For a period of time, she is required to assume the "sick role." Derive a goal related to this circumstance interfering with her student role. The nursing diagnosis on which to base this goal is role conflict related to hospitaliza-

tion and confinement as a result of injury and need to keep up with study requirements at school. Note the goal components of behavior, change expected, and time frame.

8. Suggest interventions that would help her accomplish the previously stated goal.

9. Identify behavior that would indicate that the nursing interventions have been successful and the goals have been achieved.

Feedback

1. (a) RT, (b) IR, (c) DR, (d) RT, (e) IR, (f) RT, (g) DR

2. (c) Ineffective instrumental behaviors

3. (a) 2, (b) 4, (c) 3, (d) 3 or 4, (e) 1, (f) 3, (g) 2, (h) 2

4. (a) RD, (b) RD, (c) RT, (d) RT, (e) RT, (f) RD, (g) RT, (h) RT, (i) RD

5. (a) ineffective role transition
   (b) prolonged role distance
   (c) role conflict
   (d) role failure
   (e) role ambiguity
   (f) outgroup stereotyping

6. Nursing diagnosis example: Effective pattern of student role performance associate with presence of all role performance requirements.

7. Example of a goal: During her time of immobilization (time frame), the student will continue (change expected) to work on assignments (behavior) as she feels physically able.

8. Suggested interventions: friends could be asked to take notes for her during class, teachers could be contacted for assignment information, requests could be made to have exams deferred, a laptop computer could be accessed to enable work on assignments

9. Possible evaluation indicators: assignments would be completed on schedule, exam would be rescheduled for a realistic date in the future, courses would be completed in an appropriate time frame, no courses would have been dropped

▶ **REFERENCES**

Bales, R. (1958). Task roles and social roles in problem-solving groups. In Maccoby, E., Newcomb, T., & Hartly, E. (Eds.), *Readings in social psychology* (3rd ed., pp. 437–447). New York: Holt.

Banton, M. (1965). *Roles: An introduction to the study of social relations.* New York: Basic Books.

Biddle, B. J., & Thomas, E. J. (Eds.). (1979). *Role theory: Concepts and research.* Huntington, NY: Kreiger Publishing.

Brehm, S. S., & Kassin, S.M. (1996). *Social psychology* (3rd ed.). Boston: Houghton Mifflin.

Chinn, P. L. (1995). *Peace and power: Building communities for the future* (4th ed.). New York: Natioal League for Nursing Press.

Clark, B. A., & Strauss, S. S. (1992). Nursing role supplementation for adolescent parents: Prescriptive nursing practice. *Journal of Pediatric Nursing, 7(5),* 312–318.

Dovidio, J. F., & Gaertner, S. L. (Eds.). (1986). *Prejudice, discrimination, and racism: Theory and research.* Orlando, FL: Academic Press.

Eagly, A. H. (1987). *Sex differences in social behavior: A social-role interpretation.* Hillsdale, NJ: Erlbaum.

Ekman, P., & O'Sullivan, M. (1991). Who can catch a liar? *American Psychologist, 46,* 913–920.

Erikson, E. H. (1963). *Childhood and society* (2nd ed.). New York: Norton.

Erikson, H., Tomlin, E., & Swain, M. A. (1988). *Modeling and role modeling: A theory and paradigm for nursing.* Lexington, SC: Press of Lexington.

Fiske, S. T., & Neuberg, S. L. (1990). A continuum of impression formation from category-based to individuating processes: Influences of information and motivation on attention and interpretation. In Zanna, M.P. (Ed.), *Advances in experimental social psychology* (pp. 1–74). New York: Academic Press.

Goode, W. J. (1960). A theory of role strain. *American Psychological Review, 25,* 483–496.

Handel, W. (1979). Normative expectations and the emergence of meaning as solutions to problems: Convergence of structural and interactionist views. *American Journal of Sociology, 84(4),* 855–881.

Hass, R. G., Katz, I., Rizzo, N., Bailey, J., & Moore, L. (1992). When racial ambivalence evokes negative affect, using a disguised measure of mood. *Personality and Social Psychology Bulletin, 18,* 786–797.

Linton, R. (1945). *Cultural background of personality.* New York: Appleton-Century.

Malaznik, N. (1976). Theory of role function. In Roy, Sr. C. (Ed.), *Introduction to nursing: An adaptation model* (pp. 245–264). Englewood Cliffs, NJ: Prentice-Hall.

McMahon, E. M. (1993). *Beyond the myth of dominance: An alternative to a violent society.* Kansas City, MO: Sheed & Ward.

Mead, G. H. (1934). *Mind, self, and society.* Chicago: University of Chicago Press.

Meleis, A. I. (1975). Role insufficiency and role supplementation: A conceptual framework. *Nursing Research, 24(4),* 264–271.

Merton, R. K. (1957). The role-set: Problems in sociological theory. *British Journal of Sociology, 8,* 106–120.

Merton, R. K. (1968). *Social theory and social structure.* New York: Free Press.

Nuwayhid, K. A. (1991). Role transition, distance, and conflict. In Roy, Sr. C., & Andrews, H. (Eds.), *The Roy Adaptation Model: The definitive statement.* Norwalk, CT: Appleton & Lange.

Nuwayhid, K. A. (1984). Role function: Theory and development. In Roy, Sr. C. (Ed.), *Introduction to nursing: An adaptation model* (2nd ed., pp. 284–305). Englewood Cliffs, NJ: Prentice-Hall.

Parsons, T. (1964). *The social system.* New York: The Free Press.

Parsons, T., & Shils, E. (Eds.). (1951). *Toward a general theory of action.* Cambridge, MA: Harvard University Press.

Patterson, M. L. (1996). Social behavior and social cognition: A parallel process approach. In Nye, J. I., & Brower, A. M. (Eds.), *What's social about social cognition? Research on socially shared cognition in small groups* (pp. 87–105). Thousand Oaks, CA: Sage Publications.

Randell, B. (1976). Development of role function. In Roy, Sr. C. (Ed.), *Introduction to nursing: An adaptation model* (pp. 256–264). Englewood Cliffs, NJ: Prentice-Hall.

Rantz, M. J., & LeMone, P. (Eds.). (1997). *Classification of nursing diagnoses: Proceedings of the 12th conference NANDA.* Glendale, CA: CINAHL Information Systems.

Roy, Sr. C. (1967). Role cues and mothers of hospitalized children. *Nursing Research, 16,* 178–182.

Roy, Sr. C. (1988). An explication of the philosophical assumptions of the Roy Adaptation Model. *Nursing Science Quarterly, 1(1),* 26–34.

Roy, Sr. C. (1997a). Future of the Roy model: Challenge to redefine adaptation. *Nursing Science Quarterly, 10(1),* 42–48.

Roy, Sr. C. (1997b). Knowledge as universal cosmic imperative. In *Proceedings of nursing knowledge impact conference 1996* (pp. 95–118). Chestnut Hill, MA: Boston College Press.

Roy, Sr. C., & Roberts, S. L. (Eds.). (1981). *Theory construction in nursing: An adaptation model.* Englewood Cliffs, NJ: Prentice Hall.

Schofield, A. (1976). Problems of role function. In Roy, Sr. C. (Ed.), *Introduction to nursing: An adaptation model* (pp. 265–287). Englewood Cliffs, NJ: Prentice-Hall.

Stangor, C., & Lange, J. (1994). Mental representations of social groups: Advances in understanding stereotypes and stereotyping. *Advances in Experimental Social Psychology, 26,* 357–416.

Tuckman, B.W. (1965). Developmental sequence in small groups. *Psychological Bulletin, 63,* 384–399.

Turner, R. (1962). Role-taking process versus conformity. In Rose, A. (Ed.), *Human behavior and social processes.* Boston: Houghton Mifflin.

Turner, R. H. (1979). Role-taking, role standpoint and reference group behavior. In Biddle, B. J., & Thomas, E. J. (Eds.), *Role theory: Concepts and research* (pp. 151–159). Huntington, NY: Kreiger Publishing.

U.S. Bureau of the Census. (1994). *Statistical abstract of the United States: 1994.* Washington, DC: The Reference Press.

Worchel, S. (1996). Emphasizing the social nature of groups in a developmental framework. In Nye, J. L., & Brower, A. M. (Eds.), *What's social about social cognition? Research on socially shared cognition in small groups* (pp. 261–281). Thousand Oaks, CA: Sage Publications.

Zohar, D., & Marshall, I. (1994). *The quantum society: Mind, physics, and a new social vision.* New York: Quill/Morrow.

16

INTERDEPENDENCE MODE

The final adaptive mode to be introduced is the interdependence mode. This mode, like the role function mode, involves interaction with others. Interdependence, however, focuses on close relationships of people, as individuals and groups, rather than roles in society. The interdependence mode is one in which the need for relational integrity, associated with affection, development and maturation, and resources, is met. The Roy Adaptation Model notes that each individual or collective human system strives for relational integrity by adequacy and mastery in each of these areas. In the interdependence mode, that sense of adequacy is experienced through satisfying and sufficient interrelationships with others and with the environment.

This chapter provides an overview of the interdependence mode with a focus on three integrated processes associated with affection, development of relationships, and resource adequacy. Relationships involving both individuals and collectives are addressed. Illustrations of compensatory adaptive processes related to interdependence are provided and examples of compromised processes of interdependence are explored. Finally, guidelines for planning nursing care by formulating diagnoses, establishing goals, selecting interventions, and evaluating nursing care are described.

▶ OBJECTIVES

After studying this chapter, the reader will be able to do the following:

1. Describe the interdependence mode according to the Roy Adaptation Model.

2. Identify important first-level assessment parameters (behaviors) for the interdependence mode.

3. Identify second-level assessment factors (stimuli) that influence the interdependence mode.

4. Describe one compensatory process related to the interdependence mode.

5. Name and describe two situations of compromised processes of interdependence.

6. Develop a nursing diagnosis, given a situation related to interdependence.

7. Derive goals for a given situation illustrating ineffective interdependence in a given situation.

8. Describe nursing interventions commonly implemented in situations of ineffective interdependence.

9. Propose approaches to determine the effectiveness of nursing interventions.

▶ KEY CONCEPTS DEFINED

Affectional adequacy: One of three processes associated with the basic need of relational integrity; the need to give and receive love, respect, and value satisfied through effective relations and communication.

Context: External (economic, social, political, cultural, belief, family systems) and internal (mission, vision, values, principles, goals, plans) influences within relationships; also viewed as stimuli.

Developmental adequacy: One of three components associated with the basic need of relational integrity; learning and maturation in relationships achieved through developmental processes.

Infrastructure: The affectional, resource, and developmental processes that exist within a relationship; process that determines adaptation levels.

Interdependence: The close relationships of people aimed at satisfying needs for affection, development, and resources to achieve relational integrity.

People: The third component of the interdependence model; the participants in the relationship and particularly their coping abilities.

Relational integrity: The basic need of the interdependence mode; the feeling of security in relationships.

Resource adequacy: One of three processes associated with the basic need of relational integrity; the need for food, clothing, shelter, health, and security achieved through interdependent processes.

Significant others: The individuals to whom the most meaning or importance is given.

Support systems: Persons, groups, organizations with whom one associates in order to achieve affectional, developmental, and resource requirements.

► INTERDEPENDENCE PROCESSES

Interdependence is defined as the close relationships of people aimed at satisfying needs for affection, development, and resources to achieve relational integrity—the basic need of the interdependence mode. It is through affectional, developmental, and resource processes that one continues to grow as a person and as a contributing member of society.

The quest for adequacy in relationships is part of today's culture. Intact families try to spend time together, divorced people seek new relationships, social groups for young and old proliferate, and organizations expand and contract. There is a preponderance of self-help books on "satisfying relationships." Movies and novels focus on the struggles of intimate and loving relationships. However, the times reflect that fewer people are married, more are living alone, and social interaction through volunteer activities is less than a decade ago. Demographic and societal changes, including the aging population, family breakdown, cultural integration, and transition in communities, indicate that new ways of achieving relational adequacy will be sought. For example, immigrant young people, particularly boys, alone in a foreign country, tend to form gangs to fulfill their need for relational adequacy and security when their families are absent and they are isolated in a culturally strange environment.

Much has been written about relationships and their influence on quality and length of life. Some literature ties "length of life" and "the good life" to relationships with others or social support (see, for example, Cohen, 1985; Dimond & Jones, 1983; Gottlieb, 1981; and Greenblatt, Beccera, & Serafetinides, 1982; Roy, 1981). House, Landis, and Umberson (1988) reviewed the literature noting a relationship between social interaction and health. The classic study of Spitz (1945) showed that infants who were deprived of touch or affection simply wasted away and died. For years, it has been known that married people live longer and are healthier, and often happier, than unmarried people. The "social contact index" (Berkman, 1978) often used in these studies takes into account whether the individual is married, has close contacts with friends and relatives, belongs to a religious group, or has organizational links. People who have contacts in only one of these categories appear to have a greater risk of dying than those who have contacts in more than one category.

Interdependent relationships involve the willingness and ability to give to and accept from others aspects of all that one has to offer: love, respect, value, nurturing, knowledge, skills, commitments, material possessions, time, and talents. People who demonstrate adaptive interdependence have a comfortable balance between their needs for affiliation (dependence) and achievement (independence). They have learned to live successfully in a world of other people, animals, objects, the environment, and a God figure.

Interdependence needs are met through social interaction on many levels. From the individual perspective, relationships are developed with significant others and support systems. As the perspective broadens, extended families, clubs, networks, associations, organizations, bureaucracies, and political parties, for example, occupy positions in interdependent relationships. On the broadest level is the interrelationship of humanity with creation as a whole.

Productive and rewarding relationship processes meet needs related to affection (love, respect, value, nurturance, care, attention, affirmation, belonging, approval, and understanding); developmental needs associated with learning and maturation in relationships; as well as basic resource requirements such as food, clothing, shelter, health, and security. These three processes form the basis for assessment of the interdependence behavior.

Interdependent relationships are divided into two categories, significant others and support systems. *Significant others* are the individuals to whom the most meaning or importance is given. The significant others for a person may be parents, spouse, friends, family members, God, or even an animal. These significant others are loved, respected, and valued, and in turn, they love, respect, and value to a degree greater than in other relationships. Significant others can be identified by answering the question of who are the most important people in my life. For most people, the significant others are relatively stable and remain for periods of time. Individuals usually can identify at least one person who is the significant other. In some situations, material possessions or money become more significant than other people. However, in these instances, the love, respect, and value is not reciprocal and ineffective interdependence results.

Support systems include people, groups, and organizations with which one associates in order to accomplish goals or to achieve some purpose. The meanings of relationships with support systems do not usually carry the same intensity as those of relationships with significant others. Consider the example of an adult woman who might consider her spouse and children as significant others and a friend at work and her bridge club as support systems. A place of work, itself, becomes part of a person's support system. At times of illness, the nurse can occupy a position in a support system for an individual who requires health care. Thus, interrelationships, whether they are with significant others or support systems, become an important consideration in the nurse–patient relationship.

Involved in interdependent relationships is the giving to and receiving from others aspects of that which we have to offer as persons, such as love, respect, value, nurturing, knowledge, skills, commitment, time, talents, and material possessions. This is evident in friendships, family relationships, groups, larger organizations, or any collective in society. Such relationships involve both giving and receiving of something, love and nurturing in parent–child relationships, work in return for pay in employment relationships, participation in return for security and belonging in youth gang relationships, as simplistic examples.

Interdependent relationships, whether they be with significant others (such as the family) or with support systems (relations, friends, clubs, associations, work groups, or components of larger social service systems) can be viewed in terms of an interdependence model, adapted from Andrews et al. (1994) and consisting of three interrelated components: context, infrastructure, and people (see Fig. 16–1).

The *context* is a particular set of both external and internal stimuli influencing the relationship. Externally, factors such as the economic, social, political, cultural, belief, and family systems influence the relationship. Internally, the mission (purpose of existence) of the relationship, its vision (where it is headed), the associated values (enduring beliefs), principles (guidelines for

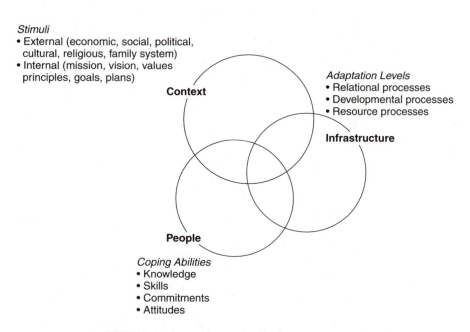

FIGURE 16–1. Interdependence mode with subareas and components.

action), and goals, formalized or not, influence the actions and accomplishments of participants in the relationship.

The *infrastructure* component pertains to the processes involved in adaptation, that is, affectional, developmental, and resource processes that exist within the relationship. These are the affectional, developmental, and resource processes that affect adaptation levels. These processes involve formal or informal procedures, activity, and systems that are part of the interaction. For example, a family may have decided to school their children at home. This system differs from that associated with public or private school education. In relational processes, people must coordinate their activities with others through communication. This holds true in relations with significant others and with support systems.

The *people* component addresses the participants themselves and their cognitive coping abilities, such as knowledge level, skills, commitments, and attitudes. Does the new hospice nurse have the knowledge required to successfully be with the patient and family through the dying process? Is the hospice administrator committed to preserving good working relationships among staff? Does the hospice support staff have the necessary skills to accomplish the goals of their jobs? Do family members adhere to the values and principles of the family unit? Knowledge, skills, commitments, and attitudes are important considerations in interdependent relationships of all descriptions, whether they are with significant others or support systems.

An important consideration when evaluating the effectiveness of these components in achieving the goals of the relationship and, ultimately, effective adaptation is the congruence and alignment of these three interrelated components. Disruption occurs if any one component is not compatible with or does not complement the other. Ineffective adaptation is the outcome. For example, if a young person (people) transgresses the family's values and guidelines (context), the entire family experiences tumult and lack of integrity. If the example set by parents (people) differs from their instruction (context, values, and principles), the outcome will be ineffective adaptation. From the perspective of an organization, if its principles (context) advocate empowerment of staff and decentralized decision making, but the managers (people) are not committed and do not demonstrate a supportive attitude, conflict will occur. As well, the organization's infrastructure is an important factor in enabling such principles. An example is whether or not the organization rewards initiative on the part of staff.

Kane (1988) reported beginning work toward a conceptual model of family social support and presented three interaction factors: reciprocity, advice and feedback, and emotional involvement. This work on reciprocity is based on the earlier work of Cobb (1976) that described an individual as involved in a network of mutual obligation. This belonging is noted by the sharing of resources with others and the giving and receiving of help. Advice and feedback relates to the quality and quantity of communication between the family and its network. Kane also drew on the work of Caplan (1974), who emphasized the importance of relationships with significant others to work

TABLE 16–1 PRINCIPLES OF EFFECTIVE RELATIONSHIPS

Listen Generously
Listen for the contribution and commitment of the other person, suspending assessments, judgments, and opinions about what he or she is saying. This does not mean that we agree or disagree with what is being said, but that we are committed to the legitimacy and value of the other's view.

Talk Straight
Speak honestly in a way that forwards the action as opposed to reacting to or attacking what is being said. This includes learning to make clear and direct requests.

Be for Each Other
Believe and commit to the premise that we are all in this together and that no one individual can win at the expense of another. This is the basis for trust and for making it safe for each other to take risks without fear of censure or being undermined by one's colleagues.

Honor Each Other's Commitments
Respect each other's commitments including one's own.

Appreciate and Acknowledge Each Other
Each member in the relationship commits to continuously acknowledge and appreciate the contributions of others and the team itself, even when things do not work out. It also means requesting and receiving acknowledgment from others if it is missing.

Be Concerned for Inclusion
Ask the question "Who else should be included or has a stake in what we are talking about?"

Be Concerned for Alignment
Participate in every conversation with a commitment to build alignment. Alignment does not mean consensus or universal agreement. It means that everyone is either "committed to" or "able to support" the commitments of others. No one is committed against the direction in which we are moving.

---

through the issues of living. Kane (1988) noted that communication is done through a process of giving advice and feedback. Emotional involvement includes the concepts of intimacy and trust. This final factor includes emotional bonds such as love, caring, warmth, and compassion.

The importance of communication in the achievement of effective relationships was also described by others. Koch and Haugk (1992, p. 18) observed that, "Without communication in a personal relationship, you risk collapse of that relationship." Selman and Andrews (1994) claimed that relationship issues are inseparable from communication issues, and in most cases are the same thing. Since relationships exist for a purpose, there must be a way of accomplishing the goals and plans associated with that purpose. Communication is that vehicle. As Selman and Andrews (1994, p. 54) observed:

> Success in realizing intentions is accomplished through relationships with others. The future is continually being created through conversations with others—by asking for or making commitments, by making requests and promises. Any potential future exists only as a possibility unless and until it is realized through action. From this perspective, commitments are actions. Successful coordination in relationships is the coordination of commitments.

> As the vision and commitments [in interrelationships] grow, so do the relationship breakdowns. This is both inevitable and healthy—an indication that the real underlying patterns and negative behavioral mechanisms are beginning to surface. These mechanisms normally are concealed, buried . . . ; they often thwart the best intentions to change. When they are uncovered, breakdowns in relationship are no longer taken for granted or covered over with platitudes. Rather, practices for getting to the bedrock question of what constitutes a "good relationship" begin to develop—that is, what are an individual's commitments, and how can one learn to develop and continuously improve effective relationships?

Selman and Andrews (1994) presented seven principles of effective relationships that have proven valuable, both in relationships with significant others and in interaction with support systems. These are identified and defined in Table 16–1. As they are applied, the effectiveness of relationships is markedly enhanced.

The basic need of the interdependence mode is relational integrity—the feeling of security in relationships. As previously noted, three processes are involved in achievement of relational integrity: *affectional adequacy* (the giving and receiving of attributes and assets), *developmental adequacy* (learning in and maturation of relationships), and *resource adequacy* (needs such as food, clothing, shelter, health, and security).

▶ AFFECTIONAL ADEQUACY: PROCESS AND ASSESSMENT

Affectional adequacy involves the willingness and ability to give to and receive from others aspects of all one has to offer as a person: love, respect, value, nurturance, knowledge, skills, commitments, talents, possessions, time, loyalty, for example. Affectional adequacy incorporates the need to be nurtured and to nurture in terms of care, attention, affection, affirmation, belonging, approval, and understanding. These needs are met primarily by establishing in-depth relationships with other people. Behaviors that demonstrate this exchange of personal attributes and assets are called receptive (receiving) and contributive (giving) behaviors (Randell, Tedrow, & Van Landingham, 1982).

Receiving behaviors are those that indicate that a person is receiving, taking in, or assimilating that offered by another. Receiving behaviors include allowing another to care for and protect oneself, accepting a thoughtful gesture, and receiving physical or psychological support. Giving behaviors are those of giving or supplying nurturance to another person. Examples include caring for another, touching, providing physical and psychological support, and performing thoughtful gestures. These giving and receiving behaviors reflect the circular relationship between a person and others (individuals or collectives) in the environment. People who successfully maintain relationships have developed the ability to recognize and deal with their own love and support needs, as well as those of other people.

The process of achieving affectional adequacy includes many components of interaction such as language skills, nonverbal communication skills, and the ability to recognize the feelings and attitudes of others. The development of sympathy and caring, as well as sharing, is inherent in this process. This development begins early and continues throughout a person's life. Focus on learning and maturation in relationships is further addressed in the section on developmental adequacy.

Just as there are relational dynamics in friendships and family relationships, there are group dynamics. Giving and receiving behaviors are evident in group dynamics, for example, in a work group in a health care setting. In return for time and application of knowledge, staff members receive a wage, educational benefits, opportunities to affiliate with others, and experience in their discipline of focus. Many factors influence the nature of dynamics within this collective. Of primary importance are the previously described context, infrastructure, and people components.

There is much information in the literature about relationships and group dynamics. The reader is referred to sources on organizational behavior, organizational development, and group dynamics if a more in-depth understanding of interrelationships and collective human systems is required. Before examining the other relational processes, the first- and second-level assessment of affectional adequacy is explored.

Assessment of Behavior

The nurse begins assessment in the interdependence mode when first meeting the person and is keenly attuned to behaviors that the person might reveal spontaneously. After creating a comfortable milieu, the nurse proceeds with an in-depth assessment of behaviors related to affectional adequacy. These focus on the identification of significant others and support systems and the giving and receiving behaviors evident in these relationships.

Significant Others and Support Systems

The nurse first addresses the two major categories of interdependent relationships, significant others and support systems. Who does the person name as significant others? Who or what are his or her support systems and to what extent does he or she depend on them? With what groups, associations, or organizations is the person involved? What significance do they hold in terms of time commitments and associated responsibilities? Does the person work? All of this information is significant in terms of interdependence and affectional adequacy.

Giving and Receiving

What giving behaviors are evident; what receiving behaviors are evident? Some questions that can be helpful in the identification of giving and receiving behaviors are as follows. How do you express your caring to the significant other? How does the significant other express caring and affection to you? It is important to observe nonverbal behaviors when others are present with the person. Do they touch each other, look at each other, give gifts, share jokes or stories? An example of giving behaviors on the part of a wife could be the statement, "I tell him often that I love him," or "I always make his lunch." Receiving behaviors could include statements such as, "I love the way he rubs my back," or "Look at the beautiful roses he brought me," or "He calls me from work several times a day."

Giving and receiving behaviors are also evident in assessment of group and collective dynamics. Perhaps a person has been receiving home care services to assist in coping with a disability. The services provided to the client constitute the commodity being received; the payment for the services (giving behavior) may be channeled through the health insurance company (another agency in the picture).

Assessment of Stimuli

Stimuli that are important when assessing affectional adequacy from both individual and collective points of view include the following.

1. Expectations of relationships and awareness of needs
2. Nurturing ability of both parties
3. Levels of self-esteem
4. Levels and kinds of interaction skills
5. Presence of others in the physical environment
6. Knowledge about relationships and the behaviors that enhance them
7. Developmental age and tasks
8. In terms of collectives, an understanding of the interdependent relationships in terms of context, infrastructure, and people

Exploration of this complexity constitutes advanced nursing practice.

Expectations

The expectations of the persons who are involved in a relationship affect the quality of the relationship. If the person expects that affection is expressed by physical proximity, spending time together, physical contact, and remembering birthdays, it is important that the other person in the relationship be aware of and respond to these expectations. When two people in a relationship can define their expectations clearly and communicate them, the relationship is enhanced. Once each person is aware of expectations and needs of self and the others, it is essential that they all act on this information in a consistent fashion.

Nurturing Ability

The nurturing ability of each person in the relationship also contributes to the quality of the relationship. Nurturing involves providing growth-producing care and attention. A person who experienced early bonding as an infant and tactile and verbal loving as a child will usually be able to move into adult love relationships with ease. They have experienced a high-quality love relationship and know what it feels like and what the characteristics are. An adult who experienced delayed bonding or minimal bonding in a parent–child relationship that was characterized by distance, separation, and verbal negating will probably need help in learning how to build a friendship or love relationship. Likewise, traumatic experiences in the early years, for example, loss of a parent or abuse by a trusted adult, can interfere with later effective nurturing ability.

Level of Self-esteem

The level of self-esteem, as related to the self-concept mode, is an influencing factor for interdependent relationships. People tend to choose friendships and love relationships with persons who have a similar level of self-esteem that is, people who have low self-esteem choose friends with low self-esteem. They then are reinforced in the feelings of negative self-worth and the circular process continues. Similarly, when two people, both of whom experience high self-esteem, develop a caring relationship, the reinforcement for the other serves to enhance the already high level of self-esteem. A person's level of self-esteem influences the degree to which the person feels that he or she can go out to others. Likewise, self-esteem is a basic contextual factor when interdependent circumstances in life change, for example, the permanent separation from one who has been a significant other. Level of self-esteem influences the person's ability to adapt in such situations.

Communication Skills

The level and type of communication skills are closely related to affectional adequacy and relational integrity. If the person has open communication, is flexible, can articulate clearly, and is sensitive to other people's verbal and nonverbal behavior, the relationship is facilitated. If one of the partners does not have interaction skills at the level desired, those skills can be learned with help. Learning begins with recognition that one needs to communicate more effectively. Many self-help books are available on this subject. Feedback from a knowledgeable person as changes are initiated is an important factor.

Presence

Presence in the physical environment influences interdependent relationships. If friends or a couple are separated often and for long periods, it is more difficult to maintain the relationship. The impact of presence on bonding between a mother and child has been mentioned previously. It is evident that attachment occurs more readily when the mother and baby have frequent and early access to each other. Any relationship (individual or collective) is maintained more effectively when proximity is possible.

Context, Infrastructure, People

The effectiveness of collective interrelationships is influenced extensively by the context, infrastructure, and people as described in the interrelationship model. For in-depth understanding of the factors influencing the collective, it is important to assess the internal and external influences described within the context. Mission, vision, values, principles, and goals influence behaviors within the collective. It is also important to comprehend the infrastructure in terms of system, processes, and procedures through which action is accomplished. In addition, the people in terms of their cognitive strategies of knowledge, skills, and commitments are important considerations.

This depth of assessment of behaviors as related to collective human systems pertains to advanced analysis of the collective under consideration. Such analysis would be expected only in situations of advanced system assessment where the nurse is interested in the health, well-being, and adaptation of the collective itself.

▶ DEVELOPMENTAL ADEQUACY: PROCESS AND ASSESSMENT

Developmental adequacy refers to the processes associated with learning and maturation in interrelationships, be they individual (involving two people) or collective (involving families, groups, associations, organizations, or networks, for example). Each undergoes development and transition in terms of dependency and independency throughout the life span. The appropriateness of this balance as learning and maturation proceed influences adaptation and the ability to achieve relational integrity.

Randell, Tedrow, and Van Landingham (1982) believe that, when a baby is born, two adaptive modes are operational, the physiologic mode and the interdependence mode. Many studies document the infant's need for touch, physical contact, the bonding process, and love. Out of the interactions that are primarily affectional or nurturing in nature arises the beginning of self-concept; finally, roles are learned. These authors further suggest that, with the living out of one's life, the modes are given up in reverse sequence. For example, people who are admitted to convalescent centers in their final years give up many of their previously held roles. Sometimes even the identity of their self-concept becomes less apparent if the person moves to senility or a state of coma. A form of the interdependence mode, the receiving part of interaction, and the physiologic mode remain operational.

According to this view, a person begins and ends life as a physiologic and interdependent being. There are exceptions to this continuum, such as sudden death or a long productive life with minimal deterioration of functioning. This general picture of the development and relinquishing of the four adaptive modes is illustrated in Figure 16–2.

Many sociological and psychological theorists have studied the development of relationships in terms of dependence and independence. The works of Erikson (1963), Selman (1980), Fromm (1956), Havighurst (1953), and Maslow (1954) provide an understanding of the development and maintenance of relational integrity. Selman (1980) provided a description of five stages of friendship that are similar to Erikson's work but apply more specifi-

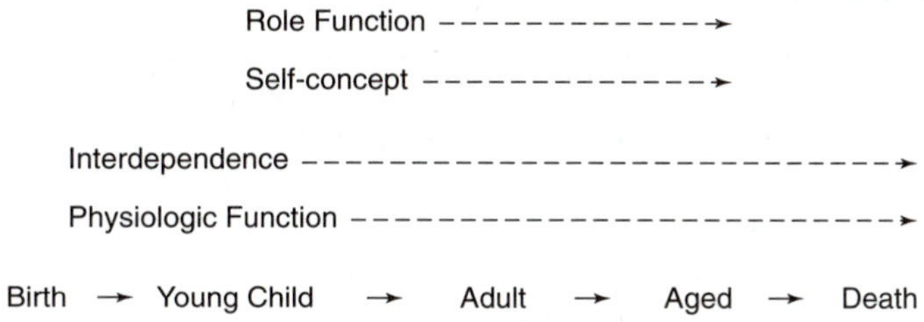

Role Function – – – – – – – – – – – – →

Self-concept – – – – – – – – – – – – →

Interdependence – →

Physiologic Function – →

Birth → Young Child → Adult → Aged → Death

FIGURE 16–2. Four adaptive modes for the individual from birth to death.

cally to affectional needs. The stages and their characteristics are listed in Table 16–2.

A friendship builds out of some commonly held beliefs, values, and interests. Some people experience the growth of a friendship from which an adult love relationship can develop. Fromm (1956) talked about love being a

TABLE 16–2   THE FIVE STAGES OF FRIENDSHIP

Stage	Age (Years)	Characteristics
0	3–7	*Monetary Playmate:* The child has difficulty distinguishing between a physical action, such as grabbing a toy, and the psychological intention behind this action. Friends are valued for their material and physical attributes, and defined by proximity.
1	4–9	*One-way Assistance:* At this stage, the child can differentiate between his or her own perspective and those of others. However, the child does not yet understand that dealing with others involves give-and-take between people. In a "good" friendship, one party does what the other party wants to do.
2	6–12	*Two-way Fair Weather Cooperation:* The child has the ability to see that interpersonal perspectives are reciprocal, each person taking into account the other's perspective. Conceptions of friendship include a concern for what each person thinks about the other. It is much more a two-way street. The limitation of this stage is that the child still sees the basic purpose of friendship as serving many separate self-interests, rather than mutual interests.
3	9–15	*Intimate, Mutually Shared Relationships:* Not only can the child take the other's point of view, but by now he or she can also step outside the friendship and take a generalized third-person perspective on it. With the ability to take a third-person perspective, the child can move from viewing friendship as a reciprocal cooperation for each person's self-interests to seeing it as a collaboration with others for mutual and common interests. That is, friends share feelings, help each other to resolve personal and interpersonal conflicts, and help each other solve personal problems.
4	15 on	*Autonomous Interdependent Friendships:* The individual sees relationships as complex and often overlapping systems. In a friendship, the adolescent or adult is aware that people have many needs and that in a good friendship each partner gives strong emotional and psychological support to the other, but also allows the friend to develop independent relationships. Respecting needs for both dependency and autonomy is seen as being essential to friendship.

Selman, R. C. (1980) The growth of interpersonal understanding: Development and clinical analyses. *New York: Academic Press.*

feeling and an action. Love has the characteristics of knowing, caring about, respecting, and feeling responsibility toward the receiver of love. Each of us has a need to be loved and supported and to love and support. The love relationship is an intense interaction with close identification with the loved one. As such, the joy and pain, as well as stresses and happiness, of the other, are experienced by both people in the relationship. The love relationship includes a friendship with the other person.

Havighurst (1953) described developmental tasks for the infant to the mature adult. Each stage of life includes tasks related to establishing and maintaining relational integrity.

Collectives, too, proceed through developmental stages as new groups are formed. From the collective perspective, the context, infrastructure, and people are important components that must be addressed. The extent to which these develop as complementary and in alignment influences the effectiveness of the collective in goal achievement.

Within groups, isolated or as part of a larger entity, developmental stages have been described. Many are familiar with Tuckman and Jensen's (1977, p. 419) description of "forming, storming, norming, performing, and adjourning"—the stages of a collective throughout its life span, as it becomes effective in accomplishing its goals and ultimately relinquishing being a relating group. Another approach to stages of group development was described in Chapter 15.

Several developmental perspectives have been applied to interrelationships in the work place. Creative Nursing Management (1992) observed that employees progress developmentally in a cycle similar to that described by Erikson (1963). This suggests that leadership approaches must complement the employees' needs, requirements, and capabilities as they progress from being a novice (dependency) to becoming more experienced and confident (independency) in their work. A well-known approach to examining development of nursing practice from novice to expert that can be helpful to nurses at all stages of their careers has been described by Benner (1984).

Assessment of Behavior

Understanding processes of developmental adequacy associated with learning and maturation in interrelationships, whether individual (involving two people) or collective (involving families or other groups) is useful for assessment of the interdependence mode. In particular, the nurse assesses behavior in relation to developmental processes and includes consideration of the developmental stage of the individual or collective, and evidence of dependency and independency.

Developmental Stage

Of initial importance in assessment of developmental adequacy of the individual or collective is the current developmental stage. What is the gender, age, and maturity level of the individual? At what stage is the family—childless, small children, teenagers, grown children? Are the individuals involved in the relationship comfortable with and confident in each other?

For the collective, how long has it been in existence? Is it rigidly or loosely structured? Is its purpose clear to those participating? Is transition occurring?

Dependency

Dependency as it pertains to interdependent relationships refers to the extent to which the person looks to or relies on others for support, attention, affection. To what extent does the person rely on significant others or support systems to meet the necessities of daily living? For example, young children tend to be dependent on their parents for preparation of meals, help with dressing, and protection in an unsafe situation. As individuals mature, their dependency lessens. An elderly man may have been dependent on his wife to prepare his meals. If she is no longer able to fulfill that responsibility, he may not feel capable of or have the initiative to accomplish the associated tasks. It is thus important to understand to what extent and for what activities an individual depends on others.

Dependency also involves attention and affection seeking. Is the person demonstrating any behavior that indicates that he or she is seeking attention or affection? As an individual matures, attention and affection are sought from different sources. Whereas parents were the chief source of both for young children, soon friends and teachers enter that sphere. As individuals enter the workplace, their contacts broaden further to involve other significant others and support systems. During a contact with the health care system, individuals may look to the nurse to fulfill some of these needs.

Dependency in interrelationships of collectives is also considered. In situations of families, there may be dependence on relatives for support. For example, grandparents may have a role in the care of young children. Larger organizations may be dependent on a government agency for funding.

Independency

Independency refers to the situations in which the person or collective takes initiative for independent achievement. It is important for the nurse to understand in what areas the person possesses the necessary knowledge, skills, capabilities, and attitudes to be independent. As much as possible, independence is encouraged and supported, with the recognition that the more the person uses his or her capacities and capabilities, the more effective adaptation will be.

At times, achievement behavior associated with independence becomes exaggerated, and aggression, rivalry, hostility, competitiveness, disengagement, dominance, exhibition, and rejection can result. Aggression has been described as the energy or tension behind the need for achievement. Patterns of control over the aggressive drive have been described as important focal stimuli for adaptation problems in the interdependence mode (Ellison, 1976). Roy and Roberts (1981) noted the significance of balancing dependency and aggressive drives in social situations. Lack of effective control of aggression and related behaviors are manifestations of ineffective adaptation associated with interdependence.

Independence also applies to collectives, families, networks, and associations, for example. Families who farm as an occupation demonstrate more independence in terms of generating their own food supply than do families dependent on urban retail outlets. Self-standing organizations often have more independence than organizations that are tied to or dependent on another agency for their mandate to operate or their funding.

Assessment of Stimuli

Assessment of the factors influencing the development of interrelationships includes the developmental stage of the individual or collective, significant changes that have impact on the integrity of the self-concept, and knowledge about relationship development. Each of these is important in understanding developmental adequacy.

Developmental Stage

In the case of developmental adequacy, developmental stage is considered to be both a behavior and a stimulus. Erikson's (1963) eight developmental crises are often manifest in terms of interdependent relationships and the development and maturation of these relationships. For example, in the stage of identity versus identity diffusion, the peer group and models of leadership are important. The development of trust versus mistrust is a stimulus to receiving behaviors in the interdependence mode.

Two other theories that are particularly relevant to understanding how interdependence behavior develops are those described by Havighurst (1953) and Selman (1980). The reader is encouraged to consult the primary sources for further information about these perspectives.

Groups and organizations proceed through developmental stages, as well. When they are just being formed, issues related to mission, vision, values, principles of operation, and initial plans must be addressed. A structure and its associated systems, processes, and procedures must be created and people must be in place to accomplish the objectives. As Smith and Berg (1990) described, groups struggle with ambivalence, contradiction, paralysis, and movement throughout the course of group life. A great deal is written about group effectiveness, productivity, and success. All of these processes relate to developmental adequacy.

Significant Changes

There are times in each person's development that radical life changes occur. These include events such as divorce, serious illness, death of a significant other, and change in support system. Their impact on the person's interdependence and adaptation as a whole is enormous. The person's ability to cope with them results in either effective or ineffective adaptation.

Groups and collectives are also influenced by significant changes. Examples of such include mergers or separations, funding cutbacks, changes in leadership, or organizational problems in general.

Integrity of Self-concept

Dunning (1976, p. 309) suggested that one of the most important factors influencing the development of interdependence is the developing self-concept of the individual which is, in turn, influenced by affection and reinforcement received from others. Through this process, the person develops a style of coping with affiliative and achievement needs which is predominantly dependent, independent, or interdependent.

Members of groups and collectives also possess a self-concept, or group identity, relating to the group itself. Family members hold perceptions of how successful or dysfunctional they are. Association members feel adequate or inadequate in terms of the mission and objectives of their group. "School spirit" is regarded as an indicator of the self-concept of the associated body of students and in some cases is described as perceptible on entering the doors. Staff in certain hospitals, and perhaps the larger community, views certain health care agencies as "flagships" for the industry. Each of these illustrates collective self-concept, which then affects the developmental adequacy of the relating group.

Knowledge About Relationships

Knowledge about friendship and how to build and maintain a relationship is an important stimulus. There are many theoretical discussion of friendship available. McGinnis (1980) described five activities that can deepen a friendship.

1. To put friendships or relationships first or give them top priority
2. To talk about and express affection for the other person
3. To create space in the friendship so that both people can maintain their identity and autonomy
4. To cultivate the art of affirmation, making sure that the other person knows what is valued about them
5. To accept own and the other person's anger on a temporary basis

When a person has developed nurturing ability and has significant knowledge regarding the dynamics of friendship, there is a greater possibility of an in-depth, long-lasting relationship.

From the broader perspective, knowledge about transition in collectives and organizational dynamics is an important influence on development. As more is understood about group dynamics and factors that influence these, development in organizations and other collectives can become more effective and efficient.

► RESOURCE ADEQUACY: PROCESS AND ASSESSMENT

The interdependence mode identifies *resource adequacy* as the need for food, clothing, shelter, health, and security achieved through interdependent processes, the third important process in the achieving of relational integrity. Maslow (1954) provided a hierarchy of needs (physiologic needs, safety needs, need for belongingness and love, esteem needs) organized in terms of the degree to which satisfaction of each is a prerequisite to the search for satisfaction of the next. This suggests that, unless the physiologic and safety requirements are met, the individual's attention is not directed toward higher order needs involving relationships with others. The application of this understanding to interdependence points to the importance of resource adequacy to support effectiveness in relationships. The implication is that physiologic needs must be met before higher order needs can be addressed.

Acknowledging that individuals' requirements for material resources vary greatly from person to person and group to group, it must be recognized that a certain level of resources is necessary to support and maintain relationships and to enable them to develop, mature, and achieve their mission. Unless requirements associated with food, clothing, and shelter are met, a given relationship will struggle. Interestingly, it is often through relationships that these needs are met.

Even in groups and larger organizations there has been traditional emphasis on physical facilities, organizational structure, materials and supplies, and information processes as basic to functioning. Contemporary organizational theory is now recognizing and addressing the crucial aspect of effective relationships in the equation. A philosophic approach such as quality management is a case in point.

Broader in scope is the contemporary emphasis on the interrelationship of humanity with the environment. Recognizing this complex integration and interdependence, social conscience regarding respect for and preservation of the environment has become a matter of substantial social concern. Protection of the environment, in its broadest sense, ultimately preserves and promotes resource adequacy and, in turn, the ability to satisfy basic physiologic and safety needs, so that higher order needs can be addressed.

Assessment of Behavior

It is often through interdependent relationships that resource adequacy is achieved. In turn, resource adequacy is fundamental to the ability to achieve relational integrity. This circular interrelationship is an example of the complexity and "kaleidoscopic" nature of the person as described in the Roy Adaptation Model. Behaviors in one mode may be stimuli for another. The focus of assessment of behavior related to resource adequacy focuses on one indicator: physiologic–physical status as an indicator of the extent to which basic needs are being met.

Physiologic–Physical Integrity

For the individual, an important behavioral assessment relates to the person's physiologic status—evidence that basic needs are being met. In particular, needs for nutrition, protection, and activity and rest provide indicators of physiologic integrity as supported by adequate food, clothing, and shelter.

Does the person have adequate clothing? Does he or she have a home and is it secure? Does he or she have access to nutritious food? Do significant others or support systems play a role in the supplying of basic needs?

Physical integrity of collectives is also an important consideration. As presented in Chapter 4, physical facilities are an important component for collective human systems. This includes a physical plant (shelter for the family, a meeting place for a group, and an organizational physical facility for the operation, for example). Also included in this component are the operational resources required to fulfill the purpose of the group. In a family situation, food and clothing are examples of operational resources. In an organization, supplies and equipment constitute physical resources. Some aggregate human systems have need for technologic resources, as well. A community requires a communication system and maintenance equipment. All of these physical commodities contribute to meeting the need of resource adequacy in the physical mode.

Assessment of Stimuli

The stimuli that have the primary effect on the adequacy of resources for individuals and for collectives are primarily monetary resources and assisting relationships. Without money, it becomes difficult to supply basic needs. Further, interdependent relationships may have a focus on assisting with meeting basic resources requirements.

Monetary Resources

The satisfaction of basic needs and, in turn, physiologic–physical integrity, are largely dependent on the financial resources available to the individual or the collective system. Without money, food and clothing cannot be purchased and rent and utilities cannot be supplied. Inadequate levels of resources compromise the ability of the collective to continue to operate. In a family situation, if there is not an adequate income, it will be difficult to provide food for the family members. If an organization is not healthy financially, eventually, it will be unable to pay employees, purchase operating supplies, or, ultimately, remain in business.

Capital resources are also an important aspect of financial adequacy for most collective human adaptive systems. Capital resources pertain to the significant and infrequent purchases that can be required to support ongoing integrity of the collective. In a family situation, this may be a major health care expenditure on behalf of a member or the purchase of a house for the family. For a group, a baseball team, for example, it may be the purchase of uniforms so that the team can be involved in a competition league. Organizations, communities, and societal groups often have major requirements for capital resources to support their ongoing and orderly operation.

If inadequate funding persists over time, the integrity of the entire system is compromised and ineffective behaviors result.

Assisting Relationships

Individuals and collective human systems often are associated with others that assist in meeting basic needs. This assistance can take the form of family support systems, social service systems, and other organizations. Consider the examples of younger families, or elderly parents, who receive financial assistance from more prosperous relatives to assist with the meeting of basic needs. Social service systems have been developed to assist individuals and families with needs in times of hardship or crisis. In some situations, organizations provide for other organizations. The complex relationships between organized crime and legitimate business in Eastern Europe is an interesting consideration. In this example, businesses contract with the criminal element for protection in return for a proportion of earnings. Without such an arrangement, the business would be unable to operate. Perhaps government subsidies for faltering businesses or service agencies could also be viewed as one organization providing for the basic needs of another organization in order to ensure continued operation.

There is an abundance of literature pertaining to relationships and their effectiveness, structure, problems, and keys to success. The reader is referred to sociology, psychology, and organizational literature for further information.

► COMPENSATORY ADAPTIVE PROCESSES

Viewed as human adaptive system (see Chap. 2), both individuals and collectives have innate and acquired ways of responding to the changing environment. Further, Roy conceptualizes these complex adaptive dynamics as the coping processes of the regulator and cognator subsystems for the individual and the stabilizer and innovator for the collective. Compensatory processes represent the adaptation level at which the cognator–regulator or innovator–stabilizer have been activated by a challenge to the integrated life processes.

Compensatory processes associated with interdependence often involve support systems. Individual and collective human systems often call on these for assistance when affectional, developmental, or resource challenges occur. Two illustrations of interdependence compensatory adaptive responses are provided: a mentorship program for disadvantaged young people and programs to assist those affected by alcohol abuse.

Many social service programs have arisen in response to a need to provide assistance to individuals and collectives in the achievement of relational integrity, that is, affectional, developmental, and resource adequacy. Agencies participating in and supporting such initiatives often include the business community, labor associations, school districts, and civic councils. One such program is a mentorship program for disadvantaged young people. This program provides an opportunity for employed adults to mentor students at their workplace. The mentor functions as a positive role model for the student and encourages that individual to develop to his or her fullest potential and to develop a vision for the future. Mentorship is an attempt to encourage young people in disadvantaged situations to stay in school and to be successful in life. The impact of such a program is reflected in the following quotation from a high school principal: "Today schools and educators are asked to take on so many responsibilities in nurturing and developing young people, but we cannot do it by ourselves. We are grateful for the support provided by all the partners in [the program] as we challenge our students to seek their greatest potential."

Another example of a support system that is assisting families in compensatory processes is focused on a major interdependence problem, alcohol abuse. The Al-Anon Family Group Headquarters, Inc. is an organization designed to support those whose lives have been affected by someone else's drinking. There is also an arm of the organization directed at the needs of teens in such a situation. For the person who has the desire to overcome alcohol dependency, Alcoholics Anonymous is an agency with branches throughout North America. Through interdependent relationships with individuals experiencing the same dependency problem, mutual support and encouragement have helped many individuals to gain control of their situation.

► COMPROMISED PROCESSES OF INTERDEPENDENCE

When integrated and compensatory life processes are inadequate, the third adaptation level of compromised processes results. Adaptation problems (compromised processes of adaptation) can be caused by difficulties in any or all of the processes of interdependence since affectional adequacy, developmental adequacy, and resource adequacy are all interrelated. Five examples of compromised processes of interdependence are discussed in this section. They are separation anxiety, loneliness, substance abuse, aggression (from the individual perspective), and the problem of pollution (from the societal perspective).

Separation Anxiety

Separation anxiety is the painful uneasiness of mind related to separation from a significant other. Since the focal stimulus for this condition is the actual or threatened separation from a significant other, it is isolated as a compromised process of the interdependence mode. Separation anxiety is first experienced in infancy, and the person then has the potential for experiencing it throughout the life span. There are developmental crises in the person's life that create a vulnerable period for anxiety related to separation. These developmental crises are addressed in the works of Mahler (1979), Bowlby (1969, 1973), Robertson (1953), and Erikson (1963).

The infant is separated physiologically at birth from the mother with the cutting of the umbilical cord. The beginning of emotional separation occurs during later stages of development. Before emotional separation can occur, emotional bonding or attachment with the significant other must occur (Klaus & Kennel, 1981). Bonding is a term that describes a reciprocal joining or unity. It begins for the woman as she experiences pregnancy and proceeds through the tasks of pregnancy. Bonding probably begins for the fetus during this time, but is accelerated during and immediately following birth. By the time the child is ready to enter school, a process of bonding and attachment, followed by a stage of separation and becoming a distinct separate individual, has occurred. It is after that attachment phase, and during the separation–individuation phase, that separation anxiety first occurs and is most intense.

Mahler (1979) described three phases of the attachment–separation process that are experienced in sequence. The first phase, autism, occurs during the first few weeks of life. The infant does not differentiate the self from the environment, but does learn to differentiate between pain and pleasure. The second phase, the symbiotic phase, refers to the attachment to the mother. At this time, about 1 month of age, the infant does not differentiate the self from the nonself but does attach to the mother. Mahler's third phase, the separation–individuation process, begins soon after the symbiotic or attachment phase.

There is a four-part progression that occurs during the separation–individuation process. Separation refers to separation from the constant caregiver (usually the mother). Individuation refers to clearly becoming a self. The first subphase is termed differentiation and emerges as the infant becomes mobile by creeping, walking, climbing, and exploring self and the environment. The infant stays near the mother and enjoys playing games with objects and people that repeatedly disappear and reappear, such as "where did it go?" and "peek-a-boo." The next subphase is termed practicing, during which the child explores the environment near the mother and develops motor skills. The child in this stage accepts strangers readily as long as the mother is near and the stranger does not approach. The next subphase, rapprochement, is one in which the child actively resists separation. It is manifested by the toddler using negative behavior, such as repeatedly saying "no" or self-identity behavior such as saying "me" and "mine." There is an intense period of growth in the formation of the self-concept mode during the rapprochement phase. The separation from the mother is for longer periods, but the toddler continues to return to her frequently. The self-concept and interdependence modes are interconnected closely at this point of the toddler's life. The final subphase, object constancy, occurs from 18 to 36 months of age. The child develops intrapsychic symbols for the significant other. This development enables the child to begin separating without the overwhelming fear of abandonment.

Early work in separation anxiety was done by Robertson (1953) and Bowlby (1969). These authors described the infant between 3 and 6 months of age as recognizing the mother as an individual. They defined the period of 18 to 24 months as a time of peak dependency on the caregiver. The child at this time is possessively and passionately attached to the mother. The child is overwhelmed when separated from the mother. Bowlby and Robertson documented on film the behavior of children who were separated at the time of hospitalization. They defined three stages of separation anxiety through which children proceed if their significant other is separated from them. They are protest, despair, and denial (detachment).

In the protest stage, children are acutely aware of their need for their mothers. They will do anything and do it vigorously to recapture their mothers. They do believe that their energetic protesting behaviors will, in fact, return their mothers to their sides.

The next state of separation occurs in a few hours or days, the stage of despair. During this stage, children are actively mourning the loss of the significant other and they withdraw. While mourning, each child remains preoccupied with the loss of the mother and remains vigilant for her return. It is the quiet phase of separation anxiety. The child is passive and will perform self-comforting activities such as thumb-sucking or clinging to a favorite toy.

The final phase of denial (detachment) is moved into slowly. At this point, children repress the need for their mothers and begin to be interested in the environment. Children begin to seek comfort in food and support from anyone who will give it to them. A stranger viewing a child at this stage would tend to remark on how well-adjusted the child has become.

When the parents return, the child who has gone only as far as the stage of despair will usually reject the parents initially and then respond to them slowly. The attachment is reestablished slowly as the child and significant other are reunited. Passing through these stages to a resolution hopefully will lead to a more comfortable separation another time.

Although separation experiences are essential to the development of the individual, they should be minimized during periods of increased stress, such as hospitalization. These early works of Robertson and Bowlby were helpful in the movement of extending visiting hours in pediatric hospitals and instituting policies of rooming-in for parents and families so that they can stay with the child at this time.

Erikson (1963) identified eight developmental crises, or stages, that are to be mastered sequentially through the life span. These were identified in Chapter 14. The tasks of infancy and early childhood relevant here are building trust and achieving autonomy. Thus, another theorist described the attachment and separation through which the child must proceed to attain a separate identity.

Ainsworth (1964) and Mead (1971) explored child behavior in other cultures. Ainsworth studied children and parents in Uganda and Mead, in Samoa. Both cultures have extended family units with many adults in the child's environment. Both researchers documented that the infant did not attach as intensely to the mother and therefore did not experience the degree of separation anxiety that children do who are reared in a society without extended families.

Another crisis period for separation anxiety occurs for the school-aged child with the beginning and the end of the school year. Phenomena identified as "school phobias" are frequently separation anxiety. Ezor (1980) studied the separation anxiety related to school. The adolescent experiences separation anxiety with high frequency. This chaotic period is not unlike the toddler period, with an emphasis on clarifying one's identity and again separating from one's parents. Separation from the peer group also causes anxiety.

The adult can experience separation anxiety. An example of adult separation anxiety is the couple who is separating for a long period for a business or a family commitment. During the process of saying good-bye, the stages of protest, despair, and denial (detachment) can be experienced. Protest is manifested by such statements as "I wish you weren't going," or, "I'd like to be going with you." Feelings related to the protest stage are feelings of anxiety surrounding the actual separation and the projected time alone. The despair state can be manifested by behaviors of listlessness and lack of interest in the environment or anger behaviors. Many couples experience feelings and behaviors of anger that are unexpected and disturbing to them as they separate. Most adults move into detachment quickly, maintain the relationship in whatever way is possible, and look forward to being reunited and the resolution stage.

When living in a highly mobile society, adults and children terminate from their support systems with some frequency. Stanford's (1977) work with groups, especially cohesive groups, reported on separation anxiety as a group comes to a closure. If a person has given importance to the group, many of the behaviors identified by Stanford will be evident.

Although Stanford's work was with students, it appears that his observations can relate to individuals in the general population who are terminating with a group. Stanford's behaviors of termination anxiety are as follows.

1. *Increased conflict:* Students may start bickering with one another for no apparent reason, or at least no significant reason. It is almost as though they were trying to prove to themselves that "I don't really like these people, or else I wouldn't be fighting with them. And since I don't like them, it won't be painful for me to leave them."

2. *Breakdown of group skills:* Working together on a task, the group may suddenly exhibit what appears to be a complete lack of skills, and they may violate all the norms that were established previously. It is almost as though they were saying to themselves and the teachers, "You see, we really didn't change much this year. We're still like every other class. And since this is like every other class, it won't be so hard to leave."

3. *Lethargy:* Some students begin to show less and less interest in their work, as if to say, "What does it matter any more? If we're going to have to break up, what's the use of continuing to work?" Their lethargy may also be a symptom of depression indicating feelings of sadness about the imminent breakup of the group.

4. *Frantic attempts to work well:* Conversely, some groups may actually increase their productivity, taking on more and more projects and rushing to do everything they can before the term ends. They may display impeccable group skills, working far more effectively than ever before. Implicit in this behavior may be the message, "If we're a model class, maybe the teacher will like us so much we won't have to leave. Maybe our group can continue forever."

Thus separation anxiety can be demonstrated throughout the life span, all caused by a temporary separation from the significant other or a support system.

Loneliness

From the aged individual to the infant, from the economically privileged person to the more deprived, loneliness exists as a common adaptation problem. No one is immunized against loneliness. It is a lifelong struggle for everyone to maintain relational integrity. Even the person who has mutually satisfying relationships experiences periods of loneliness and alienation.

The person who does not attain affectional adequacy and who, for the greater part, may have no or very few satisfying relationships suffers great emotional pain. Alienation is a condition or feeling of being estranged or separated from self and others. Alienation feelings develop when significant others are not meeting what is expected as suppliers of affiliation. This deprivation of presence or contact leads to a feeling of not being needed, valued, or appreciated by others, and therein lies the root of loneliness.

Alienation is a serious problem in contemporary society. Many social theorists have written on its pervasiveness in North American life and on the contextual factors that affect this pattern. Among these are the diminishing of the family as the basic unit of society, mobility, urbanization, and computerization. Early childhood experiences of affectional adequacy or inadequacy can further contribute to interdependence adaptation. Socially, friends seem to be transient, families are physically separated, and after all, "Who does care what happens to me?" Many more persons end up living in the streets because they have no human ties that can be of help in a housing crisis. That alienation exists is undeniable. Particularly because of the contemporary situation, people in our society have a good to excellent chance of developing one of the variants of alienation. The major types of alienation were described by Seeman (1959) as powerlessness, meaninglessness, normlessness, isolation, and self-estrangement. Any of these types of alienation can cause the individual to feel further separated from others.

Some individuals can handle these alienated feelings by innovative ways of building relationships. An example of this is the young adult who appraises the situation and says that things are not good, not the way one would like to have them, but recognizes that they do not have to remain as such. The individual proceeds to become involved in changing things and building relationships.

People can use less positive means to deal with alienated feelings. These avenues involve a dependency on things or others to ward off alienated feelings. There is a pattern of using "something" to act as a bridge to relationships. These patterns include the following.

1. Dependency on a lifestyle that emphasizes withdrawal and retreatism to feel secure.

2. Dependency on performing ritualistic behaviors to deal with anxieties of alienation (chain-smoking, overeating, psychosomatic illness, or any activity that is done to excess to stay busy).
3. Rebelling against society by joining an alternate cultural group with subsequent dependency on it (drug culture, alcoholic state, sexual variancy groups, for example).
4. Dependency on situations retaining the status quo. This individual sees no possibility for change and considers turning against the world as the only way to deal with alienation.

Some of these alternatives can be so ineffective as to stimulate self-concept disruption. An example of this would be the individual who chooses to withdraw from the real world and stay in a fantasy existence. This condition is referred to as self-alienation and can involve a total collapse of the self-concept.

Substance Abuse

Substance abuse, as it relates to the individual, is a pressing concern associated with dependency behaviors and ineffective relational integrity. Contemporary society is highly drug oriented with increasing numbers of individuals becoming involved in various forms of substance abuse. The roots, dynamics, and effects of these problems are complex. However, literature in the field cites connections between these problems and what the Roy Adaptation Model calls unmet interdependence needs. The complexities of modern society in industrially developed countries has brought about high levels of stress at the same time that close relationships with others are less available to help individuals cope. The breathtaking rate of change, the erosion of family life, and the threat of internal and external hostile political forces are but a few of the factors causing stress. In these situations, the basic need for relating to others in mutual love, respect, and valuing is intensified. When this need goes unmet through a lack of meaningful significant others and support systems, the person can develop a condition known as insatiable longing.

Insatiable longing is a vague yearning or gnawing sensation that keeps a person in a constant state of anticipation, which is never fulfilled and cannot be fulfilled in an ordinary way. The individual with insatiable longing is vulnerable to addiction or being taken over by some substance or activity. People can become dependent on almost anything—morphine, phenobarbital, cocaine, marijuana, alcohol, food, or even work or hobbies (Brown & Fowler, 1969). Once people are in the condition of insatiable longing, they are also prone to frustration, anxiety, and depression. Life's experiences for these individuals easily become exhausting and unmanageable, and dependence on drugs results when more effective coping mechanisms are not available within the person's cognitive domain.

Aggression

When a person does not have an effective pattern of control over aggression, a generalized pattern of behavior develops that indicates a need to control others. The problem of aggression stems from an unmet need for balance in dependency and independency. Where an overemphasis on dependency exists, passive behavior tends to predominate; if independency is overbalanced, aggression becomes evident. In understanding aggression, it is helpful to first explore the notion of passive behavior. Koch and Haugk (1992, p. 16) describe passive behavior as "behavior that moves against the self." This includes physical passivity, personal withdrawal from the situation, or verbal passivity, the tendency to keep quiet or to withhold feedback. "Passive performers frequently give up important parts of their own personalities to avoid disapproval or criticism so others will like them" (Koch & Haugk, 1992, p. 17).

Aggressive behavior, on the other hand, moves against others. Aggressive people have few internal restraints and few external limits. The expression of aggression can be physical, nonverbal, verbal, or in a pattern labeled passive aggression and decribed as follows.

1. *Physican aggression.* Koch and Haugk (1992, p. 19) point out, "You are all too familiar with physical acts of aggression as you read the daily news reports of abused spouses, abused children, and abused older persons. You hear of murders, assaults, drive-by shootings and gang warfare. You doubtless know more than you want to know about physical aggression."

2. *Nonverbal aggression.* Aggressive patterns in interrelationships can also develop nonverbally. "Individuals move against others simply by the expression on their faces or by the gestures they use, or their tone of voice" (Koch & Haugk, 1992, p. 20). Has a decision you made while driving ever irritated another driver? Other instances of nonverbal aggression include sneers, looks of scorn, rolling the eyes, or an exasperated sigh. All of these are an effort to move against another person by trying to establish superiority over them.

3. *Verbal aggression.* Verbal aggression constitutes moving against others with words as weapons. It can take the form of insults, put-downs, profanity, blaming, or sarcasm. Each of these is an attempt to humiliate or demean another person in an attempt to manipulate or dominate an encounter.

4. *Passive aggression.* Koch and Haugk (1992, p. 22) describe passive aggression as subtle, "an underhanded way of moving against another person or manipulating others to get one's own way." Passive aggression can take the form of procrastinating, forgetting, dawdling, pouting, silent treatment, or manipulative tears. For example, the person who uses the "silent treatment" is trying to punish the other person by withholding the love and affection associated with relational integrity.

All of this is contrasted with assertive behavior in interrelationships. Assertive behavior is defined by Koch and Haugk (1992, p. 23) as "a constructive way of living and relating to other people . . . that reflects concern about being honest, direct, open, and natural in relations with others."

Pollution

The adaptation problem of pollution represents a compromised process of interdependence from a much broader perspective, that of society as a whole. It was mentioned previously that relational integrity with the environment is vital to resource adequacy, particularly as it relates to basic physiologic and safety needs. Unfortunately, in many places of the world, pollution of the environment is causing astronomical resource and health concerns.

Consider the following quotation from an international study of the Gorbachev Foundation Joint Trust Fund (1997, p. 50):

> As McCullum (1996) reported, "In addition to Chernobyl [the successor states have] . . . other environmental problems to bear. Industrial areas suffer high levels of air and water pollution with resulting health-related problems. The infrastructure, such as the public water systems, are in a state of neglect, with disasters such as the breakage of the water filtration system in Kharkiv in June 1995, which resulted in sewage flowing into the city water system and the emergence of cholera."
>
> Other concerns pertain to the purity of food, the conditions under which it is produced, shipped and marketed. There are reports that bountiful crops fail to reach consumers because the mechanisms for shipment are inefficient and primitive. In many cities, water from the tap is not drinkable and water treatment systems are unreliable and rare.
>
> Speculations have been raised regarding the relationship of air quality to the incidence of respiratory disease evident in the population. Other non-communicable diseases are attributed to industrial hazards and contamination.

This is a description of environmental problems and their health impact. This situation is not unique to Eastern Europe. Pollution has become a mammoth problem that is of concern beyond the boundaries of the countries affected. In fact, many modern industrialized countries are involved in processes to determine how best to deal with the challenge to clean up pollution.

Adaptation problems of societal proportions become issues for advanced nursing practice in collaboration with other disciplines. The American International Health Alliance (Washington, D.C.) is an example of an interdisciplinary body engaged in efforts to assist in the promotion of health and the advancement of nursing practice in Eastern Europe and the former Soviet states.

▶ PLANNING NURSING CARE

In applying the nursing process to the integrated processes of interdependence, the nurse makes a careful assessment of behaviors and stimuli. In assessing factors influencing interdependence, regulator and cognator effectiveness in initiating compensatory processes are considered. The presence of compromised processes of adaptation is also an important matter. Based on this thorough first- and second-level assessment, the nurse formulates nursing diagnoses, sets goals, selects interventions, and evaluates care.

Throughout this section on planning nursing care, the situation of Mr. and Mrs. E. is used for illustrative purposes. Although many perspectives could be taken with this case, the focus will be on the three processes associated with interdependence and the achievement of relational integrity.

Mr. and Mrs. E. are a couple in their mid-70s. They are both physically healthy and continue to live in their own residence. However, over the past 5 years, Mr. E. has demonstrated a progressive deterioration in mental capacity. His memory is failing, he has decreased judgment, and often he has difficulty making decisions. At times he is disoriented and does not recognize familiar people. Mrs. E. also describes mood swings and changes in his personality. She stated, "He was always such a loving husband. We had a very good relationship. I can't understand what gets into him!" In fact, at times he becomes aggressive. For example, when their son was attempting to help Mr. E. with his bath, he became hostile and struck him.

Mr. E. was examined by his physician over a year ago and it was suggested that he had many of the symptoms of Alzheimer's disease. At that time, Mrs. E. determined to keep her husband with her at home as long as possible. However, now she needs help. She is working with the nurse practitioner to determine what can be done to enable him to continue residing at home.

When asked about her significant others, Mrs. E. identified that in addition to her husband, she has a son and a daughter, whose families live within a half-hour drive from their home. Once a week, their daughter brings a meal and some baked goods. On Saturdays, the grandchildren take Mrs. E shopping for groceries while Mr. E.'s favorite grandson takes him for a walk. Mr. and Mrs. E. had been very involved with their church until recently, when Mr. E.'s condition worsened. Many of their friends continue to stop by for a visit, often bringing baked items or flowers.

During her career, Mrs. E. had been a nurse. She was confident in her ability to deal with her husband but is now beginning to feel that she cannot handle him all the time, particularly when he does not sleep through the night. She has concerns about how to support him, as his functional abilities continue to decrease. Mrs. E. is also voicing concerns about her husband's safety in the environment. She has to keep him locked in the house most of the time and this increases his restlessness and agitation. Mrs. E. recently asked the nurse if there was more that could be done to enhance the security of the environment to prevent potential problems.

Nursing Diagnosis

Development of nursing diagnoses associated with interdependence is accomplished in the same way as in the other modes. One method involves the statement of the behaviors together with the influencing stimuli; another method makes use of summary labels.

Nursing diagnoses can reflect either adaptive or ineffective behaviors. In the case of Mr. and Mrs. E., a sample adaptive nursing diagnosis states, "Commitment to at-home care for mentally impaired husband related to deep affection for him, confidence in own capabilities, and assistance provided by significant others and support systems."

In the case of ineffective behaviors, a multitude of nursing diagnoses may result. The interdependence mode is closely interrelated with the other modes; therefore, a disturbance in one is likely to precipitate disturbances in others. For example, for Mr. E., a diagnosis might be "Increased agitation, restlessness, and risk of mishap due to environment that does not provide the required freedom or security." The interdependent relationship between the individual and the environment is evident in this diagnosis.

Two diagnoses that focus on Mrs. E. are "Fatigue and exhaustion due to sleep disturbances of Mr. E." and "Concern about ability to cope with husband's decreasing functional abilities related to lack of knowledge about effective approaches and actions to support a mentally impaired individual."

It is also possible to construct a nursing diagnosis using a summary label that captures clusters of behaviors. This method is used by experienced nurses to communicate significant amounts of information in one phrase. As identified in Chapter 3, there are six indicators of positive interdependence adaptation identified as summary labels in the Roy Adaptation Model. They are affectional adequacy, stable pattern of giving and receiving, effective pattern of dependency and independency, effective coping strategies for separation and loneliness, developmental adequacy, and resource adequacy.

Likewise, five commonly recurring adaptation problems are identified: ineffective pattern of giving and receiving, ineffective pattern of dependency and independency, separation anxiety, loneliness, ineffective development of relationships, and inadequate resources.

A nursing diagnosis using a summary label reads, "Inadequate resources in home environment to ensure adaptive interrelationship between environment and its effect on Mr. E." Both the behavior and the stimuli stated in this example of a nursing diagnosis communicate a wealth of information to an individual experienced in adaptation problems associated with interdependence. However, for the inexperienced person, the more detailed expression of behaviors and stimuli is more meaningful.

In Table 16–3, the Roy model nursing diagnostic categories for the integrated processes of interdependence are shown in relation to nursing diagnosis labels approved by the North American Nursing Diagnosis Association (Rantz & LeMone, 1997).

Goal Setting

Each step of the nursing process focuses on the individual's or collective system's behavior, the stimuli influencing that behavior, or both. With the nursing diagnosis, the statement developed included both behaviors and stimuli.

TABLE 16–3 NURSING DIAGNOSTIC CATEGORIES FOR INTERDEPENDENCE

Positive Indicators of Adaptation	Common Adaptation Problems	NANDA Diagnostic Labels
• Affectional adequacy • Stable pattern of giving and receiving • Effective pattern of dependency and independency • Effective coping strategies for separation and loneliness • Developmental adequacy • Resource adequacy	• Ineffective pattern of giving and receiving • Ineffective pattern of dependency and independency • Separation anxiety • Loneliness • Ineffective development of relationships • Inadequate resources	• Social isolation • Impaired social interaction • Relocation stress syndrome • Altered family processes • Risk for violence: self directed or directed at others • Risk for loneliness • Ineffective individual coping • Defensive coping • Impaired adjustment • Ineffective community coping • Potential for enhanced community coping • Ineffective family coping: disabling • Ineffective family coping: compromised • Family coping: potential for growth • Altered family process: alcoholism

With the goal setting step, the focus is on behavior. Each goal identifies a behavior that is to be addressed.

Many interdependence problems have a chronic as well as an acute phase. Thus, the goal setting process includes both long- and short-term goals, each of which states the behavior of focus, the change expected, and the time frame in which the goal is to be achieved.

The following statements provide examples of possible goals for the situation described previously: "Within 1 week, Mr. E. will demonstrate fewer episodes of aggression," or, "Within 1 month, Mrs. E. and her family will express an increased sense of security and support as they care for Mr. E.," or "Following enhancement of their home environment to provide for appropriate environmental influences, Mr. and Mrs. E. will confirm through their testimony and behavior an enhanced quality of life."

In order to be effective in guiding progress, goals must be established in collaboration with the persons involved. As with each step of the nursing process, the individuals, where possible, must be active participants to ensure that accurate and relevant information is obtained, that it is interpreted appropriately into nursing diagnoses, and that achievable and relevant goals are established. This is the only way that interventions can be determined that will assist in achieving relational integrity.

After formulating goals, the nurse proceeds to the identification of nursing interventions, the next step of the nursing process as described in the Roy Adaptation Model.

Intervention

The intervention step of the nursing process according to the Roy Adaptation Model focuses on the stimuli affecting the behavior identified in the goal setting step. The intervention step is thus the management of stimuli and this involves either altering, increasing, decreasing, removing, or maintaining them.

In the previous situation involving Mr. and Mrs. E., the problem of Mr. E.'s aggressive behavior was addressed in the first goal. As Fabiano (1993) describes, aggressive outbursts in mentally impaired individuals are often circumstantial in origin. The key to controlling aggressive behavior is in discovering the underlying problem and determining what can be done to prevent its recurrence. The manner in which the person is approached is often to blame. Four factors related to approach that tend to produce agitation and subsequent aggression are interrogation, forced eye contact, intimidating posture, and restraint. Fabiano (1993) recommends that the caregiver sit at a right angle to the person so that eye contact is optional and the person does not feel trapped; communicate at eye level so as to avoid intimidation; touch the person (holding the person on their dominant side will avoid injury in the event of aggression); and use a soft level of speech. Above all, the caregiver must read the person's behavior. If the person shrugs when his or her shoulder is touched, do not persist; aggressive behavior will result. By informing caregivers of these points related to approach, much aggressive behavior can be prevented. The same analysis can be conducted for other factors that seem to be initiating the aggression.

A second goal pertained to Mrs. E.'s stress and fatigue related to Mr. E.'s sleep disturbances. In this situation, a suitable intervention may be to enroll Mr. E. in a night care program where he could go for the night to receive care and monitoring in a safe environment while Mrs. E. sleeps at home. By enhancing her support systems, Mrs. E. can continue to provide the majority of the care for Mr. E. at home and still have adequate rest.

Yet another goal identified enhancement of the home environment to provide increased security and support. Zeisel, Hyde, and Levkoff (1994) described eight parameters of environment design that promote safety, security, and quality of life for people with Alzheimer's disease: exit control, wandering paths, individual private and personal places, common space structured to accommodate a variety of activities, outdoor freedom, residential scale, autonomy support, and sensory comprehension (noise management and meaningfulness). Attention to these parameters provides for greater safety and security for both the person and the caregivers, improved quality of life for the person, less stress for the caregivers, and greater control for the person over his or her life.

Through some minor renovations to their home, many of these objectives were accomplished for Mr. and Mrs. E. Three sides of their yard were fenced. Installing a fence with a locked gate on the front of their yard allowed Mr. E. to spend time out of doors. The home was located in a quite district, so the environment was relatively free of traffic noise and other chaos. Mrs. E.

developed visual cues throughout the house to assist Mr. E. with orientation. When she understood the impact of change, she avoided moving furniture or otherwise altering the surroundings in the home.

At the suggestion of the nurse, Mrs. E. made contact with the Alzheimer's society in her area as a further support in helping her care for her husband. She found that the information and advice from others involved with the disease was of great assistance in helping her understand what further steps could be taken to enhance her husband's quality of life.

All of the above interventions focus on stimuli (approach, disturbances of sleep, environmental influences, knowledge levels) that are contributing to interdependence problems for Mr. E. or his family. The next step of the nursing process returns to focus on the behaviors evident in the situation.

Evaluation

Evaluation involves judging the effectiveness of the nursing interventions in relation to the person's or collective system's adaptive behavior, that is, whether the behaviors stated in the goals have been achieved. The nursing interventions are effective if the behavior is in accordance with the stated goal. If the goal has not been achieved, the nurse identifies alternative interventions or approaches by reassessing the behavior and stimuli and continuing with the other steps of the nursing process.

In considering the previously identified goal, "Within 1 week, Mr. E. will demonstrate fewer episodes of aggression," the intervention of informing caregivers about the factors that contribute to aggressive episodes would have been successful if their revised approach to him produces less agitation and subsequent aggression. If Mrs. E. reported that her husband was aggressive three times as opposed to 10 times within the same time period, the intervention would be judged successful.

The second goal stated, "Within 1 month, Mrs. E. and her family will express an increased sense of security and support as they care for Mr. E." The interventions related to this goal focused on some enhancements around their home. Mrs. E. reported, "Now that my husband can go outside whenever he desires, he is not as restless and agitated. He appears to have an increased level of orientation and increased awareness of others."

Another goal focused on Mrs. E.'s level of fatigue and stress. The proposed intervention involved a night care program at a nearby care center. Unfortunately, that arrangement did not work well for Mrs. E. The night program began at 8 PM and often Mr. E. was asleep before that. It was also inconvenient for Mrs. E. to get him to the program's location at that time and he could not be accommodated at an earlier hour. Thus, the problem of stress and fatigue was not resolved. In reassessment of the situation, it was decided to try a rotation of home care personnel during the night so that Mrs. E. could sleep. This is provided through their health insurance for 5 nights a week. The son and daughter will provide the coverage for the other 2 nights. This approach will be assessed after a period of implementation, perhaps in 2 weeks.

The final goal stated, "Following enhancement of their home environment to provide for appropriate environmental influences, Mr. and Mrs. E. will confirm through their testimony and behavior and enhanced quality of life." It may be possible to evaluate this goal for Mrs. E. through the use of a quality of life assessment tool. Mr. E. may demonstrate outcomes such as decreased restlessness, decreased socially inappropriate behavior, decreased use of psychotropic medication, maintenance or increase in weight, regained sense of humor, or increased awareness, for example.

It is important to recognize that the nursing process and the six steps are ongoing, simultaneous, and overlapping. Although they have been separated and dealt with in an artificially linear manner for discussion purposes, often intervention is occurring at the same time as first- and second-level assessment is proceeding. Likewise, evaluation occurs on an ongoing basis, being held in mind even when nursing diagnoses are being established and as goals are being formulated.

▶ SUMMARY

This chapter has focused on the application of the Roy Adaptation Model to the interdependence mode. An overview of the three processes, affectional adequacy, developmental adequacy, and resource adequacy, associated with relational integrity was provided along with the identification of parameters for assessment of behaviors and stimuli. Illustration of compensatory responses related to interdependence were described and examples of five compromised processes (sensation anxiety, loneliness, substance abuse, aggression, and pollution) were provided. Finally, guidelines for planning nursing care through the formulation of nursing diagnoses, goals, and interventions were explored and evaluation of nursing care was described.

▶ EXERCISES FOR APPLICATION

1. In relation to an organization that you are familiar with, identify the external factors (context) that influence the function and roles of the organization.

2. What is the mission and vision (context) associated with your educational institution?

3. Think of an interrelationship situation that was ineffective. Which of the principles of effective relationship would have helped to improve the situation?

► ASSESSMENT OF UNDERSTANDING

Questions

1. The basic need of the interdependence mode is _____ _____ which is viewed as consisting of _____, _____, and _____ adequacy.

2. Classify the following behaviors as being related to affectional adequacy (A), developmental adequacy (D), or resource adequacy (R).
    (a) _____ giving and receiving behaviors
    (b) _____ physiologic–physical integrity
    (c) _____ significant others and support systems
    (d) _____ developmental stage
    (e) _____ dependency and independency

3. List stimuli associated with each of the aspects of relational integrity.
    (a) affectional adequacy

    _____

    _____

    _____

    (b) developmental adequacy

    _____

    _____

    _____

    (c) resource adequacy

    _____

    _____

4. Which of the following could be considered compensatory processes related to interdependence?
    (a) volunteer work in a hospital
    (b) joining a bridge club
    (c) obtaining food from a food bank
    (d) applying for social assistance
    (e) a lay caregiving ministry at a local church

5. Name three compromised processes of interdependence.
    (a) _____
    (b) _____
    (c) _____

Situation:

A child in second grade, upon transferring to a new school, breaks into tears after being left in her new classroom by her mother.

6. Formulate a nursing diagnosis for the above situation using two methods.
   (a) _____

   (b) _____

7. Construct a goal for the child described in the above situation.
   _____

8. Since interventions are focused on stimuli, what interventions could be used to alleviate the situation described above, considering the following stimuli:
   (a) departure of the mother
   (b) classroom of unknown children
   (c) strange teacher

9. How would you evaluate achievement of the goal you established in item 7?
   _____

Feedback

1. relational integrity, affectional, developmental, resource

2. (a) A, (b) R, (c) A, (d) D, (e) D

3. (a) Any three of: expectations, nurturing ability, level of self-esteem, communication skills, presence, context, infrastructure, people.
   (b) Any three of: developmental stage, significant changes, integrity of self-concept, knowledge about relationships.
   (c) monetary resources, assisting relationships.

4. All of the items could be considered compensatory processes related to interdependence.

5. Any three of the following: separation anxiety, loneliness, substance abuse, aggression, pollution.

6. Examples of nursing diagnoses:
   (a) Crying related to strange environment and departure of significant other.
   (b) Separation anxiety related to being left by mother in a strange setting and absence of support system in new class.

7. Examples of goals:
   (a) Within 15 minutes, the child will have settled and will be calm in classroom environment.
   (b) During lunch hour, the child will make friends with two girls from her class.

8. Examples of interventions related to the stimuli identified could include:
   (a) Departure of the mother: Invite the mother to accompany the child into the classroom for a time (perhaps 15 minutes) to establish familiarity and comfort.
   (b) Classroom of unknown children: Assign another student who will act as a buddy for the child for the first week.
   (c) Strange teacher: Introduce the child to the teacher on another occasion, preferably before the actual classroom encounter. [This is an anticipatory goal. It would not work in a situation such as that described but it might help avoid a similar situation in the future.]

9. The goals would have been achieved if the following behaviors were evident.
   (a) Within 15 minutes, the child was composed and the crying had ceased.
   (b) After the lunch break, the child reported meeting two new children.

▶ REFERENCES

Ainsworth, M. D. (1964). Patterns of attachment shown by the infant in interaction with his mother. *Merrill Palmer Quarterly, 10(1),* 51–58.

Andrews, H. A., Cook, L. M., Davidson, J. M., Schurman, D. P., Taylor, E. W., & Wensel, R. H. (Eds.). (1994). *Organizational transformation in health care: A work in progress.* San Francisco: Jossey-Bass.

Benner, P. (1984). *From novice to expert: Excellence and power in clinical nursing practice.* Menlo Park, CA: Addison-Wesley.

Berkman, B. (1978). Mental health and the aging: A review of the literature for clinical social workers. *Clinical Social Work Journal, 6,* 230–245.

Bowlby, J. (1969). *Attachment and loss: Attachment* (Vol. 1). New York: Basic Books.

Bowlby, J. (1973). *Attachment and loss: Separation: Anxiety and anger* (Vol. 2). New York: Basic Books.

Brown, M. M., & Fowler, G. R. (1969). *Psychodynamic nursing: A biosocial orientation.* Philadelphia: Saunders.

Caplan, G. (Ed.). (1974). *Support systems and community mental health.* New York: Behavioral Publications.

Cobb, S. (1976). Social support as a moderator of life stress. *Psychosomatic Medicine, 38,* 300–312.

Cohen, S. S. L. (1985). *Social support and health.* New York: Academic Press.

Creative Nursing Management. (1992). *Leaders empower staff.* Minneapolis, MN: Creative Nursing Management.

Dimond, M., & Jones, S. L. (1983). Social support: A review and theoretical integration. In Chinn, P. L. (Ed.), *Advances in nursing theory development* (pp. 235–249). Rockville, MD: Aspen.

Dunning, J. (1976). Development of interdependence. In Roy, Sr. C. (Ed.), *Introduction to nursing: An adaptation model* (pp. 303–312). Englewood Cliffs, NJ: Prentice Hall.

Ellison, E. (1976). Problem of interdependence: Aggression. In Roy, Sr. C. (Ed.), *Introduction to nursing: An adaptation model* (pp. 330–341). Englewood Cliffs, NJ: Prentice Hall.

Erikson, E. H. (1963). *Childhood and society* (2nd ed.), New York: Norton.

Ezor, P. R. (1980). *Student teacher: Separation anxiety.* Unpublished manuscript. Mount St. Mary's College, Los Angeles.

Fabiano, L. (1993). Dealing with aggression. *Caring for the Alzheimer's victim* (Video series). Seagrave, Ontario, Canada: FCS Media Production.

Fromm, E. (1956). *The art of loving.* New York: Harper & Row.

Gottlieb, B. H. (Ed.). (1981). *Social networks and social support.* Beverly Hills, CA: Sage.

Greenblatt, M., Beccera, R., & Serafetinides, E. A. (1982). Social networks and mental health: An overview. *American Journal of Psychiatry, 8,* 977–984.

Havighurst, R. J. (1953). *Human development and education.* New York: Longman.

House, J., Landis, K., & Umberson, D. (1988). Social relationship and health. *Science, 241,* 540–545.

Grant MacEwan Community College, Siberian Branch of the Russian Medical Academy of Medical Science, Siberian Business Development Corporation, & The University of Calgary—Gorbachev Foundation Joint Trust Fund. (1997). *Reform of the Novosibirsk Health Care System.* Edmonton, Alberta: Grant MacEwan Community College.

Kane, C. R. (1988). Family social support: Toward a conceptual model. *Advances in Nursing Science, 10(2),* 188–225.

Klaus, M. H., & Kennel, J. H. (1981). *Parent–infant bonding* (2nd ed.). St. Louis: Mosby.

Koch, R. N., & Haugk, K. C. (1992). *Speaking the truth in love.* St. Louis: Stephen Ministries.

Mahler, M. S. (1979). *The selected papers of Margaret Mahler: Separation–individuation* (Vol. 2). New York: Jason Aronson.

Maslow, A. H. (1954). *Motivation and personality.* New York: Harper & Row.

McCullum, R. (1996). Vision of a new health system for Ukraine. *Canada–Ukraine Monitor, 4(1),* 24.

McGinnis, L. (1980). *The friendship factor: How to get close to the people you care for.* Minneapolis, MN: Augsburg Publishing.

Mead, M. (1971). *Coming of age in Samoa.* New York: Morrow.

Randell, B., Tedrow, M., & Van Landingham, J. (1982). *Adaptation nursing: The Roy conceptual model applied.* St. Louis: Mosby.

Rantz, M. J., & LeMone, P. (1997). *Classifications of nursing diagnoses: Proceedings of the twelfth conference NANDA.* Glendale, CA: CINAHL Information Systems.

Robertson, H. (1953). Some responses of young children to loss of maternal care. *Nursing Times, 49.*

Roy, Sr. C. (1981). A systems model of nursing care and its effect on quality of human life. In Lakser, G. E. (Ed.), *Applied systems and cybernetics* (Vol. IV, pp. 1705–1714). New York: Pergamon Press.

Roy, Sr. C., & Roberts, S. L. (1981). Interdependence. In Roy, Sr. C. & Roberts, S. L. (Eds.), *Theory construction in nursing: An adaptation model* (pp. 272–282). Englewood Cliffs, NJ: Prentice Hall.

Seeman, M. (1959). On the meaning of alienation. *American Sociological Review, 24(6),* 783–791.

Selman, J. C., & Andrews, H. A. (1994). Effective relationships: Rethinking the fundamentals. In Andrews, H. A., Cook, L. M., Davidson, J. M., Schurman, D. P., Taylor, E. W., & Wensel, R. H. (Eds.), *Organizational transformation in health care: A work in progress* (pp. 53–69). San Francisco: Jossey-Bass.

Selman, R. C. (1980). *The growth of interpersonal understanding: Development and clinical analyses.* New York: Academic Press.

Smith, K. K., & Berg, D. N. (1990). *Paradoxes of group life: Understanding conflict, paralysis, and movement in group dynamics.* San Francisco: Jossey Bass.

Spitz, R. A. (1945). Hospitalism: An inquiry into the genesis of psychiatric conditions in early childhood. In Fenechel, O., Greenacre, P., Hartmann, H., Jackson, E. B., Kris, E., Kubie, L. S., Lewin, B. D., Putnam, M. C., & Spitz, R. A. (Eds.), *The psychoanalytic study of the child* (pp. 53–74). New York: International Universities Press.

Stanford, G. (1977). *Developing effective classroom groups.* New York: Hart.

Tuckman, B. W., & Jenson, M. A. (1977). Stages of small group revisited. *Group and Organization Studies, 2(4),* 419–427.

Zeisel, J., Hyde, J., & Levkoff, S. (1994). Best practices: An environment–behavior (E–B) model for Alzheimer special care units. *The American Journal of Alzheimer's Care and Related Disorders & Research,* March/April, 4–21.

▶ **ADDITIONAL REFERENCES**

Hall, G. R. (1991). This hospital patient has Alzheimer's. *American Journal of Nursing,* October, 45–50.

Perkins, B. (1992). Alzheimer's disease: Ten ways to cope. *Dialog,* Spring/Summer, 41–43.

Tueth, M. J. (1995). How to manage depression and psychosis in Alzheimer's disease. *Geriatrics, 50(1),* 43–49.

III PART

THE ROY ADAPTATION MODEL IN PRACTICE AND RESEARCH

The Roy Adaptation Model has been described throughout this text as a systematic framework for nursing activities. It guides the activities of the nursing process, which includes two levels of assessment (behaviors and stimuli), nursing diagnosis, goal setting, intervention, and evaluation. Furthermore, the model serves as a basis for knowledge development. Part III focuses on the application of the model in these two important areas: practice and research.

As health care is experiencing unprecedented change and ever-increasing complexity, expectations for high-quality, effective, and coordinated care and services are evident in both consumer and provider groups. In response to this challenge, Connerley, Ristau, Lindberg, and McFarland point out in Chapter 17: "Model implementation offers the opportunity for designing a structured, organized approach to patient care delivery, with the potential for increased efficiency and effectiveness." Since the Roy Adaptation Model provides a structure for thinking about patient care and for organizing nursing work focused on comprehensive and holistic care, enhanced outcomes associated with care delivery are possible. Chapter 17 describes the process and outcomes of implementing the Roy Adaptation Model as a basis for nursing practice as experienced at St. Joseph Regional Medical Center in Lewiston, Idaho.

In Chapter 18, Dr. Roy reviews how the Roy Adaptation Model contributes to nursing as a scholarly practice discipline by guiding research in the two aspects of nursing knowledge development: basic science and clinical science. Following a brief exploration of strategies for knowledge development, examples are provided of research by Dr. Roy and numerous other investigators who based their research on the Roy Adaptation Model. The latter work is summarized in a model-based synthesis project of 163 studies published from 1970 to 1994 (Roy, Sr. C., Pollock, S., Massey, V., Lauchner, K., Velsco-Whetsell, M., Frederickson, K., Barone, S., & Carson, M. [1998]. *The Roy Adaptation Model-based research: Twenty-five years of contributions to nursing science.* Indianapolis, IN: Sigma Theta Tau International).

17

THE ROY MODEL IN NURSING PRACTICE

Health care systems continue to experience increased complexity in organization, purpose, and services during this era of rapid change. Consumer and provider expectations regarding health care are rooted in the desire for high-quality, caring, effective, and coordinated services. Nursing as a profession has a historic commitment to the value of providing care through a holistic perspective. Through the use of the Roy model, health care facilities can realize clarity in provider roles and can strengthen interdisciplinary collaboration and effectiveness in the organization and delivery of health care. The use of this model assists in organizing the components of a complex health care system while centering service on each individual as a whole person.

This chapter describes the process and outcomes of implementing the Roy Adaptation Model as a basis for nursing practice throughout St. Joseph Regional Medical Center (SJRMC) in Lewiston, Idaho. SJRMC, a 145-bed Catholic-sponsored hospital, and a member of Carondelet Health Systems, is a full-service health care facility located in a rural environment. Services include traditional inpatient programs and diagnostic services, as well as trauma, oncology, home care, mental health, and subacute services. The hospital uses a participatory leadership and management style and embraces the leadership precepts of collaboration, *subsidarity*, accountability, and commitment to continuous improvement.

The process of implementation of a model is a major undertaking requiring commitment and perseverance. To achieve full internalization required a period of several years. In this chapter, an exploration of the integrated processes of nursing models in practice is provided with particular emphasis on the theory underlying the decision to implement a model and the content and process associated with the change. Then, the Roy Adaptation Model nursing process itself is used as a framework to describe the process experienced at SJRMC as the model was implemented as the basis for practice.

▶ OBJECTIVES

After studying this chapter, the reader will be able to do the following:

1. Describe the potential benefits of model-based nursing practice.

2. Identify conditions and strategies that support the transition to model-based practice.

3. Name the aspects of nursing practice that are influenced by the implementation of model-based practice.

4. Use systems theory to provide examples of the inputs, throughputs, and outputs of the transition to model-based practice.

5. Identify suggested criteria for model selection.

6. Name the critical components of the implementation process as described in this chapter.

7. Select sources for evaluative information about the outcomes of model-based practice.

▶ KEY CONCEPTS DEFINED

Creative goals: Goal statements which individualize how each respective unit will meet the expressive goals. Creative goals are similar to the concept of equifinality in general systems theory. In the implementation project, this allowed adaptation of the model to each unique area of nursing practice (Carper, 1978; Chinn & Jacobs, 1987).

Expressive goals: Goal statements which articulate the purpose of a given project. In the implementation project described in this chapter, expressive goals addressed the outcome of hospital-wide implementation of the Roy Adaptation Model (Carper, 1978; Chinn & Jacobs, 1987).

Model-based nursing practice: Use of a nursing model as a systematic approach to guide practice, education, and research.

Planned change: Strategic actions toward desired objectives.

Subsidiarity: Calls for vesting decision making, authority, and responsibility as close as possible to the point where the impact of the decision will be felt and at the point where individuals are most competent to make the decision.

Vision: A new view of the future.

► NURSING MODELS IN PRACTICE

Nursing models are descriptive representations of nursing practice. They provide a guide for nurses as they assist people, through the use of the nursing process, to adapt effectively to life's challenges. A model provides nurses with direction for gathering information, assessing and interpreting behaviors and the factors influencing them, and then designing interventions to achieve goals aimed at effective adaptation. By defining and describing the universal elements of nursing, a model provides nursing with a structure to guide practice, research, and education.

Model-based nursing practice results in a systematic approach to organizing knowledge, so that the art and science of nursing is orderly, logical, communicable, and prescriptive. Use of models is now extending beyond research and academic settings to clinical practice sites. The clinical application of a model improves nursing practice by the integration of theory into the everyday processes of patient care and nursing administration (Allison, McLaughlin, & Walker, 1991; Rogers et al., 1991; Weiss, Hastings, Holly, & Craig, 1994). Model implementation offers the opportunity for designing a structured, organized approach to patient care delivery, with the potential for increased efficiency and effectiveness. A nursing model also assists in defining nursing roles and goals, identifying essential elements for patient databases, prescribing assessment parameters, directing nursing interventions, and providing the means for effective communication in and about nursing practice (Mayberry, 1991).

Nurses have found that model-based practice benefits both nurses and patients (Mastal, Hammond, & Roberts, 1982). According to Weiss et al. (1994), a model provides a structure for thinking about patient care and direction for organizing nursing work focused on comprehensive and holistic care for patients and families. The experience of Rogers et al. (1991) revealed that, although the model implementation process is complex and extensive, many beneficial outcomes are achieved, primarily the harmonious expression in practice of nursing values, beliefs, and assumptions related to human beings, health, environment, and nursing.

► MODEL IMPLEMENTATION: THEORY AND PROCESS

Successful model implementation requires the presence of multiple positive conditions and the use of a variety of strategies and processes to support change. Paramount among these is support and recognition of the value of defining the role of nursing in the organization. Other factors include recognition of value, education, model selection, commitment and support, vision, the change process, environmental factors, and systems approach.

Recognition of Value

An environment of trust must be pervasively present for nurses and other caregivers to make major changes in role interpretation, expression, and approach to practice. Traditional patterns of role enactment are reconstructed in the transformation to a model-based practice. The understanding and valuing of a model for practice is often present in nurses who have had exposure to advanced practice concepts; however, many nurses have a limited understanding of the utility of a model beyond the academic setting. A perception may be that models are disruptive, unnecessary, time-consuming, or useless. This can contribute to negativism when a nursing model is introduced. As Grahame (1987) observed, responses can include blocking implementation of the model, returning to practice as usual, or making humorous remarks about the model.

Education

A variety of educational activities prior to the formal implementation effort is vital to ensure that nurses have opportunities to gain knowledge and form positive attitudes about models and the benefits of model application in practice. Such educational efforts require careful timing and communication of all activities to support successful implementation.

Model Selection

Selection of the appropriate model is essential. There must be consideration of model suitability in terms of involved areas of service and potential applications. Far more important is ensuring that the model is congruent with the mission, philosophy, values, and culture of the organization. Acceptability of the concepts and terminology by nurses and other providers should be considered, as well, in order to avoid jargon that may have little meaning to nurses or other health care disciplines.

Commitment and Support

Mayberry (1991) suggested that success or failure of implementation can be linked to the commitment and support given to the full range of implementation activities and to the clarity and sincerity of communication about the chosen model. With rapid change occurring in health care, the firm belief that a model will serve as a stabilizing environmental force must be present. As this belief is shared by management and a core of care providers, the leaders of the model implementation project will be able to generate enthusiasm, participative energy, and support in the applied use of the model. Early demonstration that the model is an asset in designing and organizing approaches to the delivery of patient care is necessary to maintain the commitment for practice transformation.

Vision

Transformation frequently occurs because of vision and visionary leadership. McFarland (1993) described *vision* as the opportunity to turn the kaleidoscope of the past and the present to a new view of the future. This new view helps to develop and clarify the goals and specify the means for accomplishing organizational objectives (Robbins & Duncan, 1987).

The vision of the formal leader is essential for achievement of any planned change, including successful model implementation. Visionary leadership helps to actualize the vision by allowing the vision to drive the agenda of change including the allocation of resources (McFarland, 1993). Kouzes and Posner (1993) pointed, as well, to the importance of credibility and acceptance of the leadership—when present, they stimulate others to give more of their time, talent, and support.

The nursing management team of SJRMC shared a vision that model-based practice would positively influence the delivery of nursing care. This vision of high-quality care, provided from a common knowledge base, served as a beacon for implementation of the Roy model.

Planned Change

Application of change theory augments the process of vision attainment. In a world buffeted by change and faced daily by new threats to safety, Gardner (1993) believes that the only way to conserve is by innovation. Innovation itself requires change. Thus, successful implementation of a nursing model must occur in a context of planned change.

Planned change involves strategic actions toward desired objectives. As Tappen (1995) pointed out, formal leadership is instrumental in providing guidance to influence the direction of change. Planned change contrasts sharply with the unconsciousness of unplanned change which occurs to maintain homeostasis. Many theories and models of planned change exist. Nurses and nurse leaders should evaluate models of change and select an approach to support achievement of the desired objectives.

Involvement

The degree of individual and institutional change that is required with system-wide model implementation cannot be underestimated. Change occurs on several levels, personal, professional, and organizational. As early as possible in a planned change process, those affected by the change need to be involved in planning (Marquis & Huston, 1996).

Understanding and predicting people's responses to change of this magnitude is prerequisite to success. Open-mindedness and sensitivity to the responses and adaptations of individuals and groups is essential for the internal changes necessary for model implementation.

Environmental Factors

Organizations serve as the center for the delivery of health care. Three premises about organizations and change are: they exist in an environment that is constantly changing organizations should change systematically; and they must have formalized mechanisms by which environmental forces can be interpreted and new priorities determined. If this does not exist, the organization cannot change or adapt effectively and may cease to exist. If these formalized mechanisms are well established, innovation and effective adaptation can be occurring continuously (Veninga, 1982). This contributes to long-term stability.

At SJRMC, nursing leadership views the Roy Adaptation Model as a mechanism through which external change can be managed. The model serves as the framework for the development of policies and procedures regarding practice and practitioners, all of which are constantly adapted to respond the external requirements. Successful implementation and ongoing application of a model results in increased stability and an orderly methodology for adaptation to a rapidly changing environment.

Systems Perspective

As general systems theory contributes to the basis for the Roy Adaptation Model (Roy & Andrews, 1991), so did it influence model-based practice implementation at SJRMC. Important characteristics of systems theory include inputs, throughputs, outputs, feedback, and the principle that the whole is greater than the sum of the parts. As von Bertalanfy noted, phenomena of organized complexity must be explained with regard to the whole—"in regard to the entire set of relations between the components" (Braziller, 1972, p. 5).

The model implementation project was continuously influenced by systems theory and its application to the change process. System inputs, throughputs, outputs, and feedback were identified and utilized as the basis of change activities. Input included identified goals, information, and opinions obtained from nurses and other members of the health care team; regulatory issues; and required resources. Throughput included a participatory approach, formation of an implementation committee, role clarification, and educational activities. Output included changes in procedures, documentation tools, a model-based clinical ladder, and, most importantly, an essential change in the thought process of nurses providing care. Feedback was obtained throughout the process and was used to make adjustments as implementation progressed.

The model implementation process at SJRMC illustrates the application of systems theory to promote planned change. The changes associated with model implementation occurred throughout the medical center. As expected with systems theory, the process was dynamic and the outcome of the whole was greater than the sum of the parts.

▶ DESCRIPTION OF THE PROJECT

Earlier discussion in this text explored the application of the Roy Adaptation Model in situations of collective human systems. The framework for the following description of the model implementation process at SJRMC is Roy's six-step nursing process, providing an illustration of application of the model to collective systems. Following brief explanation of the background relating to model implementation, first- and second-level assessment of nursing at

SJRHC is provided, diagnoses are illustrated, goals and interventions are addressed, and evaluation is explored.

Background

The decision to implement a nursing practice model at SJRMC was initially made in 1989. Although there was not a great deal of support in the literature for model-based practice, description of comprehensive application of one model in practice was beginning to occur. The nursing management and leadership team at SJRMC shared a vision that collaboration, professional respect, adaptation to change, and continuity would be enhanced through implementation of a practice model used by all nurses.

Preliminary activities were initiated to prepare for implementation. Through a participative approach, a formal philosophy of nursing was developed. The philosophy contained mutually owned beliefs about nursing present in the culture.

A participatory approach was also utilized in selection of the model. Since the nurse manager and leadership team at SJRMC had varied educational backgrounds and levels of preparation, a review of theories and models was initiated to acquire a common knowledge level. The criteria for model selection were determined, and then the Roy Adaptation Model was identified as meeting the criteria. The selection criteria included the following.

- Congruence with medical center and nursing department mission and philosophy.
- Understandable process and orientation of the model, complementary to that of other health care disciplines.
- Applicability across the health care continuum.
- Consistency with regulatory requirements associated with nursing or patient assessment and care processes.
- Enough flexibility to provide a framework for practice, management and leadership, and educational roles within the medical center.

Assessment of Behavior and Stimuli

Initially, the need to bring about a change in the expression of nursing practice was recognized internally within the Medical Center. It was apparent that, to fully actualize the change, external expertise would be required. Consultation with a faculty member at the Lewis-Clark State College Division of Nursing was obtained for the initial stages of model implementation. This individual had a special interest and expertise in nursing theory and its application.

The Roy Adaptation Model itself was used as the framework for assessing the behavior and stimuli within the environment. The assessment revealed a variety of internal system forces and external events that served as catalysts and reinforcers for model implementation.

Behaviors included the following.

- Motivated, bright nursing staff, many of whom were returning to school for baccalaureate or advanced nursing degrees.
- Use of multiple assessment tools and forms.
- Lack of standardization in communication.
- Eclectic interpretation of the role of the nurse.
- Lack of formal expression of nursing practice.

Other specific behaviors that pointed to the need for model-based practice are contained in Table 17–1 in the column labeled "challenges."

Stimuli were assessed as the following.

- Recognition of the need to standardize, organize, and unify the expression of nursing practice.
- A goal to prepare nurses to fulfill their role as coordinators of patient care.
- A need to appropriately interpret and measure the effectiveness of nursing roles.
- The need to clarify the role of the nurse for other members of the interdisciplinary health care team.
- The need to demonstrate the value of nurses' knowledge base and their contribution to health care, internally and externally.
- A need to create an environment where the requirements of the Idaho Nurse Practice Act could be achieved through a holistic expression of nursing practice.
- A need to operationalize the philosophy of nursing and the Center's belief in holistic caring.
- Requirements of the Joint Commission on the Accreditation of Healthcare Organizations for a written definition of nursing care.
- Existing internal conditions associated with practice, documentation, and professionalism.
- The shared vision of the nursing management and leadership that model-based practice would strengthen the nursing profession.

Diagnosis

The diagnosis step of the Roy model nursing process calls for an interpretive statement associating the observed behaviors with their most relevant influencing stimuli. For example, one nursing diagnosis relating to the roles of the nurse is, "eclectic interpretation of the role of the nurse related to a lack of standardization, organization, and unity in the expression of nursing practice." A diagnosis that is related to goal 4 in Table 17–1 can be stated, "proliferation of unique forms and documentation systems contributing to replication of work due to lack of a standardized system of documentation."

Careful analysis and interpretation of assessment data led to the goals identified in column one of Table 17–1. An analysis of the behaviors and stimuli reinforced the decision to implement the model and created forward momentum.

TABLE 17-1 EXPRESSIVE GOALS

Expressive Goal	Challenges	Interventions	Outcome
1. Fulfill role expectations of nurses as coordinators of patient care.	Lack of awareness of interdependence of all disciplines Care "schedule" driven	Education Outcome-oriented approach to planning care	Improved efficiency and coordination of care Increased patient satisfaction Improved communication of goals and outcomes
2. Utilize knowledge base to support adaptive behaviors of patients and nurses.	Incomplete application of knowledge base Belief in curing vs healing Knowledge deficit related to nursing diagnosis Inadequate understanding of concept of progress toward a goal	Applied concept of adaptive behavior to patients and nurses Education and monitoring to promote understanding and use of nursing diagnosis with progress assessed and documented	Integration of model-based system which included assessment of adaptation for patients and staff Developed standards of care and outcomes for nursing diagnosis Regular assessment of progress toward goal and outcome
3. Increase understanding of the role and contribution of nursing.	Misunderstanding and confusion regarding the role of the professional nurse	Development of standardized nursing position description, with specialty interpretations Development of clinical ladder Involvement of other disciplines in discussion regarding nursing and in development of documentation system	Improved role clarity Increased understanding of interdisciplinary nature of patient care Increased appreciation of nursing contribution to care
4. Demonstrate use of nursing process and model in documentation form and tools.	Nursing process interpreted as linear phenomenon Nursing process not always utilized or reflected in documentation	Development of "cycle" representation of nursing Intensive education on nursing process Integration of process concept in all aspects of clinical and management roles Nursing process demonstrated in documentation system	Excellent understanding and utilization of nursing process Developed admission forms, patient care flow sheets, and patient teaching guides, consistent with model and nursing process Improvements in accuracy and efficiency of documentation of nursing care Improved outcomes of care
5. Achieve consistency in practice across the continuum and through the facility by formally redefining evaluating effectiveness of nursing roles.	Specialty-based definition and interpretation of nursing roles Lack of consistency in the demonstration of nursing care	Education Consistent application of a framework across the facility	Clinical ladder based on common framework, yet expresses unique aspects of clinical specialties Standardized role expectations and evaluations across the facility

Goals

Outcome statements were developed to address the ineffective behaviors and their influencing factors, and to predict outcomes of implementation. These were formulated as expressive and creative goals. *Expressive goals* are those that articulate the purpose of a given project. The use of the term "expressive" in this context differs from its use related to roles in Chapter 15. In the implementation project described, expressive goals addressed the outcome of hospital-wide implementation of the Roy Adaptation Model (Carper, 1978; Chinn & Jacobs, 1987). These address such factors as the role of nurses, the application of their knowledge base, the perception of nursing by other disciplines, documentation, and consistency of nursing practice. Expressive goals are numbered 1 to 5 in Table 17–1.

An example of an expressive goal is goal 2: Utilizing the knowledge base to support adaptive behaviors of patients and nurses, for example, is illustrated by nurses' ongoing understanding of the value of a care delivery system guided by a defined process. Daily, nurses assess patients' progress toward expected outcomes and continue or change plans for care based on the patients' progress or lack of progress. In one instance, a registered nurse was overheard explaining the role of a registered nurse to a student. She guided the student through assessment and evaluation of patient progress. The nurse articulated the accountability registered nurses have in assuring individualized holistic patient care. It is apparent by these types of day-to-day observations that the application of the model has provided a framework while simultaneously empowering nurses to express compassionate and holistic nursing care.

Creative goals are those that individualize how each respective unit will meet the expressive goals. Creative goals are similar to the concept of equifinality in general systems theory. In the implementation project, creative goals allowed adaptation of the model to each unique area of nursing practice (Carper, 1978; Chinn & Jacobs, 1987). For example, the first creative goal states, "Improve communication between nursing and other health care disciplines." Creative goals are numbered 1 to 4 in Table 17–2.

A particular illustration of accomplishing goal 3 was noted in a community symposium held following implementation of the model with Sr. Callista Roy as a guest and participant. Nurses throughout SJRMC and students of local nursing programs had the opportunity to showcase their interpretations and operationalization of the Roy model in practice. Model-based projects included a prenatal education program, clinical practice nurses' position descriptions and clinical ladder, integrated documentation system, and a framework for a nurse practice fair.

Intervention

The intervention step was actually the process of model implementation. Planning for implementation was initiated with the development of a small leadership team with representation from administration, middle management, and education. The team was committed to a dynamic planning

TABLE 17–2 CREATIVE GOALS

Creative Goal	Challenges	Interventions	Outcome
1. Improve communication between nursing and other health care disciplines.	Lack of a common language No formal screening criteria for interdisciplinary referrals Knowledge deficit related to nursing diagnosis Eclectic, specialty-based approach to nursing process and documentation	Education on nursing diagnosis Formal referral criteria developed and integrated into assessment form Interdisciplinary input into model-based assessment tools Standardize definition on nursing process based on model Interdisciplinary documentation forms	Developed a referral system based on screening criteria Improved coordination of care Timely and appropriate interdisciplinary referrals Improved understanding of nursing role Enhanced knowledge and application of nursing diagnosis
2. Operationalize philosophy and fulfillment of beliefs regarding care of whole person.	Lack of meaningful psychological cue for in-depth assessment Interview skills undeveloped Predominant competence in assessment limited to physiologic mode	Role-play interview techniques Development of assessment tool Required individual assessment of personal self-concept Focused study on each mode integrated into professional practice fair	Nursing care based on holistic approach Enhanced appreciation of need for holisic approach by other disciplines Increased understanding of impact of self-concept, role function, and interdependence on healing
3. Achieve higher level of pride in the profession of nursing.	Predominant medical model Lack of understanding of professional nursing independent and interdependent roles	All activities including education, committee involvement, awards, recognition, and role modeling focused on valuing of nursing Teleconference with Sr. Callista Roy Symposium, with Sr. Roy, to showcase achievements	Improved understanding and enhanced valuing of nursing's contribution to patient care Nurses more confident and competent in patient advocacy
4. Minimize redundancy in facets of documentation and describing nursing care.	No standardization of assessment and documentation Repetitive documentation Nursing specialties developed unique forms and systems, contributing to replication of work	Education Standardized framework for documentation system Carefully constructed documentation system that builds on database vs repeat database	Increased trust among nursing professionals Standardized documentation framework Improved continuity of care and documentation Increased patient satisfaction

process, recognizing that flexibility and creativity were essential. It was impossible at this stage to create an accurate blueprint for implementation, or to even accurately predict time frames, because learning needed to occur at every point. Critical components for successful implementation were identified and included management development, education, critical mass, early application, as well as other factors.

Management Development

Manager support and commitment were considered crucial to successful implementation. Thus, actions were initiated that focused on the development of knowledge, expertise, and commitment of managers. Strategies that were implemented to maintain commitment were primarily oriented toward education, communication, and clearly stated expectations. Promoting a high degree of confidence regarding model application was achieved by initial formal education programs, ongoing informal information exchange, and initiation of a biweekly process meeting, which provided opportunities to share success stories and address obstacles. A stated objective was, "to create a learning environment for managers that would enable them to be viewed as knowledgeable resources for personnel during change phases." Accountability for learning and achieving a successful implementation was integrated into performance expectations.

Education

Initial mandatory education programs were provided for all staff to introduce the model and its application in clinical practice. Throughout the project, knowledge deficits were identified and addressed. Education was provided about key concepts of the model, nursing diagnosis, interview skills, and effective approaches for patient education. Multiple methods for learning about the nursing model were made available to the staff. A study to evaluate internalization and factors that promote or impede internalization was completed approximately 18 months following the introduction of a model-based assessment tool (Lindberg, 1993). Findings indicated that nurses with extensive experience in a hospital-based practice have more difficulty in acquiring expertise in assessment, diagnosis, and intervention in the self-concept and role function modes. These same nurses quickly internalize and utilize the physiologic and interdependence modes. New graduates and nurses with less than 3 years of experience acquire confidence and competence quickly and equally in all four modes. This study suggested that nurses may adapt to the predominant medical model of most hospital settings.

Of particular interest in this study was the evaluation of how learning occurred. Table 17–3 lists the characteristics of the sample and the percentage who benefited from each learning strategy. The greatest learning took

TABLE 17–3   INTERNALIZATION OF LEARNING OF ROY ADAPTATION MODEL FOR NURSING PRACTICE

Sample Characteristics

Education Level		Years of Experience	
LPN	15%	Mean	11.37
RN	83.2%	Median	10
Aides	1.9%		

How Learning Occurred

	Yes	No
Read book	24%	76%
Read journal articles	59.6%	40.4%
Ask other nurses	90.4%	9.6%
Discuss with peers	94.9%	5.1%

place when interpretation and application of the model were discussed with peers and members of the core implementation group (94.9 percent). In addition, "asking other nurses" occurred frequently, that is, with 90.4 percent of the sample. These findings have implications for planning and education when considering or initiating model implementation.

Critical Mass

It was recognized that a critical mass of "true believers" was essential to bring about the transformation of nursing practice. Therefore, a 30-member core group was established, comprised of representatives from all areas where nursing is practiced. The members of the core group were the energizers of the project and acted as departmental resources for interpretation and implementation of the model. Activities to support the core group included learning activities, providing reading materials, and a teleconference with Sr. Callista Roy. College credit was available for individuals who participated in the core group and contributed to the education of their colleagues. Members of the core group were responsible for establishing communication books, providing updates on progress and change during departmental meetings, and obtaining feedback regarding changes to the documentation system. This process ensured the establishment of mechanisms to assure a high degree of participation, motivation, commitment, and communication between the implementation team and all levels of users.

Early Clinical Application

Newly learned information must be applied quickly to achieve integration. The benefits of model-based practice have to be experienced by nurses to sustain energy and commitment. The core group was requested to develop a model-based nursing assessment tool for early implementation and evaluation. This form and other components of the documentation system were developed and implemented on a trial basis, with mechanisms to receive feedback and constructive criticism. Mutual trust was demonstrated during early form implementation by listening and rapidly responding to concerns. Frequent departmental rounds were made. Feedback was obtained and evaluated, and appropriate adaptations of tools initiated.

Other important factors for model-based practice are interpretation of the nursing process in terms of the practice model, and definition of clinical nurse roles based on the model, including comprehensive integration of the framework into structure and process activities.

Nursing Process

Nursing process was recognized as the basis of the practice of nursing. Nursing process as described in the Roy Adaptation Model was visualized as a dynamic continuum rather than the typical linear progression (Fig. 17–1). When visualized on a continuum, the patient's progress toward treatment goals becomes a driving force within the process. Education about the Roy model nursing process was conducted. A documentation system based on the model was developed to guide care providers through the continuum.

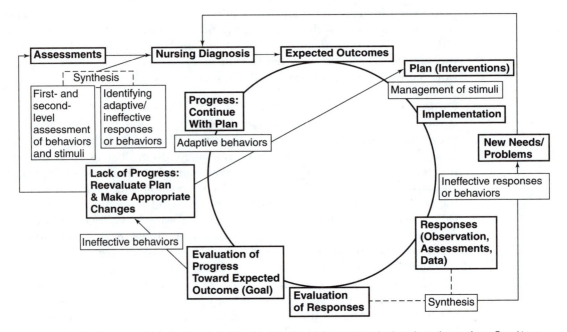

FIGURE 17–1. Nursing process interpreted in context of Roy Adaptation Model. Demonstrates the dynamic continuum of care. Found to enhance critical thinking. *(Courtesy of St. Joseph Regional Medical Center, Lewiston, Idaho.)*

Nursing Roles

The implementation of a nursing model provided a method to more clearly delineate the unique contribution of nurses to patient care. To ensure complete expression of the nursing profession, nursing roles must be focused on the application of nursing knowledge.

At SJRMC, all clinical nursing position descriptions were interpreted in the context of physiologic, self-concept, role function, and interdependence modes. Evaluation tools were developed consistent with the job description and role expectations of nurses practicing in a model-based environment. The evaluation tools, written in model format, also recognized the transformation process from novice to expert practitioner consistent with the work of Benner (1984). A four-step clinical ladder was developed with each step specifying growth in use of the Roy Adaptation Model and development in professional expertise (see Table 17–4). As noted earlier, the nurses most comfortable in the medically based hospital environment had the greatest difficulty in acquiring competence and comfort in application of the psychosocial modes (Lindberg, 1993).

In summary, the implementation phase has many components, occurs over a long time span, and actually continues before, during, and after the project. Tables 17–1 and 17–2 provide further explanation of the interventions that were associated with each of the goals developed for the transition to model-based practice. The next phase of the process is evaluation.

TABLE 17–4 FOUR-STEP CLINICAL LADDER: FRAMEWORK FOR DEVELOPMENT OF EVALUATION TOOLS[a]

General Position Description: Primary Duties	Evaluation Criteria		
	RN II *Competent/Basic Provider*	RN III *Proficient*	RN IV *Expert*
1. Delivers and/or coordinates the delivery of patient care by using the nursing process of assessment, expected outcome identification, intervention, and evaluation of care.	A. Completes patient assessments according to departmental standards. B. Participates in formulation of a plan of care based on individual patient needs. C. Delivers patient care following departmental and divisional policies and procedures. D. Interprets patient responses and communicates to appropriate person.	A. Completes admission assessment, reassessment according to department standards. B. Develops, implements, evaluates, and revises the plan of care for assigned patients. C. Delivers patient care following departmental and divisional policies and procedures. D. Interprets patient responses to care and collaboratively modifies plan or approach to care.	A. Completes admission assessment, reassessments according to department standards. B. Develops, implements, evaluates, and revises the plan of care for assigned patients. C. Delivers patient care following departmental and divisional policies and procedures. D. Interprets patient responses to care and collaboratively. Modifies plan or approach to care. E. Provides direction and assistance to others in assessing, formulating, and modifying plan of care.
2. Demonstrates knowledge and/or proficiency in management and delivery of patient care in assigned area of clinical practice.	A. Considers patient's current level of function and adaptation in four modes in the delivery of care. B. Differentiates alterations from normal parameters using appropriate assessment tools, ie, auscultation, palpation. C. Carries out established techniques for safe administration of medications and parenteral fluids. Includes transfusion, infusion pump, venopunctures, intravenous site maintenance, and infusion therapy. D. Maintains competency in basic care provider, including urinary catheterization, oximetry, reagent testing, auto blood pressure, TPN, tube feedings, and department-required skills for RN II.	A. Considers patient's current level of function and adaptation in four modes in the delivery of care. B. Differentiates alterations from normal parameters using appropriate assessment tools, ie, auscultation, palpation, assists colleagues in data interpretation. C. Carries out established techniques for safe administration of medications and parenteral fluids. Includes transfusions, infusion pump, venopunctures, intravenous site maintenance, and infusion therapy. D. Maintains competency in basic care provider, including urinary catheterization, oximetry, reagent testing, auto blood pressure, TPN, tube feedings, and department-required skills for RN III.	A. Considers patient's current level of function and adaptation in four modes in the delivery of care. B. Differentiates alterations from normal parameters using appropriate assessment tools, ie, auscultation, palpation. Provides guidance to their personnel in improving their observations, the alertness to specific patient problems, and possible approaches to those problems. C. Carries out established techniques for safe administration of medications and parenteral fluids. Includes transfusions, infusion pump, venopunctures, intravenous site maintenance, and infusion therapy. D. Maintains competency in urinary catheterization,

TABLE 17–4   FOUR-STEP CLINICAL LADDER: FRAMEWORK FOR DEVELOPMENT OF EVALUATION TOOLS(CONT.)

General Position Description Primary Duties	Evaluation Criteria		
	RN II Competent/Basic Provider	RN III Proficient	RN IV Expert
		E. Prioritizes the plan of nursing care with sensitivity to patient needs and differentiates situations that require immediate and nonimmediate action and responds accordingly.	oximetry, reagent testing, auto blood pressure, TPN, tube feedings, and department-required skills. E. Serves as a consultant and advisor regarding unit-specific competency. F. Demonstrates ability to modify nursing approach innovatively in changing conditions, needs, and goals of the patient.

[a]Demonstrates integration of Roy Adaptation Model and Benner's novice-to-expert progression.

Evaluation

Implementation of a model, once undertaken, is an ongoing process. Simultaneously, SJRMC utilized many sources of information to evaluate model effectiveness: practicing nurses, physicians, other interdisciplinary team members, patient feedback about nursing care, quality outcome data, and surveyors. This information identified opportunities for new applications, adaptations, and refinement of earlier steps of implementation. Insight into actual or potential knowledge and practice deficits as well as opportunities to develop educational programs consistent with the model were obtained from the evaluation data. Educational materials consistent with the Roy framework promoted ongoing synthesis of the model into approaches to thinking, caring and problem-solving capabilities of nurses.

Model-based nursing has influenced patient care, the documentation system, and communication, while empowering nurses. Holistic nursing care is provided with patient and family participation, and patient assessments throughout the medical center consistently include all four modes as described by Roy. The daily documentation is clear and concise and allows a 24-hour view of patient assessment and responses to care. Outcomes are written with evidence of patient and family participation, and progress toward goals (or lack thereof) is easy to follow. Patient teaching guidelines that consider the four modes have been developed. Communication in both inpatient and outpatient programs is based on the four modes and the person's adaptation. In addition, interdisciplinary communication has improved as holistic care is practiced on a more consistent basis. Nurses now are able to identify and describe their practice and the influence they have on patient outcomes.

Education focuses on patient care and model-based nursing practice. Skills fairs have become nursing practice fairs with the focus changing from tasks and procedures to nursing process—how to plan and implement patient care based on the model. Nursing orientation and ongoing nursing education are also based on the model.

Throughout the implementation process, outcomes were measured and changes were made based on the findings. Outcome measurements included surveys of what nurses believed about patient care and nursing practice. Data were collected at each point of change in the implementation process to identify problems or concerns and user satisfaction. Students enrolled in nursing programs have conducted several research projects on the value and impact of model-based practice at SJRMC. The work completed by these students provided an external objective validation of the progress and value of the implementation of a model in a clinical setting.

Ongoing monitoring of outcomes is focused on patient adaptive responses and this information guides practice improvements. Performance improvement is measured by continuous monitoring of the nursing process, patient education, pain, patient satisfaction, and other important indicators of the quality of care. The Roy Adaptation Model of nursing, which promotes positive adaptation to a changing environment, complements the SJRMC commitment to continuous improvement of service.

Tables 17–1 and 17–2 provide a further summary of the outcomes associated with each of the nine creative and expressive goals.

► SUMMARY

The implementation of the model has been a transformation process that has unified the delivery of nursing care throughout the SJRMC. The full transformation to a holistic approach to service can be achieved if there is harmony in values and philosophy of the participants and the philosophic basis and assumptions of the chosen model. Only then does it become a part of each individual's beliefs.

The SJRMC dynamic implementation process has provided both predicted and unforeseen opportunities for application of the model and subsequent improvement of nursing care. Use of a model has been found to guide clinical, management, and educational practice. There have been many positive achievements and outcomes identified throughout this chapter. In addition, there have been many subtle but observable benefits including pride, enhanced continuity, accountability, and greater harmony in the interdisciplinary delivery of patient care.

Implementation of a model is a journey. In the future, the Roy Adaptation Model will be a significant influence on the SJRMC development of an interdisciplinary patient care model. The model will influence curriculum modifications and provide learning opportunities for students exploring nursing theory.

The work and effort at SJRMC supports the ongoing theory development originated by Sr. Callista Roy. SJRMC will continue to explore applications of the model, embracing each point of change as a learning opportunity and valuing the model as the foundation for practice in the future.

► EXERCISES FOR APPLICATION

1. As you have the opportunity to be involved in a setting where nursing care is delivered, inquire about the model that is used as a basis for practice.

2. Are there other areas of practice that would benefit from the use of a model such as that developed by Roy? Could it be of use in the school system? Explain the possibilities.

► ASSESSMENT OF UNDERSTANDING

Questions

1. Which of the following statements describe potential benefits of model-based nursing practice?
   (a) provides direction for data gathering
   (b) enables nurses to use the medical model more effectively
   (c) is a systematic approach to organizing knowledge
   (d) provides a means of effective communication
   (e) assists in role definition
   (f) ensures that all disciplines use the same framework

2. Name four conditions or strategies that support the transition to model-based practice.
   (a) _____
   (b) _____
   (c) _____
   (d) _____

3. Identify five aspects of nursing practice that are influenced by the implementation of a nursing model as the basis for practice.
   (a) _____
   (b) _____
   (c) _____
   (d) _____
   (e) _____

4. Systems theory can be used to view the process of nursing model implementation in practice. Label the following factors as inputs (I), throughputs (T), or outputs (O).
   (a) _____ goals

(b) _____ change in procedures
(c) _____ regulatory requirements
(d) _____ educational activities
(e) _____ documentation tools
(f) _____ participatory approach
(g) _____ staff input

5. Which of the following are suggested criteria for the selection of an appropriate model to be implemented in a practice setting?
   (a) congruence with mission and philosophy
   (b) understandable for other disciplines
   (c) applicable across the health care continuum
   (d) consistent with regulatory requirements
   (e) applicable in nursing practice, management, and education

6. The authors identify critical components that contribute to successful implementation of a model in practice. Complete the following statements identifying these components.
   (a) _____ development
   (b) development of a _____ mass
   (c) _____ education
   (d) early _____ application

7. Identify four sources of information that can be used in the evaluation of the outcomes of model implementation in practice.
   (a) _____
   (b) _____
   (c) _____
   (d) _____

Feedback

1. a, c, d, e

2. Any four of: administrative support, education, model selection, supportive communication, early success, vision.

3. Any five of: patient care, role descriptions, documentation, communication, family involvement, education, evaluation.

4. (a) I, (b) O, (c) I, (d) T, (e) Q, (f) T, (g) I

5. all of the responses

6. (a) management
   (b) critical
   (c) staff
   (d) clinical

7. Any four of the following: practicing nurses, physicians, other team members, patients, surveyors, family members, quality outcome data.

▶ **REFERENCES**

Allison, S. E., McLaughlin, K., & Walker, D. (1991). Nursing theory: A tool to put nursing back into nursing administration. *Nursing Administration Quarterly, 15(3),* 72–75.

Benner, P. (1984). *From novice to expert: Excellence and power in clinical nursing practice.* Menlo Park, CA: Addison-Wesley.

Braziller, G. (1972). In Laszlo, E. (Ed.), *The relevance of general systems theory: Papers presented to Ludwig von Bertalanfy on his seventieth birthday.* New York: Braziller.

Carper, B. A. (1978). Fundamental patterns of knowing in nursing. *Advances in Nursing Science, 1(1),* 13–23.

Chinn, P., & Jacobs, M. (1987). *Theory and nursing* (2nd ed.). St. Louis: Mosby.

Gardner, J. (1993). *Self renewal.* New York: Harper & Row.

Grahame, C. (1987). Frontline revolt. *Nursing Times, 83(16),* 60.

Kouzes, J., & Posner, B. (1993). *Credibility.* San Francisco: Jossey-Bass.

Lindberg, C. (1993). Communication between nursing departments concerning clients after implementing the Roy Adaptation Model of nursing. (Research report.) Lewis-Clark State College, Lewiston, ID: Author.

Marquis, B., & Huston, C. (1996). *Leadership roles and management functions in nursing.* Philadelphia: Lippincott.

Mastal, M., Hammond, H., & Roberts, M. P. (1982). Theory into practice: A pilot implementation. *The Journal of Nursing Administration, 12,* 9–15.

Mayberry, A. (1991). Merging nursing theories, models and nursing practice: More than an administrative challenge. *Nursing Administrative Quarterly, 15(3),* 44–53.

McFarland, M. R. (1993). The process of vision development described by six college and university presidents. (Doctoral dissertation, Gonzaga University, 1993.) *Dissertation Abstracts International,* DAI-A 54/04 (pp. 1256–1386).

Robbins & Duncan, R. (1987). The role of the CEO and top management in the creation and implementation of strategic vision. In Hambrick, D. (Ed.), *The executive effect: Concepts and methods for the study of top managers.* Greenwich, CT: JAI Press.

Rogers, M., Paul Jones, L., Clarke, J., Mackay, C., Potter, M., & Ward, W. (1991). The use of the Roy Adaptation Model in nursing administration. *Candian Journal of Nursing Administration,* June, 21–26.

Roy, Sr. C., & Andrews, H.A. (1991). *The Roy Adaptation Model: The definitive statement.* Norwalk, CT: Appleton & Lange.

Tappen, R. M. (1995). *Nursing leadership and management* (3rd ed.). Philadelphia: Davis.

Veninga, R. L. (1982). *The human side of health administration.* Englewood Cliffs, NJ: Prentice Hall.

Weiss, M. E., Hastings, W. J., Holly, D. C., & Craig, D. I. (1994). Using Roy's Adaptation Model in practice: Nursing perspectives. *Nursing Science Quarterly, 7(2),* 80–86.

18

THE ROY ADAPTATION MODEL IN NURSING RESEARCH

Nursing, as both a profession and a scholarly discipline, is rooted in knowledge for nursing practice. Throughout history, family members have used their cultural traditions and understanding of the other person to help increase wellness, prevent illness, assist with recovery, and comfort the suffering and dying. Today, nursing has clearly emerged as a discipline that focuses on developing an understanding of the human processes that promote health. The social concern of nursing as a profession is to contribute to health by focusing on life processes of people integrated with their environments. Knowledge for nursing practice, then, seeks to understand how to promote interactions of persons and environment that, in turn, promote health. Caring and clinical reasoning are skills used in nursing practice to fulfill the social mandate of the profession.

This chapter describes how the Roy Adaptation Model contributes to nursing as a scholarly practice discipline by guiding research in these two aspects of knowledge development for clinical practice, that is, understanding basic life processes that promote health *(basic nursing science)* and understanding how persons cope with health and illness and what can be done to enhance adaptive coping *(clinical nursing science)*. Examples are provided from research by Roy and a research synthesis project involving critical analysis of 163 studies by numerous investigators who based their research on the Roy Adaptation Model and published between 1970 and 1994 (Roy, Pollock, et al., 1998).

▶ OBJECTIVES

After studying this chapter, the reader will be able to do the following:

1. Differentiate between science and art as it pertains to nursing knowledge.

2. Identify ways in which nursing conceptual models contribute to the development of nursing knowledge.

3. Label model concepts as being associated with basic nursing knowledge or clinical nursing knowledge.

4. Differentiate between qualitative and quantitative research approaches.

5. Name four strategies for knowledge development that have been used over the past 30 years to develop and refine the Roy Adaptation Model.

6. Develop research questions illustrating basic nursing research and clinical nursing research.

▶ KEY CONCEPTS DEFINED

Basic nursing science: Understanding of the basic life processes that promote health.

Clinical nursing science: Understanding how human systems cope with health and illness and what can be done to promote adaptive coping.

Deductive: Using a general theory to provide a tentative hypothesis for a given situation.

Inductive: Identifying individual experiences that can be interpreted to provide generalizations of human experiences.

Knowledge development strategies: Specific approaches that can use nursing model concepts and include model construction, theory development (concept analysis, synthesis, and derivation of propositional statements), philosophical explication, and research (qualitative and quantitative).

Qualitative research: Views reality as emerging and relative; approach is inductive.

Quantitative research: Views reality as discovered and measured; approach is deductive.

▶ PERSPECTIVE FOR NURSING RESEARCH

Nursing is a science and an art. Science deals with understanding both the how and why questions. How does something work, why does it not, and how can we help it work? Art deals with understanding and expressing the realities of life. When a child takes a small plant apart, only the parts that make it up are evident, not how it works. Biology looks deeper to explain how and why the plant grows. When an artist such as Monet paints a water lily, both the artist and the viewer of the art know the plant in a way not known in biologic science. Through science and art, one knows and appreciates oneself, others, and the world.

Basic knowledge, in both arts and sciences, looks deeply and closely at being; such knowledge aims to understand and express the essence of what is there and how it works. Nursing has such basic knowledge, just as do other disciplines. Nursing models provide a perspective from which to view and develop the basic knowledge of the discipline. The conceptual models for nursing that have emerged over the past decades have the task of probing the reality of nursing to add to our knowledge for practice through research, and to direct nursing education in the science and art of nursing. Each of the several widely used nursing models (for example, those of Peplau, Orem, Johnson, Rogers, Roy, Newman, Leininger, and others) is a vehicle for developing the basic science of nursing as well as the practice discipline.

Roy (1988a) described a general perspective for nursing knowledge as including the basic science of nursing, namely, focus on human life processes from which life patterns emerge. Secondly, this perspective for nursing knowledge places emphasis on the related clinical science of nursing, including midrange theories of intervention and strategies related to enhancing positive life processes and patterns.

According to the Roy Adaptation Model, basic knowledge is understanding people adapting within their various life situations. The model conceptualizes the person as having cognator and regulator coping strategies that act to promote adaptation in each of the four adaptive modes: physiologic, self-concept, role function, and interdependence. Within the adaptive modes, adaptation levels are integrated, compensatory, or compromised. Basic nursing knowledge derived from this model seeks to understand and appreciate the how's and why's of people functioning as adaptive systems. When people are studied in groups, the group is viewed as an adaptive system, with stabilizer and innovator adaptive strategies promoting adaptation in physical, group identity, role function, and interdependence adaptive modes.

Nursing is also a practice discipline. Therefore nursing knowledge based on a model includes a clinical art and science. Nursing has a long tradition of caring. Through the years, this has been called by various names, such as the interpersonal process (Peplau, 1952), empathy (Travelbee, 1971), caring need (Leininger, 1981), and now such terms as the transpersonal caring relationship (Watson, 1985) and caring in the human health experience (Newman, Sime, & Corcoran-Perry, 1991). The notes of a famous New England writer working as a nurse during the American Civil War in the 19th century reflect the values of this tradition. Louisa May Alcott (1863, pp. 51–52) wrote in *Hospital Sketches: An Army Nurse's True Account of Her Experience During the Civil War:*

A few minutes later, as I came in again, with fresh rollers, I saw John sitting erect, with no one to support him, while the surgeon dressed his back. I had never hitherto seen it done; for, having simpler wounds to attend to, and knowing the fidelity of the attendant, I had left John to him, thinking it might be more agreeable and safe; for both strength and experience were needed in his case. . . . John looked lonely and forsaken just then, as he sat with bent head, hands folded on his knee, and no outward sign of suffering, till, looking nearer, I saw great tears roll down and drop upon the floor. It was a new sight there; for, though I had seen many suffer, some swore, some groaned, most endured silently, but none wept. Yet it did not seem weak, only very touching, and straightway my fear vanished, my heart opened wide and took him in, as, gathering the bent head in my arms, as freely as if he had been a little child, I said, "Let me help you bear it, John."

The clinical art and science of nursing according to the Roy Adaptation Model uses the basic knowledge of adapting persons to understand people in situations of health and illness. This understanding is translated to practical clinical knowledge as nurses seek to discover ways of enhancing adaptation. The basis for the clinical art and science of nursing is the knowledge of human processes related to adaptive strategies and modes in situations of health and illness as well as the planning of nursing care with individual people and groups to enhance their own adaptation.

Knowledge is developed through research in many ways. Formal research can be designed to describe phenomena (what), to correlate two or more phenomena (what and how), and to experiment with the effects of one phenomena on another (how and why). Within each of these general types of research, there are two broad categories of research design that can answer a research question.

A *qualitative research* approach views reality as emerging and relative. The basic approach to knowledge is *inductive,* that is, identifying individual experiences that can be interpreted to provide generalizations of human experience. For example, how does this woman experience pregnancy? How does she feel and why? If this experience is compared with that of other women, are there common themes that describe the experience?

A *quantitative research* approach sees reality as discovered and measured. Knowledge is *deductive,* that is, a general theory is used to provide a tentative hypothesis for a given situation. For example, based on theories of body image, do predicted changes occur in pregnant women? How are these changes affected by various factors described in the general theory? Nurses increasingly use several types of research designs and are aware of the complementarity of each. Qualitative analysis of field observations can be, for example, the basis of defining the variables for a correlational quantitative study. In one study, many observations and interviews of mothers with their children in the playroom of a hospital led to the concept of role adequacy that was used in a pre- and postintervention observation tool to measure changes in the level of role adequacy of mothers of hospitalized children (Roy, 1967).

Using many approaches, and with increasing resources such as the National Institute of Nursing Research, nursing research has advanced greatly in the past few decades and will make even greater progress in the 21st century. As noted earlier, nursing models make their contribution to knowledge development by providing a perspective for research. Furthermore, the phenomena to study and the research questions to be asked are derived from the elements and assumptions of the model.

The specific elements of the Roy Adaptation Model have been described throughout this text. In Chapter 2, the initial philosophic and scientific assumptions of the model were outlined in Table 2–1. Expanded notions of systems theory and adaptation were then combined into one set of scientific assumptions in Table 2–2 and further articulation of the philosophic assumptions was summarized in Table 2–3. The model clearly identifies persons, as individuals and groups, as the phenomena for study. Whereas the biologist views the person as a living organism with functions such as ingestion and reproduction in common with other living organisms, the nurse using the Roy Adaptation Model views the person as unique among all living organisms. Rather than being a living system acting to maintain itself, the person participates in the purposefulness of human existence in a universe that is creative. Furthermore, the model's view of person differs from psychology and sociology. As a discipline, psychology studies individual behavior as explained by cognition and feeling, whereas the view of person taken by sociology is the behavior of individuals and groups explained by understanding organized groups. Based on the philosophic assumptions of the nursing model, persons are seen as coextensive with their physical and social environments. The nurse takes a values-based stance, focusing on awareness, enlightenment, and faith.

The broad perspective of nursing knowledge described is basic to identifying and conducting research for nursing. The Roy Adaptation Model has a clear perspective for developing the basic and clinical art and science of nursing. Further specification of the model's focus for research is delineated by descriptions of the person and environment. Research by Roy and that reported by other investigators as completed, in progress, and to be accomplished can be placed within this broad perspective to outline one view of the basic and clinical science of nursing.

► STRATEGIES FOR KNOWLEDGE DEVELOPMENT

Over the past 30 years, *knowledge development* based on the Roy Adaptation Model has integrated several *strategies:* model construction; theory development, including concept analysis, synthesis, and derivation of propositional statements; philosophic explication; and research, both qualitative and quantitative. The model was originally described in the literature by Roy (1970). At Mount St. Mary's College, Los Angeles, Roy worked with colleagues to elaborate the elements of the model in two widely used editions of the definitive text on the model (Roy, 1976, 1984a). Specific concepts were developed through both literature review and clinical experience, as well as reviews by content experts. (See chapters in each edition and the list of special acknowledgments for contributions of individual authors.) This present definitive statement of the model, as well as an earlier edition (Roy & Andrews, 1991), updates and refines these model elements so as to be useful to educators and students at all levels, and to nurses in clinical practice. The development of essential elements of the model is basic to each of the other strategies of knowledge development, including research. Theory development based on the model included the concept development already described, as well as early use of inductive processes and the later classic deductive work by Roy and Roberts (1981). Originally, the four adaptive modes were defined and described by sampling 500 incidents of patient behavior in all areas of nursing practice (Roy, 1971). Content analysis with inductive clustering was used to derive the smallest number of categories that covered all cases. Confirmation of label codes was sought from the literature. Then the categories, with minor revisions based on clinical experience, were subjected to 10 years of testing in nursing practice by 1,500 faculty members and students. Criteria of significance, usefulness, and completeness were met (Roy, 1981). At the same time, numerous other educational and practice institutions were implementing the basic model elements, including the four adaptive modes as organizing concepts. Those implementing the model were reaching similar conclusions about the adequacy of the adaptive modes.

Using a format for deductive theorizing described by Burr (1973) and extensive literature review, Roy and Roberts (1981) derived a total of 97 propositions that described relationships between and among the concepts of the regulator, cognator, and the four adaptive modes. More in-depth theorizing and research related to cognator and regulator were begun when Roy was involved in postdoctoral studies and clinical research in neuroscience nursing. A nursing model for cognitive information processing has been published (Roy, 1988b; in press). Roy used the cognitive processing model to derive and test hypotheses for recovery from mild and moderate head injury (Roy, 1989). Additional theoretical work was continued in Roy's (1990) clarification of her view of adaptation and of health as both processes and states. Furthermore, Roy has redefined adaptation in keeping with scientific and philosophic assumptions for the 21st century (Roy, 1997a).

The philosophic basis for Roy's later work began during a baccalaureate program where she earned a Bachelor in Arts degree in nursing. Roy's course of study included significant course work in the liberal arts and a substantial program in philosophy and theology. The opportunity to explicate the philosophic assumptions of the model came with an invitation to give the inaugural address of a distinguished nurse lecture series (Roy, 1984b) on values for science. In individual analysis, and in discussion with colleague philosophers at Mount St. Mary's, Roy continued to articulate distinctions related to the model that were not clear to the early critics, who equated Roy's use of term stimuli from Helson's work (1964) with the stimulus–response connections of behaviorism. The philosophic aspect of the development of the model is most fully treated in two articles a decade apart (Roy, 1988a, 1997a). In the decade between the two papers, Roy's interest in earth science, cosmology, and creation spirituality grew. Roy was particularly affected by the works of de Chardin (1966, 1969) and Berry (Berry, 1991; Swimme & Berry, 1994). As a teacher and mentor, Roy was challenged to think ever more deeply about the nature of knowledge in nursing by talented doctoral students at Boston College School of Nursing. Likewise, she was affected by colleagues at a series of nursing knowledge development conferences in the Northeast (Jones & Roy, 1997b; University of Rhode Island, 1996), and in the Faith and Science Exchange of the Boston Theological Institute (Smith-Moran, 1997).

Given the generic perspective for nursing knowledge described earlier, a structure for knowledge based on the Roy Adaptation Model was derived. Table 18–1 shows the broad categories of the basic and clinical science of nursing. Major subdivisions of the basic science of nursing are the person or group as an adaptive system and adaptation related to health. In looking at the person or group, both adaptive processes and the adaptive modes are a focus. Topics to consider within the adaptive processes are: cognator and regulator activity for the individual, and stabilizer and innovator activity for a group; stability of adaptive patterns; and the dynamics of evolving adaptive patterns. In looking at the adaptive modes, study focuses on development, interrelatedness, and cultural and other contextual and residual influences. The second major category, adaptation related to health, is divided into research related to person and environment interaction, and integrity and inte-

TABLE 18–1 STRUCTURE OF KNOWLEDGE BASED ON THE ROY ADAPTATION MODEL

Basic Nursing Science
- Person or group as adaptive system
  Adaptive processes
    Cognator–regulator activity
    Stabilizer–innovator activity
    Stability of adaptive patterns
    Dynamics of evolving adaptive patterns
  Adaptive modes
    Development
    Interrelatedness
    Cultural and other influences
- Adaptation related to health
  Person and environment interaction
  Integration of adaptive modes

Clinical Nursing Science
- Changes in cognator–regulator or stabilizer–innovator effectiveness
- Changes within and among adaptive modes
- Nursing care to promote adaptive processes
  In times of transition
  During environmental changes
  During acute and chronic illness, injury, treatment, and technologic threats

gration of the adaptive modes. This forms the framework for the study of the basic nursing science.

Clinical nursing science according to the Roy Adaptation Model involves three major categories: changes in cognator–regulator or stabilizer–innovator effectiveness, changes within and among adaptive modes, and nursing care to promote adaptive processes. The latter particularly relate to times of transition; environmental changes; acute and chronic illness, injury, and treatment; and technologic threats.

Roy has contributed to knowledge based on the Roy Adaptation Model by using each of the several strategies for developing knowledge, including research. In addition, however, the model has an important role in guiding research of many investigators for both a basic science of nursing and a clinical science of nursing. Of particular use to describe the role of the model in guiding research and contributing to nursing knowledge is a recently completed research synthesis project by Roy and colleagues (Roy, Pollock, et al., 1998). Each of these perspectives is described in the following sections.

► MODEL-BASED RESEARCH BY ROY

Major studies by Roy illustrate some of the categories from the structure of knowledge based on the Roy Adaptation Model. Examples of basic nursing research and clinical nursing are provided. Further, the variety of methods used at various stages of knowledge development are illustrated.

Basic Nursing Science Examples

Two examples from Roy's earlier work (1975, 1977), are used to illustrate studies related to basic nursing science. One is related to knowledge of persons as adaptive systems and the other is related to adaptation and health. In the first example, the general research aim was to explore how the cognator coping processes act to promote adaptation and how they relate to the four adaptive modes. Three methods were used to explore this basic question.

Initially, literature on coping processes was reviewed from the perspective of the adaptive modes. Grids were prepared that displayed different authors' views on each of the modes in such a way that relationships among the views could be synthesized.

The second step in exploring cognator processes was to obtain a closer view of them acting in a given context. Ten patients on a medical unit of an acute care hospital were interviewed. Half of the patients were scheduled for diagnostic tests the next day. The other half had been in the hospital for at least 5 days. Patients were asked open-ended questions about coping with diagnostic tests and about coping with the experience of hospitalization. Then, individual patient responses were analyzed and coded into categories that seemed to express the specific cognator activity, such as "selective attention—differential focus on a good outcome" and "affective isolation." Regulator activity was also noted when reported or observed.

In the third approach to identifying coping processes, an analysis was done of 76 written recordings of the process of nursing care. The recordings were made by students in seven schools using the Roy Adaptation Model and where Roy or a colleague had consulted on curriculum implementation. Although the formats and length of the recordings of care differed, the common nursing framework made it possible to prepare charts for analysis of the patient data in three categories: patient behavior; focal, contextual, and residual stimuli; and inferred coping process.

After naming the inferred coping processes for each patient incident, a count was made of the number of times the strategy was used across the patient sample. A list of synthesized categories was devised by organizing and combining categories from the literature and the two clinical samples until the smallest number of categories was reached which represented all situations observed. At that point, 41 different coping processes were tentatively identified, 18 related to self-concept, 16 concerned role function, and 11 related to interdependence. Four categories were repeated once or more across the modes. This was seen as a beginning effort to move the study of cognator and regulator activity beyond the descriptions presented by Roy in 1970.

In the second research example, the relationship of adaptation to health was looked at as part of a larger study of decision making, powerlessness, and adaptation (Roy, 1977). It was hypothesized that levels of wellness would be greater with higher levels of adaptation. The design of the study involved systematic controlled comparisons using survey data collected by the investigator in six hospitals across the United States. Two hundred eight patients met study criteria and completed data collection.

Instruments to measure adaptation included an Affect Adjective Check List for anxiety (Zuckerman & Lubin, 1965) and a 49-item hospital events card sort and distress scale (Roy, 1977) that compared how much the events bothered the patient early in the hospitalization and on the day before discharge. In addition, physiologic data from the chart were collected and the patients were interviewed about usual patterns to ascertain adaptation in the physiologic mode components. Wellness was described as rate of recovery and general physical welfare. Common measures of wellness evident in the literature, such as days in hospital, use of medications prescribed for use as needed, complications, self-report of degree of independence, and rate of return to work were used. Data were analyzed with Somer's D asymmetric measure of association for ordinal variables (Nie, Hull, Jenkins, Steinbrenner, & Bent, 1975, p. 229). In the total sample, some of the measures of physiologic adaptation were related to levels of wellness, but there was no evidence of a relationship between psychosocial adaptation and any of the measures of level of wellness. In analysis of different hospitals and lengths of stays in the hospital, however, there was such a relationship in the least acute setting and for the longer stay patients. Thus, it was suggested that adaptation can have an effect on level of wellness in less acute situations and over a longer period of time. It also was noted that the measures of levels of wellness were limited and not entirely appropriate to measure the dynamic and holistic concept of health as it has been defined in the Roy model.

Clinical Nursing Science Examples

The clinical nursing science based on the Roy Adaptation Model is divided into changes in cognator–regulator and stabilizer–innovator effectiveness, changes within and among the adaptive modes, and nursing care to promote adaptive processes. Studies in the third category focus particularly on times of transition; environmental changes; acute and chronic illness, injury, and treatment; and technologic threats. Roy's more recent research is clinical nursing science research. Two clinical research examples are provided to show the process of research and knowledge development that arises from basic nursing science of adaptive processes. The research first describes changes in adaptation in given situations, and then devises and tests nursing interventions to promote adaptive processes within this context.

As noted earlier, to move forward the theoretical work on cognator adaptive processes (Roy & McLeod, 1981), a model of cognitive information processing was developed (Roy, 1988b). A program of research was initiated to contribute to further understanding of basic human cognitive processes (how people take in and process environmental interactions, and how nurses can help people use these processes to positively affect their health status). Specifically, these studies aimed to develop knowledge relevant to nursing care and the recovery of patients with neurologic conditions.

The two specific aims of the first study (Roy, 1985) were the following. The first aim was to describe the direction and degree of change of simultaneous and successive modes of information processing in patients with mild and moderate closed head injuries at four points in time over the first 6 months of recovery. The study also sought to identify the relationship of specific demographic and medical factors to the nature and degree of change in information processing.

The methodology involved a descriptive repeated measures design. Data were collected for each participant at times that would maximize evidence of the dynamic changes in information processing taking place during recovery from head injury, that is, when the patient was first verbally responsive and at 1 week, 1 month, and 6 months after injury. The data included cognitive testing of simultaneous and successive information processing, clinical measures, and demographic data related to the factors that influenced information processing. Seven theoretically and empirically sound processing tests were selected and pilot tested for use at the bedside of an injured patient. Participants included 50 patients with mild and moderate head injury as defined by scores on the Glasgow Coma Scale (Mitchell, 1988) and the Galveston Orientation and Amnesia Test (Sisson, 1988). Plotting of mean scores and analysis of variance with repeated measures showed a clear pattern of change over time. Scores improved over the 6 months and

the variance among scores decreased. Furthermore, the pattern of information-processing deficits was more pronounced for successive and planning
functions than for simultaneous processing. Patients with a more extensive
history of drug and alcohol use scored lower on all measures, and these differences were significant on three of the nine measures. Still, the overall pattern of change resembled the changes for the group as a whole. There was
support for the notion that the first month following mild head injury is a
critical period for recovery.

The second study drew upon the findings of the first. It had two aims including to develop and implement information-processing practice protocols.
The second goal was to determine whether or not there was a difference in
the change of information-processing scores during the first 6 months of recovery from mild and moderate head injury for patients who received information-processing interventions as compared with matched participants who
recovered without such interventions.

Criteria for admission of participants were the same as in the initial
study and the matched controls were taken from that study. The intervention
protocol was devised from the understanding of information processing and
of the changes that were described in the first study. It was then submitted to
a multidisciplinary review panel for review, critique, and consensus. The protocol involved information-processing practice sessions held twice a day in
the hospital for 10 to 20 minutes and twice a week at home for up to 1 hour.
At least eight practice sessions were held during the first month of recovery,
with a prescribed distribution of approximately 20 percent simultaneous
tasks, 30 percent successive tasks, and 50 percent planning tasks attained over
time as the patient progressed. The sessions were planned individually for the
patient and conducted by a neuroscience clinical nurse specialist using simple and complex exercise materials in each of the three categories of information processing. Outcome measures of information processing, time
points, and conditions for testing were the same as described for the first
study.

Data on the initial nine matched pairs showed some promising trends.
First, the intervention protocol proved useful in information-processing practice and appropriate for clinical use. Second, when matched scores were compared on graphs, the recovery curves for the treated group had steeper
slopes, particularly between the first two data points, indicating greater improvement of performance. Changes in the untreated group on the other
hand appeared more gradual. Processing practice, developed from basic and
clinical nursing science, may enhance information processing for those who
have had changes in this ability through injury. Finally, the return rate of subjects to ensure complete data sets was brought to an acceptable level. As the
number of participants in this research is increased, the data can be subjected to repeated measures analysis of variance to determine differences
over time and between groups. As well, a two-stage model of regression analysis could be applied to determine differences in the slopes between scores at
different times and between scores of the two groups.

More recently, Roy's clinical research has focused on relating cognitive abilities and adapting to chronic illness. This work has included development of an instrument, the Cognitive Adaptation Processing Scale (CAPS). Roy's conceptual and empirical work resulted in a pool of 73 items that can be used to measure adaptation strategies. The survey instrument is undergoing psychometric evaluation while being used in conjunction with other tools in samples of patients with spinal cord injury, the elderly with hearing loss and same-day surgery, and those who have had neurosurgery resulting in sensory and motor deficits. An effort will be made to relate cognitive abilities measured by the Das–Luria battery and a revised form of the Cognitive Adaptation Processing Scale. This approach to Roy model-based research aims to understand better the person as an adaptive system and the person's use of cognator processes.

▶ MODEL-BASED RESEARCH SYNTHESIS PROJECT

The Roy Adaptation Model–based research synthesis project illustrates some of the categories from the structure of knowledge and identifies contributions of the model to nursing science.

The Boston-Based Adaptation in Nursing Research Society (BBARNS) began in 1991 with a small group of scholars who presented and published joint papers on the research that each had done using the Roy model to guide individual studies. It was noted that a synthesis of findings of several authors using the same model goes beyond the work of any one individual (Pollock, Frederickson, Carson, Massey, & Roy, 1994). The investigators formed the BBARNS group with broadly stated purposes to advance nursing practice by developing basic and clinical nursing knowledge based on the model, and to provide scholarly networks to facilitate and disseminate the model-based research. Recognizing the benefits of looking across studies based on the model and noting that a significant number of studies had been reported in the literature, the group planned a project to locate, critique, and synthesize English-language research based on the Roy Adaptation Model.

Since a project of integrating model-based research had not been published before, the BBARNS group developed a method for critical analysis and synthesis of model-based research. The project, from developing the method, identifying and locating the literature, conducting the critical review, and presenting the findings in a research monograph, spanned 4 years (Roy, Pollock, et al., 1998).

A total of 163 studies, appearing in 44 journals, plus *Dissertation Abstracts International* and *Masters Abstracts International,* met the criteria for inclusion in the review. There were 94 research articles in journals and the specialty journals by far had the highest representation, particularly maternal and child health and women's health journals. Research journals were next with 16 percent of the identified reports. Journals published outside the United States also had one of the higher proportions with 11 percent of studies in journals from other countries. There were 77 dissertations and theses from a total of 35 universities and colleges in the United States and Canada.

Studies were grouped by the major focus of the research, although many studies covered several model concepts. Sections of the review were organized according to seven major concepts of the Roy Adaptation Model: multiple modes and adaptive processes ($n = 36$), physiologic ($n = 21$), self-concept ($n = 18$), role function ($n = 21$), interdependence ($n = 20$) modes, stimuli ($n = 19$), and interventions ($n = 28$).

The research team developed guidelines for critical analysis to provide a summary of the strengths and limitations of the reported research. Five major categories were used: internal validity, external validity, measurement, data analysis, and interpretation of results. Criteria were modified for quantitative, qualitative, and instrument development studies and a scoring system was adopted to provide a summated rating of criteria used for critical analysis. A second step in the critical review was to evaluate within each study the linkages to the model. The linkages between the concepts of the Roy Adaptation Model and research variables, between the model and the empirical measures, and between the findings and the model were evaluated as either explicit, implied, or absent (Fawcett, 1995; Moody, 1990). Studies meeting criteria for adequate methods and model linkages ($n = 116$) were used to test propositions derived from the model.

The process of testing propositions from the model was a major step in the synthesis of knowledge from research based on the Roy Adaptation Model. The BBARNS investigators derived 12 generic propositions from Roy's published work, particularly Roy and Roberts (1981) (see Table 18–2). As research studies were analyzed, the findings of each study were used to state ancillary and practice propositions. Ancillary propositions are subsidiaries, or special instances, of the general propositions, some of which are stated in terms directly relevant for practice. Research support for an ancillary proposition lends support to the theoretical statement of the general proposition.

TABLE 18–2 GENERIC PROPOSITIONS DERIVED FROM THE ROY ADAPTATION MODEL

1. At the individual level, regulator and cognator processes affect innate and acquired ways of adapting.
2. At the group level, stabilizer and innovator processes affect adaptation.
3. The characteristics of the internal and external stimuli influence adaptive responses.
4. The characteristics of the internal and external stimuli influence the adequacy of cognitive and emotional processes.
5. The adequacy of cognator and regulator processes will affect adaptive responses.
6. Adaptation in one mode is affected by adaptation in other modes through cognator and regulator connectives.
7. The pooled effect of focal, contextual, and residual stimuli determines the adaptation level.
8. Adaptation is influenced by the integration of the person with the environment.
9. The variable of time influences the process of adaptation.
10. The variable of perception influences the process of adaptation.
11. Perception influences adaptation through linking the regulator and cognator subsystems.
12. Nursing assessment and interventions relate to identifying and managing input to adaptive systems.

Selected results of analysis from studies on adaptive modes and processes are used to illustrate the testing of propositions. Thirty-five of the 36 studies assigned to this section were critically analyzed as acceptable for use in testing propositions. Nine of the general propositions listed in Table 18–2 were tested in the 35 research reports. Under each general proposition, more specific propositions were derived related to adaptive modes and processes. For example, the first two general propositions relate the internal processes of individuals and groups and the effect of innate and acquired ways of adapting. Five ancillary propositions, three at the individual level and two for groups, were derived from the evidence of the studies on adaptive modes and processes.

Generalizing from six studies, the first ancillary proposition notes that "patterns of unique cognator processing can be identified in given patient groups" (Roy et al., 1998). In the studies reviewed, rich descriptions of the cognator processes of adapting are given for families with children with muscular disease (Gagliardi, 1991), HIV-positive women (Florence, Lutzen, & Alexius, 1994), chronically ill children (Pittman, 1993), hearing-impaired elderly (Zhan, 1994), women who became mothers after breast cancer (Dow, 1993), and patients in hospice care (Dobratz, 1991). The results of the studies provide clear support for the general proposition.

A second ancillary proposition notes that "cognitive processing affects self-concept and self-concept may affect cognitive processing" (Roy et al., 1998). Examples from the research show that cognitive adaptation processing affected self-consistency (Zhan, 1993) and decision making affected levels of perceived powerlessness in some patients (Roy, 1977). However, decision making did not always affect powerlessness and the proposition was not supported by some of the data from this study. Further, a reciprocal relationship of self-concept influencing cognitive processing was noted in several studies. In summary, this ancillary proposition was supported in data from five out of six studies addressing the issue. Thus, the ancillary proposition adds new theoretical insights about the cognator related to the adaptive modes. The original general proposition is both enhanced, empirically supported, and validated in practice.

Roy has highlighted the significance of perception to adaptation in several publications (Roy, 1988b; Roy & Roberts, 1981). Two studies, using the same sample of patients, supported the ancillary proposition that "perception affects adaptation" (Frederickson, Jackson, Strauman, & Strauman, 1991; Jackson, Strauman, Frederickson, & Strauman, 1991; Roy et al., 1998).

Two researchers addressed group level adaptive processes. Lutjens' (1991, 1992) study supported the general proposition by specifying and testing the ancillary proposition that "a combination of nursing and medical factors best predicts patients' length of stay" (Roy, Pollock, et al., 1988). The study used an explanatory model for how various factors in the health organization contributed to patient length of stay, viewed as a manifestation of an adaptive system. Similarly, Rich (1992) found specific relationships between decreased organizational resources and increased burnout in nurses. Thus, the second ancillary proposition related to group adaptive processes notes that "organizational resources have a negative relationship to the phenomenon of nurse burnout" (Roy, Pollock, et al., 1998).

From the entire research review, it can be noted that, related to the first general proposition, there were 35 tests of derived ancillary propositions. Of these, 33 supported and 2 did not support the general proposition. The number of times the ancillary propositions were empirically supported implies that the general proposition is clear enough for utilization in nursing research and that new knowledge is developed when it is tested from different perspectives in differing research samples.

It is also noted that the examples of synthesized nursing knowledge identified relate to the categories included in the Basic Nursing Science Examples section earlier in the chapter. Specifically, the general and ancillary propositions relate to persons and groups as adaptive systems and the dynamics of the adaptive modes with the central adaptive processes. In the total research review, 94 (63 percent) of ancillary propositions were identified as basic nursing science knowledge. On the other hand, 55 (37 percent) were considered contributing to clinical nursing science. It seems appropriate that, in the early stages of research based on the model, that is, the first 25 years, descriptive basic nursing science is the greater focus.

Another significant aspect of the integrated review of research was the applications of findings to nursing practice. The investigators used three categories in assessing potential of research findings for use in practice. Although the authors of the monograph note that caution is to be used in making such recommendations without replication of studies, they determined that some studies had a high potential for implementation (category one). This category included positive findings from studies that met the criteria for methodological adequacy, and that did not pose risks to patients. For example, studies identifying relevant stimuli to assess in given situations were in this category. Category two included studies that needed further clinical evaluation before implementation. It was recommended that the findings of these studies could be referred to teams of advanced practice nurses in the relevant area of practice for evaluation as to potential effectiveness relative to the risk involved. Finally, there were studies that clearly warranted further research before implementation (category three). This category applied to findings that were negative or equivocal, or that were promising, but posed a significant risk to patients and thus needed replication and clarification before being used in practice.

Selected examples from the 60 studies that have a high potential for application to practice are taken from the studies related to the model concepts of adaptive modes and processes. Scherubel (1986) found a relationship between family environment and the post-hospital course of adaptation for patients following coronary bypass surgery. Families exhibiting cohesion, achievement orientation, and strong moral or religious values were associated with positive adaptive responses. Although descriptive correlational studies do not immediately indicate intervention strategies, they do identify positive factors that can be assessed and supported by nurses.

The works by Broeder (1985), Stohmyer, Noroian, Patterson, & Carlin (1993), Barone (1994), and Dobratz (1993) all identify factors affecting the process of adaptation that nurses can take into account in planning nursing care. Broeder described how children felt scared by illustrations of a nurse in isolation attire and all identified procedures as the most stressful experience while in isolation. Although the nurse cannot change these factors, it is possible to help the children become familiar with the environment and help them express and handle their misunderstandings, fears, and stressors. In caring for patients with multiple trauma, the 6-month follow-up descriptive data by Stohmyer et al. can be useful to nurses in helping the patient anticipate and plan for problems that occurred in most of the patients studied, that is, self-devaluation, guilt, depression, hostility, body-image distortion, and anxiety. Barone's work highlights the importance of integrating patients' use of escape–avoidance coping strategies and maintaining hope of recovery shortly after sustaining a spinal cord injury. Further, the nurse can recognize that the older the person with a spinal cord injury, the more time and intervention required for psychosocial adaptation, and that those with paraplegia may achieve greater levels of physiologic adaptation. Similarly, Dobratz (1993) identified contextual stimuli that affect psychosocial adaptation in hospice patients. In particular, it is valuable for both the nurse and family caregiver to know that social support and pain can be managed and affect adaptation.

Examples of findings in category two, indicating the need for further evaluation before implementation, are found in the qualitative data analyzed in four studies. Dobratz (1991), Zhan (1993), Dow (1993), and Florence et al. (1994) provide rich accounts of the process of adaptation using cognator strategies. The patterns summarized from the data represent plausible representations of the patient situations. The observations, however, were made on a limited number of participants, and thus the patterns need to be subjected to further evaluation by clinicians or researchers to judge their fit for describing cognitive processing to achieve adaptation in the populations they represent.

An example of a study that was rated in category three, needing further study, was that conducted by Shuler (1991). The researcher found a small and nonsignificant percentage of the variance in physical and psychosocial adjustment to illness was accounted for by social isolation, loneliness, and self-concept. Given the weakness of the relationships and vagueness of the variables, further concept analysis and testing are warranted before the study can be the basis for implementations in practice.

▶ ISSUES RELATED TO RESEARCH BASED ON THE ROY MODEL

In analyzing Roy Adaptation Model–based nursing research through the years, and in reviewing the research synthesis project, some issues are noted that affect knowledge development and future directions for research based on the model. The question was raised early on as to whether an understanding of the model was used to generate research questions, or whether some elements of the model were used to organize certain variables, either during design of the project or in data analysis. Any of these approaches are considered valid. However, it was noted (Roy & Andrews, 1991) that a point would be reached when using the model for data analysis only would be recognized as redundant with little new understanding being added. For example, if patient or family needs are described according to the four adaptive modes, little new information is added to the basic model assumption that adaptive and ineffective behaviors can be described in four modes. In fact, in the research synthesis project, the potential of the model to direct research questions was recognized increasingly in the years 1970 through 1994.

A second issue is related, that is, linking model concepts to the variables of the study, to the empirical measures, and to the findings of the study. Evaluation of the linkages of the Roy Adaptation Model to these three aspects of the research was a key point in the synthesis project. It is encouraging to note that in studies evaluated for links to the model, research variables were linked to the model explicitly in 104 instances out of 117, or 89 percent of the time. In the remaining 11 percent of cases, the links of the model to research variables were implied. Similarly, in linking the model to empirical measures, the investigators judged the links explicit 79 percent of the time and implied 20 percent of the time. In only two cases (a little over 1 percent) was the link considered absent. In linking the model to their studies, investigators included in this phase of the research synthesis project were somewhat less likely to discuss their findings in relation to the model. That is, 77 percent did so explicitly, 10 percent implied the link, and in 15 cases, or 13 percent, the link was absent. These observations seem to indicate that the role of the model in directing research has become increasingly strong. Further, this synthesis of research can help future investigators to make explicit links to the model throughout the research process.

Another issue that is raised in relation to model-based research is the choice of methods used to answer the research question. Some authors divide theorists' works into those using qualitative methods and those using quantitative methods. Roy maintains that such divisions are misleading. As noted earlier, in the examples given from Roy's research, multiple methods are used at every stage of the work of developing knowledge based on this particular model, and further, this is likely the case with other models. Likewise in the research synthesis project, a variety of research methods were described. Frequently, studies used multiple methods; however, each study was assigned to a major design category. The majority ($n = 137$) were classified as quantitative, with 16 using primarily qualitative designs, and 10 being primarily instrument development studies. In particular, for many of the quantitative studies, the researchers used strategies such as interview schedules and open-ended questionnaires to obtain qualitative data about model concepts.

A major issue in research with the Roy Adaptation Model is that conceptual development has far outstripped methodologic development. How does the investigator measure holistically variables related to persons and groups? The notion of individual patterns is strongly represented by the assumptions of the Roy model. But the assumption of unique wholes presents difficulties in describing commonalities that allow understanding beyond a given human experience. In fact, the challenge of studying holism now challenges the clinical investigator using the Roy model to seek ways to understand infinite diversity, common destiny, systems progressing to higher levels of complex self-organization, the common patterns and integral relations of persons and the earth, and personal accountability for deriving, sustaining, and transforming the universe.

Holistic research, within the person and environment paradigm of the model, is particularly difficult when the investigator is deriving appropriate outcome measures. As noted in the study addressing adaptation related to levels of wellness, Roy (1977) felt that the measures of wellness were inadequate, rather than that the relationship did not exist. The dimensions measured did not validly represent the conceptual definition of health within the model that implies a process of being and becoming integrated and whole. The methodology, then, will be designed to tap the manifestation of the human experience of being whole and integrated.

In the synthesis study, there is some evidence of directions that can lead to more holistic research. A number of studies have begun to identify the dynamics of evolving adaptive patterns. Stages of adaptation were described clearly in dying patients (Dobratz, 1991), in women having children after breast cancer (Dow, 1993), and in families with chronically ill children (Gagliardi, 1991; Gibson, 1994). Some influencing factors were identified in each study; however, complex research designs using qualitative and quantitative approaches in diverse populations are needed to reach purposeful and imaginative generalizations from the dynamics of adaptive patterns in individuals. As to progress in holistic research by investigations across the four adaptive modes, 15 studies in the synthesis sample demonstrated the interrelatedness of the adaptive modes.

An issue in studying model-based research is the challenge of compiling a complete list of publications, and identifying work in progress is even more difficult. A report in the Bulletin of the Medical Librarians Association (Johnson, 1989) noted that 75 percent of the clinical studies applying a specific nursing conceptual framework will be missed by using conventional subject and textword search in MEDLINE or CINAHL databases. Database searches have improved, as manifested by the relative success of the BBARNS project in locating citations. Further, it is hoped that the publication of the synthesis project will provide the impetus to use Internet capabilities for researchers to be connected while designing their research and in sharing results. In addition, the completed research can be more readily available through such projects as Sigma Theta Tau International's on-line journal and efforts to make studies available for implementation in practice.

TABLE 18–3 RECOMMENDED FOCI FOR NURSING RESEARCH BASED ON THE ROY ADAPTATION MODEL

Basic Nursing Science
1. Groups as adaptive systems.
2. Age and gender as part of pooled effect on adaptation.
3. Levels of adaptation as integrated, compensatory, and compromised.
4. Dynamics of evolving adaptive patterns.
5. Reciprocal relationships of adaptive modes and processes.
6. Factors influencing adaptive mode development, particularly the effect of culture.
7. Extension of major concepts to all age groups and commonly occurring situations of health and illness.
8. Interdependence mode adaptation in children.
9. Relationship of adaptation to health.
10. Conceptual, theoretical, and empirical basis of perception in integrating the adaptive modes.

Clinical Nursing Science
11. Protocols to identify patient and family perceptions in commonly occurring clinical situations.
12. Appropriate timing for effectiveness of given nursing interventions.
13. Appropriate time interval to measure adaptation as an outcome in differing situations.
14. Specific stimuli to manage for effectiveness of given nursing interventions.
15. Programs of research to design and test interventions to promote adaptive processes in given patient populations.
16. Intervention studies that deal directly with cognator and regulator processes.

Source: Roy, Sr. C., Pollock, S., Massey, V., Lauchner, K., Velasco-Whetsell, M., Frederickson, K., Barone, S., and Carson, M. (1998). The Roy Adaptation Model-based research: Twenty-five years of contributions to nursing science. *Indianapolis, IN: Sigma Theta Tau International. (Used with permission.)*

► RECOMMENDATIONS FOR FUTURE RESEARCH BASED ON THE MODEL

In both sets of studies, those by Roy and those from the research synthesis project, the need for longitudinal studies, for refinement and replication, and for programs of research is noted. Research in nursing and research based on the Roy model structure of knowledge are beyond simply accumulating more facts. The opportunity to seek meaning and understanding is provided. The philosophic and scientific assumptions, the essential elements of the model, and published research efforts can guide further research. The research synthesis project recommended 16 foci for nursing research based on the Roy Adaptation Model, based on the analysis, evaluation, and synthesis of 163 studies published over 25 years. The recommended foci are listed in Table 18–3.

► SUMMARY

In this chapter, the Roy Adaptation Model in nursing research was described from the viewpoint of the theorist. A broad perspective of nursing knowledge included the relationship between a basic nursing science and a clinical nursing science. The structure of knowledge based on the Roy Adaptation Model was derived from this broad perspective. Within this, specific categories for research were identified. Several of Roy's research projects were described to illustrate knowledge development in specific categories, and also to show clinical studies related to understanding of basic nursing science. A recently completed project of synthesizing nursing research based on the Roy Adaptation Model, published in English from 1970 through 1994, was also used to provide examples of model-based research and their contributions to nursing science. Issues were raised that look to the future of knowledge development based on the model. Finally foci for future research were identified based on the examination of published studies.

▶ EXERCISES FOR APPLICATION

1. Develop a research question addressing an aspect of clinical nursing science derived from the Roy Adaptation Model. Describe how you would plan to investigate the question.

2. Find a research report that uses the Roy Adaptation Model as a basis. Describe the approach taken (qualitative versus quantitative) and the component of knowledge (basic knowledge versus clinical knowledge) chosen as the focus of the study.

▶ ASSESSMENT OF UNDERSTANDING

Questions

1. Identify the following questions as pertaining to the science (S) or art (A) associated with nursing knowledge.
   (a) _____ How does it work?
   (b) _____ How can we help it work?
   (c) _____ How can I understand what is happening?
   (d) _____ How can we express this reality?
   (e) _____ Why does it not work?

2. In what three ways can nursing models be used to contribute to the development of nursing knowledge?
   (a) _____
   (b) _____
   (c) _____

3. Label the following model concepts as associated with basic (B) nursing knowledge or clinical (C) nursing knowledge.
   (a) _____ human processes in health and illness
   (b) _____ cognator and regulator activity
   (c) _____ managing stimuli
   (d) _____ planning nursing care
   (e) _____ behaviors and stimuli

4. Classify the following statements as qualitative (QL) or quantitative (QN) in their approach to knowledge development.
   (a) _____ reality as emerging and relative
   (b) _____ deductive reasoning
   (c) _____ generalizes from individual experiences
   (d) _____ inductive approach
   (e) _____ measurement of reality
   (f) _____ provides tentative hypothesis

5. Name four strategies for knowledge development that have been used over the past 30 years to develop and refine the Roy Adaptation Model.
   (a) _____
   (b) _____
   (c) _____
   (d) _____

Feedback

1. (a) S, (b) S, (c) A, (d) A, (e) S

2. (a) provide a perspective for research
   (b) provide the basis for the phenomena to be studied and the research question to be asked
   (c) direct education

3. (a) C, (b) B, (c) C, (d) C, (e) B

4. (a) QL, (b) QN, (c) QL, (d) QL, (e) QN, (f) QN

5. (a) model construction
   (b) theory development
   (c) philosophic explication
   (d) research (qualitative and quantitative)

▶ REFERENCES

Alcott, L. M. (1963). *Hospital sketches: An army nurse's true account of her experience during the Civil War.* Concord, MA (Edition Cambridge, MA: Applewood Books, 1986.)

Barone, S. H. (1994). Adaptation to spinal cord injury (Doctoral dissertation, Boston College, 1993). *Dissertation Abstracts International, 54,* 3547B.

Berry, T. (1991). *Befriending the earth.* Mystic, CT: 23rd Publications.

Broeder, J. L. (1985). School-age children's perceptions of isolation after hospital discharge. *Maternal Child Nursing Journal, 14,* 153–174.

Burr, W. R. (1973). *Theory construction and the sociology of the family.* New York: Wiley.

de Chardin, P. T. (1966). *Man's place in nature.* New York: Harper & Row.

de Chardin, P. T. (1969). *Human energy.* New York: Harcourt Brace Jovanovich.

Dobratz, M. C. (1991). Patterns of psychological adaptation in death and dying: A causal model and exploratory study (Doctoral dissertation, University of San Diego, 1990). *Dissertation Abstracts International, 51,* 3320B.

Dobratz, M. C. (1993). Causal influences of psychological adaptation in dying. *Western Journal of Nursing Research, 15,* 708–729.

Dow, K. H. M. (1993). An analysis of the experience of surviving and having children after breast cancer (Doctoral dissertation, Boston College, 1992). *Dissertation Abstracts International, 53,* 5641B.

Fawcett, J. (1995). *Analysis and evaluation of conceptual models of nursing.* Philadelphia: Davis.

Florence, M. E., Lutzen, K., & Alexius, B. (1994). Adaptation of heterosexually infected HIV-positive women: A Swedish pilot study. *Health Care for Women International, 15,* 265–273.

Frederickson, K., Jackson, B. S., Strauman, T., & Strauman, J. (1991). Testing hypotheses derived from the Roy Adaptation Model. *Nursing Science Quarterly, 4,* 168–174.

Gagliardi, B. A. (1991). The impact of Duchenne muscular dystrophy on families. *Orthopaedic Nursing, 10(5),* 41–49.

Gibson, C. H. (1994). A study of empowerment in mothers of chronically ill children (Doctoral dissertation, Boston College, 1993). *Dissertation Abstracts International, 54,* 4078B.

Helson, H. (1964). *Adaptation level theory.* New York: Harper & Row.

Jackson, B. S., Strauman, J., Frederickson, K., & Strauman, T. (1991). Long-term biopsychosocial effects of interleukin-2 therapy. *Oncology Nursing Forum, 18,* 683–690.

Johnson, E. D. (1989). In search of application of nursing theories: The nursing citation index. *Bulletin Medical Librarians Association, 72(2),* 176–184.

Leininger, M. (1981). *Caring: An essential human need.* Thorofare, NJ: Slack.

Lutjens, L. R. J. (1991). Relationships between medical condition, nursing condition, nursing intensity, medical severity, and length of stay in hospitalized medical-surgical adults using the theory of social organizations as adaptive systems (Doctoral dissertation, Wayne State University, 1990). *Dissertation Abstracts International, 52,* 1354B.

Lutjens, L. R. J. (1992). Derivation and testing of tenets of a theory of social organizations as adaptive systems. *Nursing Science Quarterly, 5,* 62–71.

Mitchell, P. H. (1988). Consciousness: An overview. In Mitchell, P. H., Hodges, L. C., Muwaswes, M., & Walleck, C. A. (Eds.), *American Association of Neuroscience Nurses' Neuroscience nursing: Phenomena and practice* (pp. 57–66). Norwalk, CT: Appleton & Lange.

Moody, L. E. (1990). *Advancing nursing science through research* (Vol. 1). Newbury Park, CA: Sage.

Newman, M. A., Sime, A. M., & Corcoran-Perry, S. A. (1991). The focus of the discipline of nursing. *Advances in Nursing Science, 14,* 1–6.

Nie, N. H., Hull, C. H., Jenkins, J. G., Steinbrenner, K., & Bent, D. H. (1975). *SPSS: Statistical package for the social sciences* (2nd ed.). New York: McGraw-Hill.

Peplau, H. (1952). *Interpersonal relations in nursing.* New York: Putnam.

Pittman, K. P. (1993). A Q-analysis of the enabling characteristics of chronically ill school-age children for the promotion of personal wellness (Doctoral dissertation, Boston College, 1992). *Dissertation Abstracts International, 52,* 4593B.

Pollock, S. E., Frederickson, K., Carson, M. A., Massey, V. H., & Roy, C. (1994). Contributions to nursing science: Synthesis of findings from adaptation model research. *Scholarly Inquiry for Nursing Practice, 8(4),* 361–372.

Rich, V. L. (1992). The use of personal, organizational, and coping resources in the prevention of staff nurse burnout: A test of a model (Doctoral dissertation, University of Pittsburgh, 1991). *Dissertation Abstracts International, 52,* 3532B.

Roy, Sr. C. (1967). Role cues and mothers of hospitalized children. *Nursing Research, 16(2),* 178–182.

Roy, Sr. C. (1970). Adaptation: A conceptual framework for nursing. *Nursing Outlook, 18(3),* 43–45.

Roy, Sr. C. (1971). Adaptation: A basis for nursing practice. *Nursing Outlook, 19(4),* 254–257.

Roy, Sr. C. (1975). *Psycho-social adaptation and the coping mechanisms.* Unpublished manuscript.

Roy, Sr. C. (1976). *Introduction to nursing: An adaptation model* . Englewood Cliffs, NJ: Prentice Hall.

Roy, Sr. C. (1977). Decision-making by the physically ill and adaptation during illness. University of California, Los Angeles (Dissertation). Ann Arbor: University Microfilms International.

Roy, Sr. C. (1981). Roy Adaptation Model: Evaluating ten years of progress and setting future goals. In Roy, C. (Ed.), *Proceedings of the Third International Conference on the Roy Adaptation Model in Nursing* (pp. 1–10). Los Angeles, CA: Mount St. Mary's College.

Roy, Sr. C. (1984a). *Introduction to nursing: An adaptation model.* Englewood Cliffs, NJ: Prentice Hall.

Roy, Sr. C. (1984b). *Values for science: A clinical nurse scholar's perspective.* Paper presented at the Geraldine Crawford Distinguished Nursing Lecture Series, University of San Francisco.

Roy, Sr. C. (1985). *Cognitive processing in patients with closed head injury.* Poster session, 18th Annual Communicating Nursing Research Conference, Western Society for Research in Nursing, Seattle, WA.

Roy, Sr. C. (1988a). An explication of the philosophical assumptions of the Roy Adaptation Model. *Nursing Science Quarterly, 1(1),* 26–34.

Roy, Sr. C. (1988b). Alterations in cognitive processing. In Mitchell, P. H., Hodges, L. C., Muwaswes, M., & Walleck, C. A. (Eds.), *American Association of Neuroscience Nurses' neuroscience nursing: Phenomena and practice.* Norwalk, CT: Appleton & Lange.

Roy, Sr. C. (1989). Nursing care in theory and practice: Early interventions in brain injury. In Harris, R. D., Burns, R. J., & Rees, R. J. (Eds.), *Recovery from brain injury: Expectations, needs and processes* (pp. 95–110). Adelaide, South Australia: Institute for the Study of Learning Difficulties.

Roy, Sr. C. (1990). Theorist's response to "Strengthening the Roy Adaptation Model through conceptual clarification." *Nursing Science Quarterly, 3(2),* 64–66.

Roy, Sr. C. (1997a). Future of the Roy model: Challenge to redefine adaptation. *Nursing Science Quarterly, 10(1),* 42–48.

Roy, Sr. C. (1997b). Knowledge as universal cosmic imperative. In Jones, B., & Roy, C. (Eds.), *Knowledge Conference 1996 Proceedings, Developing Knowledge for Nursing Practice: Three Philosophical Modes for Linking Theory and Practice* (pp. 95–117). Chestnut Hill, MA: BC Press.

Roy, Sr. C. (in press). Alterations in cognitive processing. In Stewart-Amidei, C., Kunkel, J., Bronstein, K. (Eds.), *American Association of Neuroscience Nurses' Neuroscience nursing: Human responses to neurologic dysfunction* (2nd ed.). Philadelphia: Saunders.

Roy, Sr. C., & Andrews, H. (1991). The Roy Adaptation Model: The definitive statement. Norwalk, CT: Appleton & Lange.

Roy, Sr. C., & McLeod, D. (1981). Theory of the person as an adaptive system. In Roy, C., & Roberts, S. (Eds.), *Theory construction in nursing: An adaptation model* (pp. 49–69). Englewood Cliffs, NJ: Prentice Hall.

Roy, Sr. C., & Roberts, S. (Eds.). (1981). *Theory construction in nursing: An adaptation model.* Englewood Cliffs, NJ: Prentice Hall.

Roy, Sr. C., Pollock, S., Massey, V., Lauchner, K., Velsco-Whetsell, M., Frederickson, K., Barone, S., & Carson, M. (1998). *The Roy Adaptation Model-based research: Twenty-five years of contributions to nursing science.* Indianapolis, IN: Sigma Theta Tau International.

Scherubel, J. C. M. (1986). Description of adaptation patterns following an acute cardiac event (Doctoral dissertation, University of Illinois at Chicago, 1985). *Dissertation Abstracts International, 46,* 2627B.

Shuler, P. J. (1991). Physical and psychosocial adaptation, social location, loneliness, and self-concept of individuals with cancer (Doctoral dissertation, The Catholic University of America, 1990). *Dissertation Abstracts International, 51,* 2289B.

Sisson, R. (1988). Alterations in memory. In Mitchell, P. H. , Hodges, L. C., Muwaswes, M., & Walleck, C. A. (Eds.), *American Association of Neuroscience Nurses' Neuroscience nursing: Phenomena and practice* (pp. 171–183). Norwalk, CT: Appleton & Lange.

Smith-Moran, B. (1997). *The Journal of Faith and Science Exchange.* Newton Centre, MA: The Boston Theological Institute.

Strohmyer, L. L., Noroian, E. L., Patterson, L. M., & Carlin, B. P. (1993). Adaptation six months after multiple trauma: A pilot study. *Journal of Neuroscience Nursing, 25,* 30–37.

Swimme, B., & Berry, T. (1994). *The universe story.* San Fransicso: Harper.

Travelbee, J. (1971). *Interpersonal aspects in nursing* (2nd ed.). Philadelphia: Davis.

University of Rhode Island College of Nursing. (1996). *Proceedings of the Conference on Building a Cumulative Knowledge Base for Nursing from Fragmentation to Congruence of Philosophy, Theory, Methods of Inquiry and Practice.* Kingston, RI: University of Rhode Island College of Nursing.

Watson, J. (1985). *Nursing: Human science and human care.* Norwalk, CT: Appleton & Lange.

Zhan, L. (1994). Cognitive adaptation processing and self consistency in the hearing impaired elderly (Doctoral dissertation, Boston College, 1993). *Dissertation Abstracts International, 54,* 4086B.

Zuckerman, M., & Lubin, B. (1965). *Manual for the affect adjective check list.* San Diego, CA: Educational and Industrial Testing Service.

► ADDITIONAL REFERENCES

Armer, J. M. (1989). Factors influencing relocation adjustment among community-based rural elderly (Doctoral dissertation, University of Rochester, 1998). *Dissertation Abstracts International, 50,* 1321B.

Limandri, B. (1986). Research and practice with abused women: Use of the Roy Adaptation Model as an exploratory framework. *Advances in Nursing Science, 8(4),* 52–61.

Norris, S., Campbell, L., & Brenkert, S. (1982). Nursing procedures and alterations in transcutaneous oxygen tension in premature infants. *Nursing Research, 31,* 330–336.

Phillips, J. A., & Brown, K. C. (1992). Industrial workers on rotating shift pattern: Adaptation and injury status. *American Association Occupational Health Nurses Journal, 40,* 468–476.

Pollock, S. E. (1986). Human responses to chronic illness: Physiologic and psychosocial adaptation. *Nursing Research, 35,* 90–95.

Smith, C. E., Garvis, M. S., & Martinson, I. M. (1983). Content analysis of interviews using a nursing model: A look at parents adapting to the impact of childhood cancer. *Cancer Nursing, 6,* 269–275.

INDEX

Page numbers followed by f indicate figure. Pages numbers followed by t indicate table.